SIXTH EDITION

Handbook of
Kidney
Transplantation

Edited by
Gabriel M. Danovitch, MD

Medical Director, Kidney and Pancreas Transplant Program
Ronald Reagan Medical Center at UCLA
John J. Kuiper Chair of Nephrology and Renal Transplantation
Distinguished Professor of Medicine
David Geffen School of Medicine at UCLA
Los Angeles, California

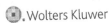. Wolters Kluwer

Philadelphia · Baltimore · New York · London
Buenos Aires · Hong Kong · Sydney · Tokyo

Acquisitions Editor: Kate Heaney
Product Development Editor: Leanne Vandetty
Production Project Manager: Kim Cox
Design Coordinator: Stephen Druding
Manufacturing Coordinator: Beth Welsh
Marketing Manager: Rachel Mante Leung
Prepress Vendor: S4Carlisle Publishing Services

Sixth Edition

9 8 7 6 5

Printed in the United States of America

Library of Congress Cataloging-in-Publication Data

Names: Danovitch, Gabriel M., editor.
Title: Handbook of kidney transplantation / edited by Gabriel M. Danovitch.
Description: Sixth edition. | Philadelphia, PA : Wolters Kluwer, [2017] | Includes bibliographical references.
Identifiers: LCCN 2017003544 | ISBN 9781496326157
Subjects: | MESH: Kidney Transplantation
Classification: LCC RD575 | NLM WJ 368 | DDC 617.4/610592—dc23 LC record available at https://lccn.loc.gov/2017003544

LWW.com

Dedicated to the UCLA Kidney Transplant Program that has been my clinical and academic home for over three decades, and to my many friends and colleagues at UCLA that it is my enduring pleasure and privilege to work alongside.

And to Nava, my beloved companion on this journey, who made it all possible.

The modern era of transplantation can be said to have begun with two momentous events in the early 1950s. In 1953, Peter Medawar and his colleagues at University College London described actively acquired immunologic tolerance in rats, thus heralding the science of transplant immunology and an ongoing search for a similar, reproducible phenomenon in humans. The modern era of clinical transplantation began on December 23, 1954, when Joseph Murray and his colleagues at Harvard performed the first kidney transplantation between identical twin brothers. Both of these pioneers were rewarded with the Nobel Prize for their contributions. In many ways, the promise of these discoveries has been fulfilled in the over 60 years that have followed. The mere fact that organ transplantation is the subject of a handbook series such as this reflects the extent to which it has become normative medical practice. Hundreds of thousands of lives have been saved, and quality years have replaced years of suffering. Our understanding of the complex immunobiology of the immune response has advanced and has brought widespread benefits well beyond the field of organ transplantation. A broad armamentarium of immunosuppressive medications is now available, and innovative surgical techniques serve to expand the donor pool and minimize morbidity. National and international organ-sharing organizations are an accepted part of the medical landscape of the developed world.

Modern organ transplantation can be visualized as a complex edifice that rests on a triangular base: in one corner is the basic research that is the lifeblood of improvement and innovation; in another corner is clinical transplant medicine, a relatively new medical subspecialty that requires compulsive, detail-oriented clinical care and both organ-specific and broad medical expertise; in the third corner are the ethical and cultural underpinnings of the whole transplantation endeavor, an endeavor that is utterly dependent on a well-developed sense of shared humanity and community and on absolute trust among medical staff, patients, and families. Trust is the bedrock of societal acceptance of organ donation, from both the living and the dead. The generosity and altruism of organ donors and their families can provide an enlightening antidote to our sometimes cruel and fragmented world.

Yet the success of clinical transplantation—with low mortality, high graft survival, and a low incidence of rejection episodes—has, paradoxically, made it more difficult to prove the benefit of new approaches. Because the demand for organs greatly outstretches supply, patients with advanced kidney disease who do not have a living donor may be faced with an interminable, and often morbid, wait for an organ from a deceased donor. The need for living donors has, on the one hand, provided a stimulus to develop ingenious new approaches to facilitate donation, and on the other hand, spawned an illegal, exploitive, global market in purchased organs. The Declaration of Istanbul on Organ Trafficking and Transplant Tourism (see Chapter 23) serves to codify the protection of the health and welfare of living donors while promoting the effective and healthy practice of deceased donation all over the globe. The chronic shortage of transplantable organs is unlikely to be solved without dramatic progress in the prevention of end-stage organ failure. Clinical xenotransplantation, a procedure that promised to provide the ultimate answer to the organ donor shortage, remains remote. Regenerative techniques and "organ printing" may yet provide an inexhaustible supply of organs, but not for a while!

This sixth edition of the *Handbook of Kidney Transplantation* has been thoroughly updated and revised to reflect the most current knowledge and practice in the field. Like its predecessors, its mission is to make the clinical practice of kidney transplantation fully accessible to all those who are entrusted with the care of our long-suffering patients.

—Gabriel M. Danovitch, March 2017

CONTRIBUTORS

Basmah Abdalla, MD
Assistant Professor
Kidney and Pancreas Transplant Program
Department of Medicine
David Geffen School of Medicine at UCLA
Los Angeles, California

Suphamai Bunnapradist, MD
Director of Research
Kidney and Pancreas Transplant Program
Professor Department of Medicine
David Geffen School of Medicine at UCLA
Los Angeles, California

J. Michael Cecka, PhD
Professor Emeritus
Department of Pathology and Laboratory Medicine
David Geffen School of Medicine at UCLA
UCLA Immunogenetics Center
Los Angeles, California

Eileen Tsai Chambers, MD
Associate Professor of Pediatrics
Duke University Medical Center
Pediatric Kidney Transplant Medical Director
Durham, North Carolina

Nick G. Cowan, MD
Fellow in Kidney Transplantation
Department of Urology
David Geffen School of Medicine at UCLA
Los Angeles, California

Hehua Dai, MD
Research Instructor
Department of Surgery
Thomas E. Starzl Transplantation Institute
University of Pittsburgh
Pittsburgh, Pennsylvania

Gabriel M. Danovitch, MD
Medical Director
Kidney and Pancreas Transplant Program
Distinguished Professor, Department of Medicine
David Geffen School of Medicine at UCLA
Los Angeles, California

Itai Danovitch, MD, MBA
Chair Department of Psychiatry Clinical Services
Associate Professor
Department of Psychiatry and Neurobehavioral Sciences
David Geffen School of Medicine at UCLA
Cedars-Sinai Medical Center
Los Angeles, California

Francis L. Delmonico, MD
Academician
Pontifical Academy of Sciences
World Health Organization
Advisory for Human Transplantation
Professor of Surgery Harvard Medical School
Massachusetts General Hospital
Chief Medical Officer
New England Donor Services
Boston, Massachusetts

Susan Weil Ernst, RD, CSR
Renal Dietitian Emeritus
Kidney Transplant Program
David Geffen School of Medicine at UCLA
Los Angeles, California

Robert B. Ettenger, MD
Director Emeritus
Renal Transplantation Service
Professor Emeritus
Department of Pediatrics
Mattel Children's Hospital at UCLA
Los Angeles, California

Fabrizio Fabrizi, MD
Staff Nephrologist
Division of Nephrology and Dialysis
Maggiore Hospital
Milan, Italy

Rudolph A. García-Gallont, MD
Surgical Director
Transplant Units
San Juan de Dios and Roosevelt Hospital
Guatemala City, Guatemala

Prasad Garimella, MD
Chief Operating Officer
OneLegacy
Organ Procurement Organization
Los Angeles, California

Mareena George, MS, RD
Renal Dietitian
Kidney Transplant Program
David Geffen School of Medicine at UCLA
Los Angeles, California

Alexandra Glazier, JD, MPH
President and CEO
New England Donor Services
Boston, Massachussetts

H. Albin Gritsch, MD
Surgical Director
Kidney and Pancreas Transplant Program
Professor Department of Urology
David Geffen School of Medicine at UCLA
Los Angeles, California

Mark Haas, MD
Professor of Pathology
David Geffen School of Medicine at UCLA
Cedars-Sinai Medical Center
Los Angeles, California

Mara Hersh-Rifkin, MSW
Clinical Social Worker
Department of Medical Center Care Coordination
Kidney and Pancreas Transplant Program
Los Angeles, California

Edmund Huang, MD
Associate Professor
Kidney Transplant Program
Cedars Sinai Medical Center
Los Angeles, California

Rami Jandali, BA, MHA
OneLegacy
Organ Procurement Organization
Los Angeles, California

Bertram L. Kasiske, MD
Professor and Chair
Division of Renal Diseases and Hypertension
University of Minnesota Medical School
Minneapolis, Minnesota

Bernard M. Kubak, MD, PhD
Professor
Department Medicine/Infectious Diseases
David Geffen School of Medicine at UCLA
Los Angeles, California

Fadi G. Lakkis, MD
Frank and Athena Sarris Chair in Transplantation Biology
Professor of Surgery, Immunology, and Medicine
Scientific Director
Thomas E. Starzl Transplantation Institute
University of Pittsburgh
Pittsburgh, Pennsylvania

Gerald S. Lipshutz, MD, MS
Professor of Surgery
Director Pancreas Transplant Program
Departments of Surgery and Urology
David Geffen School of Medicine at UCLA
Los Angeles, California

Erik L. Lum, MD
Assistant Professor, Division of Nephrology
Department of Medicine
Kidney and Pancreas Transplant Program
David Geffen School of Medicine at UCLA
Los Angeles, California

Paul Martin, MD
Professor and Chief
Division of Hepatology
Center for Liver Diseases
Leonard M. Miller School of Medicine at the University of Miami
Miami, Florida

Suzanne McGuire, RN, BSN
Senior Living Donor Coordinator
Connie Frank Kidney Transplant Clinic
Ronald Reagan Medical Center at UCLA
Los Angeles, California

Tom Mone, BA, MS
CEO
OneLegacy
Organ Procurement Organization
Los Angeles, California

Elmi Muller, MD
Professor and Chair
Department of Surgery
Groote Schuur Hospital
University of Cape Town
Cape Town, South Africa

Cynthia C. Nast, MD
Professor of Pathology
David Geffen School of Medicine at UCLA
Cedars-Sinai Medical Center
Los Angeles, California

Helen M. Nelson, RN, BSN
Senior Vice President
Organ Donation Services
New England Donor Services
Boston, Massachusetts

Meghan H. Pearl, MD
Clinical Instructor
Department of Pediatrics
David Geffen School of Medicine at UCLA
Los Angeles, California

Phuong-Thu T. Pham, MD
Professor of Medicine
Director of Outpatient Services
Kidney Transplant Program
Department of Medicine
David Geffen School of Medicine at UCLA
Los Angeles, California

Nagesh Ragavendra, MD
Professor Emeritus
Department of Radiological Sciences
David Geffen School of Medicine at UCLA
Los Angeles, California

Rajalingam Raja, PhD
Professor of Clinical Surgery
Department of Surgery
Director Immunogenetics and Transplantation Laboratory
University of California, San Francisco
San Francisco, California

Steve S. Raman, MD, FSAR, FSIR
Professor of Radiology, Urology, and Surgery
Director of Abdominal Imaging Fellowship
David Geffen School of Medicine at UCLA
Los Angeles, California

Anjay Rastogi, MD, PhD
Medical Director
Living Kidney Donor Evaluation Program
Professor
Department of Medicine
David Geffen School of Medicine at UCLA
Los Angeles, California

Uttam Reddy, MD
Assistant Professor
Medical Director, Kidney Transplant Program
University of Irvine Medical Center
Irvine, California

Elaine F. Reed, PhD
Professor
Department of Pathology and Laboratory Medicine
Director, UCLA Imunogenetics Center
David Geffen School of Medicine of UCLA
Los Angeles, California

Joanna M. Schaenman, MD, PhD
Associate Professor
Division of Infectious Diseases
David Geffen School of Medicine at UCLA
Los Angeles, California

Akhil Shenoy, MD, MPH
Assistant Professor
Department of Psychiatry
Mount Sinai School of Medicine
New York, New York

Theodore M. Sievers, D. Pharm
Clinical Transplant Pharmacist
UCLA Medical Center
Los Angeles, California

Jeffrey L. Veale, MD
Associate Professor
Department of Urology
Director Paired Donation Program
David Geffen School of Medicine at UCLA
Los Angeles, California

Amy Waterman, PhD
Associate Professor in Residence
Division of Nephrology
Director Transplant Research and Education Center
David Geffen School of Medicine at UCLA
Los Angeles, California

Qiuheng Jennifer Zhang, PhD
Associate Professor
Department of Pathology
UCLA Immunogenetics Center
David Geffen School of Medicine at UCLA
Los Angeles, California

CONTENTS

1

Options for Patients with Advanced Kidney Disease

Gabriel M. Danovitch

Before 1970, therapeutic options for patients with end-stage kidney disease (ESKD) were quite limited. Only a few patients received regular dialysis because few dialysis facilities had been established. Patients underwent extensive medical screening to determine their eligibility for ongoing therapy, and treatment was offered only to patients who had renal failure as the predominant clinical management issue. Kidney transplantation was in the early stages of development as a viable therapeutic option. Transplant immunology and immunosuppressive therapy were in their infancy, and for most patients, a diagnosis of chronic kidney disease (CKD) was a death sentence.

In the decades that followed, the availability of care for patients with kidney failure grew rapidly throughout the developed world. In the United States, the passage of Medicare entitlement legislation in 1972 to pay for renal replacement therapy (RRT—maintenance dialysis and renal transplantation), provided the major stimulus for this expansion. In the so-called developed world, RRT services are now available, in principle if not always in practice, for all those in need. In the developing world, such services are still sporadic. It has been estimated that in South Asia, more than 90% of patients with ESKD die within months of diagnosis, and in most parts of Africa, the reality is even starker (see Chapter 22).

Despite numerous medical and technical advances, patients with kidney failure who are treated with dialysis often remain unwell. Constitutional symptoms of fatigue and malaise persist despite better management of anemia with erythropoietin stimulating agents. Progressive cardiovascular disease (CVD), peripheral and autonomic neuropathy, bone disease, and sexual dysfunction are common, even in patients who are judged to be treated adequately with dialysis. Patients may become dependent on family members or others for physical, emotional, and financial assistance. Rehabilitation, particularly vocational rehabilitation, remains poor. Such findings are not unexpected, however, because even efficient hemodialysis regimens provide less than 15% of the small-solute removal of two normally functioning kidneys. Removal of higher-molecular-weight solutes is even less efficient.

For most patients with kidney failure, kidney transplantation has the greatest potential for restoring a healthy, productive life. Kidney transplantation does not, however, occur in a clinical vacuum. Virtually all transplant recipients have been exposed to the adverse consequences of CKD. Practitioners of kidney transplantation must consider the clinical impact of CKD on the overall health of renal transplant candidates when this therapeutic option is first considered. They must also remain cognizant of the potential long-term consequences of previous and current CKD (see Chapter 8) during what may be decades of clinical follow-up after successful renal transplantation (see Chapter 11). For updated reviews of the medical literature relating to ESKD and dialysis and transplantation, readers are referred to the American Society of Nephrology Self-Assessment Program (NephSAP) (see "Selected Readings").

STAGES OF CHRONIC KIDNEY DISEASE: THE BIG PICTURE

The nomenclature, staging, and prognosis of CKD as defined by the 2012 Kidney Disease: Improving Global Outcomes (KDIGO) Clinical Practice Guidelines are shown in Figure 1.1. A similar classification has been defined by the National Kidney Foundation Disease Outcome Quality Initiative (K/DOQI). The purpose of these classifications is to permit more accurate assessments of the frequency and severity of CKD in the general population, enabling more effective targeting of treatment recommendations. Note that the classifications are based on estimated values for glomerular filtration rate (GFR) and albuminuria and that the terms *kidney failure* and *ESKD* are used for patients with values less than 15 mL/min.

The United States Renal Data Systems (USRDS) reports annually on the prevalence of CKD in the US population, analyzing data from the National Health and Nutrition Examination Survey (NHANES). It

Prognosis of CKD by GFR and albuminuria categories: KDIGO 2012			Persistent albuminuria categories Description and range		
			A1	**A2**	**A3**
			Normal to mildly increased	Moderately increased	Severely increased
			<30 mg/g <3 mg/mmol	30–300 mg/g 3–30 mg/mmol	>300 mg/g >30 mg/mmol
GFR categories (mL/min/1.73 m²) Description and range	G1	Normal or high	≥90		
	G2	Mildly decreased	60–89		
	G3a	Mildly to moderately decreased	45–59		
	G3b	Moderately to severely decreased	30–44		
	G4	Severely decreased	15–29		
	G5	Kidney failure	<15		

Green, low risk (if no other markers of kidney disease, no CKD); Yellow, moderately increased risk; Orange, high risk; Red, very high risk.

FIGURE 1.1 Current Chronic Disease (CKD) nomenclature as used by KDIGO. CKD is defined as abnormalities of kidney structure or function, present for >3 months, with implications for health, and CKD is classified based on cause, GFR category, and albuminuria category (CGA). (Reprinted from Kidney Disease: Improving Global Outcomes (KDIGO) CKD Work Group. KDIGO 2012 Clinical Practice Guideline for the Evaluation and Management of Chronic Kidney Disease. Kidney Inter Suppl 2013;3:1–150, with permission from Elsevier.)

has been estimated that the overall prevalence of CKD in the general population is approximately 15%, with almost half reporting a diagnosis of diabetes and/or CVD. The prevalence of CKD with respect to its stages is shown in Figure 1.2. As of 2016, over approximately 700,000 individuals had overt kidney failure, or ESKD, a number that represents only the "tip of the iceberg" of progressive CKD. Fortunately, the incidence of ESKD has declined somewhat in the last decade, and the incidence of newly diagnosed diabetes has fallen by 20%. It is also evident from Figure 1.1 that most, if not all, kidney transplant recipients can be regarded as having some degree of CKD because their kidney function is rarely normal, whereas living kidney donors, whose GFR may be mildly reduced, are at low risk of developing CKD (see Chapter 7).

A discussion of the management of CKD in the general population is beyond the scope of this text. Strict blood pressure control and the use of angiotensin-converting enzyme inhibitors and receptor blockers, both in diabetic patients and in those with proteinuria from other glomerular diseases, are standard practice. There is less certainty, however, about the benefits of these agents in patients without significant proteinuria. Low-protein diets, with or without amino acid supplementation, may delay the onset of kidney failure or death in patients with established CKD, but there is insufficient evidence to recommend restricting

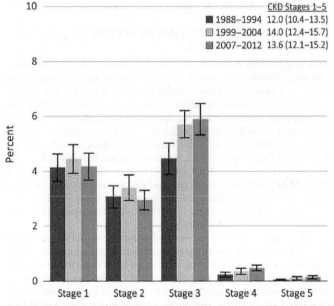

FIGURE 1.2 Prevalence of CKD by stage among NHANES participants, 1988 to 2012. Data Source: National Health and Nutrition Examination Survey (NHANES), 1988 to 1994, 1999 to 2004 and 2007 to 2012 participants aged 20 and older. Whisker lines indicate 95% confidence intervals. (Reprinted from Saran R, Li Y, Robinson B, et al. US Renal Data System 2015 Annual Data Report: epidemiology of kidney disease in the United States. Am J Kidney Dis 2016;67(3, suppl 1):S1–S434, with permission from Elsevier.)

dietary protein intake to less than 0.8 g/kg/day on a routine basis, and malnutrition is a real concern (see Chapter 20). Lipid-lowering agents and lifestyle changes, particularly smoking cessation, and reduction in red-meat intake may slow disease progression. New agents, such as empagliflozin, a sodium–glucose cotransporter 2 inhibitor, may slow the development of CKD in type 2 diabetes. Many of the concerns and treatment recommendations pertaining to the long-term management of kidney transplant recipients, which are discussed in Chapter 11, also apply to patients with CKD.

Estimation of Glomerular Filtration Rate

Measurements of GFR provide an overall assessment of kidney function in both the transplant and nontransplant settings. The GFR is measured best by the clearance of an ideal filtration marker such as inulin or with radiolabeled filtration markers (see Chapter 14). In clinical practice, GFR is usually estimated from measurements of creatinine clearance or serum creatinine levels to circumvent the need for timed urine specimen collections. Several equations have been developed to estimate GFR after accounting for variations in age, sex, body weight, and race. These include the Cockcroft–Gault, Modification of Diet in Renal Disease (MDRD), and the 2009 CKD-EPI equations. Further accuracy may be achieved by adding measurement of the serum cystatin C level. Although these equations are valuable in large cohorts of patients, their validity in individual patients is inconsistent.

DEMOGRAPHICS OF THE END-STAGE KIDNEY DISEASE POPULATION: UNITED STATES

Each year, the USRDS provides updated demographic information about patients with kidney disease who are treated with either dialysis or renal transplantation in the United States. Excerpts of this massive report, presented in an easily accessible fashion, are published annually in the January issue of the *American Journal of Kidney Diseases* (see "Selected Readings"). According to the 2015 report, as of December 2013, about 470,000 patients were receiving maintenance dialysis in the United States, and about 200,000 had a functioning transplant (Table 1.1). The increase in the number of dialysis patients has slowed somewhat, and this number now increases at an annual rate of about 4%. By the year 2020, the number of dialysis patients is expected to approach 500,000. Those who live with ESKD are 1% of the U.S. Medicare population but account for 7% of the Medicare budget.

Approximately 40% of patients receiving regular dialysis are older than 65 years, and the mean age of those beginning treatment is greater than 60 years; these numbers are projected to increase in the next decade. This phenomenon has been described as the "gerontologizing" of nephrology, and accounts for the frequency of aged patients being evaluated for, awaiting, and undergoing renal transplantation (see Chapter 8). In the ESKD population, men slightly outnumber women, and more than 30% are African American. The prevalence of African Americans in the ESKD population thus exceeds by threefold their percentage in the general population of the United States. Much of this increased incidence is because of the frequency of the *APOL1* gene,

TABLE 1.1 Number and Percentage of Prevalent Cases of Hemodialysis, Peritoneal Dialysis, and Transplantation by Age, Sex, Race, Ethnicity, and Primary ESRD Diagnosis, in the US Population, 2013

	Total	HD n	HD %	PD n	PD %	Transplant n	Transplant %
Age							
0–21	9,979	1,993	20.0	1,206	12.1	6,780	67.9
22–44	100,836	50,973	50.6	8,751	8.7	41,112	40.8
45–64	292,344	174,610	59.7	20,051	6.9	97,683	33.4
65–74	149,225	102,609	68.8	9,368	6.3	37,248	25.0
75+	107,485	91,164	84.8	5,882	5.5	10,439	9.7
Sex							
Male	378,185	238,277	63.0	24,602	6.5	115,306	30.5
Female	281,604	183,009	65.0	20,651	7.3	77,944	27.7
Race							
White	407,377	239,192	58.7	30,323	7.4	137,862	33.8
Black/African American	202,843	153,406	75.6	11,169	5.5	38,268	18.9
Native American	7,188	5,000	69.6	438	6.1	1,750	24.3
Asian	36,882	22,548	61.1	3,195	8.7	11,139	30.2
Other/Unknown	5,579	1,203	21.6	133	2.4	4,243	76.1
Ethnicity							
Hispanic	111,622	76,790	68.8	6,901	6.2	27,931	25.0
Non-Hispanic	548,247	344,559	62.8	38,357	7.0	165,331	30.2
Primary Cause of ESRD							
Diabetes	247,257	187,520	75.8	16,060	6.5	43,677	17.7
Hypertension	165,634	122,624	74.0	11,962	7.2	31,048	18.7
Glomerulonephritis	107,853	45,012	41.7	8,557	7.9	54,284	50.3
Cystic kidney	30,977	9,810	31.7	1,990	6.4	19,177	61.9
Other/Unknown	108,148	56,383	52.1	6,689	6.2	45,076	41.7
All	659,869	421,349	63.9	45,258	6.9	193,262	29.3

Data Source: Special analyses, USRDS ESRD Database. The numbers in this table exclude "Other PD" and "Uncertain Dialysis."
ESRD, end-stage renal disease; HD, hemodialysis; PD, peritoneal dialysis.
(Reprinted from Saran R, Li Y, Robinson B, et al. US Renal Data System 2015 Annual Data Report: epidemiology of kidney disease in the United States. Am J Kidney Dis 2016;67(3, suppl 1):S1–S434, with permission from Elsevier.)

which occurs exclusively in African Americans and is associated with a more rapid decline in GFR. The gene is believed to have been perpetuated by the resistance it provides to disease-causing trypanosomes.

Evidence also links poverty to CKD, either as a direct impact of poverty on CKD or indirectly through the increased health care burden linked to poverty-associated diabetes and hypertension. The poor and socially deprived have a greater prevalence of ESKD. Access to renal care, dialysis, and transplantation may also be affected by social deprivation. Poverty and social deprivation are emerging as major risk markers for CKD in both developing and developed countries (see Chapter 22). Much of the excess risk for CKD ascribed to ethnicity is essentially economic in nature.

Despite improvements in the clinical management of both diabetes mellitus and hypertension, these two diagnostic categories remain by far the most common causes of ESKD. In Hispanic, Native American, and Pacific Island patients, the burden of diabetes is particularly heavy. Older patients and those with diabetes are more likely to be accepted for dialysis in the United States than in other countries. Moreover, patients now beginning dialysis in the United States have more comorbid medical conditions than those accepted for treatment in the 1980s. Congestive heart failure is present in 35% of the incident dialysis population, whereas coronary artery disease can be found in up to 40% of the incident dialysis population in some published reports.

There has been a slow but steady increase in the number of deceased donor kidney transplants performed each year: approximately 8,500 in 2002 and over 12,000 in 2016. This increase reflects the efforts of the Organ Donation and Transplantation Breakthrough Collaborative (see Chapter 5), statewide registration for organ donation such that 60% of adults in the United States are registered organ donors, and repeated positive public relations messages such that 95% of the US adult population expresses approval for the concept of deceased organ donation. The annual number of living donor transplants has remained steady in the years 2011 to 2016 at approximately 5,600 despite an increase in the number of transplants from living donors who are not biologically related to the recipient (Fig. 1.3 and Chapter 7). The number of patients who are awaiting deceased donor renal transplantation is progressively rising, reaching more than approximately 100,000 by mid-2016. About one-third of these patients have been designated "inactive," and the "active" transplant waiting list has remained relatively stable (see Chapter 5). There

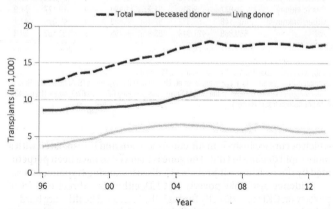

FIGURE 1.3 Number of kidney transplants, 1996 to 2013. Data Source: National Health and Nutrition Examination Survey (NHANES), 1988 to 1994, 1999 to 2004 and 2007 to 2012 participants aged 20 and older. (Reprinted from Saran R, Li Y, Robinson B, et al. US Renal Data System 2015 Annual Data Report: epidemiology of kidney disease in the United States. Am J Kidney Dis 2016;67(3, suppl 1):S1–S434, with permission from Elsevier.)

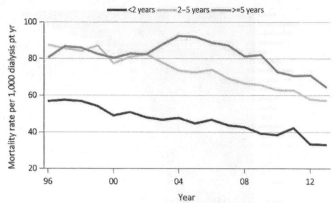

FIGURE 1.4 Annual mortality rates for dialysis patients on the kidney transplant waiting list by time on the list, 1996 to 2013. Annual mortality rates of dialysis patients on the kidney transplant waiting list per 1,000 dialysis patient years at risk, by patient vintage. Data Source: National Health and Nutrition Examination Survey (NHANES), 1988 to 1994, 1999 to 2004 and 2007 to 2012 participants aged 20 and older. (Reprinted from Saran R, Li Y, Robinson B, et al. US Renal Data System 2015 Annual Data Report: epidemiology of kidney disease in the United States. Am J Kidney Dis 2016;67(3, suppl 1):S1–S434, with permission from Elsevier.)

are likely many ESKD patients who are potential transplant candidates but have not been referred to transplant programs, so there remains a massive gap between the supply of and the demand for deceased donor kidneys. Consequently, the average waiting time for a deceased donor transplant has increased substantially, and it is now measured in years for most patients (see Chapters 5 and 8). The increasing incidence of CKD and ESKD, in a background of a national "epidemic" of obesity, diabetes, and inadequately treated hypertension, makes it unlikely that waiting time for a transplant will be eradicated in the absence of more effective CKD prevention and radical advances in the development of artificial organs. The mortality rate for patients on the waiting list increases as the time on the list gets longer (Fig. 1.4), and the longer the wait the worse is the outcome of the transplant (see Chapter 8).

DEMOGRAPHICS OF THE END-STAGE KIDNEY DISEASE POPULATION: WORLDWIDE

The worldwide ESKD population is estimated to be greater than 2 million persons. The highest prevalence and incidence rates for ESKD are reported from Taiwan, Japan, Mexico, and the United States. The high rate in the United States (Fig. 1.5) reflects, in part, the high incidence of ESKD in African Americans. Other factors, particularly limitations on the availability of dialysis, also play a role. Age is an important factor for patient selection in some countries, whereas in the United States, there is no age restriction for providing dialysis, and this largely explains the steady rise in the average age of the US dialysis population. Modalities for the management of ESKD vary among countries. For example, in the United Kingdom, Australia, and Canada,

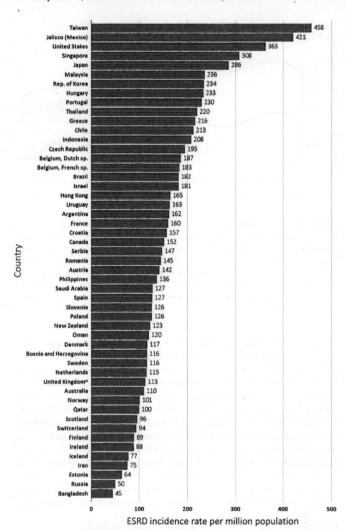

FIGURE 1.5 Incidence of treated ESRD, per million population, by country, 2013. Data Source: Special analyses, USRDS ESRD Database. Data presented only for countries from which relevant information was available. All rates are unadjusted. (Reprinted from Saran R, Li Y, Robinson B, et al. US Renal Data System 2015 Annual Data Report: epidemiology of kidney disease in the United States. Am J Kidney Dis 2016;67(3, suppl 1):S1–S434, with permission from Elsevier.)

home dialysis is used extensively, whereas this therapeutic approach is uncommon in Japan and the United States. Renal transplantation rates from both deceased and living donors vary considerably among developed countries (See Chapter 22 and Fig. 22.1). Legal constraints and cultural barriers to the acceptance of brain-death criteria or living donation are important determinants of national transplantation rates.

TREATMENT OPTIONS FOR END-STAGE RENAL DISEASE: HEMODIALYSIS

Hemodialysis is the predominant technique for treating ESRD throughout the world. In the United States, most patients start their ESRD care with hemodialysis. The procedure can be done either in a medical facility specifically designed for this purpose or in the patient's home. When performed in a dialysis facility, hemodialysis treatments typically range in length from 2.5 to 5 hours, and they are usually done 3 times a week. For highly motivated patients with a suitable living environment and a willing assistant, usually a spouse, hemodialysis can be done at home, freeing the patient from the need to visit a dialysis center and to adhere to a rigid treatment schedule.

During dialysis, solutes are removed by diffusion across a semipermeable membrane within a dialyzer, or artificial kidney, from blood circulated through an extracorporeal circuit. Fluid retained during the interval between treatments is removed by regulating the hydrostatic pressure across the membrane of the dialyzer. Most hemodialysis machines now control fluid removal, or ultrafiltration, using volumetric systems controlled by electronic microcircuits to ensure accurate and predictable results.

Hemodialysis is generally well tolerated, although ultrafiltration can cause hypotension, nausea, and muscle cramps. Older patients and those with established CVD may tolerate the procedure less well. Vascular access failure from repeated cannulation procedures and the need for intermittent heparinization to prevent clotting in the extracorporeal blood circuit are additional concerns, particularly in diabetic patients. The intermittent nature of hemodialysis, which results in rapid changes in extracellular fluid volume, blood solute concentrations, and plasma osmolality, may contribute to fatigue and malaise after treatment. This reality has led to attempts to increase the frequency and thus overall solute and fluid removal capabilities of hemodialysis. Increasing the number of treatments to five or six per week, increasing the time per treatment, and using daily nocturnal dialysis are approaches currently under intense study. These approaches are generally performed at home because they are not easily accommodated in the schedule of a dialysis center. Most dialysis membranes are now synthetic and provide a reasonably efficient removal of low-molecular-weight solutes.

Urea clearances of 180 to 200 mL/min are readily achieved during hemodialysis. Despite the favorable water permeability of synthetic membranes, the clearance of middle- and higher-molecular-weight toxins remains a fraction of that achieved for small substances. Although the minute-by-minute removal of low-molecular-weight solutes during hemodialysis may actually exceed that provided by normal endogenous renal function, the intermittent nature of hemodialysis as employed in clinical practice substantially undermines the overall efficiency of this form of renal replacement therapy. Even for patients receiving 12 to 15 hours of hemodialysis per week, adequate solute clearance is provided for less than 10% of a 168-hour week. During the remaining 153 to 156 hours of each week, no additional solute removal is achieved unless there is some residual endogenous renal function. This residual function needs to be considered when recommending native kidney nephrectomy before transplantation (see Chapter 8).

Guidelines for implementing and monitoring dialysis prescriptions in the United States have increasingly recognized the critical role of cumulative weekly procedure length as a key element for maintaining hemodialysis adequacy. The amount of dialysis achieved can be measured objectively by the term Kt/V, where K represents the rate of urea clearance by the dialyzer; t represents the duration, in minutes, of the treatment session; and V represents the volume of distribution for urea. Longer dialysis sessions and more frequent treatments have been reported to provide better blood pressure, extracellular volume, and metabolic control in patients with kidney failure. More dialysis reduces the substantial disparity between the amount of solute removal provided by the standard thrice-weekly hemodialysis schedule and that achieved by normal endogenous renal function. The impact of alternative dialysis regimens on long-term clinical outcomes is not yet known. Readers are referred to the K/DOQI guidelines, published and updated by the National Kidney Foundation, which are an invaluable resource for the management of patients with ESKD.

The hemodialysis procedure requires access to the patient's circulation to provide continuous blood flow to the extracorporeal dialysis circuit. For ongoing hemodialysis therapy, an autologous arteriovenous (A-V) fistula is the most reliable type of vascular access and the one associated with the best prognosis. Long-term patency is greatest with A-V fistulas, and the incidence rates of thrombosis and infection are low. A-V grafts that use synthetic materials are often placed in elderly patients and in diabetic patients whose native blood vessels may be inadequate for the creation of a functional A-V fistula that matures into a functioning access. Complication rates are considerably higher, however, with grafts than with fistulas. Thrombosis is a recurrent problem, and it frequently occurs because of stenosis at the venous end of the graft, where it forms an anastomosis with the native vein. Infections and the formation of pseudoaneurysms are more common with grafts than with fistulas. Temporary venous dialysis catheters are used to establish vascular access when hemodialysis must be started urgently. Other venous catheters, designed to be used over longer intervals, are frequently used as a method for providing vascular access for patients undergoing regular hemodialysis, particularly when treatment is first begun or when permanent access sites require surgical revision. Reliance on these approaches should be limited, however, and permanent access should be established using A-V fistulas or A-V grafts as soon as ESKD is deemed inevitable.

Stenotic lesions in large proximal veins in the thorax are an increasingly recognized complication of indwelling venous dialysis access catheters. These may involve the subclavian and innominate veins and the superior vena cava. Their presence can interfere with successful placement of permanent vascular access by producing venous hypertension that interferes with venous blood return from A-V fistulas or grafts. The sustained use of venous dialysis access catheters should be avoided. Early referral of patients with CKD to nephrologic care and elective placement of dialysis access, preferably in the form of an arterial autologous fistula, reduces morbidity. This becomes particularly important for patients who do not have a living kidney donor and who are thus likely to experience a prolonged wait on the deceased donor transplant waiting list (see Chapter 8). As a rule, a fistula should be placed at least 6 months before the anticipated start of hemodialysis treatments.

Peritoneal Dialysis

Peritoneal dialysis is an alternative to hemodialysis that exploits the fluid and solute transport characteristics of the peritoneum as an endogenous dialysis membrane. In the United States, approximately 10% of patients start dialysis with this technique. In many countries, peritoneal dialysis is more popular. "Assisted" peritoneal dialysis refers to the popularization of the procedure, particularly for the elderly, by daily visits by a trained health care professional. Peritoneal dialysis can be done either as *continuous ambulatory peritoneal dialysis* (CAPD) or as *continuous cycling peritoneal dialysis* (CCPD). Access to the peritoneal cavity is achieved by surgically placing a silastic catheter (often called a Tenckhoff catheter) of varying design through the abdominal wall. Surgery is done several weeks before treatment begins, and patients are trained subsequently to perform their own dialysis procedures.

Peritoneal dialysis is accomplished by instilling a specified volume of peritoneal dialysis fluid, typically between 1,500 and 3,000 mL, into the abdominal cavity by gravity-induced flow, allowing the fluid to remain in the abdomen for a defined period, and then draining and discarding it. During each dwell period, both solute removal and ultrafiltration are achieved. Solute removal occurs by diffusion down a concentration gradient from the extracellular fluid into peritoneal dialysate, with the peritoneal membrane acting as a functional semipermeable dialysis membrane. The efficiency of removal of small solutes is relatively low compared with hemodialysis, whereas the clearance of higher-molecular-weight solutes is somewhat better. Ultrafiltration is accomplished by osmotic water movement from the extracellular fluid compartment into hypertonic peritoneal dialysate that contains a high concentration of dextrose, ranging from 1.50 to 4.25 g%. The lower rates of solute removal that characterize peritoneal dialysis are offset by prolonged treatment times. For CCPD, an automated cycling device is used to regulate and monitor the dialysate flow into and out of the abdominal cavity.

Four to ten dialysis exchanges, ranging from 1 to 3 L each, are done nightly over 8 to 10 hours. A variable amount of dialysate is left in the abdomen during the day to provide additional solute and fluid removal. For CAPD, dialysis is done 24 hours a day, 7 days a week, using manual exchanges of peritoneal dialysate 4 or 5 times per day. Peritoneal dialysis has certain advantages over hemodialysis, including the maintenance of relatively constant blood or serum levels of urea nitrogen, creatinine, sodium, and potassium. Hematocrit levels are often higher than for patients receiving hemodialysis, and gradual and continuous ultrafiltration may provide better blood pressure control. Because it is a form of self-care, peritoneal dialysis promotes patient independence. The major complication of peritoneal dialysis is bacterial

TABLE 1.2	Comparison of Hemodialysis and Peritoneal Dialysis	
Advantages		**Disadvantages**
Hemodialysis		
Short treatment time		Need for heparin
Highly efficient for small-solute removal		Need for vascular access
Socialization occurs in the dialysis center		Hypotension with fluid removal
More frequent contact with health care professionals		Poor blood pressure control
		Need to follow diet and treatment schedule
Peritoneal Dialysis		
Steady-state chemistries		Peritonitis
Higher hematocrit		Obesity
Better blood pressure control		Hypertriglyceridemia
Dialysate source of nutrition		Malnutrition
Intraperitoneal insulin administration		Hernia formation
Self-care and flexible form of therapy		Back pain
Highly efficient for large solute removal		Caretaker fatigue
Liberalization of diet		

peritonitis. Its frequency varies considerably among patients and among treatment facilities, but it occurs with an average frequency of one episode per patient per year. When bacterial peritonitis is diagnosed promptly and treatment is begun immediately, infections are generally not severe and resolve within a few days with appropriate antibiotic therapy. Episodes of peritonitis are an ongoing threat, however, to the long-term success of peritoneal dialysis, and they can lead to scarring of the peritoneal cavity and to the loss of the peritoneum as an effective dialysis membrane. In the past, gram-positive organisms, such as *Staphylococcus epidermidis* or *Staphylococcus aureus,* accounted for most cases of peritonitis, but almost half of episodes are now caused by gram-negative bacteria. Fungal peritonitis typically causes extensive intra-abdominal scarring and fibrosis, and it often leads to the failure of peritoneal dialysis as an effective mode of treatment.

With few exceptions, hemodialysis has no medical advantage over peritoneal dialysis. Both effectively manage the consequence of uremia. Matters of individual lifestyle and other psychosocial issues should be considered when selecting a particular mode of dialysis (Table 1.2). Home hemodialysis provides an opportunity for independence and rehabilitation, but it can be a cause of substantial emotional stress for the dialysis assistant and other family members. In some home settings, neither hemodialysis nor peritoneal dialysis is advisable. In-center hemodialysis can provide ongoing social interaction and structure for older, single, patients who have few friends or family members available to provide support.

Long-Term Complications of Dialysis

As survival for patients on regular dialysis improves, a number of debilitating complications of either long-term renal failure or protracted dialysis may develop, even in well-rehabilitated and medically adherent patients.

As the waiting time for deceased donor renal transplants inexorably increases (see Chapter 5 and Fig. 1.4), these complications are more likely to manifest clinically. Their presence may affect the medical indications for transplantation, and they may influence the choice of renal transplantation as a therapeutic option (see Chapter 8). The longer patients receive dialysis, the greater the risk for post-transplant morbidity, mortality, and graft loss. The following discussion concentrates on those long-term complications that are most relevant to the post-transplant course.

Vascular Disease

The incidence of CVD in the CKD population has been described as reaching epidemic proportions. Even in the early stages of CKD, factors that contribute to the excess risk for CVD can be identified. Nearly all patients at some time during their clinical course develop hypertension, and many require multiple antihypertensive medications. The incidence of hypertension and diabetes as primary causes of CKD is increasing more rapidly than that of other diagnoses. Both traditional and novel risk factors account for the high incidence of CVD that is deemed responsible for close to 50% of all dialysis deaths.

Patients with kidney disease have a greater risk for developing left ventricular hypertrophy (LVH) than those in the general population, even in the early stages of CKD. The prevalence of LVH varies directly with the degree of renal dysfunction. At the time that regular dialysis is begun, 50% to 80% of patients have LVH, and the prevalence of coronary artery disease may reach 40%. Patients receiving regular dialysis have an adjusted death rate from all causes that is estimated to be 3.5 times higher than that in the general population, and the overall first-year mortality rate of hemodialysis patients in the United States is more than 20%. CVD accounts for 50% of this mortality at a rate that is 10 to 20 times greater than that in the general population. Hypertensive patients have worse outcomes after dialysis, and patients with LVH have a twofold to threefold higher death rate from cardiac causes.

Progressive calcification of the coronary arteries occurs over the years spent on dialysis and can be recognized even in young adult dialysis patients. Soft tissue calcification may also affect heart valves and the pelvic and peripheral vasculature. Vascular calcification is recognized increasingly as a complication of long-term dialysis. Mortality rates after myocardial infarction in dialysis patients are substantially higher than in the general population, a finding that probably reflects the severity of underlying CVD. The passage of time in patients receiving regular dialysis reflects ongoing exposure to multiple cardiovascular risk factors, and worsening myocardial function has been described, particularly during the first year of treatment. Although much attention is given to the cardiac manifestation of vascular disease, 10% of dialysis patients have peripheral vascular disease, and 15% cerebrovascular disease. All these observations may explain the consistent finding that post-transplantation prognosis worsens the longer patients are treated with dialysis before renal transplantation.

Anemia

The routine administration of recombinant erythropoietin (epoetin alfa) to treat the anemia of CKD and ESRD has had an enormously beneficial impact on morbidity. Fatigue, depression, cognitive impairment, sexual dysfunction, and LVH all improve with adequate treatment of anemia. The degree to which anemia is corrected is, to a large extent, determined in the United States by Medicare reimbursement policies that govern the target level of hemoglobin. Readers are referred to the K/DOQI anemia guidelines for updated recommendations. Successful treatment of anemia in dialysis patients is closely linked to replenishment of iron stores. Darbepoetin alfa (Aranesp) is a protein that stimulates erythropoiesis and is closely related to erythropoietin. Because its terminal half-life is about threefold longer than that of epoetin alfa, darbepoetin alfa can be administered less frequently.

Renal Osteodystrophy

Secondary hyperparathyroidism and high-turnover bone disease often develop in patients with ESKD. Several factors contribute to excess parathyroid hormone (PTH) secretion in patients with renal failure. These factors include hypocalcemia, diminished renal calcitriol production, skeletal resistance to the calcemic actions of PTH, alterations in the regulation of *pre-pro-PTH* gene transcription, reduced expression of receptors for vitamin D and calcium in the parathyroid glands, and hyperphosphatemia caused by diminished renal phosphorus excretion. Progressive parathyroid gland hyperplasia occurs often. Severely affected patients experience bone pain, skeletal fracture, and substantial disability. Hypercalcemia and soft tissue and vascular calcifications may develop. Treatment with one of several vitamin D sterols may lower plasma PTH levels and restore bone formation and bone-remodeling rates toward normal. Episodes of hypercalcemia and hyperphosphatemia occur frequently, however, during vitamin D therapy. Newer therapeutic agents, such as calcimimetic compounds, may offer an alternative for controlling excess PTH secretion in patients undergoing dialysis without aggravating disturbances in calcium and phosphorus metabolism.

Low-turnover lesions of renal osteodystrophy include osteomalacia and adynamic bone. In the past, osteomalacia was found in patients with tissue aluminum accumulation, but aluminum-related bone disease is now uncommon. Most ESKD patients with osteomalacia have evidence of vitamin D deficiency, mineral deficiency, or both. The adynamic lesion of renal osteodystrophy occurs in patients with normal or only modestly elevated serum PTH levels. It can also be a manifestation of aluminum toxicity, and affected patients have severe bone pain, muscle weakness, and fractures. Adults with adynamic bone may be at increased risk for vertebral fracture. The impact of transplantation on uremic bone disease is discussed in Chapter 11.

Uremic Neuropathy

Peripheral neuropathy is a feature of chronic renal failure, and encephalopathy will develop if appropriate renal replacement therapy is not begun. A mild stable sensory neuropathy is common even in nondiabetic dialysis patients; it is usually largely sensory and detected clinically by impaired vibration and position sense. It may be a source of pain and "restless legs." Neuropathy can recover dramatically after successful transplantation. It may also improve substantially after intensification of dialysis treatment.

Severe encephalopathy is rare in patients who receive adequate amounts of dialysis. Impairments in the ability to concentrate and minor memory loss represent more subtle manifestations of cognitive impairment in dialysis patients, and improvement after transplantation is gratifying. Autonomic neuropathy in nondiabetic patients receiving dialysis can be recognized by impaired heart rate variability, and it may account for variations in blood pressure during dialysis procedures. Autonomic dysfunction is also reversible after renal transplantation. Neuropathy contributes to sexual dysfunction in many dialysis patients. About half of men suffer from erectile dysfunction; menstrual disturbances and infertility are common in women. Improvement after transplantation is variable and is discussed in Chapter 11.

Acquired Cystic Disease and Cancer of the Kidney and Urinary Tract
Patients on all forms of maintenance dialysis are at increased risk for cancer, especially of the kidney and urinary tract. The risk increases with time. Kidney cancer rates are elevated nearly fourfold. The pattern of risk is consistent with causation through acquired cystic disease. Urothelial cancer risk is increased by about 50%, presumably as a result of the carcinogenic effects of certain primary renal diseases. The incidence of acquired cystic disease rises progressively with increasing duration of CKD and time on dialysis. The incidence of multiple cysts has been reported to be 7% in those with CKD and 22% in those on maintenance dialysis. The condition is characterized by multiple, usually bilateral, renal cysts in small, contracted kidneys and is, therefore, easily distinguishable from adult polycystic kidney disease. Cysts may become infected, bleed, or cause localized pain, and they can undergo malignant transformation. Suspicious cysts should be imaged at regular intervals, and concern about malignant transformation may be an indication for pretransplant nephrectomy. The capacity for malignant transformation should not be forgotten in the post-transplantation period.

Dialysis Access Failure
Early referral before the initiation of regular hemodialysis is required and is essential for establishing optimal long-term vascular access. For patients managed with hemodialysis, reliable vascular access is a life-sustaining aspect of medical care. Vascular access failure not only threatens the near-term well-being of patients but also has long-term implications with regard to the success of ongoing renal replacement therapy. Access-related morbidity accounts for almost 25% of all hospital stays for ESKD patients and for close to 20% of the cost of ESKD care. As discussed previously, A-V fistulas are the gold standard for long-term vascular access for hemodialysis. A-V grafts almost invariably undergo thrombosis; their 3-year cumulative patency rate has been estimated to be about 50%. Because the number of sites that can be used for permanent vascular access placement is limited, the choice of A-V grafts for long-term vascular access conveys the risk for ultimately losing all remaining vascular access sites, rendering further hemodialysis technically impossible.

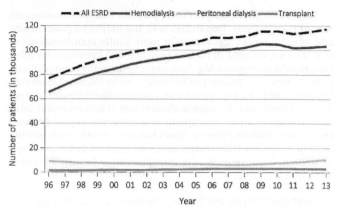

FIGURE 1.6 Trends in the annual number of ESRD incident cases (in thousands) by modality, in the US population, 1996 to 2013. Data Source: Special analyses, USRDS ESRD Database. (Reprinted from Saran R, Li Y, Robinson B, et al. US Renal Data System 2015 Annual Data Report: epidemiology of kidney disease in the United States. Am J Kidney Dis 2016;67(3, suppl 1):S1–S434, with permission from Elsevier.)

TREATMENT OPTIONS FOR END-STAGE RENAL DISEASE: TRANSPLANTATION

The relative prevalence of the major ESKD treatment options between 1996 and 2013 in the United States is shown in Figure 1.6. Deceased donor transplantation accounts for about half of all kidney transplantations in the United States, the remainder being from living donors (Fig. 1.3). The rate of renal transplantation varies considerably among patient groups. Transplant rates are lower in older patients, who represent a relatively high-risk group (see Chapter 8). Transplant rates have tended to be lower in African American ESKD patients, partly for reasons that constrain access to deceased donor organs (see Chapter 5). Mean 1-year graft survival for all types of living donor transplants is over 95%. In many centers, it is greater than 90% for all match grades of deceased donor transplants. The question patients frequently ask—"how long will my transplant last"—is a very difficult one to answer. In terms of half-life, it is approximately 10 years for a transplant from a deceased donor and 15 years for a transplant from a living donor (Fig. 1.7). Providing half-life estimates to patients, however, can cause confusion and distress, since the range survival is so great and patients tend to "latch on" to numerical estimates that may not be relevant to them.

Patient Survival
Difficulties with Data Analysis
To help select the most appropriate therapeutic option for patients with advanced CKD, clinicians and patients are understandably interested in comparative survival rates among various treatment modalities. Such comparisons are difficult, however, because data in the literature often do not reflect the fact that patients change treatment modalities frequently and that the characteristics of patients selected for each

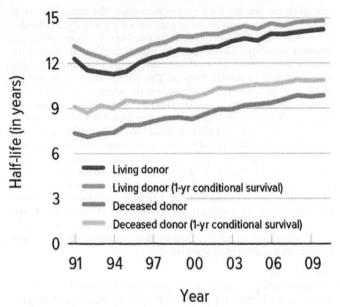

FIGURE 1.7 Half-lives for adult kidney transplant recipients. Data Source: See Hart A, Smith M, Skeans A, et al. OPTN/SRTR Annual Data Report 2014: kidney. Am J Transplant 2016;(suppl 1):18. (Reprinted from Matas AJ, Smith JM, Skeans MA, et al. OPTN/SRTR 2012 Annual Data Report: kidney. Am J Transplant 2014;14(suppl 1):11–44, with permission.)

modality may differ substantially when therapy is begun. For dialysis patients, a number of comorbid factors can adversely affect survival; these include increased age, diabetes, coronary artery disease, peripheral vascular disease, chronic obstructive pulmonary disease, and cancer. Overall, African Americans have a better survival rate on dialysis than do non–African Americans, as do obese patients, whereas certain renal diagnoses, such as amyloidosis, multiple myeloma, and renal cell cancer, are associated with poorer prognoses. Poor nutritional status, as measured by serum albumin and prealbumin levels, has been increasingly recognized as an important predictor of survival during long-term dialysis (see Chapter 20). Exclusion of consideration of these factors limits the accuracy of comparisons among therapeutic modalities. The concept of *reversed epidemiology* describes the phenomenon whereby factors associated with a poor prognosis in individuals free of renal disease (e.g., obesity, hyperlipidemia, and hypertension) may be associated with an improved prognosis in dialysis patients.

Comparison of Treatment Modalities

Most of the data comparing survival rates for patients treated with hemodialysis, CAPD, and deceased donor kidney transplantation suggest that an individual's state of health before treatment, rather than the treatment modality itself, is the most important factor in determining survival. Healthier dialysis patients are more likely to be placed on the waiting list for transplantation. The annual mortality rate for dialysis patients awaiting a transplant is about 6%, a value that is several-fold lower than the overall mortality rate among all dialysis patients. Waitlisted dialysis patients enjoy a further reduction in the relative risk for death if they subsequently receive a transplant rather than continue to receive dialysis. This phenomenon is illustrated graphically in Figure 1.6, which records the relative risk for death for dialysis patients who were placed on a deceased donor transplant waiting list. The long-term survival rates were better for transplant recipients who received either an "ideal" or a "marginal" donor kidney (see Chapter 5). This survival benefit can be recognized within the first post-transplantation year despite the higher mortality rates associated with the surgical procedure and with immunosuppressive therapy. The magnitude of the survival benefit varies according to the quality of the transplanted kidney and the patient characteristics at the time of placement on the waiting list. It is most marked for young diabetic patients. As a gross approximation, it can be said that with a high-quality donor kidney has the capacity to about double the anticipated life span of a waitlisted dialysis patient.

Cost of Therapy

The annual cost of medical care for patients undergoing chronic hemodialysis in the United States is about $75,000. Medical costs during the first year after renal transplantation are considerably higher and are estimated to be nearly $100,000. The cost of care is less after the first post-transplantation year compared with the cost of dialysis despite the annual cost—about $10,000—of immunosuppressive therapy (see Chapter 21). The mean cumulative costs of dialysis and transplantation are about the same for the first 4 years of therapy. Thereafter, overall costs are lower after successful renal transplantation.

Quality of Life. Most studies demonstrate that the quality of life (QOL) of patients receiving peritoneal dialysis exceeds that of patients receiving hemodialysis in a dialysis center. Home hemodialysis patients reportedly have a high QOL, although selection factors, such as the level of patient motivation and the patient's overall health status at the beginning of treatment, make it difficult to attribute this benefit to the modality alone. Most dialysis patients select renal transplantation with the hope of improving their QOL, and recipients of successful transplantations consistently report a better QOL than do patients undergoing either peritoneal dialysis or home hemodialysis. Life satisfaction, physical and emotional well-being, and the ability to return to work are all significantly better in transplant recipients than in dialysis patients. Transplantation often corrects or improves some complications of uremia that are typically not reversed fully by dialysis; these include anemia, peripheral neuropathy, autonomic neuropathy, and sexual dysfunction (see Chapter 11). The QOL for recipients of living donor transplants compares favorably with that seen in the general population. QOL surveys of dialysis and transplant patients suggest that, as a gross approximation, dialysis patients value a year of life on dialysis at 80% of a year of life with a functioning transplant.

INITIATION OF END-STAGE RENAL DISEASE THERAPY

An in-depth discussion of the indications for starting renal replacement therapy is beyond the scope of this text. Most patients with progressive renal failure develop symptoms of kidney failure and will require treatment for ESKD when the GFR falls to below 15 mL/min or the serum creatinine level increases to more than 10 mg/dL. Many patients, particularly those with diabetes, develop symptoms at lower serum creatinine levels and at higher GFR values. Hemodialysis or peritoneal dialysis access should be arranged sufficiently far in advance so that treatment can be started when needed, rather than on an urgent or emergency basis. Patients can then be spared the suffering and risk that are inevitably associated with advanced CKD. Because permanent vascular access for hemodialysis requires 4 to 8 weeks to mature, placement should be undertaken early so that the use of temporary venous catheters for dialysis access can be avoided. For peritoneal dialysis, peritoneal catheter placement can be delayed until dialysis is more imminent because only 2 to 4 weeks is required before the access can be used. Early referral of CKD patients to the care of a nephrologist about doubles the chance of being placed on the waiting list and of receiving a transplant before the commencement of dialysis. Patients who start dialysis emergently, or who have not had predialysis nephrologic care, have a worse prognosis.

The decision to start dialysis is a clinical one, however, and should be based on the plasma levels of creatinine, urea nitrogen, and selected electrolytes as well as on a careful assessment of uremic symptoms. Predialysis or preemptive transplantation is discussed in Chapter 8. It is the preferred therapeutic modality for ESKD in terms of morbidity, mortality, and long-term graft survival, but only 6% of ESKD patients receive preemptive transplantation. The allocation algorithm for deceased donor transplants (see Chapter 5) allows patients who have not yet started dialysis to accrue waiting-time points when their eGFR is 20 mL/min or less. The very long waiting time for deceased donor organs makes it unlikely, however, that a predialysis patient without a living donor will be allocated a kidney. Predialysis patients who are placed on the deceased donor transplant waiting list and those prepared for living donor transplantation should be warned explicitly not to delay establishing access for dialysis should it become necessary before a donor organ is available. Such an approach avoids the need for an unduly hurried pretransplant preparation that can be dangerous and emotionally stressful both for patients and caregivers.

Selected Readings

Choi M, Fried L. Chronic kidney disease and progression. NephSAP 2015;14:5.

Hart A, Smith M, Skeans A, et al. OPTN/SRTR Annual Data Report 2014: kidney. Am J Transplant 2016;(suppl 1):18.

Inker L, Astor B, Fox C, et al. KDOQI US Commentary on the 2012 KDIGO Clinical Practice Guideline for the Evaluation and Management of CKD. Am J Kidney Dis 2014;63:713–735.

Iyasere O, Brown E, Johansson J, et al. Quality of life and physical function in older patients on dialysis: a comparison of assisted peritoneal dialysis with hemodialysis. Clin J Am Soc Nephrol 2016;11:423–430.

Kidney Disease: Improving Global Outcomes (KDIGO) CKD Work Group. KDIGO 2012 Clinical Practice Guideline for the Evaluation and Management of Chronic Kidney Disease. Kidney Inter Suppl 2013;3:1–150.

Radhakrishnan J, Remuzzi G, Saran R, et al. Taming the chronic kidney disease epidemic: a global view of surveillance efforts. Kidney Int 2014;86:246–250.

Salomon D. A CRISPR way to block PERVs—engineering organs for transplantation. N Engl J Med 2016;374:1089–1091.

Saran R, Li Y, Robinson B, et al. US Renal Data System 2015 Annual Data Report: epidemiology of kidney disease in the United States. Am J Kidney Dis 2016;67(3, suppl 1):S1–S434.

Thomas B, Wulf S, Bibkov B, et al. Maintenance dialysis throughout the world in years 1990 and 2010. J Am Soc Nephrol 2015;26:2621–2633.

Vella J, Wiseman A. Transplantation. NephSAP 2015;14:5.

Wetmore J, Collins A. Meeting the world's need for maintenance hemodialysis. J Am Soc Nephrol 2015;26:2601–2603.

2

Transplantation Immunobiology

Hehua Dai and Fadi G. Lakkis

Transplantation Immunobiology is the study of the mechanisms that underlie graft rejection. It owes its scientific roots to the discovery of blood groups in the early 1900s by Karl Landsteiner in Vienna and the elucidation of the cellular mechanisms of graft rejection by Peter Medawar in London, and Jacques Miller in Melbourne, less than 50 years later. Their seminal discoveries paved the way for the first successful kidney transplant between identical twins in Boston in 1954 and, shortly thereafter, the development of anti-rejection drugs that enabled kidney transplantation between genetically dissimilar individuals. The rest, of course, is history.

The goal of this chapter is to describe the principal immunologic pathways that cause graft rejection. We begin by providing basic concepts and definitions and then discuss the cellular and molecular players responsible for initiating and mediating the rejection process. Knowledge gained should assist the reader with understanding the fundamental tenets of histocompatibility testing (tissue typing and crossmatching, see Chapter 3), the diagnosis and classification of rejection (see Chapters 10, 11, and 15), and the mechanisms of action of immunosuppressive drugs (see Chapter 6).

BASIC CONCEPTS AND DEFINITIONS

Cells, tissues, or organs transplanted between genetically indistinguishable individuals (identical twins) are not rejected. The slightest genetic difference between the donor and recipient, however, is sufficient to cause graft rejection, necessitating the administration of continuous immunosuppression to the recipient. The greater the genetic disparity, the greater are the likelihood and severity of rejection. Rejection is, therefore, the end-result of the recipient's immune response to genetically determined elements present in the transplanted organ. These elements are usually proteins that are dissimilar between the donor and the recipient. They are known as transplantation antigens or *alloantigens*. The transplanted organ itself is referred to as an allogeneic graft, or more simply as the *allograft*, and the immune response mounted against it as the *alloimmune* response. Since "allo" in ancient Greek means "other," it is used in clinical transplantation to represent all matters related to organs transplanted between members of the same species. In contrast, the prefix "xeno," which means "foreign," is used to denote transplantation between members of different species (for example, from pigs to humans)—thus, the terms *xenoantigens*, *xenografts*, and *xenotransplantation*.

Distinct organs have different propensities for rejection, either because they elicit unequal alloimmune responses or because they have distinct susceptibilities to immune-mediated damage. This is reflected in the amount of immunosuppression required to maintain long-term graft survival and function. Liver allografts need the least immunosuppression and last the longest; lungs and small bowel allografts require the most immunosuppression and last the least; and heart and kidney transplants are somewhere in between. It has also been observed that kidney allografts transplanted simultaneously with a liver (or heart) from the same donor are less prone to rejection than kidneys transplanted alone or those transplanted after an organ from a different donor. Likewise, kidney allografts obtained from living unrelated donors enjoy superior function and survival than equally matched kidneys from deceased donors. These curious but important clinical observations result from fundamental features of the alloimmune response that will be addressed below.

OVERVIEW OF ALLOGRAFT REJECTION

Understanding the mechanisms of allograft rejection may seem at first blush a daunting task owing to the myriad types of cells and molecules that participate in the immune response and that crowd the pages of immunology textbooks like hieroglyphics on an ancient Egyptian tomb. The truth of the matter, however, is that transplant rejection hinges on a single key cell, the *T lymphocyte*. Experimental animals that lack T lymphocytes do not reject allografts. Similarly, profound depletion of T lymphocytes in humans prevents rejection until T lymphocytes, even a few, have returned to the circulation. It is, therefore, not surprising that immunosuppressive drugs that have achieved great success in organ transplantation, the calcineurin inhibitors (CNIs—cyclosporin and tacrolimus) and the anti-metabolites (azathioprine and mycophenolic acid), target T-lymphocyte activation and proliferation. An exception to the T-cell requirement for graft rejection is the immediate, hyperacute rejection of organs between ABO-incompatible individuals. In this case, allograft damage is caused by preexisting recipient antibodies against donor blood group antigens that are produced independently of T lymphocytes. We will revisit this type of rejection later.

T lymphocytes act as soldiers as well as orchestrators of the alloimmune response. Upon recognition of donor alloantigens introduced by the graft, recipient T lymphocytes differentiate into *cytotoxic* or *helper* lymphocytes. The former directly kill graft cells that display alloantigens on their surfaces, whereas the latter provide help to other immune cells via specialized membrane receptors or secreted proteins known as *cytokines*. Helper T lymphocytes induce *B lymphocytes* to produce antibodies against the allograft (*alloantibodies*) and cause inflammation by recruiting and activating myeloid cells such as *neutrophils* and *monocytes*. Alloantibodies inflict graft injury by triggering the *complement* cascade or by stimulating *macrophages* and *natural killer (NK) cells*, another type of lymphoid cell. Allograft rejection, therefore, is a cascade of damaging events initiated first and foremost by the recognition of foreign donor alloantigens by recipient T lymphocytes.

In the following sections we will explain what alloantigens are and how they are presented to T lymphocytes, the steps required for T-lymphocyte activation and differentiation, and the subsequent cellular and molecular processes that eventually result in graft rejection. Later we will address how immune responses are controlled by *regulatory lymphocyte* subsets and discuss the concept of *immunologic tolerance*, which will hopefully be exploited one day to minimize the use of pharmacologic immunosuppression in organ transplant recipients.

TRANSPLANTATION ANTIGENS

Human Leukocyte Antigens

The principal alloantigens responsible for triggering T-lymphocyte activation are the *human leukocyte antigens (HLA)*, also known by the generic name *major histocompatibility complex (MHC)* molecules. HLA are glycoproteins encoded by a family of adjacent (linked) genes on human chromosome 6 (Fig. 2.1). They consist of two families: HLA class I and HLA class II. HLA class I molecules comprise several groups, HLA-A to -G, but the most clinically relevant or *classical* are HLA-A, -B, and -C. They are present on the surface of all nucleated cells and platelets but are not present on RBCs. HLA class II expression, on the other hand, is restricted to B lymphocytes, certain myeloid cells, and a subset of activated T lymphocytes. The most clinically relevant groups are HLA-DP, -DQ, and -DR. Myeloid cells that express HLA class II molecules are *antigen-presenting cells (APC)* equipped to engulf and process antigens for presentation to T lymphocytes. They include *dendritic*

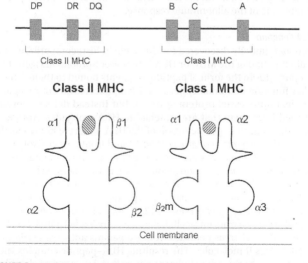

FIGURE 2.1 MHC/HLA structure. Map of the HLA genes found on chromosome 6 of humans is shown in the top panel. Schematic representations of MHC/HLA class I and MHC class II molecules are shown in the bottom panels. Hatched circles represent peptides bound to the peptide-biding grooves of MHC/HLA molecules.

cells and macrophages. They will be discussed in greater detail later. Human endothelial cells also express HLA class II during inflammation, particularly in response to the cytokine *interferon-gamma (IFNγ)*.

HLA proteins are among the most *polymorphic* (diverse) in humans. Any given HLA gene, say HLA-A, is present in many different forms or *alleles* in the human population with each allele coding for a distinct HLA-A protein; for example, HLA-A1, -A2, -A3, etc. At last count, more than 14,000 HLA alleles have been identified (>3,000 at the HLA-A locus alone), making the likelihood that two unrelated individuals share the same HLA molecules quite low. Since a person inherits two alleles of each HLA class I and class II gene, one from their father and one from their mother, and both alleles are expressed as proteins (*co-dominant inheritance*), children share 50% of their HLA molecules with either parent (so-called 1-haplotype match). Siblings, on the other hand, have a 25% chance of being HLA identical (2-haplotype match), 50% chance of being 1-haplotype matched, and 25% chance of being completely mismatched. Recombination (gene crossover) events during meiosis render these proportions less exact. The co-dominant inheritance of HLA genes and the fact that most people are heterozygous at HLA loci, imply that in the majority of individuals, cells will carry two distinct molecules of each HLA type. For example, if the HLA-A, -B, and -DR loci were typed in a prospective donor/recipient pair, as is commonly the case in clinical practice (see Chapter 3), the donor and recipient would be mismatched at anywhere between 0 and 6 of the typed HLA alleles. Therefore, the highly polymorphic nature of HLA and their ubiquitous expression in the body are important reasons why HLA are quintessential histocompatibility antigens, in a way the fingerprint of the graft. Later, it will become clear why they are also such potent stimulators of the alloimmune response.

HLA Function

Although initially discovered for their role in histocompatibility, the main function of the MHC or HLA is to present protein antigens to T lymphocytes in the form of peptide fragments bound to them. This is a key function in immunity because T lymphocytes do not recognize whole, unprocessed protein antigens, but instead detect peptides derived from them that are attached to HLA molecules. Antigenic peptides bind to a specific region of the HLA molecule known as the *peptide-binding region* or *groove* (Fig. 2.1 and front cover). Exogenous antigens that enter cells are hydrolyzed into peptides in endosomes and lysosomes, whereas endogenous antigens are processed by proteasomes. Peptide loading onto HLA molecules occurs in the endoplasmic reticulum with the help of specialized proteins known as *transporters associated with antigen processing (TAP)*. Usually, but not exclusively, peptides derived from intracellular antigens are loaded onto HLA class I molecules, whereas peptides from exogenous antigens are bound to HLA class II molecules. The resulting HLA–peptide complex then translocates to the cell membrane where it is detected by T lymphocytes. HLA molecules not loaded with peptides are degraded within the cell. Binding of the HLA–peptide complex to a specific receptor on T lymphocytes—the *T-cell receptor for antigen (TCR)*—triggers T-lymphocyte activation (more about that later). It is generally accepted that MHC molecules became polymorphic over evolutionary time to maximize the chance of binding the widest array of microbial peptides possible, thus conferring immunity against most infections—clearly a selective advantage to the host. An unintended downside of MHC polymorphism, however, is the creation of a strong barrier against transplantation. By varying in amino acid sequence, MHC molecules have become transplantation antigens themselves, serving as initiators and targets of the alloimmune response.

HLA Structure

HLA class I molecules consist of one polymorphic polypeptide chain designated *alpha* (also known as the heavy chain because it is richly glycosylated) encoded by genes in the HLA complex, and a monomorphic *β_2-microglobulin* chain encoded by a gene on chromosome 15 far from the HLA complex (Fig. 2.1). The polymorphic sides of the α1 and α2 domains of the alpha chain form the small groove where antigenic peptides are bound. Antigenic peptides, limited to 8 to 10 amino acids in length, along with the surrounding regions of the MHC class I groove are recognized by TCRs on *CD8$^+$ T lymphocytes*. CD8$^+$ T lymphocytes are the T-lymphocyte subset most often responsible for cytotoxic functions; therefore, they are also known as *cytotoxic T lymphocytes (CTL)*. The CD8 molecule is a trans-membrane protein on T lymphocytes that binds to the monomorphic α3 domain of the alpha chain and strengthens the interaction between the HLA class I–peptide complex and the TCR. The β_2-microglobulin chain, on the other hand, stabilizes the structure of the HLA class I molecule itself. Genetically engineered mice deficient in β_2-microglobulin lack MHC class I molecules on their cells.

HLA class II molecules consist of two polymorphic chains, *alpha* and *beta*, encoded by genes in the HLA complex (Fig. 2.1). The peptide-binding groove is formed by domains of both chains but has an open configuration that allows binding of peptides 14 to 20 amino acids in length. HLA class II–peptide complexes are recognized by TCRs of *CD4$^+$ T lymphocytes*, which are the lymphocytes most often responsible for helper functions: they are also known as *T helper (Th) lymphocytes*. By binding to the α2 domain, the CD4 molecule strengthens the interaction between the HLA class II–peptide complex and the TCR. Because CD4$^+$ T lymphocytes play a key role in orchestrating the alloimmune response, including providing help for alloantibody production, matching at HLA class II loci between donors and recipients is particularly advantageous for long-term allograft survival.

Nonclassical HLA

Nonclassical HLA molecules are HLA class I–like proteins that have limited polymorphism. They have aroused interest among kidney transplant specialists because they modulate NK-cell function and, in addition, are targets of alloantibodies. One prominent example is *HLA-G*. It is highly expressed in the placenta where it contributes to fetal tolerance by inhibiting maternal NK cells. HLA-G binds to an inhibitory receptor on NK cells that belongs to the *Killer-cell Immunoglobulin-like Receptor (KIR)* family. Increased levels of circulating HLA-G in kidney transplant recipients are associated with lower risk of graft rejection. Conversely, the nonclassical HLA molecules *MICA* and *MICB* (which stand for MHC class I polypeptide-related sequence A and B, respectively) stimulate NK cells and some T-lymphocyte subsets. Presence of anti-MICA or -MICB antibodies in the recipient correlates with increased incidence of rejection and graft loss.

Minor Histocompatibility Antigens

Even organs transplanted between HLA-matched individuals (for example, between two-haplotype matched siblings) are not safe from rejection. This is because any protein that is present in the graft but not the recipient, or that is sufficiently dissimilar (polymorphic) between the graft and the recipient, will behave as a foreign, transplantation antigen. Such non-HLA transplantation antigens are called minor histocompatibility antigens (*mHA*). A single mHA disparity is not as potent at inducing alloimmunity as a single HLA disparity (thus, the designation "minor"), but since many mHA mismatches exist between donors and recipients, the cumulative anti-mHA response is significant. A particular mHA that has garnered attention in transplantation is the H-Y antigen present only in males of the species. Clinical data suggest that it possibly compromises the survival of male renal allografts transplanted to female recipients. The role of mHA in graft-versus-host disease is well established as the vast majority of hematopoietic stem cell transplants are performed between HLA-matched individuals, making the contribution of mHA more noticeable. Polymorphic mitochondrial proteins are another type of mHA that can trigger alloimmunity. This is particularly relevant to transplanting-induced pluripotent stem (iPS) cells generated by nuclear transfer, wherein the nucleus is "self" but the mitochondria are foreign.

Blood Group Antigens

ABO incompatibility is a potent barrier to organ transplantation for two reasons. First, ABO antigens are not restricted to RBCs but are present on all cells. Second, humans generate antibodies against foreign blood group antigens during early infancy. These antibodies arise in response to ABO-like carbohydrate antigens present on gut commensals. Moreover, anti-ABO antibodies, which are of the IgM isotype, are produced by the *B1* or *innate B-lymphocyte* subset that functions independent of T lymphocyte's help. Therefore, the preexistence of anti-A or anti-B antibodies in the recipient (for example, in a blood group O patient) leads to the *hyperacute rejection* of grafts transplanted from A, B, or AB blood group donors. This type of antibody-mediated rejection is characterized by endothelial cell destruction and hemorrhagic necrosis of the graft, within minutes or hours of transplantation. It is an extremely rare clinical entity nowadays because of careful ABO matching and desensitization of ABO-mismatched kidney recipients prior to transplantation. Note that preexisting anti-donor HLA antibodies can also cause hyperacute rejection but diligent screening of recipients for such antibodies has all but eradicated this problem. Nevertheless, as we shall see later, preexisting anti-donor HLA antibodies (known as donor-specific antibodies or DSA) or those that form *de novo* after transplantation are an important cause of later graft injury and loss.

There are two exceptions to the ABO-incompatibility rule. First, is the transplantation of A2 kidneys across ABO barriers because A2 blood group individuals express low levels of the A antigen on their tissues. Second, is the transplantation of livers or hearts to infants because infants have low titers of anti-A or -B antibodies and, in addition, become tolerant to these antigens after transplantation. Unlike the ABO system, Rh incompatibility is not a histocompatibility barrier since the major Rh antigen responsible for allosensitization after blood exposure, RhD, is not present on nonerythroid cells.

ALLORECOGNITION

The central event in the initiation of the alloimmune response is the recognition of donor alloantigens by recipient T lymphocytes—a phenomenon referred to in transplantation as *allorecognition*. Allorecognition depends on the presence in the recipient of *alloreactive* T lymphocytes that express T-cell receptors (TCR) capable of binding alloantigens and on the presentation of alloantigens by specialized antigen-presenting cells (APCs).

Allorecognition by T Lymphocytes

T lymphocytes express on their membranes TCRs that recognize antigenic peptides bound to HLA molecules. TCRs are randomly generated during ontogeny via a gene rearrangement process, leading to a vastly diverse repertoire of TCRs that recognizes millions of foreign antigens. A given T lymphocyte, however, expresses a handful of different TCRs on its surface, allowing it to respond to a limited number of antigens. Normally, anywhere between 0.01% and 0.1% or less of an individual's T lymphocytes recognize and respond to a given microbial antigen but, in the setting of transplantation, approximately 2% to 10% of T lymphocytes react to the mismatched organ. There are two main reasons for the high prevalence (*precursor frequency*) of alloreactive T lymphocytes. First, TCRs recognize alloantigens via two pathways: direct and indirect (Fig. 2.2). *Direct allorecognition* refers to the recognition by TCRs of intact donor HLA proteins that are foreign (allogeneic) to the recipient, whereas *indirect allorecognition* refers to the recognition by TCRs of donor alloantigens (whether HLA or mHA) that are processed by recipient APCs and presented as small peptides bound to self- (recipient) HLA molecules—the same pathway responsible for presenting microbial antigens. T lymphocytes that recognize alloantigens via the direct pathway are quite prevalent (they outnumber indirectly alloreactive T lymphocytes by approximately 100 fold) because of an intrinsic bias of the immune system to generate TCRs that recognize HLA molecules in general and because of the cross-reactivity of TCRs. The bias occurs during T-cell development in the thymus where immature T lymphocytes that bind HLA molecules are favored to survive and undergo further selection and maturation. *Cross-reactivity* refers to the fact that many T lymphocytes bearing TCRs specific to microbial antigens (microbial peptides bound to self-MHC/HLA) also recognize

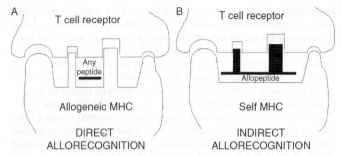

FIGURE 2.2 Allorecognition pathways. The T-cell receptor (TCR) on T lymphocytes recognizes either intact allogeneic MHC/HLA molecules (**A:** direct allorecognition) or allopeptides bound to the groove of self-MHC/HLA molecules (**B:** indirect allorecognition). T lymphocytes capable of direct allorecognition represent the majority of recipient T lymphocytes that respond to the transplanted organ.

intact, nonself (allogeneic) MHC/HLA molecules complexed to either self- or nonself peptides (Fig. 2.2). The second reason for the high frequency and potency of alloreactive T lymphocytes is the conspicuous presence of *memory T lymphocytes* in the alloreactive T-lymphocyte repertoire of humans. Memory T lymphocytes share the same antigenic specificity as their naïve precursors but are present in much higher frequency and have a much greater proliferative capacity once activated by antigen. They will be discussed in a separate section later in the chapter because of the prominent role they play in alloimmunity.

Antigen-Presenting Cells

T-lymphocyte activation depends on close contact between the APC and the T lymphocyte since the APC not only provides the means by which HLA–peptide complexes are presented to TCRs but, as will be discussed in the next section, provides the necessary signals required for T-lymphocyte proliferation and differentiation. *Dendritic cells (DC)*, macrophages, B lymphocytes, and activated human endothelial cells are all known to function as APCs, but DCs are by far the most potent. DCs are myeloid cells that derive from a precursor in the bone marrow, but also arise from monocytes during inflammation. DCs are present in a quiescent (immature) state throughout the body in both primary (bone marrow and thymus) and secondary (spleen, lymph nodes, and mucosa-associated) lymphoid organs as well as in the organs that are commonly transplanted in the clinic: the kidney, liver, heart, lung, and pancreas. Upon encountering microbial or inflammatory stimuli, DCs enter a maturation process during which they upregulate HLA; the machinery required for engulfing protein antigens and processing them into small peptides and packaging them in the peptide-binding grooves of HLA; membrane proteins that co-stimulate T lymphocytes; and the cytokines necessary for T-lymphocyte differentiation. Therefore, DCs transform into an exquisite cellular device for activating T lymphocytes. Naïve T lymphocytes encounter and are activated by antigen-presenting DCs in secondary lymphoid tissues (the lymph nodes, spleen, and mucosa-associated lymphoid tissues). In contrast, memory T lymphocytes can be activated by DCs throughout the body. The current consensus is that DCs play a key role in alloimmunity, but other APCs such as B lymphocytes and macrophages also contribute; for example, during later phases of the alloimmune response.

Transplantation poses an interesting immunologic scenario because two types of DCs that can activate recipient T lymphocytes are present: donor-type DCs that accompany the transplanted organ and, of course, the recipient's own DCs. It has been assumed for many years that donor DCs are responsible for the bulk of alloimmune activation because they carry intact, donor HLA molecules and therefore stimulate the highly prevalent directly-alloreactive T-lymphocyte population. Recipient DCs, on the other hand, were assigned the less central role of indirectly presenting processed donor antigens to a much less prevalent population of alloreactive recipient T lymphocytes. Recent evidence, however, indicates that donor DCs, which exit the graft in bulk and migrate to the recipient's secondary lymphoid organs within hours after transplantation, are in fact extremely short-lived but quickly transfer their antigenic cargo consisting mostly of donor HLA to recipient DCs. Recipient DCs then take on the task of activating recipient T lymphocytes via both the direct and indirect allorecognition pathways. Recipient DCs can also acquire donor HLA from micro-vesicles released from the graft into the circulation at the time of transplantation. The process of transferring intact donor HLA molecules to recipient DCs is referred to as *cross-dressing*. The presentation by cross-dressed, recipient DCs of donor HLA to directly alloreactive T lymphocytes is referred to as the *semi-direct allorecognition pathway*. Therefore, donor DCs are akin to fleeting cargo ships that deliver donor HLA and other alloantigens to recipient DCs, which then stimulate the alloimmune response via both the direct and indirect allorecognition pathways. Within few days of transplantation, allografts are repopulated with DCs derived from recipient monocytes. Recent experimental data suggest that these DCs continue to play a role in the rejection process by engaging effector T lymphocytes that enter the graft.

T-LYMPHOCYTE ACTIVATION

Full-fledged activation of alloreactive T lymphocytes depends on three signals (Fig. 2.3). *Signal 1* is delivered by binding of TCRs on T lymphocytes to HLA–peptide complexes on APCs. Signal 1 is necessary but not sufficient for T-lymphocyte proliferation and differentiation. *Signal 2* is delivered by binding of specialized accessory molecules on APCs to their receptors on T lymphocytes. Along with signal 1, signal 2 causes T-lymphocyte proliferation and differentiation. Finally, cytokines produced by APCs deliver *signal 3*, which determines the differentiation pathway of T lymphocytes into specialized subsets. These signals and the types and functions of T-lymphocyte subsets that are generated are described below.

Signal 1: TCR Signaling

Binding of antigen (HLA–peptide complex) to the TCR triggers a signaling cascade that leads to T-lymphocyte activation. These signals are not transduced through the TCR proper, but through the adjacent *CD3 complex*, a group of invariant (nonpolymorphic) protein chains that associate with the TCR. CD4 and CD8 co-receptors on T lymphocytes also participate in the activation signal mediated by the TCR–CD3 cluster by binding to the same MHC molecule that engages the TCR. Antibodies that target one or more proteins in the CD3 complex block T-lymphocyte activation. An example is OKT3, the first monoclonal antibody used in clinical medicine, and since withdrawn (see Chapter 6), that was used to treat severe acute allograft rejection. The activation signal transduced by the TCR–CD3 cluster is dependent on *tyrosine kinases* (*Lck, ZAP-70,* and *Fyn*) that cause the recruitment and activation of the enzyme *phospholipase C-γ (PLC-γ)*. PLC-γ catalyzes the breakdown of the membrane lipid phosphatidylinositol biphosphate (PIP_2) to generate two second-messengers: Diacylglycerol (DAG) and inositol 1,4,5-triphosphate (IP_3). DAG activates the *protein kinase C (PKC)* and *mitogen-activated protein (MAP) kinase* pathways, whereas IP_3 triggers the *calcineurin* pathway by increasing intracellular calcium concentration. Together, the PKC, MAP kinase, and calcineurin pathways ultimately activate key *transcription factors* (*NFkB, NFAT,* and *AP-1*) that induce the transcription of cytokine genes required for T-lymphocyte proliferation and differentiation. The calcineurin pathway is the target of the CNIs (see Chapter 6). CNIs bind to specialized proteins in the cell known as *immunophilins—cyclophilin* in the case of cyclosporin and *FK-binding protein* (*FKBP*) in the case of tacrolimus. The drug–immunophilin complex then blocks the activation of calcineurin by the calcium-dependent enzyme *calmodulin*.

Signal 2: Co-Stimulation

In addition to signal 1, T lymphocytes must receive a second signal to undergo full proliferation and differentiation into *effector* lymphocytes, which include either cytotoxic or helper cells. Signal 2 is delivered by engagement of *co-stimulatory receptors* on T lymphocytes by their ligands on APCs (Fig. 2.3). Failure to provide the second signal results in aborted T-lymphocyte activation, which causes T-lymphocyte *deletion* (death) or *anergy*. The latter is a prolonged state of refractoriness to stimulation by antigen. Co-stimulatory molecules are either absent or are constitutively expressed on naïve T lymphocytes, but are induced or upregulated upon activation of T lymphocytes with antigen. This ensures that stimulation of T lymphocytes that have already encountered antigen is further amplified, while unintended activation of bystander T lymphocytes is not. What follows is a summary of the main co-stimulatory pathways involved in T-lymphocyte activation.

Integrins

Extended interaction between the DC presenting the alloantigen and the alloreactive T lymphocyte is necessary for sustained TCR signaling. Prolonged, stable interaction between the two is made possible by cell-adhesion molecules known as *integrins*. The integrins *LFA-1* and *CD2 (LFA-3)* on T lymphocytes bind to their ligands *ICAM-1/ICAM-2* and *CD58*, respectively, on DCs (Fig. 2.3). LFA-1 and CD2 mediate initial, transient adhesion between naïve T lymphocytes and DCs, but once a T lymphocyte encounters the DC presenting the antigen it recognizes, signaling via the TCR alters the molecular conformation of the integrins

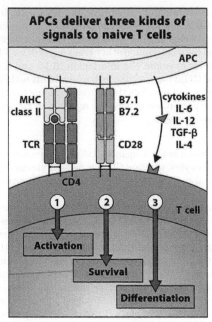

FIGURE 2.3 Signals required for T-lymphocyte activation, proliferation, and differentiation. *Signal 1* is delivered by binding of the TCR on T lymphocytes to the MHC–peptide complex on APCs. CD4 or CD8 in T lymphocytes strengthens this interaction by binding to a nonpolymorphic region of MHC class II or class I, respectively. Signal 1 is necessary but not sufficient for T-lymphocyte proliferation and differentiation. *Signal 2* is delivered by binding of specialized co-stimulatory molecules on APCs to their receptors on T lymphocytes. Along with signal 1, signal 2 causes T-lymphocyte proliferation. Finally, cytokines produced by APCs deliver *signal 3*, which determines the differentiation pathway of T lymphocytes into specialized subsets (see Fig. 2.4). Co-stimulatory molecules and cytokines shown are only a few examples of several others. (Reprinted from Murphy K, Weaver C. *Janeway's Immunobiology.* 9th ed. New York: Garland Science; 2016, with permission.)

(inside-out-signaling) and enhances their affinity and avidity to their ligands. LFA-1 and CD2 also deliver intracellular signals *(outside-in-signaling)* that contribute to T-lymphocyte activation—thus, serving as *bona fide* co-stimulatory molecules. Antibodies against LFA-1 or CD2 delay kidney transplant rejection in nonhuman primates and in the case of CD2 reduce the number of alloreactive memory T lymphocytes. The development and marketing of anti-LFA-1 (Efalizumab) and anti-CD2 antibodies (Alefacept) for clinical use in autoimmunity and transplantation have been halted owing to serious side effects such as progressive multifocal leukoencephalopathy (PML) caused by JC virus reactivation.

B7–CD28

CD28 is a co-stimulatory receptor present on all naïve T lymphocytes. It binds the co-stimulatory molecules B7.1 (CD80) and B7.2 (CD86) on mature APCs, namely DCs. A naïve T lymphocyte must engage both antigen and co-stimulatory ligands on the same APC. Intracellular signaling by CD28 augments the activation of the same enzyme triggered by the TCR cluster, PLC-γ, and potentiates the effects of antigen stimulation on the transcription of key genes required for T-lymphocyte proliferation; for example, the interleukin (IL)-2 and IL-2 receptor (IL-2R) genes. CTLA4-Ig (Belatacept), which binds with high affinity to B7 molecules and prevents them from engaging CD28, is in clinical use for the prevention of allograft rejection in kidney transplant recipients (see Chapter 6).

CD40–CD154

CD154, also known as CD40 ligand (CD40L), is expressed on activated CD4$^+$ T lymphocytes, whereas CD40 is present mainly on B lymphocytes, DCs, and macrophages. CD154 was first discovered because of its role in inducing antibody isotype switching in B lymphocytes. Isotype switching is the process by which B lymphocytes shift from producing IgM to the more effective IgG antibody isotypes. Therefore, engagement of CD40 by CD154 is an important mechanism by which CD4$^+$ T lymphocytes provide help to B lymphocytes. CD154 is also a key enhancer of T-lymphocyte stimulation, albeit in an indirect manner. By binding to CD40, it upregulates B7 expression and enhances cytokine production by DCs. This in turn leads to further co-stimulation of T lymphocytes, especially the CD8$^+$ subset. Preclinical studies have shown that antibodies that block the CD40–CD154 pathway are very effective anti-rejection agents. When tested in humans however, anti-CD154 antibodies caused serious thromboembolic side effects owing to CD154 expression on platelets. An alternate and likely safer approach to blocking the CD40–CD154 pathway is the use of anti-CD40 antibodies. These are currently undergoing clinical testing in renal transplant recipients.

Other Co-Stimulatory Pathways

Additional co-stimulatory pathways that contribute to signal 2 in T lymphocytes include *41BBL–41BB (CD137)*, *OX40L–OX40*, *CD70:CD27*, and *ICOSL–ICOS* pathways. Except for CD27, which is constitutively present on naïve T lymphocytes, 41BB, OX40, and CD70 are induced upon T-lymphocyte activation, underscoring their role in sustaining T-lymphocyte activation. Blocking these pathways inhibits allograft rejection to varying degrees in experimental animals.

Signal 3: Cytokines

Cytokines involved in T-lymphocyte activation are proteins secreted by mature APCs or the T lymphocytes themselves. They serve two main purposes in the context of T-lymphocyte activation: they stimulate T-lymphocyte proliferation and induce the differentiation of T lymphocytes into multiple effector subsets that have distinct phenotypes and functions. However, cytokines can also regulate T lymphocytes or act on other immune and nonimmune cells to either enhance or suppress inflammation. Most cytokines are known by the term *interleukin* (IL) followed by a number that refers to the order in which they were discovered. Here, we will summarize salient features of the key cytokines involved in T-lymphocyte activation and differentiation.

Interleukin-2 (IL-2)

IL-2 is the first T-lymphocyte mitogen to be discovered by virtue of its strong capacity to induce T-lymphocyte proliferation in culture (*in vitro*). IL-2 is produced by antigen-activated T lymphocytes and acts on the same lymphocytes that produce it (autocrine) or on neighboring lymphocytes (paracrine). Naïve T lymphocytes express a low-affinity form of the *interleukin-2 receptor (IL-2R)* consisting of two protein chains: gamma (γ) and beta (β). Upon activation by antigen and co-stimulatory molecules, T lymphocytes express a third chain, alpha (α) or *CD25*, which increases the affinity of the IL-2R by approximately 1,000 fold. IL-2 binding to the high-affinity IL-2R causes the proliferation (*clonal expansion*) of antigen-activated T lymphocytes (Fig. 2.3). Anti-CD25 monoclonal antibodies that block the α chain of the IL-2R are potent inhibitors of T-lymphocyte proliferation *in vitro*, but when used in humans (for example, Basiliximab employed as induction therapy in kidney transplant recipients, see Chapter 6), are relatively modest immunosuppressive agents. One explanation for this paradox is the presence of several other cytokines that also support the proliferation and survival of T lymphocytes. These include *IL-4, IL-7, IL-9, IL-15, and IL-21*. The receptors for these cytokines contain the same γ-chain present in the IL-2R and are therefore referred to as the *common γ-chain cytokine receptor family*. Antibodies that target the γ-chain should be highly immunosuppressive but would likely cause severe lymphopenia because IL-7 and IL-15 are also required for the homeostatic maintenance of naïve and memory T lymphocytes. Humans who carry mutations in the X-linked gene that codes for the common γ-chain have severe combined immunodeficiency (SCID), the "boy in a bubble" syndrome, characterized by very low numbers of T and NK lymphocytes and defective B-lymphocyte function. Signaling via the common γ-chain cytokine receptor family is mediated by a *Janus kinase (JAK)* protein tyrosine kinase, *Jak3*. Mutations that inactivate Jak3 also cause SCID in humans. JAK3 phosphorylates and activates specific transcription factors known as signal transducers and activators of transcription *(STATs)*. A JAK3 inhibitor, Tofacitinib, is currently available for the treatment of rheumatoid arthritis and psoriasis. Although it proved to be noninferior to cyclosporin in preventing rejection, it has not been approved for use in transplantation, possibly owing to increased incidence of infections when combined with other immunosuppressive agents. Another reason why blocking the IL-2Rα turned out not to be as effective in transplant recipients as expected is that IL-2 is also required for the proliferation and maintenance of a subset of CD4$^+$ T lymphocytes that have regulatory functions. Regulatory T lymphocytes, or *Treg*, express high levels of IL-2Rα and are necessary for preventing autoimmunity. In transplantation, they likely prevent rejection. More about them later.

Cytokines and T-Lymphocyte Subsets

Cytokines produced by APCs or by activated T lymphocytes direct the differentiation of proliferating T lymphocytes into multiple effector populations (Fig. 2.4). *CD4$^+$ T lymphocytes* differentiate into four major *helper* subpopulations (*Th1, Th2, Th17, T_{FH}*) and one *regulatory*

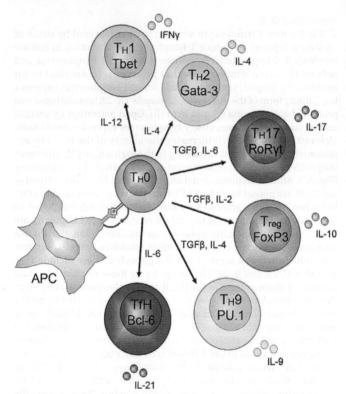

FIGURE 2.4 T helper (T_H) lymphocyte subsets. Upon activation by antigen-presenting cells (APCs), $CD4^+$ T_H lymphocytes differentiate into multiple subsets based on which cytokines are present in the milieu and on the expression of specific transcription factors in the cell nucleus (Tbet, Gata3, etc...). T_H9, not discussed in the text, represent a T-lymphocyte subpopulation that produces the cytokine IL-9. It is involved in either immunity or tolerance, but its role in transplantation is unclear. (From Russ BE, Prier JE, Rao S, et al. T-cell immunity as a tool for studying epigenetic regulation of cellular differentiation. Front Genet 2013;4:218. Copyright © 2013 Russ, Prier, Rao and Turner. https://creativecommons.org/licenses/by/3.0/legalcode)

subpopulation *(Treg)*, whereas *CD8⁺ T lymphocytes* differentiate into *cytotoxic T cells (CTL)*. CD8⁺ T lymphocytes can also acquire helper or regulatory functions along the same lines as CD4⁺ T lymphocytes and, conversely, CD4⁺ T lymphocytes can be cytotoxic. Cytokines also assist effector T lymphocytes in transitioning to long-lived *memory T lymphocytes (T_M)*. Below is a brief account of T-lymphocyte subsets and the cytokines required for their differentiation and function. Importantly, all effector T-lymphocyte subsets participate in allograft rejection, some playing a more dominant role than others.

Th1 lymphocytes are the prototypical lymphocyte subpopulation responsible for rejection. Their differentiation is driven by *IL-12* and *interferon-gamma (IFNγ)*. IL-12 is produced by activated DCs whereas

IFNγ is secreted by the Th1 lymphocytes themselves as well as other cells such as B lymphocytes. The transcription factors *STAT1* and *T-bet* are necessary for Th1 differentiation. Th1 lymphocytes produce copious amounts of IFNγ, *tumor necrosis factor-alpha (TNFα)* and *lymphotoxin (LT)*, which promote allograft rejection by activating macrophages, directly inflicting damage on graft endothelial cells, inducing production of complement-fixing IgG antibodies by B lymphocytes, and stimulating the differentiation of CD8$^+$ T lymphocytes to CTL. Blocking IFNγ alone is not a useful therapeutic strategy because IFNγ also has regulatory functions. In mice, it enhances Tregs and limits T-lymphocyte proliferation. Ustekinumab, a monoclonal antibody against the IL-12p40 subunit of IL-12 that is also shared with IL-23 (see below), has been approved by the FDA for the treatment of psoriasis. Its utility in transplantation has not been tested yet.

Th2 lymphocytes are the lymphocyte subset responsible for allergic reactions. They also contribute to allograft rejection. Their differentiation is dependent on *IL-4*, produced by a variety of cells, and on the transcription factors *STAT6* and *GATA3*. Th2 lymphocytes produce IL-4, *IL-5, IL-9, IL-10, and IL-13*, which activate eosinophils, basophils, and mast cells and enhance production of particular antibody isotypes, usually those that do not fix complement. IL-10 also has immunoregulatory properties that dampen rejection. Th2 lymphocytes are sufficient for mediating allograft rejection in experimental rodents but are much less potent than Th1 lymphocytes. In some circumstances, Th2 lymphocytes inhibit Th1 lymphocyte formation and delay rejection.

Th17 lymphocytes constitute a subpopulation that is particularly adept at responding to fungal infections. They are named after the signature cytokine they produce, *IL-17*, and contribute to allograft rejection by promoting inflammation. Differentiation of antigen-stimulated naïve T lymphocytes to the Th17 phenotype is dependent on *TGFβ, IL-6,* and *IL-21* and on the transcription factors *STAT6* and *RORγT*. The cytokine IL-23 stabilizes the Th17 lymphocyte phenotype by ensuring continued IL-17 production. IL-6 and IL-23 are produced by DCs and other activated myeloid cells. IL-23 shares a protein chain, the IL-12p40 subunit, with IL-12. IL-21 is produced by Th17 lymphocytes and functions as an autocrine growth factor. Th17 lymphocytes promote inflammation by secreting IL-17, which stimulates the production of neutrophil chemoattractants by epithelial and other stromal cells in the graft. Th17 lymphocytes also participate in the formation of *tertiary lymphoid tissues* at sites of chronic inflammation. Tertiary lymphoid tissues, which share similar architecture to lymph nodes, have been observed in renal allografts undergoing chronic rejection, suggesting that they could participate in the local immune response. A monoclonal anti-IL-17 antibody, Secukinumab, is available for use in patients with psoriasis and rheumatoid arthritis. The approval of antibodies that block the IL-17R is likely forthcoming. An anti-IL-21 monoclonal antibody is currently under evaluation in patients with autoimmune disease. It remains to be determined whether any of these novel biologic agents is of benefit to renal transplant recipients.

T$_{FH}$ (follicular helper) lymphocytes play a key role in antibody production by providing help to B lymphocytes. Their generation is dependent on IL-21 and on the transcription factor *Bcl6*. They express the chemokine receptor *CXCR5*, which guides their migration to B-cell follicles in secondary lymphocyte tissues. There they induce the differentiation of activated B lymphocytes to antibody-producing plasma cells via CD40L–CD40 interactions and the secretion of cytokines, namely IL-4 and IL-21. In transplantation, T_{FH} are important for driving the production of alloantibodies that are detrimental to graft survival. Therefore, interrupting CD40L–CD40 interactions is expected to be dually beneficial by blocking T-lymphocyte activation as well as T-lymphocyte help to B lymphocytes.

Cytotoxic T lymphocytes (CTL) bind via their TCRs to target cells expressing nonself MHC–peptide complexes and induce target cell killing by secreting *perforin* and *granzymes*. Perforin is a channel-forming protein, whereas granzymes are serine proteases that trigger programmed cell death by activating caspases. IFNγ secreted by Th1 lymphocytes and the transcription factor Tbet are necessary for CTL differentiation from activated $CD8^+$ T lymphocytes.

The Mammalian or Mechanistic Target of Rapamycin (mTOR) Pathway

An important intracellular signaling pathway involved in T-lymphocyte proliferation is the mTOR pathway that is inhibited by the immunosuppressive drug Rapamycin (also known as Sirolimus) and the closely related drug, Everolimus (see Chapter 6). mTOR is a protein kinase present in many cell types including T lymphocytes. It is involved in cell-cycle progression from the G1 to S phase (proliferation), cell survival, cell growth, and cell autophagy. mTOR functions by associating with other proteins to form two complexes: mTORC1 and mTORC2. mTORC1, the principal target of Rapamycin, is a nutrient sensor that plays a central role in regulating cell metabolism and, therefore, cell homeostasis and proliferation. mTORC2, which is inhibited by higher concentrations of Rapamycin, is involved in actin organization and cell survival. The pleiotropic functions of mTOR and its ubiquitous expression in many cell types are the likely explanations why the clinical use of Rapamycin in transplantation has been limited by variable efficacy and high incidence of side effects. For example, Rapamycin inhibits T-lymphocyte proliferation but paradoxically increases memory T-lymphocyte generation. Nevertheless, Rapamycin is sometimes administered to transplant recipients to replace or as an adjuvant to CNIs or those patients who have concomitant neoplasia. Newer, selective inhibitors of mTORC1 and mTORC2 may prove more useful in the future.

MEMORY T LYMPHOCYTES

A large number of effector lymphocytes are generated during an immune response, but most undergo *activation-induced cell death (AICD)* by apoptosis as the response progresses. The few effector lymphocytes that survive give rise to *memory T lymphocytes (T_M)*. The differentiation from effector to memory is dependent on the cytokines IL-7 and IL-15. T_M retain the antigen specificity and often the functional phenotype of their precursors. In humans, they consist of two major subsets: *central memory (T_{CM})* and *effector memory (T_{EM})*. T_{CM}, which express the chemokine receptor CCR7, circulate through both secondary lymphoid and nonlymphoid peripheral tissues and have a large proliferative capacity, whereas T_{EM}, which express the chemokine receptor CXCR3 but lack CCR7, circulate predominantly through nonlymphoid tissues and the spleen and have a higher capacity for immediate effector functions marked by IFNγ, perforin, and granzyme release. Resident memory T-lymphocyte populations (T_{RM}) that remain within nonlymphoid tissues have been described recently in the skin, lungs, and gut in mice and humans, but their relevance to transplantation has yet to be determined.

T_M have several advantages over their naïve counterparts. They are present at a much higher frequency and have a longer lifespan, wider migration pattern (they migrate to and reside in either lymphoid or nonlymphoid organs), and lower threshold for activation than their naïve predecessors. Upon re-encountering antigen, T_M lymphocytes generate a much stronger immune response (recall response) than that of naïve T lymphocytes (primary response). The recall response is only partially dependent on traditional co-stimulatory pathways such as B7-CD28 (therefore, resistant to inhibition by CTLA4-Ig [Belatacept]) and is elicited not only by DCs but also by endothelial cells. These properties of memory T lymphocytes confer a significant protective advantage against infection but are deleterious to transplanted organs if the T_M are alloreactive. Indeed, T_M constitute approximately half of the alloreactive T-lymphocyte repertoire in humans, even in naïve individuals not previously exposed to alloantigens. Humans harbor or acquire alloreactive T_M for three reasons. First, T_M generated in response to vaccination or infection are frequently *cross-reactive* with alloantigens—that is, they recognize intact nonself HLA molecules on donor cells in addition to their target microbial antigens (microbial peptides bound to self HLA). Second, alloreactive T_M arise after exposure to alloantigens in blood transfusions, prior organ transplants, or pregnancy. Third, alloreactive T_M emerge during recovery from lymphophenia; for example, following the administration of lymphocyte-depleting, induction therapy at the time of transplantation.

The ubiquitous presence of alloreactive T_M and the functional advantages they have over naïve T lymphocytes make them a formidable barrier to allograft acceptance. Patients who harbor higher frequencies of T_M against donor alloantigens have higher incidence of acute rejection. Similarly, patients receiving CTLA4-Ig (Belatacept) experience more severe rejection episodes than patients on tacrolimus, likely because CTLA4-Ig does not adequately inhibit T_M activation. Moreover, since T_M are generated during recovery from lymphopenia, transplant recipients induced with Thymoglobulin or anti-CD52 (Campath) have on average more circulating T_M than nondepleted recipients. Increased T_M for many years after lymphodepletion could explain why these induction agents, although effective at preventing rejection in the early post-transplantation period, do not enable the safe withdrawal of CNI at a later time point.

T-LYMPHOCYTE MIGRATION

Naïve T lymphocytes circulate between the blood and secondary lymphoid organs but do not enter nonlymphoid tissues. They are activated within secondary lymphoid organs. Their migration from the blood to the T-cell zones of lymph nodes occurs via specialized *high endothelial venules* and is dependent on both adhesion molecules (L-selectin and LFA-1) and chemokine receptors (CCR7). *L-selectin (CD62L)* mediates naïve T-lymphocyte rolling by binding to *addressins* on endothelial cells, while CCR7 and LFA-1 mediate firm adhesion and trans-endothelial migration by binding to the chemokine *CCL21* and the adhesion molecules ICAM-1 and 2, respectively. *CCL19*, another ligand of CCR7, helps direct naïve T lymphocytes to the T-cell zones of lymph nodes. As in lymph nodes, naïve T lymphocytes enter the spleen via the blood and are directed to the T-cell zones (periarteriolar lymphoid sheaths of the splenic white pulp) by the chemokines CCL21 and CCL19. Naïve T lymphocytes that encounter DCs presenting the alloantigens they recognize are retained within secondary lymphoid organs where they proliferate and differentiate into effector and memory T lymphocytes. Those that do not continue their journey back to the blood via efferent lymphatic channels and ultimately the thoracic duct in the case of lymph nodes, and directly back to the blood in the case of the spleen. DCs bearing alloantigens reach lymph nodes via afferent lymphatics and the spleen via the blood. Their migration there is dependent on CCR7. Alloantigens shed by the graft, usually in the form of exosomes, also reach lymph nodes and the spleen via afferent lymphatics or the blood, respectively, where they are picked up by resident DCs. Either the spleen or lymph nodes are sufficient for initiating naïve T-lymphocyte activation after kidney transplantation.

Once generated, effector and memory T lymphocytes exit secondary lymphoid organs and migrate to the allograft via the bloodstream. Their egress into the blood is dependent on sphingosine 1 receptors (S1P). Blocking S1P with the immunosuppressant *FTY720* causes the retention of effector and memory T lymphocytes within secondary lymphoid organs, preventing them from targeting the graft. Unlike naïve T lymphocytes, effector and memory T lymphocytes express high levels of the adhesion molecule *VLA-4* and the chemokine receptor *CXCR3*. VLA-4, which binds VCAM-1 on inflamed endothelial cells, is critical for effector and memory T lymphocyte's firm adhesion to and transmigration across graft vessels. The role of CXCR3 and its chemokine ligands is controversial. Recent experimental evidence shows that recognition of donor antigens by the TCR, and not chemokines by chemokine receptors, is the initial trigger for effector and memory T-lymphocyte migration into transplanted organs. Note that unlike naïve T lymphocytes, memory T lymphocytes can be activated outside secondary lymphoid organs—for example, in the graft itself.

Chemokine or chemokine receptor antagonism has failed to pass preclinical testing as a useful strategy to prevent rejection. Targeting VLA-4 with Natilizumab, although highly promising, is fraught with unacceptable risk of PML because VLA-4 is essential for immune surveillance of latent viruses by memory T lymphocytes. Although FTY720 has been approved for the treatment of multiple sclerosis, it is not approved for use in transplantation because of serious side effects that include macular edema, bradycardia, and increased risk of infection. Therefore, none of the agents that target T-lymphocyte migration are currently available for preventing or treating allograft rejection in the clinic.

B LYMPHOCYTES AND ANTIBODIES

B lymphocytes and their progeny, the plasma cells, are the immune cells responsible for antibody production. Interest in B lymphocytes and antibodies as causative agents in transplant rejection dates back to the beginnings of renal transplantation when it was realized that grafts are hyperacutely rejected by recipients who harbor preformed antibodies against donor antigens. As outlined earlier, hyperacute rejection is caused by either anti-ABO or anti-HLA antibodies. Careful ABO matching of donors and recipients and careful testing of the recipient's serum for antibodies against the donor's HLA prior to transplantation have eliminated hyperacute rejection in the clinic. More recently, however, the significance of donor-specific antibodies (DSA) that arise after transplantation has come to the fore. These antibodies, usually against donor HLA but sometimes directed against non-HLA, are associated with poor renal allograft outcomes by causing acute or chronic antibody-mediated rejection (ABMR), often in combination with an ongoing T-lymphocyte–mediated (cellular) rejection. Therefore, understanding B-lymphocyte biology is a necessary step toward tackling DSA and ABMR.

B-Lymphocyte Activation and Differentiation

Naïve B-lymphocyte activation is dependent on antigen recognition by the *B-cell receptor (BCR)* and on critical help from the T_{FH} subset of $CD4^+$ T lymphocytes inside secondary lymphoid organs. Upon binding antigen, the BCR signals to the cell's interior to trigger essential gene expression programs and, in addition, internalizes the antigen. Internalized antigen is delivered to endosomal compartments where it is degraded into peptides that are then bound to MHC class II molecules and recycled to the surface of the B lymphocyte. These MHCII–peptide complexes are recognized by $CD4^+$ T lymphocytes, leading to stable contact between the B lymphocyte and the T lymphocyte providing help to it. Since the helper T lymphocyte is activated by the same antigen as the B lymphocyte, the interaction between T and B lymphocytes is referred to as "cognate" or "linked." The chemokine receptors CCR7 on B lymphocytes and CXCR5 on T_{FH} lymphocytes are essential for bringing the two cells together at the interface between B-cell zones (or follicles) and T-cell zones in secondary lymphoid organs. The help from T lymphocytes is delivered in the form of co-stimulatory ligands (for example, CD40L on activated T lymphocytes engages CD40 on activated B lymphocytes) and cytokines (for example, IL-4, -5, and -6). B lymphocytes receive additional stimulatory signals from myeloid cell-derived cytokines such as BAFF (also known as BLys) to which monoclonal antibodies have been developed for use in SLE in humans. B lymphocytes that receive all the necessary stimulatory signals coalesce in the follicles to form *germinal centers*. There, they proliferate extensively, undergo affinity maturation, and differentiate into plasma cells and memory B lymphocytes. *Affinity maturation* is the process by which immunoglobulin genes undergo extensive somatic hypermutation that improves the affinity of the resultant antibody to its antigen. *Plasma cells* are antibody factories and, along with memory B lymphocytes, maintain long-term humoral immunity. The transcriptional repressor *BLIMP-1* is critical for B-cell differentiation to plasma cells. Plasma cells exit secondary lymphoid organs and reside for a long time in the bone marrow. They rely on IL-6 for survival. *Memory B lymphocytes,* on the other hand, populate secondary lymphoid tissues and circulate in the blood. In humans, they are marked by expression of the surface protein *CD27.* Similar to memory T lymphocytes, memory B lymphocytes respond much more vigorously than their naïve counterparts to the antigen to which they are specific and produce antibodies of higher affinity.

Antibodies

Antibodies or *immunoglobulins (Ig)* are glycosylated protein molecules present on the surface of B lymphocytes, and therefore serve as BCRs for antigen, or are secreted as B lymphocytes and plasma cells into the extracellular space where they can bind to target antigens. A single antibody molecule consists of four protein chains, two "heavy" and two "light," linked to each other by disulfide bonds. The N-terminus regions of the heavy and light chains are where the variability between one antibody molecule and another resides and, therefore, collectively make up the antigen-binding site. Five *isotypes* or classes of antibodies (IgM, IgD, IgG, IgA, and IgE) exist. They are distinguished based on the C-terminus regions of the heavy chains, which are nonvariable (constant) and therefore do not participate in binding antigen. Instead, these regions are important for the effector functions of antibodies: the means by which antibodies eliminate pathogens or cause tissue injury. Antibodies that bind to donor antigens can lead to *antibody-mediated rejection (ABMR).* They cause allograft damage in two principal ways: they activate the classical pathway of the complement system and stimulate macrophages and other immune cells by binding to *Fc receptors (FcR)* that recognize the constant regions of specific antibody classes. Complement activation via the classical pathway leads to the accumulation of *C4d,* an inactive complement component, in the tissues thus, aiding in the histologic diagnosis of ABMR. Which effector mechanism dominates is determined by the heavy-chain isotype. For example, IgM, IgG3, IgG1, and IgG2 (in decreasing order of potency) activate complement, while IgG1 and IgG3 also bind FcR to stimulate macrophages and NK cells. Note that IgM antibodies, produced early in the immune response, are of lower affinity to their antigens than IgG antibodies that arise later—thus, IgG alloantibodies are of the most concern in transplantation. The switch from IgM to IgG antibodies is referred to as *isotype switching* and is mediated by T-lymphocyte help via the CD40L–CD40 pathway and the action of cytokines. Recent observations suggest that binding of human alloantibodies to donor HLA on endothelial cells contributes to graft injury via yet another mechanism: the activation of the endothelial cells themselves.

Antibody-Independent Functions of B Lymphocytes

In addition to producing antibodies, B lymphocytes contribute directly to T-lymphocyte immunity by three known mechanisms: (1) they serve as APCs that enhance T-lymphocyte differentiation to memory T lymphocytes; (2) they function as *bona fide* cellular effectors that produce inflammatory cytokines (for example, TNFα); and (3) a subgroup of them, known as regulatory B lymphocytes (Breg) characterized by IL-10 secretion, modulate immune responses. Recent observations in experimental animals and in humans suggest that the "cellular" functions of B lymphocytes contribute significantly to the pathogenesis of allograft rejection, especially chronic rejection, or, conversely, dampen the alloimmune response and promote better allograft outcomes in some patients.

Targeting B Lymphocytes and Plasma Cells in Transplantation

Since all human B lymphocytes express the surface marker CD20, monoclonal antibodies against CD20 (Rituximab) are quite effective at depleting B lymphocytes in the circulation and to a lesser extent in lymphoid organs. Plasma cells, however, do not express CD20, providing one explanation why Rituximab has not been particularly successful at reversing DSA or ABMR in renal transplant recipients. More recently, proteasome inhibitors, originally developed for the treatment of multiple myeloma, have been employed to inhibit plasma cell function in sensitized patients or those with DSA/ABMR. Finally, B-lymphocyte depletion at the time of transplantation can increase the incidence of acute rejection because of nonselective depletion of both pathogenic and regulatory B lymphocytes. Further understanding of B-lymphocyte activation, alloantibody production, and B–T-lymphocyte interactions is needed before more precise interruption of B-lymphocyte function can be attained. A more comprehensive view of targeting B lymphocytes, plasma cells, or complement that is based on our current understanding of the immunobiology of ABMR is shown in Figure 2.5.

Natural Killer Cells

Another participant in the alloimmune response is the *NK cell*. NK cells are lymphoid cells that do not carry TCRs or BCRs but instead express complementary activating and inhibitory receptors. Activating receptors recognize ligands induced on many cell types during inflammation or infection, while inhibitory receptors bind self-MHC class I molecules. NK cells are stimulated when the balance between activating and inhibitory signals is tilted in favor of the former. Since allograft tissues express nonself MHC proteins, they do not engage inhibitory receptors on donor NK, leading to NK-cell activation. Therefore, in contrast to alloreactive T and B lymphocytes which respond to nonself, NK cells respond to *missing self*. NK cells that infiltrate allografts can also be activated by binding of alloantibodies in the graft to FcRs on NK cells. Once activated, NK cells kill their targets by secreting the same molecules utilized by CTL (perforin, granzyme, and IFNγ) and differentiate to memory cells. Despite their cytotoxic and memory functions, NK cells appear to have a secondary role in allograft rejection. Their most conspicuous role in immunity is in the setting of viral infection. Infected cells are rapidly detected by NK cells because of diminished MHC class I expression and increased expression of activating ligands.

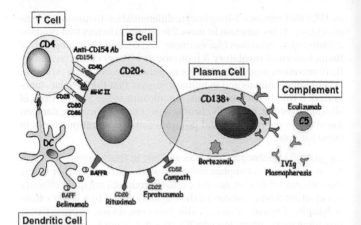

FIGURE 2.5 Potential means to prevent or treat antibody-mediated rejection based on underlying immunologic mechanisms. Multiple components of the innate and adaptive immune systems participate in the pathway that leads to alloantibody production. One or more of these components can be targeted to prevent or treat ABMR. Targeting B lymphocytes can also potentially attenuate T-lymphocyte responses because B lymphocytes function as antigen-presenting cells as well. (Reprinted from Zarkhin V, Chalasani G, Sarwal MM. The yin and yang of B cells in graft rejection and tolerance. Transplant Rev 2010;24(2):67–78, with permission from Elsevier.)

THE INNATE IMMUNE SYSTEM

The immune system consists of two integrated arms, the innate and adaptive—the latter has been the subject matter of this chapter so far. The adaptive immune system consists principally of T and B lymphocytes, which as explained earlier, express diversified receptors that recognize foreign antigens with high molecular specificity, expand clonally upon sensing antigen, and undergo affinity maturation and further differentiation to effector and memory cells. These adaptive features of lymphocytes (clonal expansion, maturation, differentiation, and memory) earned lymphocytes the well-justified moniker *adaptive immunity*. Although highly effective at providing the host with long-lasting protection against foreign intruders, the adaptive immune system is relatively sluggish in its response, requiring hours to several days to generate sufficient numbers of effector cells and even several weeks to generate high antibody (IgG) titers.

The *innate immune system,* on the other hand, comprises inflammatory cells (neutrophils, monocytes, macrophages, and dendritic cells among others) and soluble mediators (the complement system being a prime example) that respond instantly to foreign intrusion. Innate immune cells express nonrearranging, germ-line encoded receptors that recognize broad nonself patterns present usually on microbes (for example, LPS and viral DNA or RNA) but also respond to molecules released by stressed or dying cells (for example, uric acid, nuclear proteins, and DNA derived from chromosomes or mitochondria). This rapid-fire innate response serves three purposes. It mobilizes first-line defense mechanisms such as phagocytosis and the release of acute inflammatory mediators, ranging from small molecules to cytokines; causes the activation and maturation of APCs that then launch the adaptive T-lymphocyte response; and participates in the effector phase of most adaptive immune responses, providing the foot soldiers that eliminate foreign antigens and cause tissue damage or fibrosis in response to cytokines and antibodies released by lymphocytes. To illustrate the contributions of the innate immune system to transplant rejection, we will discuss the example of ischemia-reperfusion injury and the role it has in renal allograft outcomes.

ISCHEMIA-REPERFUSION INJURY

The process of depriving harvested organs from blood supply, placing them on ice, and reattaching them to the vasculature of the recipient results in an immediate inflammatory response known as ischemia-reperfusion injury that is mediated by the innate immune system, although lymphocytes have been shown to participate as well (see Chapter 10). The time duration during which the organ is outside the human body is referred to as the *cold ischemia time*, whereas the time required to complete the surgical revascularization of the organ in the recipient is the *warm ischemia time* (see Chapter 4, Part II). The inflammatory response that ensues is characterized by graft cell injury and death, activation of the complement system, and infiltration of the graft parenchyma with neutrophils and monocytes. Reactive oxygen species released by hypoxic graft cells and infiltrating immune cells are thought to play an important role in the injury process.

Ischemia-reperfusion injury is the principal cause of delayed graft function after kidney transplantation. Later, it is associated with increased incidence of acute rejection and reduced long-term allograft survival. This perhaps provides the strongest argument why living unrelated renal allografts fare significantly better than similarly mismatched cadaveric kidneys. It also highlights the need to minimize ischemia time. Significant attention has been placed lately not only on shortening the cold ischemia time but also on utilizing machine perfusion to maximize the delivery of oxygen and nutrients to the graft parenchyma. Ongoing studies are exploring whether machine perfusion at room temperature or inhibition of complement activation would reduce ischemia-reperfusion injury at the time of transplantation.

TOLERANCE AND IMMUNE REGULATION

Tolerance broadly refers to the absence of immune responses to specific antigens. During development, one of the critical functions of immune system is to prevent responses directed toward self-antigens, thus preventing autoimmune disease. This is achieved by *central tolerance* in the thymus and by *peripheral tolerance* in extrathymic lymphoid tissue. During T-lymphocyte development, most T lymphocytes found in the thymus have undesirable reactivities, and so are deleted or made unresponsive by negative selection. T lymphocytes that recognize foreign antigen in the context of self-MHC are positively selected and allowed to circulate in the blood. The process of negative selection is imperfect, so autoreactive T lymphocytes can be found in the periphery. Autoimmunity is usually prevented by the process of peripheral tolerance.

Peripheral tolerance is maintained by a number of mechanisms that include regulation by specialized lymphocyte subsets known as T_{REG} and B_{REG}, anergy, and exhaustion. T_{REG} and B_{REG} populations have been identified in rodents and humans. Regulatory lymphocytes suppress alloimmune reactions *in vitro* and prolong allograft survival in rodent transplantation models. The mechanisms by which regulatory lymphocytes suppress immune responses are varied. They include cytokines (e.g., IL-10 and TGFβ) and inhibitory membrane molecules (e.g., CTLA-4). T_{REG} in humans are $CD4^+$ T lymphocytes that express high levels of CD25 and the transcription factor Foxp3. Anergy and exhaustion refer to the state in which T or B lymphocytes become unresponsive to re-stimulation with antigen. *Anergy* occurs when naïve lymphocytes encounter antigen in the absence of critical co-stimulatory or help signals necessary for their full activation. *Exhaustion* occurs when effector or memory T lymphocytes repeatedly encounter a persistent antigen, as would occur during chronic viral infection or in the case of an allograft. Repeated antigenic stimulation induces the expression of inhibitory molecules that keep T cells hypo- or unresponsive. One example of such inhibitory molecules is *PD-1*, shown in rodents to suppress alloreactive effector T lymphocytes.

In the context of transplantation, *tolerance* can be defined as the absence of a destructive immune response to a graft, in a host with otherwise intact immunity. This generally implies that the patient is not on chronic immunosuppression yet maintains excellent graft function. This is an important goal because transplant recipients are otherwise subjected to global immunosuppression that leaves them at increased risk for infections and malignancies. In addition, current chronic immunosuppression regimens do not guarantee indefinite or even excellent long-term allograft survival. A variety of experimental approaches have tried to take advantage of basic mechanisms of tolerance in an attempt to induce transplantation tolerance. The most promising strategy so far has been to induce donor-specific tolerance by ablation or near ablation of the recipient's immune system and reconstitution with donor hematopoietic stem cells (bone marrow), thus generating either a transiently or permanently chimeric immune system that does not reject donor organs. The mechanisms of tolerance in these patients appear to be a combination of central (thymic) deletion of alloreactive T lymphocytes and peripheral regulation.

Selected Readings

Espinosa JR, Samy KP, Kirk AD. Memory T cells in organ transplantation: progress and challenges. Nat Rev Nephrol 2016;12:339–347.

Ferrer IR, Hester J, Bushell A, et al. Induction of transplantation tolerance through regulatory cells: from mice to men. Immunol Rev 2014;258:102–116.

Ford ML, Adams AB, Pearson TC. Targeting co-stimulatory pathways: transplantation and autoimmunity. Nat Rev Nephrol 2014;10:14–24.

Fuchs E. Transplantation tolerance: from theory to clinic. Immunol Rev 2014;258:64–79.

Hoffman W, Lakkis FG, Chalasani G. B cells, antibodies, and more. Clin J Am Soc Nephrol 2016;11:137–154.

Hu M, Wang YM, Wang Y, et al. Regulatory T cells in kidney disease and transplantation. Kidney Int 2016;90:502–514.

Laplante M, Sabatini DM. mTOR signaling in growth control and disease. Cell 2012;149:274–293.

Liu Z, Fan H, Jiang S. CD4$^+$ T-cell subsets in transplantation. Immunol Rev 2013;252:183–191.

Mori DN, Kreisel D, Fullerton JN, et al. Inflammatory triggers of acute rejection of organ allografts. Immunol Rev 2014;258:132–144.

Murphy K, Weaver C. *Janeway's Immunobiology.* 9th ed. New York: Garland Science; 2016.

Oberbarnscheidt MH, Lakkis FG. Innate allorecognition. Immunol Rev 2014;258:145–149.

Sheen JH, Heeger PS. Effects of complement activation on allograft injury. Curr Opin Organ Transplant 2015;20:468–475.

Woodle ES, Rothstein DM. Clinical implications of basic science discoveries: janus resurrected—two faces of B cell and plasma cell biology. Am J Transplant 2015;15:39–43.

Yatim KM, Lakkis FG. A brief journey through the immune system. Clin J Am Soc Nephrol 2015;10:1274–1281.

Zarkhin V, Chalasani G, Sarwal MM. The yin and yang of B cells in graft rejection and tolerance. Transplant Rev 2010;24:67–78.

Zhang Q, Lakkis FG. Memory T cell migration. Front Immunol 2015;6:504.

Zhuang Q, Lakkis FG. Dendritic cells and innate immunity in kidney transplantation. Kidney Int 2015;87:712–718.

3 Histocompatibility Testing, Crossmatching, Immune Monitoring

J. Michael Cecka, Qiuheng Jennifer Zhang,
Raja Rajalingam, and Elaine F. Reed

Tissues and organs transplanted from one individual to another genetically disparate individual are rejected unless immunosuppressive medications are given. The recipient's lymphocytes recognize cell-surface proteins of the grafted tissue that differ from the recipient's, and trigger immune responses leading to rejection. Human leukocyte antigens (HLA) expressed on the surface of the graft provoke the most severe immune rejection, and the gene family encoding HLA molecules has been named the major histocompatibility complex (MHC). The similarity between the constellation of HLA antigens of the donor and recipient (the degree of histocompatibility) affects long-term graft survival, and for that reason, HLA matching has been incorporated into kidney allocation. Antibodies directed against mismatched donor HLA antigens that might arise as a result of pregnancies, blood transfusions, or transplantation cause hyperacute or accelerated acute graft rejection when they are present before transplantation. Additionally, recent evidence implicates their appearance after transplantation with accelerated acute rejection and with chronic graft dysfunction and loss. This chapter describes the HLA antigens and their genetics, methods to identify them, HLA antibodies and the means to detect and characterize them, and the important roles each plays in kidney transplantation.

THE MAJOR HISTOCOMPATIBILITY COMPLEX

Human MHC Gene Cluster

The human MHC comprises about 3.6 Mb DNA (0.1% of the genome) located on chromosome 6p21.31. The MHC is the most gene-dense region of the human genome comprising more than 220 genes. The average gene density over the entire MHC region is one gene per 16 kilobases (kb). Only 50% of the genes in the MHC region appear to be expressed, and the remainder are unexpressed pseudogenes. One possible explanation for maintaining such high levels of pseudogenes could be that they are involved in generating new alleles by gene conversion, a phenomenon that has been observed at other human immune loci. About 40% of the expressed genes have immune system function.

The human MHC has been divided physically into three regions: class I (telomeric), class II (centromeric), and class III (Fig. 3.1). The HLA class I cluster comprises three classical class I genes (*HLA-A, -B,* and *-C*), three nonclassical class I genes (*HLA-E, -F,* and *-G*), two class I–like genes (MHC class I–related chain A [*MICA*] and MHC class I–related

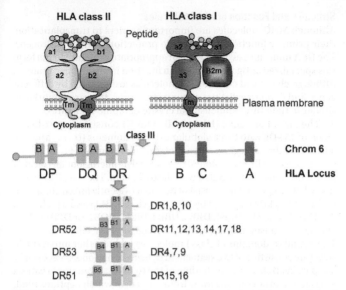

FIGURE 3.1 Schematic of the genetic organization of the classical *HLA* genes and class I and class II molecular structures.

chain B [*MICB*]), and several pseudogenes. The classical class I genes are constitutively expressed by all nucleated cells and control the activation and function of cytotoxic T lymphocytes. The expression of nonclassical class I antigens is restricted to specific tissues, while the class I–like genes are expressed under some physiologic stress conditions. The products of both nonclassical and class I–like genes serve as ligands to receptors that control the function of natural killer cells. The HLA class II cluster comprises classical class II genes (*HLA-DR, -DP*, and *-DQ*), nonclassical class II genes (*HLA-DM* and *-DO*), and several pseudogenes. The HLA-DR region contains one functional gene for the α chain (*DRA*), but has one or two functional genes for the β chain, depending on the HLA-DR type. All HLA-DR types have the *DRB1* gene, and some contain an additional functional *DRB* gene, *DRB3, DRB4,* or *DRB5*, which forms a second cell-surface heterodimer with the DRA-encoded α chain (Fig. 3.1). HLA class II molecules are constitutively expressed by antigen-presenting cells (dendritic, macrophage, and monocyte cells) and B lymphocytes, but these antigens can be induced on activated T cells and endothelial cells, including the glomerular endothelium, renal tubular cells, and capillaries. The nonclassical class II genes are not expressed on the cell surface, but form heterotetrameric complexes involved in peptide exchange and loading onto classical class II molecules. The class III region comprises genes that encode molecules involved in critical immune functions such as those encoding tumor necrosis factors, complement proteins, and heat shock proteins.

Structure and Function of HLA Molecules

Although MHC molecules are important barriers to transplantation, their primary function is to provide protection against pathogens. The HLA molecules evolved with an appropriate structure to perform this specialized antigen presentation function in an effective manner. Although class I and class II HLA molecules are encoded by different genes and comprise distinct subunit structures, they are remarkably similar in their three-dimensional crystallographic structures.

The class I antigens (HLA-A, -B, and -C) consist of an α heavy chain of 45 kDa with three globular external domains (α_1, α_2, and α_3), a transmembrane region, and an intracellular domain (Fig. 3.1). The structure is stabilized by a non-MHC encoded β_2-microglobulin (located in chromosome 15) associated with the α_3 domain. The class II antigens (HLA-DR, -DQ, and -DP) consist of two noncovalently linked chains: an α chain of 35 kDa (encoded by DRA, DQA1, or DPA1) and a β chain of 31 kDa (encoded by DRB1, DRB3, DRB4, DRB5, DQB1, or DPB1). Both chains are transmembrane with two globular extracellular domains. The α_1 and α_2 domains of class I molecules fold together into a single structure consisting of two segmented α_1 helices lying on a sheet of eight antiparallel β strands. The folding of the α_1 and α_2 domains creates a long cleft or groove facing away from the cell, in which peptides bind. Similarly, the membrane distal α_1 and β_1 domains of class II molecules form the peptide-binding cleft. The class I and class II molecules differ with regard to the ends of the groove that are closed in class I and open in class II molecules, permitting longer peptides to be accommodated on class II molecules. The HLA antigens (self) with their loaded peptides (nonself) are exposed to T cells, which recognize these compound structures (self + nonself) through their T-cell receptors and trigger immune activation against the foreign antigens. Their central role in triggering the immune system also makes the HLA antigens powerful alloantigens, as described in Chapter 2.

The Nature of HLA Polymorphism

The classical class I and class II genes encode HLA molecules, the most polymorphic proteins known to date in humans. Earlier studies using serologic typing methods identified an unprecedented number of HLA alleles at each locus. DNA sequencing revealed an even more extensive polymorphism as the serologically defined antigens included multiple allelic variants that could differ by a single nucleotide substitution. The differences among HLA proteins are localized in the antigen-binding domain, particularly enriched in positions that interact with antigenic peptides or the T-cell receptor. Class I polymorphisms are predominantly found in the first 180 amino acids of the heavy chain, and the class II polymorphisms are found in the first 90 to 95 amino acids of the α and/or β chains. This extreme polymorphism is thought to be driven and maintained by the long-standing battle for supremacy between our immune system and infectious pathogens.

Even when we limit the discussion to the products of the HLA-A, -B, and -DR loci, which are most commonly encountered in clinical kidney transplantation, there are 88 recognized antigens (defined by antibodies), encoded by nearly 7,000 distinct alleles, and the number of new alleles is still increasing. Although the number of HLA antigens, alleles, and combinations is very large, the frequencies in a given population vary considerably. The most common HLA antigen is A2, which is found in roughly 50% of individuals from populations around the world. Approximately 96% of Whites with European ancestry who express HLA-A2 have the HLA-A*02:01 allele. Northern Chinese and many Hispanics who express HLA-A2 have the HLA-A*02:06 allele. HLA-B8 is found in 30% of Scots, and the frequency declines as populations in Europe and more distant areas are analyzed, except in those areas that were colonized by the British—South Africa, India, Australia—where the frequency is higher. Thus, certain antigens and alleles are common, whereas others are very rare. Some HLA antigens are racially limited. Thus, HLA-B54 is found almost exclusively in persons from Japan and nearby Asian countries. HLA-A36 is relatively common among Blacks, but is very rare in other populations.

The additional HLA polymorphism revealed through the application of DNA technologies has provided interesting insights into the role of HLA in many autoimmune diseases, but its significance in clinical kidney transplantation remains to be seen. Allele differences between the donor and recipient of bone marrow transplants lead to graft-versus-host disease. Limited analyses of HLA allele-level mismatches among kidney transplant recipients suggest an added effect of allele-level HLA mismatches on graft survival rates, but matching at this level has not yet been attempted prospectively. Among sensitized renal candidates, there are instances where allele-specific antibody reactions occur and these pose problems in allocation or in interpretation of post-transplant donor-specific antibodies when the allele-level HLA type of the donor is unknown.

HLA Nomenclature

Obviously, keeping track of this diversity requires a specialized nomenclature. The HLA antigens were identified and characterized over a 50-year period beginning with the discovery of the MAC (now HLA-A2) antigen by Dausset in Paris in 1958. A series of international workshops beginning in 1964 and held approximately every 4 years until 1987 established a nomenclature for the HLA antigens, naming unique antigens in the sequence they were officially recognized: A1, A2, A3, Bw4, B5, Bw6, B7, B8, and so on. The antigens were identified using antisera obtained primarily from multiparous women. As the field evolved, new antisera were discovered that could "split" some HLA antigens into narrower specificities. HLA-A9 was split into HLA-A23 and -A24, and HLA-A10 was split into HLA-A25, -A26, -A34, and -A66, for example. Table 3.1 lists the broad parent antigens for splits in parentheses together with the antigen frequencies among US organ donors.

The already complicated HLA nomenclature became more complex when DNA-based typing technologies for HLA were developed in the mid-1980s. To accommodate the growing numbers of alleles that could be identified by their unique nucleotide sequences within the antigen designations, the established serologic nomenclature was modified to associate alleles with antigens whenever possible (Fig. 3.2). The first allele for HLA-A1 is HLA-A*01:01, which includes the locus

TABLE
3.1   Recognized HLA Specificities

Antigen	Donor Antigen Frequency	Antigen	Donor Antigen Frequency
HLA-A		B56(22)	1%
A1	24%	B57(17)	7%
A2	48%	B58(17)	4%
A3	22%	B59	<1%
A11	10%	B60(40)	8%
A23(9)	7%	B61(40)	4%
A24(9)	17%	B62(15)	11%
A25(10)	3%	B63(15)	1%
A26(10)	3%	B64(14)	1%
A29(19)	7%	B65(14)	4%
A30(19)	8%	B67	<1%
A31(19)	5%	B71(70)	1%
A32(19)	5%	B72(70)	2%
A33(19)	5%	B73	<1%
A34(10)	1%	B75(15)	<1%
A36	1%	B76(15)	<1%
A43	<1%	B77(15)	<1%
A66(10)	2%	B78	<1%
A68(28)	11%	B81	1%
A69(28)	<1%	B82	<1%
A74(19)	2%	**HLA-DR**	
A80	1%	DR1	17%
HLA-B		DR4	30%
B7	21%	DR7	32%
B8	17%	DR8	9%
B13	4%	DR9	3%
B18	9%	DR10	3%
B27	7%	DR11(5)	19%
B35	18%	DR12(5)	4%
B37	2%	DR13(6)	22%
B38(16)	3%	DR14(6)	7%
B39(16)	5%	DR15(2)	26%
B41	2%	DR16(2)	4%
B42	2%	DR17(3)	18%
B44(12)	24%	DR18(3)	2%
B45(12)	3%	DR 51	29%
B46	<1%	DR 52	62%
B47	1%	DR 53	50%
B48	1%	**HLA-DQ**	
B49(21)	3%	DQ2	37%
B50(21)	2%	DQ4	10%
B51(5)	10%	DQ5	36%
B52(5)	2%	DQ6	46%
B53	4%	DQ7	39%
B54(22)	<1%	DQ8	24%
B55(22)	2%	DQ9	13%

Based on CPRA calculator October 2015.

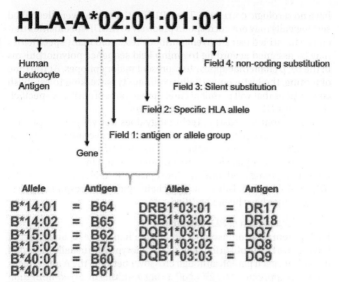

FIGURE 3.2 Current molecular nomenclature for HLA antigens.

(*A*), an asterisk (*) to indicate that the typing was performed by DNA methods, the serologic antigen (*01*), and the allele number (*01*), separated by a colon. Two additional fields (also separated by colons) may be included to accommodate synonymous substitutions that do not affect the protein sequence and to indicate nucleic acid substitutions in the introns or the untranslated 3' or 5' flanking sequences within the genes, respectively.

There are some exceptions to the naming convention that may be confusing. The HLA-B14, -B15, -B40, and HLA-DRB1*03 allele series include distinct antigens that are both immunogenic and antigenic. The HLA-B62 antigen, for example, is encoded by HLA-B*15:01, 15:04, 15:05, 15:06, 15:07, and many other B15 alleles, whereas HLA-B75 is encoded by HLA-B*15:02, 15:08, 15:11, and so on. HLA-DRB1*03:01 is HLA-DR17, whereas HLA-DRB1*03:02 is HLA-DR18. The correlation between alleles and antigens is updated periodically in the HLA Dictionary (http://www.ebi.ac.uk/ipd/imgt/hla/dictionary.html) and in the series "Nomenclature for factors of the HLA system" (published in the journal *Tissue Antigens*).The naming of HLA class II antigens is similar even though two distinct polypeptides encoded by separate genes combine to form the antigen. The HLA-DR antigens are distinguished by their DR β_1 subunit; therefore, the first allele of DR1 is DRB1*01:01. The HLA-DQ and -DP antigens comprise two polymorphic chains, α and β, which may react individually or in combination. Thus, these are named DQA1*01:01, DQB1*02:01, DPA1*01:01, and DPB1*01:01.

The naming conventions for the DQ and DP antigens are still in flux with regard to solid-organ transplants. The DQ2-6 antigens correspond to DQB1*02-DQB1*06, and the DQ7, 8, and 9 antigens are DQB1*03:01, 03:02, and 03:03, respectively. DQ α chain and combinatorial specificities have no serologic correlates. The DP1-6 antigens that were described serologically may not correspond precisely to the DP specificities that can be identified using current antibody tests, and many specificities may be assigned according to amino acid sequence polymorphisms in the DP β chain that appear to represent major epitopes. At the time of writing, the histocompatibility community is working to establish conventions that will permit accurate predictions of antibody specificities against HLA-DQ and DP heterodimers.

Unfortunately, existing technology does not yet permit precise allele-level HLA typing within time constraints for deceased donors, and as a result, the HLA nomenclature for solid-organ transplantation remains a mixture of serologic level antigen numbers and intermediate-level molecular typing to identify the most probable alleles for HLA-DRB1, -DQA1, -DQB1, and -DPB1 encoded chains and the corresponding HLA antigens that have been identified.

Family Segregation of HLA Haplotypes

Each parental chromosome 6 provides a haplotype or linked set of MHC genes to the offspring (Fig. 3.3). Haplotypes are usually inherited intact from each parent, although crossover between the A and B locus occurs in approximately 2% of offspring, resulting in a recombination (and a new haplotype). The child carries one representative antigen from each of the class I and class II loci of each parent. A child is, by definition, a one-haplotype match to each parent unless recombination has occurred.

HLA haplotypes are inherited in a Mendelian fashion. Statistically, there is a 25% chance that siblings will share the same haplotypes (two-haplotype match), a 50% chance they will share one haplotype (one-haplotype match), and a 25% chance that neither haplotype will be the same (zero-haplotype match). Even in the case of siblings who share both HLA haplotypes, 25% to 100% of other parental chromosomes may be different, and these other chromosomes include other "minor" histocompatibility antigens, which can also initiate rejection reactions.

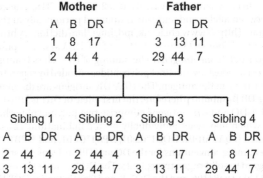

Mother			Father		
A	B	DR	A	B	DR
1	8	17	3	13	11
2	44	4	29	44	7

Sibling 1			Sibling 2			Sibling 3			Sibling 4		
A	B	DR	A	B	DR	A	B	DR	A	B	DR
2	44	4	2	44	4	1	8	17	1	8	17
3	13	11	29	44	7	3	13	11	29	44	7

FIGURE 3.3 Inheritance of haplotypes and HLA profile in four theoretical siblings. Sibling 1 is a one-haplotype match to siblings 2 and 3 and a zero-haplotype match to sibling 4.

Definition of Haplotypes and Phenotypes

Consider an individual with the following HLA profile or phenotype: A1, A24, B8, B44, DR4, DR15. From this phenotypic information alone, it is not possible to identify haplotypes because it is not known which antigens are linked on each chromosome. Consider another individual with the following HLA phenotype: A1, A3, B7, B8, DR4, DR12. If this second individual is the biologic parent, offspring, or sibling of the first individual, it becomes possible to identify a shared haplotype of the family as A1, B8, DR4. The first individual also has an unshared haplotype A24, B44, DR15, and the second individual an unshared haplotype A3, B7, DR12. These haplotypes should appear in the parents and other siblings. A kidney transplanted between these two individuals would be a one-haplotype-matched graft, and the A1, B8, and DR4 antigens would be genotypically identical in the donor and recipient because they are encoded by the same inherited genes.

If these two individuals are not related, it is not possible to identify the haplotypes. Thus, in transplants from living-unrelated or deceased donors, the haplotypes are unknown, and only the phenotypic identity of individual HLA antigens can be determined. The two individuals whose HLA phenotypes are listed would be called a three-antigen match or a three-antigen mismatch (see "HLA Matches and Mismatches," below). Sharing of minor histocompatibility antigens is serendipitous.

Linkage Disequilibrium

Although it is not possible to identify an individual's haplotypes from the phenotypic HLA-typing information alone, within racial or ethnic populations, certain HLA determinants are inherited together more often than would be expected by chance. For example, if HLA-A1 and HLA-B8 occur at gene frequencies of 16% and 10%, respectively, in a population, the probability of finding them together should be 1.6%. However, the actual occurrence rate of the HLA-A1-B8 combination is significantly above the predicted incidence (about 8%). This phenomenon represents the inheritance of haplotypes within racial groups. Existing data suggest that positive selection is operating on the haplotype and that the linked loci confer a particular selective advantage for the host.

HLA Matches and Mismatches

It is not always possible to identify two HLA specificities at each HLA locus. Consider the HLA phenotypes for the following two unrelated individuals:

1. A2, —; B27, B13; DR17, DR4
2. A2, A3; B8, B14; DR17, —

The absence of the second A-locus antigen in individual 1 and the second DR-locus antigen in individual 2 could result from a failure to identify the second antigen. Most often, however, it reflects the inheritance of the same antigen (A2 and DR17 in these cases) from both parents (the individuals are homozygous at these loci). A kidney transplanted between these two individuals would be described as a one A and one DR match, but this terminology does not take into account homozygosity in the A and DR loci of individuals 1 and 2, respectively. If individual 1 were a donor for individual 2, it would be more informative to describe the combination as a zero A, two B, and one DR mismatch. If individual 2 were a donor for individual 1, the combination would be a one A, two B, and zero DR mismatch. Antigenic differences in the donor kidney are potential targets of rejection; therefore, the convention of counting the number of donor HLA antigens that are *not* shared by the recipient provides an estimate of the antigen dose.

Identical and Fraternal Twins

The differentiation between identical twins and two-haplotype–matched fraternal twins is important because the recipient of a transplant from an identical twin requires no immunosuppression. The procedure is immunologically equivalent to an autotransplantation. Two-haplotype–matched siblings, whether they are fraternal twins or not, differ in their minor histocompatibility antigens, and immunosuppression is required. Monozygotic, or identical, twins share a single placenta and amniotic sac at birth. However, such information may be unavailable or unreliable when the patient and donor are evaluated as adults. A variety of methods have been used to identify monozygotic twins, including skin grafting from the potential twin donor to the recipient (the graft would be rejected if the twins were fraternal). Today, several genetic polymorphisms can be exploited to determine identity at many genetic loci providing a high degree of confidence that twins are identical. Extended blood groups include markers that are determined by many genes on different chromosomes. Analysis of short tandem repeats (STRs), which, as the name implies, are short nucleotide sequences that are repeated a variable number of times, provides a high probability of identifying differences between individuals. STRs are often used in monitoring engraftment of HLA-identical bone marrow transplants, so they are exquisite markers of individuality.

HLA-TYPING TECHNIQUES

The Microcytotoxicity Test

The microcytotoxicity test developed by Terasaki and McClelland in 1964 was the international standard test for HLA typing for more than 30 years. This serologic test is performed in small plastic trays with a grid of small flat-bottomed wells, each of which contains a selected antiserum to which lymphocytes from the individual to be typed are added, and incubated. Complement is added, and after another incubation, a vital dye is added to indicate the proportion of dead cells in each well when examined under the microscope. Using the products of an immune response (antibodies) to measure the targets of an immune response (HLA antigens) has a certain inherent logic. If an antigen had provoked an antibody response, its immunologic importance was demonstrated. However, the HLA-typing antisera are seldom monospecific (i.e., they do not recognize a single private specificity), so in most cases it is necessary to examine the patterns of reactivity with several antibodies to determine the HLA type.

DNA Typing Methods

Although some laboratories still use serologic HLA typing as a supplemental technique, it is now more common to type individuals by DNA-based methods. In the United States, laboratories are required to determine HLA types of transplant candidates and deceased donors by DNA-based methods. Using the extensive DNA sequence data available, oligonucleotide primers and probes that specifically hybridize to sites that are unique to an HLA locus, allele, or group of alleles have been developed and are commercially available for HLA typing. Three basic methods used in conjunction with polymerase chain reaction (PCR) employ sequence-specific oligonucleotide probes (SSOPs), sequence-specific primers (SSPs), and sequencing-based typing (SBT). SSOP is based on first amplifying genomic DNA using locus- or group-specific primers and then detecting the hybridization of specific oligonucleotide probes tagged with enzymatic or fluorescent markers to the amplified product. In commercial kits, the process is often reversed, with the probes attached to microparticles that can be hybridized with the labeled PCR product to produce a series of distinct fluorescent beads when hybridization occurs. The microparticles are read on a flow cytometer or Luminex machine and sophisticated software programs assist in interpretation of the patterns to determine the HLA type. SSP depends on DNA amplification using group- or allele-specific primers and detecting an amplified product of the correct size by gel electrophoresis. The size is determined by running an agarose gel that separates the PCR products according to their size. SBT uses gene-specific primers to sequence polymorphic regions of the gene, and alleles can be assigned based on the nucleotides identified at key positions in the sequence. Even with these molecular approaches to HLA typing, it is difficult to produce reagents that uniquely recognize each individual HLA antigen. As with serology, it is often necessary to identify patterns of primer and probe reactivity in order to determine the HLA type. Computer programs assist in the analysis of primer and probe patterns, which are more difficult to analyze unaided because of the added complexity of the *HLA* genes. It is difficult to identify HLA alleles without performing SBT, because the differences between alleles may be determined by single nucleotide differences. However, SSP and SSOP can easily provide low or intermediate levels of typing, identifying the recognized HLA antigens and major allele groups, respectively. This level of typing is sufficient for renal transplantation in most cases.

Technology is rapidly changing and the development of next-generation sequencing will eventually bring higher resolution HLA typing at all loci at decreased costs. The current platforms are limited, however, in the speed with which the typing and analyses can be performed and would not be applicable to deceased donor typing.

THE SENSITIZED PATIENT

More than one-third of patients awaiting a renal transplant in the United States are sensitized to HLA antigens. They have circulating HLA antibodies that developed from exposure to allogeneic HLA antigens during the course of pregnancies, through exposure to blood transfusions or, increasingly, because of a failed transplant. Patients who have circulating HLA antibodies are at high risk of hyperacute rejection (the immediate and usually irreversible destruction of the transplanted kidney) or of accelerated acute rejection (an early and rapid antibody-mediated rejection that is not easily controlled with immunosuppression). The presence of preformed HLA antibodies restricts the number of compatible donors for the sensitized patient to those who do not express the HLA antigens to which the patient is sensitized. Sensitized patients often must wait substantially longer for a crossmatch-compatible kidney. Assiduous attention to pretransplant lymphocyte crossmatching has virtually eliminated hyperacute rejection as a clinical threat. Very sensitive solid-phase antibody tests and the virtual crossmatch (see below) make it possible to avoid donor reactive antibodies completely for many patients today—even those who are broadly sensitized against many HLA antigens.

Origins of Alloantibodies

During pregnancy, the semi-allogeneic fetus develops and is tolerated within the mother for 9 months. At birth and during the pregnancy, the mother is exposed to paternal HLA antigens of the fetus and may become immunized and produce HLA antibodies to the mismatched HLA antigens derived from the father. Sera from multiparous women were the reagents that initially defined the HLA system. Among patients awaiting a kidney transplant, sensitization is observed in up to 40% of women with a history of pregnancy and is usually highest among those with multiple pregnancies. Transplant failure, especially when accompanied by early withdrawal of immunosuppression, results in sensitization among about 75% of those relisted for a repeat transplantation. This figure may be an underestimate since many patients are not relisted after graft loss. Exposure to allogeneic HLA antigens also occurs following blood or platelet transfusion, and the level of preformed HLA antibodies can increase as a result of viral or bacterial infections and other pro-inflammatory events.

The specificity of HLA antibodies an individual produces upon exposure to allogeneic HLA molecules is influenced by the individual's immunologic history and by the individual's own HLA type. Antibodies are generally not produced against self-HLA antigens. HLA antibodies can be directed against so-called "private" specificities such as HLA-A1, or against "public" specificities such as Bw6. Antibodies to private specificities recognize an epitope that is unique to a particular HLA molecule or a limited group or family of closely related alleles, whereas antibodies to public specificities recognize an epitope that is shared by more than one HLA molecule. Public epitopes are responsible for cross-reactivity observed in HLA alloantiserum. HLA antigens that share epitopes can be grouped into the major cross-reactive groups (CREGs) listed in Table 3.2.

The extensive sequence data on HLA alleles has been used to identify many other potential "epitopes" by comparing amino acids or amino acid clusters shared by some but not all alleles that might be expressed in an accessible area of the HLA molecule. Antisera that fit the antigenic reactivity pattern for some of these epitopes have been already been described and the tool found at http://allelefrequencies. net/hlaepitopes/hlaepitopes.asp may be used as an aid to analyze reactivity patterns in complex antisera from sensitized patients. The Bw4 and Bw6 specificities are well-defined examples of public antigens. Nearly all HLA-B antigens express either Bw4 or Bw6. The antigenic

TABLE 3.2	HLA Antigen CREGs
A1C	A1 3 11 29 30 31 32 36 74 80
A2C1	A2 B17 57 58
A10C	A25 26 29 30 31 32 33 34 66 74
A9C	A2 23 24 68 69
A28C	A2 68 69
B5C	B18 35 37 51 52 53 58 78
B7C	B7 8 13 41 42 48 60 61 81
B8C	B8 16 18 38 39 64 65
B12C	B13 37 44 45 47 49 50 60 61
B21C	B49 50 51 52 53 57 58 62 63 70 71 72 73 75 76 77 78
B22C	B7 27 42 46 54 55 56 73 81 82
B27C	B7 13 27 41 42 47 60 61
Bw4	A23 24 25 32 B13 27 37 38 44 47 49 51 52 53 57 58 59 63 77
Bw6	B7 8 18 35 39 41 42 45 46 47 48 50 54 55 56 60 61 62 64 65 67 71 72 73 75 76 78 81

determinant that defines these specificities is affected by amino acids in positions 80 and 83 of the class I molecule sequences located in the exposed part of the α_1 helix. Class I molecules with arginine at position 83 and threonine or isoleucine at position 80 are recognized by anti-Bw4 antisera and include the HLA-B13, -B17, -B27, -B37, -B38, -B44, -B47, -B49, -B51, -B52, -B53, -B57, -B58, -B59, -B63, and -B77 antigens. The HLA-A23, -A24, -A25, and -A32 antigens also have the characteristic arginine at position 83 and react with anti-Bw4 antibodies. All other B-locus antigens have glycine at position 83 and asparagine at position 80, and react with anti-Bw6 antibodies. A consequence of the "patch-work" pattern of HLA polymorphism is that an antibody generated against a particular antigen may react to a number of HLA antigens that share the same sequence motifs, leading to "cross-reactivity" of the antibody. For instance, a patient's serum carrying HLA-A2 antibodies may react with HLA-A2 as well as A68, A69, B57, and B58 since these antigens share amino acid sequence motifs with HLA-A2, but not with other HLA antigens.

THE CROSSMATCH

The first crossmatch results were reported by Patel and Terasaki in 1968, who showed that among 30 patients transplanted with a positive cytotoxicity crossmatch, 24 suffered hyperacute rejection and three others lost their grafts within the first 3 months. The crossmatch test was widely adopted by transplant programs and by the early 1970s, hyperacute rejection was rare. The authors also reported that patients who were sensitized to HLA antigens could be identified beforehand by testing the patient's serum against a panel of lymphocytes from normal individuals representative of the local donor pool. The result of these lymphocyte panel tests would also provide an estimate of how often the patient would have a positive crossmatch against donors who became available. The percent panel-reactive antibody (PRA) was the first measure of sensitization. The crossmatch tests and the methods used to measure sensitization have become more sensitive and more precise over time, resulting in more complete avoidance of preformed antibodies and improved early transplant outcomes.

The complement-dependent lymphocytotoxicity (CDC) assay was the earliest method for HLA antibody screening. The patient's serum was incubated separately with B cells and T cells from panels of donors selected to represent the known HLA class I and class II antigens, respectively. Immunoglobulin (Ig) G antibodies reactive to HLA class I and class II antigens are the most important so treatment to reduce IgM antibodies was frequently included, especially for patients with autoimmune diseases. Prolonging the complement incubation time or adding antihuman globulin (AHG) increased the sensitivity of the test and enhanced the detection of low-titer antibodies. The results were usually expressed as the percentage of panel cells killed by antibodies in the serum. Thus, on a 50-cell panel, a positive reaction against 30 donors represents a PRA of 60%.

Flow Cytometry

The flow cytometry crossmatch test (FCXM) is a very sensitive crossmatch test. The patient's serum is mixed with target cells; the cells are washed and then incubated with monoclonal mouse anti-CD3 (a pan T-cell marker) and anti-CD19 or anti-CD20 (both B-cell markers) antibodies conjugated with fluorescent dyes such as phycoerythrin (PE) or peridinin chlorophyll protein (PerCP), respectively, and an antihuman IgG antibody conjugated with fluorescein. The T cells that stain red-orange and the B cells that stain red can be gated using a flow cytometer, making the amount of yellow-green fluorescence proportional to the concentration of anti-T-cell or anti-B-cell antibodies present in the serum. Generally, a positive lymphocytotoxic crossmatch is a contraindication to kidney transplantation, whereas a positive flow cytometry crossmatch is not necessarily considered a barrier to transplantation. The flow crossmatch test can detect very low levels of circulating antibodies. Positive flow cytometry crossmatches are associated with a higher rate of early acute rejection episodes and a lower 1-year graft survival rate. Hyperacute rejection has not been reported, however, and some transplants across a positive FCXM have no early problems (if the cytotoxic crossmatch is negative). The T-cell FCXM is particularly useful for sensitized and retransplant candidates whose antibody levels may have fallen but who can mount a rapid memory response upon challenge. Low levels of circulating antibody have a more damaging effect when the deceased donor is older or the kidney quality is uncertain. The potential for false-positive reactions is responsible for much of the uncertainty about the role of the flow cytometry crossmatch. Positive, particularly weakly positive, flow crossmatch results should be supported by the patient's sensitization history or be consistent with a determination that the patient has HLA antibodies based upon the results of solid-phase assays. When the flow crossmatch detects antidonor HLA antibodies, there is a substantial risk for adverse outcomes after transplantation.

Pronase Treatment of Donor Cells

False-positive FCXMs are often caused by nonspecific immunoglobulin binding to immunoglobulin Fc receptors on lymphocytes and the degree of binding may vary among individual donors. Patients who have been treated with antibodies such as rituximab (anti-CD20 antibody) may also have false-positive FCXM results owing to the presence of the administered antibody in their serum. Pronase is a nonspecific peptidase that preferentially digests Fc receptors and other cell-surface proteins (including CD20) without substantially destroying HLA molecules under certain conditions. Pretreating donor lymphocytes with pronase reduces nonspecific binding of patient serum to lymphocytes and reduces the incidence of false-positive reactions in the FCXM. Caution is required, however, because prolonged treatment or too much enzyme will result in loss of HLA antigens. Even under optimal conditions, many cells and nuclei may be lysed during treatment releasing DNA, which causes clumping and loss of cells. This can be avoided by including DNase in the treatment.

The Virtual Crossmatch

The widespread introduction of solid-phase tests for HLA antibodies in 2003 caused a rapid change in the way sensitized patients were identified and evaluated. A virtual crossmatch can now predict actual crossmatch results based on antibody specificity and strength detected by solid-phase assays as described in the sections below (Fig. 3.4). Accurate prediction relies heavily on up-to-date HLA antibody testing of recipients and complete HLA typing of donors including HLA-A, B, C, DRB1, DRB3/4/5, DQA1, DQB1, DPA1, and DPB1. Owing to the extraordinary sensitivity and specificity of solid-phase assays, a virtual crossmatch is highly accurate. The virtual crossmatch has significantly

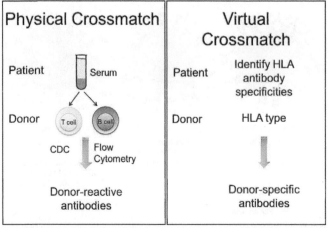

FIGURE 3.4 A comparison of the actual crossmatch test and the virtual crossmatch based on a determination of a patient's sensitization profile using solid-phase tests with purified HLA antigens and an examination of the donor's HLA type to identify DSAs.

improved organ allocation efficiency, reduced testing costs and, in many cases, cold ischemia time by reducing uncertainty and the time needed for testing after the organ arrives at the transplant center. Importantly, virtual crossmatch accuracy has facilitated kidney paired donation (KPD) programs that involve multiple transplant centers (see Chapter 7, Part IV).

Solid-Phase Assays

Solid-phase assays using affinity-purified or engineered HLA antigens are the primary tests for HLA antibodies used in most laboratories today. The tests currently fall into one of three main groups (Fig. 3.5): a mixture of affinity-purified HLA class I or class II antigens used to screen for the presence or absence of HLA antibodies: affinity-purified class I or class II antigens from individual donors used like donor cell panels to assess reactivity with individual donor phenotypes, but with the advantage of a clear separation of class I and class II antigens: and recombinant single HLA antigens attached to solid supports, permitting a very precise specificity determination. The most versatile platform uses microparticles or beads coated with purified HLA class I or class II antigens as antibody targets. The microparticles are colored to permit the discrimination of more than 100 beads simultaneously, each with distinct, chemically attached HLA antigens. Patient serum is incubated with a mixture of beads, washed and bound antibody is detected by adding fluorescently labeled antihuman IgG and measuring fluorescence in a Luminex flow cytometer or similar device (Fig. 3.6). Interpretation of the test results is based on comparisons of median fluorescence intensity (MFI) measurements of the test serum to those of positive and negative serum controls. Neither viable lymphocytes nor complement fixation is required, and the assays are robust.

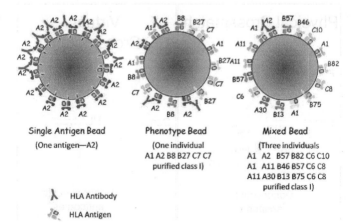

Single Antigen Bead	Phenotype Bead	Mixed Bead
(One antigen—A2)	(One individual A1 A2 B8 B27 C7 C7 purified class I)	(Three individuals A1 A2 B57 B82 C6 C10 A1 A11 B46 B57 C6 C8 A11 A30 B13 B75 C6 C8 purified class I)

ƛ   HLA Antibody

   HLA Antigen

FIGURE 3.5 Solid-phase antibody test formats. The three formats offer purified HLA antigens attached to microspheres in different combinations ranging from a single HLA antigen on each bead to a mixture of antigens from the same donor and to HLA antigens from a mixture of different donors.

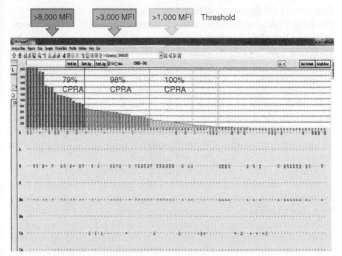

FIGURE 3.6 Antibody thresholds determine sensitization status. This histogram is the result of an HLA class I single antigen bead test. The X-axis represents individual beads, each containing a single HLA-A, -B, or -C antigen (listed below the histogram) and the Y-axis indicates the fluorescence intensity associated with each bead after binding of antibodies from a patient serum and developing with a fluorescent tagged anti-IgG antibody. Determining the threshold between a positive and negative reaction can be challenging in cases where there is no abrupt border between reactive and nonreactive beads.

The three test formats have different applications. The multibead screening test is the least sensitive and the least informative. It is used to screen blood donors for potential TRALI (transfusion-related acute lung injury)-causing HLA antibodies that are very strong and broadly reactive. This test is likely to miss weak antibodies and antibodies with a narrow specificity (i.e., B7 alone) and is of questionable utility as a screening tool to determine sensitization status in a renal transplant candidate, but might be used for subsequent screening of patients known to be unsensitized based upon a more sensitive test. The individual phenotype beads carry a mixture of HLA antigens (class I or class II) and are more similar to testing an individual's lymphocytes. These beads are more sensitive than mixed screening beads but do not allow assignment of antibody specificities because antigens may be masked in broadly reactive sera. The single antigen bead test detects reactivity with individual HLA antigens and some common alleles with high sensitivity and is used to characterize a patient's sensitization profile precisely, even when the antibody reactivity is very broad. Strategies for utilizing these tests for identifying and characterizing the sensitization profile and for monitoring changes before and after transplantation are described under "Immunologic Evaluation of Transplant Candidates" below.

Determining the Specificity of HLA Antibodies

The early PRA tests could sometimes determine the HLA target specificities (a list of HLA antigens that react with the patient's serum) by analyzing reaction patterns against the HLA types of the panel donors. However, when multiple antibodies are present in a serum, antibodies to more frequent HLA antigens mask the recognition of antibodies to less-frequent antigens. Solid-phase technologies for measuring HLA antibodies represent a major change in the sensitivity and precision of antibody identification for laboratories. Single antigen beads can precisely identify individual HLA antigen reactivities even in a complex serum containing antibodies that could not be resolved using cells or beads with multiple HLA antigens attached.

The solid-phase tests for defining HLA antibody specificity can be exquisitely sensitive and may detect antibodies that are present at very low levels that may not damage the graft. Some transplants that have been performed in the face of preexisting donor-specific HLA antibody (DSA), particularly when it is detected by a solid-phase test but not by a flow cytometric crossmatch test, are successful and have uneventful post-transplant courses while others experience delayed graft function and early antibody-mediated rejection. Testing sera at multiple dilutions shows that the degree of fluorescence shift is proportional to the titer of antibody, and this is important in determining which donor HLA antigens should be avoided to prevent hyperacute, accelerated acute antibody-mediated rejections or chronic graft damage. Laboratories have attempted to relate the strength of reactions to antibody levels that might lead to patently adverse outcomes. Of course, the patient's immunologic history also plays a role in assessing the risk of low-level antibodies. A patient with a prior graft loss or multiple pregnancies may have developed memory to mismatched HLA antigens and weak antibodies may represent the potential for a rapid increase in antibody levels after transplantation with previously mismatched HLA epitopes. The reasons for uncertainty in identifying antibodies that are clinically important may relate to the amount and specificity of antibodies, antigen expression levels in the donor, technical aspects of the production of the solid-phase reagents themselves or to features associated with the class and subclass of the antibodies, but are not well studied.

Complement Fixation and Immunoglobulin Subclass

The single antigen bead test has been modified to test for complement C1q binding, cleavage of complement component C3 to C3d and, by changing the indicator from a generic anti-IgG to a subclass-specific second antibody, to identify dominant IgG subclasses in an antigen-specific setting. These tests may reveal a more complex pattern of HLA-specific antibodies that could discriminate those antibodies which are more important clinically because of their complement-fixing capacity or some other function of the dominant subclass. Most responses include antibodies of all IgG subclasses and complement fixation can be reduced or enhanced by dilution or concentration of sera, respectively. Complement fixation is generally associated with higher titer antibodies. However, there may be utility for these tests in identifying antibodies that may be more or less a concern or antibodies that might be more easily removed by desensitization.

Unacceptable Antigens

When a patient has well-defined HLA antibodies that would result in a positive crossmatch against donors who express the target HLA specificities, the United Network for Organ Sharing (UNOS) permits the inclusion of those HLA antigens to avoid (unacceptable) as part of the patient's waitlist profile. If a patient has a clearly defined antibody to HLA-A1, potential donors expressing HLA-A1 would not be acceptable and kidneys from these donors will not be offered to that patient, thus avoiding a predictably positive crossmatch. Most transplant centers will not transplant in the face of a positive CDC or AHG crossmatch because of the high risk of hyperacute rejection. However, the results of transplantation with lower levels of antibodies may be beneficial for the broadly sensitized patient despite the anticipation that antibodies cause a higher incidence of delayed graft function, accelerated humoral rejection, and chronic allograft dysfunction. Thus, transplant centers may differ in their preference for listing unacceptable antigens that would not result in a positive CDC or AHG crossmatch, but which might cause a positive crossmatch using flow cytometry or another very sensitive crossmatch test. There is no uniformly established MFI level at which an antibody level correlates with a positive crossmatch test. Rather the probability of a positive crossmatch increases with increasing MFI such that in single antigen tests, a positive flow cytometry crossmatch is unlikely below a threshold of 2,500 MFI and very likely above a threshold of 5,000 MFI, for example. MFI thresholds may be set differently for antigens of the different HLA loci or antigens associated with large CREGs or based on the patient's history (prior transplants, pregnancies).

Calculated Panel-Reactive Antibodies

UNOS implemented a calculated PRA in December 2007 designed to address the variability in PRA reporting that had developed over the years through the use of different cell panels and different tests for HLA antibodies. The calculated panel-reactive antibody (CPRA) is calculated by determining the frequency of incompatible donor HLA phenotypes based on the unacceptable class I and class II HLA antigens that have been listed for each candidate. Since the HLA-A, -B, -C, -DR, and -DQ types of actual deceased kidney donors were used to compute the antigen frequencies, the CPRA reflects the true probability of an incompatible donor based on the unacceptable antigens that have been listed for a patient. A CPRA of 80% means that 80% of deceased donor kidneys will express at least one unacceptable HLA antigen and will not be offered to that patient. A CPRA calculated using a national donor pool may not always reflect the HLA antigen distribution of a local donor population that different regions because they differ in the racial and ethnic composition, but these variations generally do not result in substantially different CPRAs.

The same patient might have a different CPRA when listed at different transplant centers with using different thresholds for assigning unacceptable antigens. The threshold affects the CPRA as shown in Figure 3.6. A conservative center that wishes to avoid donors with HLA antigens to which a patient has DSA might select a threshold of 1,000 MFI as unacceptable, in which case the patient would have 100% CPRA.

Another center, willing to accept some risk of ABMR in exchange for more donor offers and perhaps a shorter wait for their patient might set a threshold of 8,000 MFI and base their decision to transplant on the result of the final crossmatch test. With the higher threshold, the CPRA is 79%, but there are low-level antibodies that could damage a graft that expresses one or more of the corresponding HLA antigens. The figure also illustrates a potential problem with using stringent thresholds for assigning unacceptable HLA antigens. The difference in MFI values for antigens just above and below the thresholds may not be great and upon retesting, the MFI values for some of these antigens might change enough to cross the threshold. Interpretation of these tests is not always straightforward and often requires comparing tests performed using two or more test platforms to determine whether weak reactions are consistent among different tests.

Limitations of the Virtual Crossmatch

The "virtual" crossmatch, which compares the patient's antibody profile with the donor's HLA type, has substantially reduced the need for a final "physical" crossmatch test. The CPRA now provides a virtual crossmatch for most US renal transplant candidates today. When a candidate's unacceptable antigens have been properly identified and entered into the UNOS electronic database (UNET), the unacceptable antigens predict which donors will have a positive crossmatch. Since UNOS does not offer kidneys from donors with a predicted positive crossmatch to a candidate, the crossmatch is performed by the computer. Unfortunately, there are cases when the information provided in UNET is incomplete and the virtual crossmatch is not definitive. Those patients who produce antibodies against HLA antigens that cannot be listed as unacceptable or who are offered donors whose typing is not complete cannot rely on computer-assisted donor selection.

Final Crossmatch

When sera from waiting patients are collected and tested periodically and are available in the laboratory, a final crossmatch test can usually be performed without obtaining a fresh sample from the patient. This allows the laboratory to perform final crossmatches for a deceased donor kidney before organ procurement in most cases, avoiding delays in transplantation. When the intervals between periodic sample testing are longer than a few months, the risk of undetected changes in sensitization increases. Some centers allow older sera to be used for the final crossmatch if the patient is not sensitized and has not received a recent blood transfusion.

In many cases, the virtual crossmatch can serve as the final crossmatch. Provided the patient's sensitization status is up to date and there are no ambiguous antibodies or donor antigens, the virtual crossmatch should predict the outcome of the physical crossmatch. Avoiding a last minute crossmatch test could save time in getting the transplant completed, reducing cold ischemia and allowing better scheduling. For unsensitized patients whose history is clear, the virtual crossmatch should be absolutely predictive. However, there is increasing risk in forgoing a physical crossmatch test for patients who have not been tested within 3 months of the offer, owing to the possibility of intervening sensitizing events or to changes in antibody levels that were historically determined. Likewise, patients with two or more donor-specific antibodies present at low levels (especially below the threshold of being individually unacceptable) will benefit from a physical final crossmatch test. Many broadly sensitized patients have antibodies that react with DQ α chains, DP antigens, and combinations of α and β chains that may not be effectively avoided in the virtual crossmatch test. For example, there are many more DP types than DP specificities that can be discerned in single antigen bead tests. A patient with antibodies against HLA-DPB1*04:01 might be offered a donor whose DP type is DPB1*40:01 and DPB1*105:01, neither of which can be tested directly on the single antigen bead panel. Sequences predict that the crossmatch will be positive because the DPB1*0401 is similar to DPB1*40:01, but not DPB1*105:01. Equivalences have been defined based on the HLA-DP sequence homologies to permit an educated guess at how the known DP antibodies would react with a different DP antigen, but these may not always predict accurately.

TRANSPLANTING THE SENSITIZED PATIENT

Sensitized patients remain a challenge for most transplant programs because their access to compatible donors is limited by their degree of sensitization, preformed antibodies are difficult to reduce or remove, and treatments for antibody-mediated rejection are of limited effectiveness (see Chapter 6). The patient's ABO blood type further restricts access to ABO-identical or compatible donors. The best solution for these patients is to find a compatible donor, which requires more potential donors or a longer wait as possible donors appear over time. Alternatives are discussed below and in Chapters 6 and 7.

ABO Blood Group Compatibility

The ABO blood group antigens behave as strong transplantation antigens, and transplantation across ABO barriers usually leads to irreversible hyperacute rejection. In principle, the same criteria determine kidney distribution according to ABO as do blood transfusions with group O (the universal donor) and group AB (the universal recipient). The disproportionate percentage of waiting patients who are type O or type B generally mandates that blood group identity rather than blood group compatibility determines the distribution of deceased donor kidneys. Exceptions are made for blood group AB patients who may be offered A or AB kidneys and for zero-HLA antigen mismatched kidneys, which can be offered to an ABO-compatible recipient if an ABO-identical recipient is not available. Under the new kidney allocation system (KAS, see below and Chapter 5), very broadly sensitized (98% to 100% CPRA) patients can also be offered a compatible kidney. For living-related donor transplantation, ABO compatibility is adequate.

The blood group barriers can often be overcome when there is a willing ABO-incompatible living donor by removing blood group iso-agglutinins with plasmapheresis or immunoabsorption, often in conjunction with immunosuppression (see Chapter 6). ABO-incompatible transplantations can be performed successfully in certain circumstances but is always accompanied by some level of increased cost and risk.

| TABLE 3.3 | Percent Distribution of ABO Blood Groups Among Deceased Kidney Donors in 2014 and According to Ethnicity on the Transplant Waiting List |

Blood Group	Donors	Waiting List*	White	Black	Hispanic	Asian
O	47	52	49	53	62	42
A	37	30	37	22	26	22
B	12	16	11	22	10	31
AB	4	2	3	3	2	5
n	7,763	133,817	39,980	36,892	21,080	8,814

*Waiting list including all ethnicities and donor ABO types was compiled by the UNOS research department as of October 16, 2015.

In White populations, approximately 20% of blood group A individuals can be defined as A_2; these patients have reduced levels of A antigen on graft endothelium. They permit an exception to the ABO-incompatibility barrier because A_2 kidneys can be safely transplanted into O or B recipients with low preoperative titers of isoagglutinin. Transplantation of A_2 kidneys into B or AB recipients is routine in some centers and is being encouraged under the new KAS (see Chapter 5).

Table 3.3 lists the distribution of the major ABO groups among deceased donors and different ethnic groups of potential kidney transplant recipients. If all ethnic groups contributed equally to the donor pool and all ethnic groups suffered end-stage renal disease in direct proportion to their representation in the general population, waiting times for the different ethnic groups and blood group categories would be the same. In fact, Whites contribute disproportionately to the donor pool and Blacks contribute disproportionately to the recipient pool because kidney disease is more common in Blacks. As a result, patients with blood group O or B wait longer for a blood group–identical donor.

The Kidney Allocation System

Sensitized patients have benefited from recent changes in allocation policy in the United States (see Chapter 5). The introduction of CPRA and the virtual crossmatch made allocation more efficient by avoiding futile kidney offers to patients who had donor-specific antibodies. Under this system, patients who come to the top of the list for each donor kidney are those who do not have antibodies directed against donor HLA antigens. Kidney offers that were declined because of a positive final crossmatch decreased by more than 90% since the introduction of the virtual crossmatch. Under the KAS that went into effect in December 2014, sensitized patients with a CPRA higher than 20% receive increasing priority for compatible donors on a sliding scale. For the most broadly sensitized patients, those sensitized to 98%, 99%, or 100% of donors receive top priority for a compatible kidney from the local, regional, or national pool of donors, respectively. Patients can receive an ABO-compatible kidney if no ABO-identical candidates are identified. This change resulted in a large number of broadly sensitized patients being transplanted during the first few months after the introduction of the new KAS. As many as 17% of transplants were allocated to recipients with 100% CPRA. Transplants to the very broadly sensitized patients stabilized after the first 6 months to about 10% of transplants, a figure that mirrors the percentage waiting for a transplant. The benefit may decline further as patients whose chances are closer to 1 in 100 are transplanted and the remaining patients are much less likely to find a crossmatch-compatible donor.

Desensitization of the Sensitized Patient

More than 25% of renal transplant candidates are highly sensitized. Two main approaches based on the use of intravenous immune globulin (IVIG) are currently used to reduce HLA allosensitization and facilitate transplantation in highly sensitized patients. The first therapy is based on infusion of high-dose IVIG (2 g/kg), which has been demonstrated to be a potent inhibitor of HLA antibodies and to permit transplantation with minimal risk of rejection. IVIG can also be used as therapy in the treatment of patients experiencing humoral rejection (see Chapter 6). IVIG is often administered in conjunction with plasmapheresis to reduce the circulating antibody load and with biologics and immunosuppressive medication such as rituximab and Bortezumab to limit return of antibody. There are several proposed mechanisms of action of high-dose IVIG in highly sensitized patients, including inhibition of HLA antibody in an idiotypic manner, elimination of HLA-reactive T and B cells, inhibition of cytokines involved in immunoglobulin synthesis, and blockade of T-cell activation.

A second approach uses a combined regimen of IVIG therapy and plasmapheresis. Plasmapheresis rapidly depletes donor-specific antibody and administration of IVIG blocks resynthesis of HLA antibodies. Treatment is continued until donor-specific HLA antibodies (DSAs) are no longer detected in the patient's serum. IVIG and plasmapheresis is also effective in reducing HLA allosensitization in highly sensitized patients and is a successful therapy for the treatment of humoral rejection. Combined plasmapheresis and IVIG is also reportedly effective in removing anti-A or anti-B isoagglutinins before successful transplantation across ABO blood group barriers. The precise immunomodulatory mechanisms of the combined therapy are unknown, but appear to function in a long-term, donor-specific manner.

Kidney Paired Donation

Kidney paired donation (KPD; see Chapter 7, Part IV) has achieved considerable success in transplanting sensitized patients by emphasizing matching these patients with compatible donors. Originally suggested as an option where two ABO-incompatible donor–recipient pairs could exchange their donors' kidneys for the alternate pair's compatible recipient, the concept has evolved to include pairs who are crossmatch incompatible and even pairs who are compatible, but might benefit from having an alternate donor better matched for size or HLA antigens or age. There are several programs in the United States facilitating these exchanges ranging from single centers to consortia of varying sizes and a few national programs. The most productive program to date, The National Kidney Registry had managed nearly 2000 transplants through 2016 more than 30% of which involved patients with >80% CPRA and 15% of which involved patients with >95% CPRA.

A key to success in kidney paired exchange has been active collaboration between the transplant team, coordinators and the HLA laboratory. The virtual crossmatch takes on an increased importance when pairs at several different transplant centers are involved in the exchanges. Crossmatch failures, when the patient is found to be incompatible at the last moment, are extremely disruptive. Kidney paired exchange offers participating programs an opportunity to personalize the virtual crossmatch. Instead of a one-size-fits-all approach generally used for patients awaiting a deceased donor kidney, thresholds for unacceptable antigens can be scaled depending on the likelihood of a pair finding matched donors and recipients in the pool of participants. Having advanced access to the available donors with their HLA types, centers and their laboratories can identify potential matches, evaluate their suitability, and preemptively accept or decline donors prior to match offers being made. If additional exploratory testing is needed, that can often be accommodated as well prior to an offer.

KPD is also used in conjunction with ABO-incompatible transplantation and desensitization at some centers. In these cases, the sensitized patients may not find a compatible donor in a timely manner but a less incompatible donor may be identified.

IMMUNOLOGIC EVALUATION OF TRANSPLANT CANDIDATES

Candidates for renal transplantation today fall into one of two categories: those with a potential living donor and those without. Figure 3.7 outlines the initial immunologic evaluation of these candidates. Once a patient is identified as a suitable candidate for transplantation, HLA typing and antibody-screening tests are performed using the tests outlined above. The HLA type permits assessment of donor and potential recipient pairs for degree of histocompatibility, as well as evaluation of sensitization and crossmatch results The HLA-A, -B, -C, -DR, and -DQ types are required to list a patient as a candidate for a deceased donor kidney with the US national Organ Procurement and Transplantation Network (OPTN), which is currently maintained

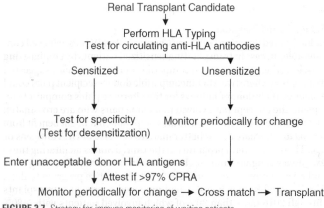

FIGURE 3.7 Strategy for immune monitoring of waiting patients.

by UNOS. The sensitization status of the patient is also determined prior to transplantation to identify those patients who are at risk for hyperacute or accelerated acute rejection. The patient's CPRA level is another important element in listing a renal candidate with UNOS, because patients with a CPRA greater than 20% receive special ranking in organ allocation and those with greater than 97% CPRA receive priority for compatible kidneys at the local (98% CPRA), regional (99% CPRA), and national (100% CPRA) levels. It is important to investigate and characterize sensitization early in the process to avoid missing a rare compatible offer for a highly sensitized patient.

The initial test of the sensitization status should be the most sensitive, the single antigen solid-phase test, to detect and characterize the HLA antibodies or to confirm their absence. Additional tests may be useful to confirm the presence of low-level antibodies or allele-specific reactivities. The phenotype bead test is often helpful to resolve these results.

Autoantibodies and other antibodies that do not pose a significant risk of hyperacute or accelerated rejection should be identified before transplantation. For patients who will wait for a deceased donor kidney or when the living donor transplant will be delayed, it is necessary to monitor changes in patterns of sensitization and reevaluate patients periodically to keep abreast of their current sensitization status.

Patients with a suitable living donor can proceed to a crossmatch against their donor(s) and, if negative, can be transplanted. When there are multiple potential donors, the evaluation of each donor can be tailored to determine whether antibodies are directed against the specific mismatched donor HLA antigens, and whether desensitization procedures could permit successful transplantation with one or more potential donors.

Role of Human Leukocyte Antigen Matching in Transplantation

The HLA antigens are strong transplant antigens that may engage large numbers of T cells (estimates of up to 100 times as many T cells as nominal protein antigens have been reported). Secondary cellular or humoral immune responses to HLA antigens may occur as a consequence of prior exposures to allogeneic HLA through pregnancy, blood transfusion, or previous transplantation. Studies have consistently shown a stepwise increase in early rejections and a decrease in long-term graft survival with increasing numbers of HLA antigen mismatches between the deceased donor and recipient. Paired kidney studies also show that when one kidney is transplanted to an HLA-matched recipient, even if it has been shipped a great distance, and the other is transplanted locally to an HLA-mismatched recipient, the HLA-matched kidney has better long-term graft survival.

Recognition of the special immunologic status of HLA-matched transplants led to the development of a national organ distribution for the sharing of donor kidneys for HLA-matched recipients. Between 1987 and 2009, kidneys matched for the HLA-A, -B, -DR antigens with an ABO-compatible candidate anywhere in the United States were mandatorily shared to increase the number of well-matched transplants and to reduce failures and patients returning to the waitlist. At the peak, about 15% of kidney transplants were performed with zero HLA-A, -B,

-DR mismatched kidneys. Allocation points were awarded to advantage candidates when a minimally mismatched kidney became available as well. The emphasis on HLA matching was modified several times in response to outcome data from the Scientific Registry of Transplant Recipients (SRTR). The current KAS provides priority for zero HLA-A, -B, -DR mismatched candidates who are sensitized (>20% CPRA) when there are no compatible highly sensitized candidates and awards one and two allocation points for candidates with zero or one HLA-DR antigen mismatch, respectively.

Among recipients of living donor transplants, however, the effect of HLA matching on long-term graft survival differs from the effect on deceased donor transplants. Although transplants between HLA-identical siblings provide the best long-term success rates (77% of these grafts will still survive at 10 years), the number of HLA antigen mismatches has little effect on the survival of mismatched grafts. Surprisingly, kidneys from genetically unrelated donors have had nearly the same long-term graft survival rates as grafts between one haplotype-matched siblings or parents and their offspring (approximately 64% at 10 years). This observation has fueled a rapid increase in the number of unrelated living donor transplants during the past decade. The results of living donor transplants are superior to those of deceased donor transplants, even for recipients of HLA-matched kidneys.

IMMUNE MONITORING

Current methods used to diagnose renal allograft rejection depend on changes in blood chemistry markers, such as creatinine levels or blood urea nitrogen (BUN). However, these markers are, at best, surrogate markers for rejection, and clearly rejection must precede the deterioration in graft function. Although diagnosis of rejection by histopathologic examination of renal biopsies remains the gold standard (see Chapter 15), there is a need for a less-invasive approach for the early detection of immunologic events leading to rejection. A promising area in the study of renal allograft rejection is the identification of noninvasive biomarkers of immune alloreactivity to the graft in the urine and blood of recipients. Monitoring the immune response to the allograft will permit the early identification of patients at risk of rejection and graft loss, optimization of drug regimens, monitoring responses to therapy following intervention, and guide the development of new immunosuppressive therapies. Immune monitoring might aid in differentiating rejection from other forms of graft dysfunction such as primary nonfunction and drug toxicity. The following outlines some of the common and newly developed cellular, humoral, genomic, and proteomic assays to assess the immune status of the transplant recipient.

Monitoring HLA Antibodies after Transplantation

Acute antibody-mediated rejection occurs during the early post-transplant period and can lead to rapid deterioration of graft function (see Chapter 10). Acute antibody-mediated rejection also increases risk of chronic rejection. The development of DSAs to class I and/or class II antigens following renal transplantation appears to be a specific marker of antibody-dependent vascular injury. The primary histopathologic feature is microvascular inflammation, which may be accompanied by the deposition of complement in the graft (see Chapter 15). DSA production also identifies transplant recipients at risk of chronic allograft rejection. Routine immune monitoring of HLA antibodies can be used to guide immunotherapy and permit early intervention. Recipients transplanted with low-level DSAs or who were desensitized should be tested early after transplant to monitor their DSA levels. A substantial increase in DSA after the transplant is associated with poor outcome, whereas a sustained decrease or disappearance of the DSA is good news. DSA that persists after transplantation may be deleterious for the graft, although some patients with persistent DSA do not develop clinical evidence of damage to the graft. Recipients of kidneys with more HLA mismatches (particularly for HLA-DR and -DQ antigens), and those with a history of nonadherence are more likely to develop DSA and more frequent monitoring could identify developing antibody responses in these patients in advance of clinical symptoms. Table 3.4 suggests a protocol for DSA monitoring in different post-transplant immunologic risk cohorts, which is supplemented by protocol biopsies in some programs.

The single antigen test is informative for post-transplant monitoring because it identifies antibodies that are reactive against the mismatched donor HLA antigens. Alternatively, DSA can be monitored by directly crossmatching recipient sera with donor lymphocytes (if they are available) using complement-dependent lymphocytotoxicity or flow cytometry methods.

Monitoring Non-HLA Antibodies after Transplantation

There is increasing recognition of the clinical importance of non-HLA antibodies following transplantation of all solid-organ types. Many of these non-HLA antibodies are directed against endothelial or epithelial cells and represent a heterogeneous group of antibodies comprising both IgM and IgG subclasses. These non-HLA antibodies are classified as either alloantibodies such as MICA or tissue-specific autoantibodies depending on whether they are directed against polymorphic antigens that differ between the host and donor, or if they represent an immune response to a self-antigen, respectively. Antibodies specific for alloantigens such as MICA and autoantigens such as agrin, angiotensin II type I receptor (AT1R) have been implicated in acute and/or chronic renal allograft injury.

TABLE
3.4 | Suggested Protocol for DSA Monitoring Post-transplant

Status Frequency of DSA Monitoring

DSA positive: Week 2, 4, and 8; 6 months; 1 year; and annually
Desensitized patients: Day 4, week 2, 4, and 8; 6 months; 1 year; and annually
DSA negative and low sensitized: 6 months, 1 year, and annually
Highly sensitized patients: 4 weeks, 6 months, 1 year, and annually

May be supplemented by protocol biopsy (see Chapter 15).

Known non-HLA targets such as AT1R antibody can be measured using ELISA assays, while cell-based crossmatch assays using endothelial cells can be used to identify non-HLA antibodies in the sera of transplant recipients. Advantages include the ability to detect antibodies specific for novel antigens, in particular, polymorphic antigens, which may differ between cell donors. However, incomplete knowledge of the non-HLA targets hampers the understanding of the clinical significance of the assay.

Biologic Basis for Immune Monitoring Assays to Allografts

The mechanisms underlying allograft rejection are not completely understood (see Chapter 2). Recipient T cells become activated upon direct recognition of HLA/peptide complexes present on the membrane of passenger dendritic cells of donor origin. This vigorous response, which appears to violate the rule of self–MHC restriction, is driven primarily by antigen mimicry. T cells activated via the direct recognition pathway are thought to be important for initiation of early acute rejection. However, these T cells play a less important role following the departure of donor dendritic cells from the graft, because upon recognition of donor HLA molecules on "nonprofessional" antigen-presenting cells (APCs) that lack costimulatory elements, they may become anergized. Studies indicate that the indirect recognition pathway, which is stimulated by allopeptides presented by professional APCs of host origin, is a major contributor to rejection, especially chronic rejection. T-helper cells engaged in the direct and indirect pathways provide lymphokines required for the proliferation and maturation of cytotoxic T cells and of HLA antibody-producing B cells. The T-helper cells may also produce cytokines, invoking a delayed-type hypersensitivity response. A semi-direct antigen presentation pathway has also been identified in which recipient APCs acquire donor MHC–peptide complexes through capture or membrane exchange and present it to recipient T cells via direct and indirect recognition pathways. Immune monitoring assays have been developed to assess alloimmune responses of the lymphocyte repertoire and functions. These include markers of cellular activation, proliferation, cytokine production, chemokine production, and cytotoxicity.

Cell-Mediated Lympholysis and Mixed Lymphocyte Culture Assays

The direct recognition pathway is thought to be the primary mediator of acute allograft rejection and can be measured *in vitro* by the strength of the antidonor mixed lymphocyte culture (MLC) assay and cell-mediated lympholysis (CML) reactivity exhibited by recipient T cells. The CML assay measures the cytotoxic T-cell reactivity to mismatched HLA class I antigens of the donor. The MLC assay measures the capacity of recipient leukocytes to respond to HLA class II differences expressed by donor leukocytes. Sequencing the T-cell receptor repertoire of alloreactive T cells generated in the MLC can be used as biomarkers to track harmful donor-specific T-cell clones in the peripheral blood of transplant recipients, whereas a reduction in alloreactive T cells after transplant may identify recipients who are either adequately immunosuppressed or tolerant. Global cellular immune response can also be measured for intracellular ATP levels in peripheral blood CD4$^+$ T cells following nonspecific stimulation with mitogens *in vitro* in solid-organ transplant patients. Although no association has been found with acute rejection, this assay has been useful in identifying patients with infection and can be used to monitor immunosuppression adherence.

Alloreactive T-Cell Precursor Frequency Analysis

The indirect recognition allorecognition pathway is thought to play an important role in mediating chronic allograft rejection. Patients who are at risk of chronic rejection of heart, renal, lung, and liver allografts can be identified by an increased capacity for indirect recognition of donor HLA allopeptides. Persistent allopeptide reactivity and epitope spreading are both characteristic of chronic allograft rejection. The precursor frequency of alloreactive T cells recognizing mismatched donor HLA antigens, measured by limiting dilution analysis (LDA), provides a means of assessing the indirect pathway. Carboxyfluorescein succinimidyl ester (CFSE) is an intracellular fluorescent label that divides equally between daughter cells following cellular division. A combination of LDA and CFSE labeling has been described to measure antigen-specific T-cell frequencies with high sensitivity and reproducibility.

T-cell precursor frequency can also be measured by an enzyme-linked immunosorbent spot assay (ELISPOT) that has the advantage of detecting cytokine-secreting antigen-specific cells. MHC multimer (Tetramer, Pentamer, or Dextramer) has recently developed to directly detect antigen-specific T and B cells by flow cytometry. Multi-parameter intracellular cytokine staining by flow cytometry has also been widely used to quantify cytokine production by lymphocyte subsets that include antigen-specific T cells and memory T cells. This method has the advantage over ELISPOT since it allows simultaneously the detection of transcription factors, cytokine production and surface phenotype of the same cell.

Gene Expression Profiling Assays

Technological advances in the field of molecular genetics allow measurement of the expression of immune activation and effector molecules involved in transplant rejection. In heart transplantation, real-time PCR-based AlloMap assay—a noninvasive 11-gene expression profiling test on blood sample—has been used for identifying patients with negative predictive value of rejection that is found to be equivalent to routine endomyocardial biopsy. Similarly, Kidney Solid-Organ Response Test (kSORT)—a 17-gene expression profiling assay focusing on kidney transplant recipients—has recently been developed to allow accurate prediction on patients with and without rejection. These gene expression markers include cytokines, chemokines, cellular cytotoxicity, and proliferation. The main limitation of monitoring expression of immune activation genes for diagnosis of rejection is that these same markers can also be elevated during viral and bacterial infections.

Microarrays have also been used to provide global insights into the mechanisms of allograft dysfunction and rejection as well as tolerance. Although the cost of this technology precludes it from being used as a routine monitoring tool at this time, genome-wide analysis by microarrays has the potential to identify novel surrogate markers of graft rejection that can be validated in a larger number of clinical samples using real-time PCR. Currently, new technology such as next-generation sequencing has been commonly used to sequence RNA directly, which offers an alternative approach for transcriptome analyses for using microarrays. The advantage over microarray technology includes higher resolution, discovery of novel transcripts, and identification of allelic expression, alternate splice variants, post-transcriptional mutations, and isoforms. Moreover, the recent developed protein arrays offer options to measure a large number of proteins or antibodies in a single assay.

Proteomic Assays

Proteomics is defined as the study of the proteome that includes all proteins encoded by genes of an organism. Proteomic assessment of biomarkers of transplant rejection and/or tolerance has typically been based on immunologic methods such as Western blot, ELISA, and luminex assays. Several studies have demonstrated the utility of measuring soluble and secreted proteins, to identify patients at risk of transplant rejection. For example, monitoring soluble CD30 levels in recipients of renal allografts has been reported to be an independent and highly predictive factor of immunologic risk. New discovery approaches have been developed using mass spectrometry that permit an unbiased approach to simultaneously analyze numerous proteins and peptides associated with pathologic processes. Recent studies employing this technology detected urinary proteins such as β_2 microglobulin and α_1 antichymotrypsin increased in patients with acute renal allograft rejection.

The immune response to the transplant is dynamic and it is unlikely that one single assay will accurately assess the immune status of the patient. We suggest that a panel of assays will be used to monitor different components of the immune response (humoral versus cellular) to provide an accurate profile of the patient. Monitoring of gene expression and proteomic profiles should enhance our understanding of transplant pathophysiology and help to identify novel biomarkers of rejection, tolerance, and targeted therapies.

Selected Readings

Genetics, Structure and Function

Bjorkman PJ, Saper MA, Samraoui B, et al. Structure of the human class I histocompatibility antigen, HLA-A2. Nature 1987;329:506–512.

Germain RN, Margulies DH. The biochemistry and cell biology of antigen processing and presentation. Annu Rev Immunol 1993;11:403–450.

Parham P, Adams EJ, Arnett KL. The origins of HLA-A,B,C polymorphism. Immunol Rev 1995;143:141–180.

The MHC Sequencing Consortium. Complete sequence and gene map of a human major histocompatibility complex. Nature 1999;401:921–923.

Nomenclature

Holdsworth R, Hurley CK, Marsh SGE, et al. The HLA Dictionary 2008: a summary of HLA-A, -B, -C, -DRB1/3/4/5, -DQB1 alleles and their association with serologically defined HLA-A, -B, -C, -DR and -DQ antigens. Tissue Antigens 2009;73:95–170.

Marsh SG. Nomenclature for factors of the HLA system, update September 2015. Tissue Antigens 2015;86(6):469–473.

HLA Typing

Erlich H. HLA DNA typing: past, present, and future. Tissue Antigens 2012;80(1):1–11.

Terasaki PI, McClelland JD. Microdroplet assay of human serum cytotoxins. Nature 1964;204:998–100.

Antibodies to HLA

Bartel G, Wahrmann M, Exner M, et al. In vitro detection of C4d-fixing HLA alloantibodies: associations with capillary C4d deposition in kidney allografts. Am J Transplant 2008;8(1):41–49.

Cecka JM. Calculated PRA (CPRA): the new measure of sensitization for transplant candidates. Am J Transplant 2010;10:26–29.

Jordan SC, Vo AA, Peng A, et al. Intravenous gammaglobulin (IVIG): a novel approach to improve transplant rates and outcomes in highly HLA-sensitized patients. Am J Transplant 2006;6(3):459–466.

Konvalinka A, Tinckam K. Utility of HLA antibody testing in kidney transplantation. J Am Soc Nephrol 2015;26(7):1489–1502.

Patel R, Terasaki PI. Significance of the positive crossmatch test in kidney transplantation. N Engl J Med 1969;280:735–739.

Sarabu N, Hricik DE. HLA-DQ mismatching: mounting evidence for a role in kidney transplant rejection. Clin J Am Soc Nephrol 2016;11:759–760.

Warren DS, Zachary AA, Sonnenday CJ, et al. Successful renal transplantation across simultaneous ABO incompatible and positive crossmatch barriers. Am J Transplant 2004;4(4):561–568.

Winters JL, Gloor JM, Pineda AA, et al. Plasma exchange conditioning for ABO-incompatible renal transplantation. J Clin Apher 2004;19(2):79–85.

Zachary AA, Montgomery RA, Ratner LE, et al. Specific and durable elimination of antibody to donor HLA antigens in renal-transplant patients. Transplantation 2003;76(10):1519–1525.

Immune Monitoring

Gloor JM, Sethi S, Stegall MD, et al. Transplant glomerulopathy: subclinical incidence and association with alloantibody. Am J Transplant 2007;7(9):2124–2132.

Hricik DE, Augustine J, Nickerson P, et al. Interferon gamma ELISPOT testing as a risk-stratifying biomarker for kidney transplant injury: results from the CTOT-01 multicenter study. Am J Transplant 2015;15(12):3166–3173.

Loupy A, Lefaucheur C, Vernerey D, et al. Complement-binding HLA antibodies and kidney-allograft survival. N Engl J Med 2013;369(13):1215–1226.

Mizutani K, Terasaki P, Bignon JD, et al. Association of kidney transplant failure and antibodies against MICA. Hum Immunol 2006;67(9):683–691.

Naesens M, Sarwal MM. Molecular diagnostics in transplantation. Nat Rev Nephrol 2010;6(10):614–628.

Safinia N, Afzali B, Atalar K, et al. T-cell alloimmunity and chronic allograft dysfunction. Kidney Int Suppl 2010;(119):S2–S12.

Terasaki PI, Junchao C. Humoral theory of transplantation: further evidence. Curr Opin Immunol 2005;17:541–545.

Viglietti S, Loupy A, Vernerey D, et al. Value of donor-specific anti-HLA antibody monitoring and characterization for risk stratification of kidney allograft loss. J Am Soc Nephrol 2017;28(2):702–715.

Wiebe C, Gibson IW, Blydt-Hansen TD, et al. Rates and determinants of progression to graft failure in kidney allograft recipients with de novo donor-specific antibody. Am J Transplant 2015;15(11):2921–2930.

Wiebe C, Nickerson P. Posttransplant monitoring of de novo human leukocyte antigen donor-specific antibodies in kidney transplantation. Curr Opin Organ Transplant 2013;18(4):470–477.

Websites

http://allelefrequencies.net/hlaepitopes/hlaepitopes.asp
http://hla.alleles.org/dictionary/index.html
www.ashi-hla.org
www.unos.org
www.ustransplant.org

4

The Science of Deceased Donor Kidney Transplantation

Helen M. Nelson, Francis L. Delmonico, Jeffrey L. Veale, and Nick G. Cowan

Though the discussion of death and its opportunities for organ donation in this chapter are dispassionate and may appear cold-hearted, the contrary is in fact the case. The circumstances of sudden death are always profoundly emotional. Organ donation can provide to those who authorize donation for themselves the knowledge that their sudden death will not be wasted. For the bereaved, it can provide much solace in the knowledge that in some way the ultimate generosity of their loved-ones permits others to live longer and better lives. None of this is lost on the professionals whose privilege it is to facilitate the donation process.

Biology requires that we will all die. But most of us will not die in circumstances that permit organ donation. Only approximately 0.5% of all deaths become eligible for organ donation and it is to this 0.5% that this chapter is devoted. Part I focuses upon the *science* of deceased organ donation to include the assessment of data categorically and consistently by recording the potential, eligible, actual, and utilized donors. The assessment of performance can be done in each hospital retrospectively by these categories to then enable prospective improvements for a sustainable deceased donation program. Part I initially addresses the process of deceased organ donation: the determination of death by neurologic function or by circulatory cessation; the identification of the potential donor; and the subsequent authorization process. This section will also include donation performance metrics to assess if donation opportunities are being maximized. Part II will briefly review the management of the deceased donor and the surgical technique of deceased donor organ recovery.

The World Health Organization (WHO) estimates that approximately 80,000 kidney transplants are performed each year in the 112 member states of the World Health Assembly with kidney transplant services. Approximately 60% of these kidney transplants are performed using kidneys recovered from a deceased donor. The supply of deceased organ donor kidneys has increased but not enough, by far, to meet the increasing demand. It has been estimated that only 10% of the annually needed kidney transplants are performed throughout the world. In the United States 13,430 deceased donor transplants were performed in 2016, an increase of 25% over the previous decade: an improvement but still far less than needed. Much of this increase was the result of death due to a tragic drug abuse and opioid addiction epidemic. During the same time period, the number of transplant candidates on the kidney waiting list increased 25%, going from 80,000 in 2009 to over 100,000 in 2014. Further details on the waitlist and its management are discussed in Chapter 8, Part B.

Part I: Death Diagnosis, Identification, Selection, and Preparation of Deceased Donors

WHEN IS SOMEONE DEAD?

For millennia there was no need to precisely define death: absence of respiration and a heartbeat was adequate. The necessity to determine the moment that death occurs is a phenomenon of the second half of the 20th century which brought with it intensive care units, the capacity for resuscitation, and deceased donor organ transplantation.

A definition of death was established in the United States in 1981 by the National Conference of Commissioners on Uniform State Laws that formulated the Uniform Determination of Death Act ([UDDA], see also Chapter 19). The UDDA states that: **"An individual who has sustained either irreversible cessation of circulatory and respiratory functions, or irreversible cessation of all functions of the entire brain, including the brain stem is dead".** Today, all 50 states and the District of Columbia follow the UDDA as a legal and medical standard of death. The UDDA provides an important framework of mechanisms of death that can be universally applied.

The UDDA criteria for brain death assess the function of the entire brain, both cerebral and brainstem. The conceptual significance of assessing brainstem function is to assure that an individual breathing spontaneously is not declared dead. In the original definition of irreversible coma by the Ad Hoc Harvard Committee in 1968, the concept included an absence of spontaneous respiration.

Dr. William Sweet, the renowned neurosurgeon of the Massachusetts General Hospital, later wrote in the New England Journal of Medicine that "it is clear that a person is not dead unless his or her brain is dead." The time-honored criteria of stoppage of the heartbeat and circulation are indicative of death only when they persist long enough for the brain to die.

The paradigm for donation and death has been ultimately emphasized as requiring absence of circulation (as stipulated by the UDDA; and thus not just the heartbeat) and by underscoring the vital function of the brain as an essential criterion of life. As opposed to other organs, the brain cannot be supported or replaced by medical technology.

The Determination of Death

The determination of death is an everyday occurrence that has social, legal, religious, and cultural consequences necessitating legal standards for declaring death. Death is a process that is usually determined on the basis of cardio-respiratory criteria, but it has now become evident that ultimately we all die when our cerebral function and all brainstem functions (inclusive of the capacity to breathe spontaneously) are irreversibly lost. The reason to make an ultimate functional assessment unique to brain function is because when it is lost (irreversibly), it is irreplaceable. If consciousness cannot be restored and one cannot breathe spontaneously (that is, without a ventilator), that person is dead. In contrast, the circulatory function of the heart can be replaced by an organ transplant, or sustained by extra corporeal devices that provide circulation; so the loss of the function of the heart, and other organs that are replaceable, does not solely constitute death.

Determining Death by an Absence of Neurologic Function
The ultimate criterion of death is the irreversible loss of brain function which can occur as the result of a devastating brain injury or the absence of circulation. The clinical criteria for the diagnosis of death by neurologic criteria are outlined in Table 4.1. In the clinical circumstance of a devastating brain injury, such as a cerebral hemorrhage or from a tumor or trauma, an edematous brain herniates through the tentorium preventing oxygenated blood circulation to the brainstem and cerebrum. Death can be declared when the criteria for death of the brain are fulfilled, but determination must include the known reason for coma. The coma is deemed irreversible with a lack of current or any future potential for awareness, wakefulness, interaction and capacity for sensory perception, or responsiveness to the external environment. There is a loss of the capacity to breathe spontaneously, evident in the absence of brainstem reflexes and confirmed by an apnea test. The commonly used term "brain-death" is an unfortunate one that may cause confusion to the lay public, since it may suggest that the dead individual may be "alive" in some other form. The term "death determined by neurologic criteria" would be preferred, but is unlikely to replace the term in common parlance.

Determining Death by an Absence of Circulation
The irreversible absence of circulation is consequential not only to the function of the vital organs such as the heart and lungs and liver, but to the brain. The permanent absence of circulation will lead to the irreversible loss of brain function. If organ donation is not to be considered during end-of-life care, then death can be declared by the absence of

TABLE 4.1	Clinical Criteria for the Diagnosis of Brain Death

Clinical Evaluation Prerequisites
- Establish irreversible and proximate cause of coma
- Exclude the presence of sedating, paralyzing, or toxic drugs
- Achieve normal or near-normal core temperature
- Absence of severe electrolyte, acid–base, or endocrine disturbance
- Achieve normal systolic blood pressure >100 mm Hg

The Clinical Evaluation (Neurologic Assessment)
- Coma—patient lacks all evidence of responsiveness
- Absence of brainstem reflexes
  - No pupillary response
  - No oculocephalic reflex
  - No corneal reflex
  - Absence of facial movement to a noxious stimuli
  - No tracheobronchial reflex
- Apnea in response to acidosis or hypercarbia

circulation and breathing because without circulation the function of the brain is inevitably lost. When donation proceeds in this manner, it is now referred to as Donation after Circulatory Death (DCD). The previous terms "donation after cardiac death" or "non–heart-beating donation" have been abandoned.

Diagnosis of Circulatory Death. A gap of scientific data persists as to the precise duration of the absence of circulation that can cause irreversible loss of brain function. As a result, the postmortem interventions that have been done for the purpose of organ donation—DCD—have been controversial, and remain so in some countries. Brain function and electrical activity are lost within seconds of the absence of circulation; what is uncertain is the duration of the absence of circulation that would prevent restoration of brain activity if the circulation is restored. Even under normothermic conditions, the brain might be able to tolerate as long as 10 to 11 minutes of circulatory arrest without any long-term sequelae should perfusion be restored. Some brain activity may be restored after long periods of circulatory arrest—perhaps up to 60 minutes.

The rare reported cases of auto-resuscitation have all occurred within the context of abandoned CPR rather than treatment withdrawal. When it did occur while the ECG was being continuously monitored, the longest reported interval between asystole and spontaneous resumption of the circulation was 7 minutes.

The Dead Donor Rule and Organ Donation

The retrieval of organs for transplantation should not cause the death of a donor. This rule is an ethical axiom of organ donation: *no organ recovery should precede the declaration of death.* Public trust in organ donation hinges upon an assurance that the medical professional will prioritize the care of the dying patient over any other objective, however noble or good.

Before the criteria for brain death were accepted in the 1970s, all deceased donor organs were recovered from patients after cardiac and circulatory death. When brain-death criteria became widely accepted, DCD organ donors decreased owing to the risks associated with ischemic damage to the kidney and due to the development of multi-organ recoveries. With the continued shortage of deceased organ donors, transplant programs and OPOs needed to reevaluate this practice. In 2006, there was a National Consensus conference on DCD that was instrumental in the promotion of DCD in the United States.

There are four basic so-called Maastricht categories of DCD donors (Table 4.2). Category I and II DCD donors, also referred to as *uncontrolled donors*, are pulseless and asystolic after adequate but failed attempts at resuscitation. Some trauma centers have developed protocols to minimize ischemia in these circumstances by rapid placement of intravenous cannulas to cool the organs after death has been declared. The option to donate is preserved until the family can be informed of the death and then counseled by the organ procurement staff. If consent to donate is obtained, the organs are recovered quickly to prevent further ischemic injury.

Uncontrolled DCD is the most common form of DCD in Spain (see Spanish Model, below). In the United States, DCD is usually

TABLE 4.2	Maastricht Categories for Non–Heart-Beating Donors

Category I: dead on arrival
Category II: unsuccessful resuscitation
Category III: awaiting cardiac death
Category IV: cardiac death in a brain-dead donor

category III or "*controlled*." These donors are comatose, irreversibly brain damaged, and respirator dependent, but are not brain dead by strict definition. At this decision point, the OPO and ICU staffs collaborate to plan the introduction of the option of donation to the family. In these circumstances, the decision to withdraw supportive care is made by the family and primary medical team, and appropriate consent for organ donation is obtained *after* the decision to withdraw support. Ventilator support is discontinued either in the operating room or in an intensive care unit, cardiac function is monitored, and death is pronounced by standard cardiac criteria after a predetermined (usually 5-minute) period of asystole. Organ recovery then proceeds expeditiously. *The organ recovery team plays no part in the diagnosis of death or medical management of the patient before asystole.* Maastricht category IV DCD donors are also known as "crashing donors," who have often become hemodynamically unstable en route to organ recovery after a diagnosis of brain death. For new classifications of DCD developed to take into account the varied circumstances of controlled and uncontrolled circulatory death, see Thuong et al. in Selected Readings.

There has been a steady increase in the number of DCD donors in the United States over the past 10 years (Fig. 4.1). If the family is supportive of donation and the patient is near brain death, the discussion may lead to the donation occurring as a donation after brain death (DBD). A robust DCD program can expand the opportunity for more kidney transplants and be additive to the number of DBD organ donors.

THE PROCESS OF DECEASED KIDNEY DONATION

The deceased donor organ donation process is a continuum from the identification of the potential organ donor through to the transplantation of renal (and other) allografts at the transplantation center and summarized in Table 4.3. To maximize the supply and quality of the deceased donor kidney pool, every step in this continuum needs to be optimized.

Donor Identification and Referral of Potential Deceased Donors

In the United States, hospitals are required by the Center for Medicare and Medicaid Services (CMS) to identify and refer all imminent deaths to the local Organ Procurement Organization ([OPO], see Chapter 5). Timely notification to the OPO is required by CMS regulation at the time of impending death, or imminent death, within 1 hour of one or more specified clinical triggers (Table 4.4). This regulation is known as "required referral" or "routine notification" and represents a unique practice internationally, and is required by law. An "imminent death"

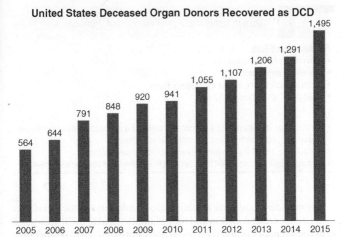

FIGURE 4.1 Deceased organ donors recovered as DCD in the United States. (Data from OPTN.transplant.hrsa.gov.)

TABLE 4.3	Deceased Donor Process: From Donor Identification to Transplantation

Donor identification
Clinical triggers
Referral to organ procurement organization
Assessment of medical suitability of the donor
Authorization for donation
Organ donor management
Organ allocation
Organ recovery surgery
Organ preservation and transportation
Organ transplantation

is defined as a mechanically ventilated, deeply comatose patient, admitted to an ICU, with catastrophic brain damage of known origin.

OPOs partner with the hospitals to provide education and services that ensure every donation opportunity is realized. Educational opportunities include identifying imminent deaths and when to refer them to the OPO, setting up a successful collaborative donation process, and clinical guidelines for maintaining the option of organ donation. These management guidelines are for patients when brain death is pending, and implemented to sustain organ function while the family is accepting the diagnosis and considering the opportunity for donation. Maintaining organ function during this time provides the greatest chance of a successful outcome in the recipient of the organs. OPOs also provide performance data to the hospital on referral rates, timely notification rates, conversion rates, and any potential organ donors who were not identified. Hospitals utilize this information to improve their donation program.

TABLE 4.4	When to Notify the Organ Procurement Organization

Any Imminent Death
- Severe acute brain injury
- Ventilator dependent
- In an intensive care unit or emergency room
- Glasgow Coma Scale (GCS) < 5

Or
- At the initial indication that a patient has suffered a nonrecoverable neurologic injury (e.g., documented loss of cranial nerve reflexes)
- As soon as a formal brain-death examination is contemplated
- Before initiating a discussion that may lead to withdrawal of life-sustaining therapy

Prompt identification of all potential organ donors is critical in efforts to maximize organ donation and transplantation and to fulfill the wishes of deceased patients and their loved ones. Potential organ donors may be identified in the emergency ward or in the critical care unit. Timely notification, as required by law, provides the OPO time to evaluate a patient's medical suitability for donation. This early notification also allows the OPO to develop a collaborative plan with the critical care team for approaching the family after they discuss end-of-life care (a "huddle"). Part of the collaborative plan will include determining if the patient is active on a Donor Registry. Over 50% of U.S. adults are registered donors, registration having taken place at the time of renewal of a driving license or through the Internet. The potential registered donor has already made the donation decision that cannot be overturned by family, though the agreement of the family is greatly to be preferred.

The WHO Critical Pathway
The WHO Critical Pathway for deceased organ donation provides a consistent and systematic approach to the process of donation after DBD and DCD. It is a reproducible tool for assessing the potential of deceased donation, evaluating performance in the deceased donation process, and identifying areas for improvement (Fig. 4.2). The Critical Pathway also provides a common scenario or trigger in which the prospective identification and referral of a possible and potential deceased organ donor can be undertaken. The definitions of possible and potential organ donors, as provided in the Critical Pathway, are important references of the clinical condition for an understanding of the timely identification and referral for organ donation.

Evaluation of a Potential Deceased Donor
The donor evaluation process begins with an assessment of medical suitability. For example, a malignancy with current metastatic disease renders the donor medically unsuitable. In light of the ongoing shortage of deceased donor kidneys, these risks of transmission of a donor malignancy or infectious disease must be weighed against the risk of continuing on dialysis to the patient awaiting transplantation. Consultation with the local OPO and hospitals is essential to ensure that potential organ donors are not inappropriately excluded.

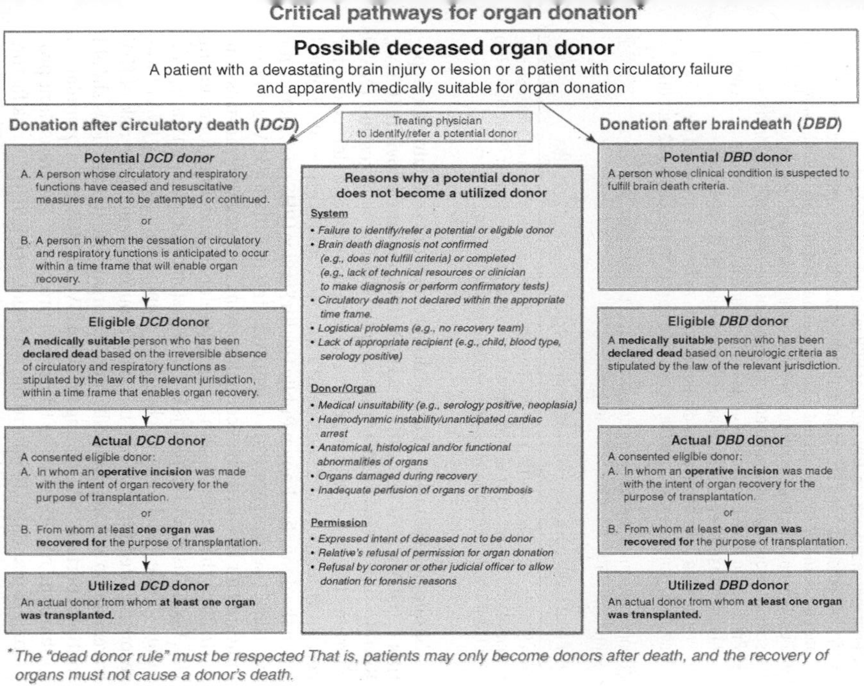

Critical pathways for organ donation*

Possible deceased organ donor

A patient with a devastating brain injury or lesion or a patient with circulatory failure and apparently medically suitable for organ donation

Treating physician to identify/refer a potential donor

Donation after circulatory death (DCD)

Potential DCD donor

A. A person whose circulatory and respiratory functions have ceased and resuscitative measures are not to be attempted or continued.

or

B. A person in whom the cessation of circulatory and respiratory functions is anticipated to occur within a time frame that will enable organ recovery.

↓

Eligible DCD donor

A **medically suitable** person who has been **declared dead** based on the irreversible absence of circulatory and respiratory functions as stipulated by the law of the relevant jurisdiction, within a time frame that enables organ recovery.

↓

Actual DCD donor

A consented eligible donor:
A. In whom an **operative incision** was made with the intent of organ recovery for the purpose of transplantation.

or

B. From whom at least **one organ was recovered for** the purpose of transplantation.

↓

Utilized DCD donor

An actual donor from whom **at least one organ was transplanted.**

Reasons why a potential donor does not become a utilized donor

System
- *Failure to identify/refer a potential or eligible donor*
- *Brain death diagnosis not confirmed (e.g., does not fulfill criteria) or completed (e.g., lack of technical resources or clinician to make diagnosis or perform confirmatory tests)*
- *Circulatory death not declared within the appropriate time frame.*
- *Logistical problems (e.g., no recovery team)*
- *Lack of appropriate recipient (e.g., child, blood type, serology positive)*

Donor/Organ
- *Medical unsuitability (i.e.g., serology positive, neoplasia)*
- *Haemodynamic instability/unanticipated cardiac arrest*
- *Anatomical, histological and/or functional abnormalities of organs*
- *Organs damaged during recovery*
- *Inadequate perfusion of organs or thrombosis*

Permission
- *Expressed intent of deceased not to be donor*
- *Relative's refusal of permission for organ donation*
- *Refusal by coroner or other judicial officer to allow donation for forensic reasons*

Donation after braindeath (DBD)

Potential DBD donor

A person whose clinical condition is suspected to fulfill brain death criteria.

↓

Eligible DBD donor

A **medically suitable** person who has been **declared dead** based on neurologic criteria as stipulated by the law of the relevant jurisdiction.

↓

Actual DBD donor

A consented eligible donor:
A. In whom an **operative incision** was made with the intent of organ recovery for the purpose of transplantation.

or

B. From whom at least **one organ was recovered for** the purpose of transplantation.

↓

Utilized DBD donor

An actual donor from whom **at least one organ was transplanted.**

*The "dead donor rule" must be respected That is, patients may only become donors after death, and the recovery of organs must not cause a donor's death.

FIGURE 4.2 Critical pathway for organ donation. (From Dominguez-Gil B, Delmonico FL, Shaheen FA, et al. The critical pathway for deceased donation: reportable uniformity in the approach to deceased donation. Transpl Int 2011;24(4):373–378, with permission from John Wiley and Sons.)

83

TABLE 4.5	United States Public Health Service Guidelines (2013) for the Reduction of Transmission of HIV, HBV, and HCV, through Organ Transplantation

Donors who meet one or more of the following 11 criteria should be identified as being at increased risk for recent HIV, HBV, and HCV infection

- People who have had sex with a person known or suspected to have HIV, HBV, or HCV infection in the preceding 12 months
- Men who have had sex with men (MSM) in the preceding 12 months
- Women who have had sex with a man with a history of MSM behavior in the preceding 12 months
- People who have had sex in exchange for money or drugs in the preceding 12 months
- People who had sex with a person who had sex in exchange for money or drugs in the preceding 12 months
- People who had sex with a person who injected drugs by intravenous, intramuscular, or subcutaneous route for nonmedical reasons in the preceding 12 months
- A child who is 18 months of age and born to mother known to be infected with, or at increased risk for, HIV, HBV, or HCV infection
- A child who has been breastfed within the preceding 12 months and the mother is known to be infected with, or at increased risk for, HIV infection
- People who have injected drugs by intravenous, intramuscular, or subcutaneous route for nonmedical reasons in the preceding 12 months
- People who have been in lockup, jail, prison, or a juvenile correctional facility for more than 72 consecutive hours in the preceding 12 months
- People who have been newly diagnosed with, or have been treated for, syphilis, gonorrhea, *Chlamydia,* or genital ulcers in the preceding 12 months

Donors who meet the following criterion should be identified as being at increased risk for recent HCV infection only:

- People who have been on hemodialysis in the preceding 12 months

(From Seem DL, Lee I, Umscheid CA, et al. PHS Guideline for reducing human immunodeficiency virus, hepatitis b virus, and hepatitis c virus transmission through organ transplantation. Public Health Rep 2013;128(4):247–343. Reprinted by Permission of SAGE Publications, Inc.)

Serologic evaluation of organ donors includes screening for hepatitis C (HCV), HIV, hepatitis B virus (HBV), cytomegalovirus (CMV), Epstein–Barr virus (EBV), and syphilis. Nucleic acid testing (NAT) shortens the "window period" (between exposure and detection) for certain viral infections such as HIV and HCV and is especially helpful when the donor has known Public Health Service (PHS) risk factors for exposure. Use of organs from donors who test positive for HIV is contraindicated for HIV-negative recipients owing to the risk of transmission.

In 2013, the Public Health Service developed guidelines for reducing HIV, Hepatitis B, and Hepatitis C transmission through organ transplantation (Table 4.5). Use of nucleic-acid amplification testing (NAT) was recommended for high-risk behavior groups to reduce the risk of HIV transmission and to potentially increase organ utilization. OPOs should routinely perform NAT testing for HIV, HBV, and HCV in this population to share the results with the transplant programs. The transplant programs are mandated to inform the potential recipient of the risk factors and potential risks and benefits of accepting the organ (see Chapter 8).

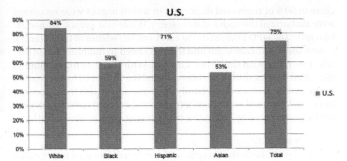

FIGURE 4.3 Variation in authorization rates based on ethnicity in the United States. (Data from Seem DL, Lee I, Umscheid CA, et al. PHS Guideline for reducing human immunodeficiency virus, hepatitis b virus, and hepatitis c virus transmission through organ transplantation. Public Health Rep 2013;128(4):247–343.)

In 2015, the U.S. Department of Health and Human Services announced that it will amend the OPTN Final Rule (42 CFR Part 121) to allow the recovery of transplantable organs from HIV-positive donors. This is a milestone in support of the federal HIV Organ Policy Equity Act (also known as the HOPE Act), which calls for study of the feasibility, effectiveness, and safety of transplanting organs from HIV-positive donors to be used for HIV-positive candidates (see Chapter 12). Recipient selection may be influenced by the donor serologic profile; for example, HCV-seropositive donor kidneys may be selected for use in HCV-seropositive patients (see Chapter 13).

Authorization for Donation

Authorization rates (previously called "consent rates") for organ donation have increased in the United States during the past 15 years by approximately 20%, with a rate of more than 75% nationwide in 2015. Some regions have authorization rates close to 90%. There is considerable variation in authorization rates based on ethnicity (see Fig. 4.3) and rates tend to be higher in English-speaking compared to non–English-speaking groups, and are higher in second-generation immigrants compared to first-generation immigrants. Success in obtaining authorization for organ donation is associated with highly trained, skilled, and sensitive staff who can spend as much time as needed to support the donor family through the process. Authorization rates are also higher when there is collaboration between the healthcare team and the OPO staff to ensure that the donation discussion occurs when the family has accepted that death is imminent and they are ready to make end-of-life decisions. Family sociodemographics (ethnicity, age, and cause of death) and prior knowledge of a potential donor's wishes to donate significantly impact the family's willingness to donate. With "first-person authorization" (prior authorization by the deceased themselves rather than the next-of-kin), there is an increase in the number of cases where the potential donor already registered their desire for donation. This can be done through a state registry, notation on a driver's license, or an advanced directive. Currently, 50% of adults in the United States are registered organ donors and in some states close to 50% of recovered donors from whom organs were recovered were authorized through a state registry. While first-person authorization gives the OPO permission to carry out the wishes of the potential donor, the healthcare team and the OPO need to maintain sensitivity when working with the donor families. With the growing number of registered donors, the healthcare team and the OPO need to be prepared for potential conflict if the family does not agree with their decision to donate. Surgical staff members involved in the recovery of organs are fully protected by law in the event of first-person authorization.

Opting-in and Opting-out

In the 40 years since the inception of organized deceased organ donation in the United States, consent to donate has been on an "opt-in" or "voluntary consent" basis, meaning either that the donor has expressly authorized donation, or that the next-of-kin do so. In the absence of consent, donation does not go forward. "Opt-out" or "presumed consent" is based, *a priori*, on the presumption that the potential donor would agree to donation which will go forward unless an objection to do so has been formally expressed. Some have suggested that an opt-in system would increase rates of deceased donation and some European countries (most recently France in 2017) have legislation that would permit it. The United States has an authorization rate which is second only, internationally, to that of Spain (see below), and although Spain has the legalized "opt-out," it does not apply it. Opt-out, if practiced, can generate an adversarial interaction with bereaved families which is obviated by opt-in. Once an individual has opted out, he or she is essentially lost to the organ donation concept. Individuals who have not opted-in may still elect to do so, as may their next-of-kin in the event of sudden demise. Opting-in is preferred to opting-out!

The Spanish Model

High organ donation rates reported in Spain are attributed to the so-called "Spanish model" of organ donation which is often used as an exemplar of an effective deceased donor organ recovery program. The Spanish model entails a highly structured, systematic approach to maximizing the identification, referral, consent rate, and management of potential deceased organ donors. Key elements of this model include compensated and well-trained staff physicians with clearly defined accountability for effectiveness in donor surveillance, and referral and aggressive pursuit of older donors. Intensive care transplant coordinators, often physicians themselves, are based at the site of the donation. Uncontrolled DCD is common practice. The Spanish-based Organizacion Nacional de Transplantes (http:/www.ont.es) does much to disseminate effective deceased donor management practices particularly throughout the Spanish-speaking world.

Measures of Performance

When comparing measures of donation performance between geographic areas, the metric "donors per million population" (DMP) has often been used. A much more meaningful method for assessing and comparing organ donation rates uses the number of medically suitable potential organ donors in a geographic area as the denominator, and the number of actual organ donors in that area as the numerator. The *"donation rate"* for this measure is eligible deaths, defined as donors aged 70 or younger who meet the criteria for death by neurologic criteria. But this only represents a subset of total potential. A better measure is the metric known as the *"CMS collaborative conversion rate."* This measure includes all DCD donors and donors over the age of 70 to both the numerator and the denominator when calculating the rate. Using this metric has been an effective tool for monitoring improvement in organ donation across all 58 U.S. OPOs. The mean conversion rate in the United States varies regionally between 60% and 90% and as of 2016, the national mean was close to 80%.

The metric *organs transplanted per donor* (OTPD) is a measurement of the effectiveness of multi-organ recovery efforts. Each deceased donor is theoretically a source of two kidneys, heart and lungs, a liver, a pancreas, and intestines. This measurement, however, does not adjust for donor characteristics such as hypertension, diabetes, or liver disease, which may impact the ability for an organ to be transplanted. A better measurement is an "observed-to-expected" (O:E) ratio yield measurement currently in place through the OPTN that adjusts for donor characteristics.

Part II: Management of the Deceased Organ Donor and Surgical Technique of Deceased Donor Organ Recovery

In the United States and most countries with an advanced organ donation infrastructure, the management of the deceased organ donor who has been declared dead by neurologic criteria (brain dead) passes from the intensive care unit staff to the staff of the OPO. Legally, the deceased donor is no longer a "person" (see Chapter 19) and the staff need not be led by physicians, but are typically specially trained coordinators working, directly or indirectly, under medical supervision. The management of the donors is complex and is designed to maximize the function, not only of the kidneys, but of organs both above and below the diaphragm. Obviating or minimizing ischemia-reperfusion injury is a major goal (see Chapter 10) made more difficult by the massive release of cytokine at the time of death ("cytokine storm"). Readers are referred to the article Kotloff et al. on Management of the Potential Organ Donor in the ICU, in Selected Readings, for a detailed account of the management of the deceased donor.

Pharmacologic Adjuncts
Deceased donors may suffer from impaired hormone physiology, tissue hypoxia, and an increased systemic inflammatory response. Donor Management Goals (DMGs) have been created to help ameliorate the effect of these responses and pharmacologic adjuncts play a part in helping to achieve these goals. Most deceased donors are given large doses of corticosteroids to deplete circulating donor lymphocytes and attenuate brain-death–induced inflammatory pathways. Additional hormone treatments including vasopressin and T3 or T4 are routinely administered, although data from randomized trials suggest marginal

benefit. For adults, 25 g of mannitol is typically given to ensure diuresis and possibly to minimize ischemic injury. There is some evidence that dopamine given intravenously before kidney manipulation may lower rates of delayed graft function. Systemic heparinization is carried out at the time of cannula placement with doses of 10,000 to 30,000 units.

Research on the optimal management of the deceased organ donor has been notoriously difficult because of logistic and legal barriers. Variations in management between OPOs have typically not been rigorously compared. An exception is the study by Niemann et al. (see Selected Readings) that showed, in a controlled trial, that mild hypothermia, as compared with normothermia, in organ donors after declaration of death determined neurologic criteria significantly reduced the rate of delayed graft function among recipients. This study represents a milestone in organ donor management research that will hopefully pave the way for further therapeutic advancements.

Surgical Technique

The principles of the operation to recover organs from the deceased organ donor are similar regardless of the organs to be removed. Wide surgical exposure is obtained. If multiple organs are to be removed, the preferred sequence is heart first, lungs second, liver (small bowel) third, pancreas fourth, and kidneys last. Each organ to be removed is dissected with its vasculature intact. A cannula is placed in the distal aorta for *in situ* cooling. At the time of aortic cross-clamping, flush and surface cooling are begun. The right and left colon are both mobilized medially, exposing each kidney which is also mobilized medially within Gerota fascia. The ureters are divided distally near their insertion into the bladder and are mobilized cephalad. Approximately 1 cm of surrounding periureteral tissue is preserved, which contains the delicate vasculature supplying blood to the ureter. The distal aorta is divided below the cannula and the inferior vena cava is divided at the confluence of the common iliac veins. To avoid damage to the renal vasculature and to prevent delayed graft function caused by vasospasm, dissection into the renal hilum is avoided. It should also be assumed that multiple renal arteries exist as a common retrieval injury is inadvertent division of an accessory renal artery. The kidneys are often removed *en bloc* with the aorta and vena cava and separated on the back table (Fig. 4.4). However, if the kidneys are from a small pediatric donor, they should not be separated. The kidneys are protected against warm ischemia by the cold flush and surface cooling with ice during the time it takes to remove the other organs.

Ischemia Times

Warm ischemia time refers to the period between circulatory arrest and commencement of cold storage. With modern *in situ* perfusion techniques, the warm ischemia time is essentially zero in brain-dead donors, although there is warm ischemia if hemodynamic deterioration or cardiac arrest occurs before harvest. A kidney may function after 60 minutes of warm ischemia, and 90 minutes in a young donor; however, rates of DGF and nonfunction increase markedly after 20 minutes.

Cold ischemia time refers to the period of cold storage or machine perfusion. Short cold ischemia times are preferred. Less than 12 hours is regarded as ideal, and less than 24 hours as acceptable. Most centers

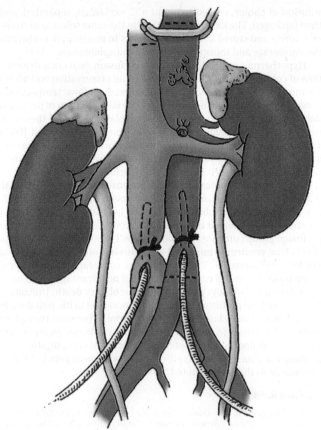

FIGURE 4.4 *En bloc* dissection for deceased donor kidney donation with cannulas in place for *in situ* perfusion. Perihilar and periureteral fat are left in place.

prefer not to use kidneys that have been in cold storage for longer than 40 hours, though kidneys from young trauma victims may function well after cold storage for even longer periods. *Rewarm time* is the period from removal of the kidney from cold storage to reperfusion. This can essentially be eliminated by wrapping the kidney in ice until completion of the vascular anastomosis.

Organ Preservation

The two dominant methods of preserving renal allografts for transplantation are cold storage and pulsatile preservation. Both methods employ hypothermia for maintenance of cellular viability and minimization of *ex vivo* ischemic injury. Cold-storage solutions include University of Wisconsin (UW) solution and histidine–tryptophan–ketoglutarate (HTK) solution, among others. Kidneys preserved in this manner are flushed *in situ* through the arterial blood supply with the preservation solution of choice, cooled to about 4°C, explanted, separated, and then packaged. The kidneys are bathed in the same solution in sterile containers and stored in wet ice in coolers to maintain hypothermia during storage and transportation until transplantation.

Hypothermic pulsatile (machine) perfusion delivers a dynamic flow of cold perfusate to the allograft during preservation and allows for monitoring of perfusion parameters such as flow, temperature, pressure, and renal vascular resistance. Serial evaluation of perfusion data can help guide the decision to transplant or discard these kidneys and may also predict outcomes. In general, flow rates of 100 to 150 mL/min or higher, and vascular resistance of 0.20 to 0.40, are considered optimal. Allografts with persistently low flow (<75 mL/min) and high resistance (>0.40) are usually declined.

The use of pulse perfusion remains inconsistent and controversial. A 2009 randomized controlled trial (see Moers et al. in Selected Readings) demonstrated an absolute reduction in delayed graft function of 6% and an improvement in 1-year graft survival of 4% in the machine perfusion group compared to cold storage. Three-year follow-up data of this trial confirmed improved graft survival of machine-perfused kidneys (91% versus 87%). Graft survival advantage was most pronounced for expanded criteria donors and no advantage was seen in the subgroup of kidneys donated after circulatory death. Utilization rates of machine perfusion have steadily increased in the past decade in the United States but remain highly variable between transplant centers. Deterrents to pulsatile perfusion include significant added recovery costs and increased potential for technical error, together with persistent doubts regarding its efficacy in organ recovery environments as complex as that in the United States.

Selected Readings

Ad Hoc Committee. A definition of irreversible coma: report of the Ad Hoc Committee of the Harvard School to Examine the Definition of Brain Death. JAMA 1968;205:337–340.

Bernat JF, D'Alessandro AM, Port FK, et al. Report of a national conference on donation after cardiac death. Am J Transplant 2006;6:281.

Dominguez-Gil B, Delmonico FL, Shaheen FAM, et al. The critical pathway for deceased donation: reportable uniformity in the approach to deceased donation. Transpl Int 2011;24:373–378.

Feng S. Optimizing graft survival by pretreatment of the donor [published online ahead of print February 17, 2017]. Clin J Am Soc Nephrol. pii: CJN.00900117; doi: 10.2215/CJN.00900117.

Hart A, Smith J, Skeans N. OPTN/SRTR Annual Data Report 2014: kidney. Am J Transplant 2016;16(suppl 2):11.

Hornby K, Hornby L, Shemie SD. A systemic review of autoresusitation after cardiac arrest. Crit Care Med 2010;38(5):1246–1253.

Jochmans I, Watson C. Taking the heat out of organ donation. N Engl J Med 2015;373:5.

Kotloff R, Blosser S, Fulda G, et al. Management of the potential organ donor in the ICU: Society of Critical Care Medicine/American College of Chest Physicians/Association of Organ Procurement Organizations Consensus Statement. Crit Care Med 2015;43:1291.

Mundt H, Yard B, Kramer B, et al. Optimized donor management and organ preservation before kidney transplantation. Transpl Int 2016;29:974.

Murphy P, Boffa C, Manara A, et al. In-hospital logistics: what are the key aspects for succeeding in each of the steps of the process of controlled donation after circulatory death. Transplant Int 2016;29:760–770.

Nelson HM, Glazier AK, Delmonico FL. Changing patterns of organ donation: brain dead donors are not lost by donation after circulatory death. Transplantation 2016;100:446.

Niemann C, Feiner J, Swain S, et al. Therapeutic hypothermia in deceased organ donors and kidney-graft function. N Engl J Med 2015;373:405.

Patel M, Zataria J, De La Cruz S, et al. The impact of meeting donor management goals on the number of organs transplanted per expanded criteria donor: a prospective study from the UNOS Region 5 Donor Management Goals Workgroup. JAMA 2014;149:969.

Robertson J. The dead donor rule. Hastings Cent Rep 1999;29(6):6–14.

Shemie SD. Clarifying the paradigm for the ethics of donation and transplantation: was "dead" really so clear before organ donation? Philos Ethics Hummanit Med 2007;2:18.

Summers D, Watson C, Pettigrew G, et al. Kidney donation after circulatory death (DCD): state of the art. Kidney Int 2015;88:241.

Third WHO Global Consultation on Organ Donation and Transplantation: striving to achieve self-sufficiency, March 23–25, 2010, Madrid, Spain. Transplantation 2011:91(suppl 11):S27.

Thuong M, Ruiz A, Evrard P, et al. New classification of donation after circulatory death donors definitions and terminology. Transpl Int 2016;29:749.

Allocation of Deceased Donor Kidneys

Tom Mone, Rami Jandali, and
Prasad Garimella

The origins of kidney allocation can be traced to the earliest days of deceased donor transplantation in the 1960s when fledgling kidney transplant programs were recovering organs for their patients and occasionally had organs with no recipients. This gave rise to voluntary sharing among cross-town and regionally adjacent programs, with little more than professional friendships to guide the sharing of organs. When the Uniform Anatomical Gift Act (UAGA) was introduced across each of the 50 states in 1968 (see Chapter 19), criteria for organ donation and recovery were defined, as was the designation of transplant doctors as a legal "beneficiary" of these organs to enable transplant to their patients. This principle recognized the ethical concept of "beneficence"—"A physician shall, while caring for a patient, regard responsibility to the patient as paramount." However, this principle does not address how to equitably share organs when the need for organs exceeded the supply, and saving the life of one patient harmed another who was passed over.

THE UNITED NETWORK FOR ORGAN SHARING

The establishment of the Organ Procurement and Transplantation Network (OPTN) through the National Organ Transplant Act of 1984 (NOTA, see Chapter 19) required the development of uniform national policies to describe how organs from deceased donors would be distributed to recipients. This was to ensure that patients awaiting a transplant anywhere in the United States would be transplanted in an established order. The United Network for Organ Sharing (UNOS) operates the OPTN under a contract with the Health Resources and Services Administration (HRSA) of the U.S. government. The so-called "final rule" issued in the year 2000 specifies the precise responsibilities of the OPTN (see McDiarmid et al. in Selected Readings).

The OPTN, through UNOS, works to balance the ethical principles of "justice," "utility," "respect for persons," and "autonomy," all of which have remained the cornerstones of organ allocation policy. Whereas *justice* seeks equality and fairness in the distribution of organs, *utility* recognizes that clinical and logistical issues inhibit and undermine the intended benefits of justice and accentuates the need for the allocation system to be efficient and to maximize the usage of every organ that is viable for transplantation. *Respect for Persons* embraces the moral requirements of honesty and fidelity to commitments made and embraces the concept of respect for *autonomy*, which holds that actions or practices tend to be right insofar as they respect or reflect the exercise of self-determination. Other critical components of organ allocation, which apply internationally, include *transparency,* which requires that data on all organ transplants performed in a given country or region be available to the general public through a governmental organization or an organization designated by a governmental authority for this purpose (UNOS, in the case of the United States), and *traceability,* with ease of identification of the source of the donor organs, being a necessary condition for the safety not only of the recipient but of the general public in the event of transmission, or suspicion of transmission, of infectious disease or malignancy.

Organ allocation is the major responsibility of UNOS. To operate the organ allocation system, the country is divided into organ procurement regions and areas (Fig. 5.1), with independent Organ Procurement Organizations (OPOs) operating according to agreed-upon distribution and sharing criteria. A donor service area (DSA) is the geographic area serviced by the OPO with its donor hospitals and transplant programs.

The offices of UNOS are in Richmond, Virginia. In addition to its permanent administrative staff, UNOS is served by a governing board, and a variety of subcommittees with members representing transplant medical professionals, transplant recipients and donor family members, and the lay public all serving voluntarily. The Members and Professional Standards Committee (MPSC) of UNOS monitors the activities of individual transplant programs and is empowered to initiate the required corrective action in the event of concerns regarding performance.

Readers are referred to the information-rich websites of the OPTN and UNOS at https://optn.transplant.hrsa.gov/ and www.unos.org.

Scientific Registry of Transplant Recipients

The Scientific Registry of Transplant Recipients (SRTR) at www.srtr.org is an ever-expanding national database of transplant statistics. Founded in 1987, the registry exists to support ongoing evaluation of the scientific and clinical status of solid-organ transplantation,

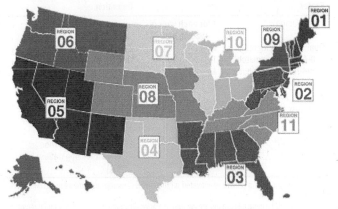

FIGURE 5.1 United Network for Organ Sharing (UNOS) regions of the United States. (From UNOS Facts and Figures. Copyright © 2015 United Network for Organ Sharing. www.unos.org.)

including kidney, heart, liver, lung, intestine, and pancreas. Data in the registry are collected by the OPTN from hospitals and OPOs across the country. The SRTR contains current and past information about the full continuum of transplant activity, related to organ donation and wait-list candidates, transplant recipients, and survival statistics. This information is used to help develop evidence-based policy, to support analysis of transplant programs and OPOs, to provide program-specific data to the MPSC (e.g., "observed vs. expected outcomes"), and to engage in research on issues of importance to the transplant community.

The SRTR is independent of UNOS and is administered by the Chronic Renal Disease group of the Minneapolis Medical Research Foundation (MMRF).

POINT SYSTEM FOR DECEASED DONOR KIDNEY ALLOCATION

To be placed on the transplant waiting list, a patient must fulfill certain listing criteria (see Chapter 8). Renal transplant recipients must either be receiving chronic dialysis or, if they are not on dialysis, have a glomerular filtration rate estimated at 20 mL/min or less.

The order in which waiting patients are offered each kidney that becomes available is determined by a set algorithm, and waiting patients are ranked by a central computer that is located in the UNOS offices. Relevant information about a potential donor is made available to transplant programs on a Web-based program called DonorNet. The ultimate decision about whether to accept an offer for a given patient rests with the responsible physician or surgeon; however, whenever an offer is declined, a reason or "refusal code" must be provided to UNOS. Table 5.1 shows the point system used to rank waiting patients that was in place from 2009 to December 2014.

TABLE 5.1	UNOS Point System for Allocation of Kidneys from Deceased Donors in Place from 2009 to December 2014	
Factor	**Points**	**Condition**
Time waiting*	1 for each year of waiting time	
Quality of HLA match	2	Zero DR mismatches
0-A, B, DR mismatch[†]	1	One DR mismatch
Panel-reactive antibody (PRA)	4	>80% PRA and negative crossmatch
Pediatric recipient priority for donors younger than 35 years		
Organ donor[‡]	4	Expanded criteria donor longest waiting patient (see text)

*Defined from the time a patient is activated on the UNOS computer. In some regions, defined by time receiving dialysis.
[†]0-A-, B-, and DR-mismatched organs are involved in national mandatory sharing program if recipient is highly sensitized or local sharing program if recipient is unsensitized.
[‡]Previous living donor in need of a kidney transplant.
(Adapted from https://optn.transplant.hrsa.gov/.)

From the outset, quantitatively measuring the comparative utility of kidney transplants has been challenging. In the earliest years, these roadblocks were due in part to limited outcomes data and because dialysis essentially equalized the benefits across patients whose lives were not immediately in jeopardy without a transplant, unlike a life-saving liver or heart transplant. Thus, kidney allocation rules were, at first, based on matching (*utility*) and waiting time (*justice*). However, recognizing that long-term survival benefit was one of the core goals of transplantation, antigen matching of donor and recipient quickly added a "lottery effect" of a zero antigen mismatch (see Chapter 3) priority that allocates a kidney to a "perfect match" recipient regardless of waiting time. Thus, utility took precedence for some 17% of kidney transplant patients who were fortunate to receive a zero-mismatched kidney and antigen matching continued to prioritize patients who had been waiting the longest when a kidney became available; patients with better antigen matching to their donors were prioritized over others with similar waiting time but poorer matches.

Over time, kidney allocation policies have been refined to address the justice issues of inequitable access to transplant of specific groups. For instance, in 2003, OPTN kidney allocation policy was changed to remove HLA-B priority points, which resulted in a 37% improvement in the likelihood of African Americans receiving a transplant if they joined the kidney transplant list on the same day as a White patient, reflecting a gain in justice.

Another rebalancing of justice and utility took place with the 2004 establishment of a "pediatric priority" that was introduced as the supply of young donor kidneys was declining due to reduced trauma deaths relative to more "marginal" or "extended criteria donor" (ECD, see below and Chapter 4) kidneys, which increased owing to policies to stimulate their transplant. The pediatric priority was intended to simultaneously tip the scales toward justice by enhancing pediatric access to transplant, while increasing utility by providing pediatric patients access to kidneys (from deceased donors under the age of 35) with longer expected graft survival. An unanticipated impact of the pediatric priority rule was that, though the number of high-quality deceased donor kidneys transplanted in children increased, the number of living donor (mainly parental) transplants fell, and the net number of transplantations in children remained approximately the same.

Expanded Criteria Donors

The term *expanded criteria donor* (ECD) kidney has been removed from the official lexicon of the terms used to describe the quality and determine the allocation of deceased donor kidneys, but it remains in the unofficial lexicon. In its time, it was preferable to the commonly used term "marginal kidney." An ECD kidney came from a deceased donor older than 60 years or aged 50 to 59 years with two additional risk factors, including a history of hypertension, death as a result of cerebrovascular accident, or an elevated terminal serum creatinine. ECD kidneys, which accounted for about 15% of deceased donor kidneys, had statistically at least a 70% increased risk for failing within 2 years compared with standard criteria donor (SCD) kidneys (expressed positively, this means that if an SCD kidney has a 2-year graft survival of 88%, an ECD kidney has an estimated survival at 2 years of about 80%). In 2003, the allocation of ECD kidneys was changed in an effort to speed their placement in an appropriate recipient so as to reduce the cold ischemia time and discard rate. ECD kidneys were offered only to those patients who had agreed to accept them, who were informed of the risk, and who understood that these kidneys were more likely to fail. ECD kidneys were allocated according to waiting time alone. As a result, it was possible to anticipate when patients were close to being allocated an ECD kidney and to ensure that they were prepared for the procedure.

The 2004 Pediatric and "ECD" policies focused the community on the topic of relative graft survival and resulted in a 10-year research and policy deliberation effort to develop a "LYFT" (Life-Years From Transplant) allocation system. This analysis relied on data from over 20 years of donation and transplantation to identify donor and recipient variables that predict graft life-years from donor–recipient matching: age being the predominant factor. LYFT was definitively driven by utility, and predicted 10,000 extra life-years from 1 year's donors, if it were relied upon solely as the allocation system. However, while LYFT was anticipated to significantly improve graft survival and life-years, and was relatively neutral across disease types and ethnic groups, most of its benefits resulted from a shift to the transplant of younger organs to younger recipients, and reduced transplant in older candidates. The U.S. government Department of Health and Human Services (HHS) Office of Civil Rights deemed organ allocation based on age to be unconstitutional. As a consequence, the UNOS Board and the transplant community set about rebalancing the ethical principles underlying kidney allocation so that it was not weighted too heavily toward utility over justice and respect for persons.

Kidney Allocation System for Deceased Donor Kidneys and Transplant Candidate Classification

The resulting Kidney Allocation System (KAS) was introduced into practice in December 2014 and is primarily intended to increase transplant graft survival. It does so by allocating kidneys with a lower Kidney Donor Profile Index (KDPI) score (longer estimated function) to recipients with low Expected Post-Transplant Survival (EPTS) scores (better post-transplant survival). The variables used to determine KDPI and EPTS are shown in Table 5.2. Note that though age is a critical component of both the KDPI and the EPTS, it is accompanied by other variables. The KDPI is a percentage score that provides a far more granular estimation of kidney quality than the binary SCD/ECD designation. The score estimates how long the kidney is likely to function when compared to other kidneys. A KDPI score of 20% means that the kidney is likely to function longer than 80% of other available kidneys. A KDPI score of 60% means that the kidney is likely to function longer than 40% of other available kidneys (see Fig. 5.2).

The EPTS score estimates how long the candidate will need a functioning kidney transplant when compared with other candidates. A person with an EPTS score of 20% is likely to need a kidney longer—live

TABLE 5.2	Factors Determining the Kidney Donor Profile Index (KDPI) and Expected Post-Transplant Survival (EPTS)*

KDPI	EPTS
Age	Age
Height and weight	Current diabetes status
Ethnicity/Race	Number of previous transplants
History of hypertension	Receiving chronic dialysis
History of diabetes	
Cause of death	
Serum creatinine	
HCV status	
Donor meets DCD criteria	

*Calculators for KDPI, EPTS are available on the websites of UNOS and OPTN. Note that lower numbers reflect higher-quality kidneys and a longer anticipated life span, respectively.

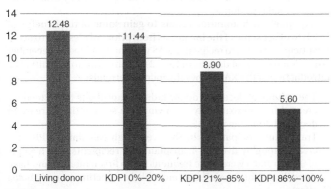

FIGURE 5.2 Estimated graft half-life of kidneys from deceased donors with varying KDPI scores and from living donors. (From Barrois B. Identification of a patient population previously not considered for organ donation. Cureus 2016;8(9):e805. Copyright © 2016, Barrois.)

longer—than 80% of other candidates. Someone with an EPTS score of 60% will likely need a kidney longer than 40% of other people.

In the KAS system, the 20% of kidneys that are expected to last the longest—those with a KDPI score of 20% or less—will first be offered to patients likely to need a transplant the longest—those with an EPTS of 20% or less. If a kidney with a KDPI of 20% or less is not accepted for any of these patients, it will then be offered to any other person who would match, regardless of their EPTS score. Kidneys with a KDPI score of 20% to 85% are allocated according to waiting time in a manner similar to the system in place prior to 2015 except that "waiting time" is now defined not by when patients are placed on the transplant list but by their *dialysis start date* or, for predialysis patients, when their eGFR is <20 mL/min.

KDPI scores ≥ 85% are similar to the previously designated "ECD" kidneys and like "ECD" kidneys, are deemed to be viable for transplant in the appropriate recipients (see Chapter 8), typically older patients, those who cannot withstand dialysis for an extended period of time, and those recipients with high EPTS score. Additionally, KDPI $\geq$ 85% are made available to a wider geographic region than all other kidneys in an attempt to locate a suitable candidate in the quickest manner possible. Modeling of the KAS predicted that the tandem use of KDPI and EPTS would produce a significant rise in the "average projected median lifespan after transplantation," as well as the "time with a functional allograft."

The KAS also prioritizes highly-sensitized patients (those with a very high calculated panel reactive antibody [CPRA]; see Chapter 3), seeking to ensure that they are transplanted. As a result, patients who are highly sensitized are now given precedence in the allocation system, thus prompting transplant centers to enhance their anti-HLA antibody screening procedures to ensure that sensitized patients receive kidneys more expeditiously, thus shifting toward justice over utility. The KAS also provides greater access to deceased donor kidneys for blood type B candidates who can safely accept a kidney from an A2 or A2B blood type donor.

Equipped with ambitious goals to gain some of the benefits of LYFT, to offset some of the inequities from prior policies, and to avoid unanticipated harm to recipients, KAS was implemented in December 2014. Comparison of data from the 12 months prior to and after the introduction of the KAS shows the following trends:

- The volume of deceased donor kidney transplants performed increased by approximately 5% owing to a substantial increase in deceased donation in 2015.
- Transplants for patients with a very high calculated CPRA increased roughly fivefold. Transplants for recipients with a CPRA of 99% to 100% were more frequent in the first 6 months and have since diminished somewhat, most likely reflecting an early bolus effect.
- Due to the longevity-matching component of KAS, fewer transplants are occurring in which the kidney is predicted to outlive the recipient. Prior to KAS, 14% of kidneys expected to last the longest (with a KDPI of 0% to 20%) went to recipients aged 65 or older, but this dropped to 5% post-KAS. While transplants have declined for patients in the 50-to-64 and 65-and-older age groups, over half of all deceased donor kidney recipients under KAS have been aged 50 or older.
- Transplants have increased substantially for patients with 5 or more years on chronic maintenance dialysis, owing to the back-dating of dialysis time for determining waiting time points under KAS.
- Transplants have increased for African Americans, who tend to stay disproportionately longer on dialysis prior to being listed for a transplant. African Americans are also more likely to have blood type B compared to other candidates, so the fivefold increase in the number of A2/A2B-to-B transplants may also be contributing to this population's increased access. However, only 3% of blood type B patients have been listed as eligible for these subtype-compatible kidneys, suggesting that further growth in this area may be attainable.
- The kidney discard rate has remained at approximately 19%. The majority of discarded kidneys had a Kidney Donor Profile Index (KDPI) between 86% and 100%. The discard rate is a source of con-

cern as potentially functioning kidneys may be being discarded
(see Steward et al in Selected Readings).

▪ Transplants for pediatric patients (age 0 to 17) declined slightly; however, this difference is not statistically significant, and pediatric access to transplants remains 5 times higher than that for most adults.
Pediatric recipients are also more often receiving kidneys expected
to last longer (lower KDPI) under KAS compared to that previously.

▪ Transplant rates for the small number of prior living donors who
are registered on the waiting list have not changed statistically and
remain sharply higher than that for all other subpopulations.

▪ More kidneys are now being shared across donor service area
(DSA) boundaries. Previously, about 20% of kidneys were transplanted outside of the recovering OPO's DSA, and this has increased to over 30% under KAS. There was a notable increase in
acceptance of kidney offers outside the recovering OPO's DSA for
candidates with a CPRA of 99% to 100%.

▪ The percentage of transplant recipients experiencing delayed graft
function (DGF) has risen from 25% to 29%, which may reflect the
increase in recipients who have been on dialysis over the longer
term. The 6-month graft survival rate has not significantly changed
and continues to exceed 95%.

These early findings are based on limited data and must be interpreted
cautiously and further tracked to assess whether observed trends will
be sustained. The effect of KAS on long-term graft survival cannot yet
be assessed, and will likely be the ultimate test of the policy change.

For 50 years, the donation and transplantation communities have
strived to find a balance in ethical principles and clinical practice
that will provide all transplant patients the maximum benefits of the
procedure. This challenge will continue owing to improvements in
clinical practice but also because of the shortage of organs available
for transplant. Efforts to reduce this shortage through increasing authorization rates, directed, chain, and paired-living donation have and
will continue to help. However, the ethical balancing act will remain
until technology provides either cures for kidney disease or alternatives to human donation.

Selected Readings

Formica R. Allocating deceased donor kidneys to sensitized candidates. Clin J Am Soc
    Nephrol 2016;11:377–378.
Gebel H, Kasiske B, Gustafson S, et al. Allocating deceased donor kidneys to candidates
    with high panel reactive antibodies. Clin J Am Soc Nephrol 2016;11:505–511.
Hall E, Massie A, Wang J, et al. Effect of eliminating priority points for HLA-B matching
    on racial disparities in kidney transplant rates. Am J Kidney Dis 2011;58:813–816.
Leichtman A. Improving the allocation system for deceased-donor kidneys. N Engl
    J Med 2011;364:1287–1289.
Massie A, Luo X, Lonze B, et al. Early changes in kidney distribution under the new
    allocation system. J Am Soc Nephrol 2016;27(8):2495–2501.
Stewart D, Kucheryavaya A, Klassen D, et al. Changes in deceased donor kidney transplan-
    tation one year after KAS implementation. Am J Transplant 2016;16(6):1834–1847.
Stewart D, Garcia V, Rosendale J, et al. Diagnosing the decades-long rise in the deceased
    donor kidney discard rate in the US [published online ahead of print October 19,
    2016]. Transplantation. doi:10.1097/TP.0000000000001539
Tambur A, Haarberg K, Friedewald J, et al. Unintended consequences of the new national
    kidney allocation policy in the United States. Am J Transplant 2015;15:2465–2469.

6
Immunosuppressive Medications and Protocols for Kidney Transplantation

Theodore M. Sievers, Erik L. Lum, and Gabriel M. Danovitch

A BRIEF HISTORY OF TRANSPLANT IMMUNOSUPPRESSION

To understand the construction of the immunosuppressive protocol and the use of immunosuppressive medications according to current standard transplantation practice, it helps to follow the development of organ transplantation and, in particular, kidney transplantation, since the 1950s. Although sporadic attempts at kidney transplantation had been made throughout the first half of the 20th century, the current era of transplantation was pioneered in 1954 at Harvard by Joseph Murray with the successful, Nobel Prize winning, living donor transplantation between the identical Herrick twins. While this case provided evidence that the technical challenges of transplantation could be overcome, the initiation of immunosuppression was necessary to provide successful transplantation for the majority of patients with kidney disease, the vast majority of whom are genetically dissimilar to their donors.

The first attempts at immunosuppression used total-body irradiation; azathioprine was introduced in the early 1960s and was soon routinely accompanied by prednisolone. The polyclonal antibody preparations antithymocyte globulin (ATG) and antilymphocyte globulin (ALG) became available in the mid-1970s. Azathioprine and prednisolone became the baseline regimen for maintenance immunosuppression following kidney transplantation, with ATG or ALG used for induction or for the treatment of steroid-resistant rejection. With this protocol, the success rate of kidney transplantation was about 50% at 1 year, acute rejection rates were approximately 60%, and the mortality rate was typically 10% to 20%.

The situation was transformed in the early 1980s with the introduction of the cyclosporine. Because the results of kidney transplantation were poor prior to its introduction, it was not hard to recognize the dramatic benefit of cyclosporine that produced statistically significant improvement in graft survival rates to greater than 80% at 1 year and a marked reduction in rejection rates to 30% to 40%. Mortality rates decreased with more effective immunosuppression, reduced use of corticosteroids, and overall improvements in surgical and medical care. The standard immunosuppressive regimen consisted of cyclosporine and prednisone, often combined with azathioprine, now used as an adjunctive agent in what was called *triple therapy*. Although the benefits of cyclosporine were clear cut, its capacity to produce both acute and chronic nephrotoxicity was soon recognized to be a major detriment. In 1985, OKT3, the first monoclonal antibody used in clinical medicine, was introduced based on its capacity to treat first acute rejection episodes, although the toxicity of the drug tended to restrict its use to episodes of rejection that were resistant to high-dose steroids and, in some programs, to use as an induction agent. With this limited armamentarium of medications—cyclosporine, azathioprine, corticosteroids, and the antibody preparations—the transplantation community entered the 1990s, achieving, with justifiable pride, success rates of up to 90% in many centers and minimal mortality. Because the number of available immunosuppressive medications was small, there was relatively little variation among the protocol options used in different programs.

Two major developments then followed. Tacrolimus was introduced into liver transplantation and eventually into kidney transplantation as an alternative to cyclosporine because of its capacity to produce equivalent patient and graft survival, and mycophenolate mofetil (MMF) was found to be a more effective agent than azathioprine by virtue of its capacity to reduce the incidence of acute rejection episodes when used with cyclosporine (and later with tacrolimus) and corticosteroids. Basiliximab and daclizumab, two humanized monoclonal antibodies, were approved for use after kidney transplantation, also based on their capacity to reduce the incidence of acute rejection episodes, and a polyclonal antibody, Thymoglobulin, available in Europe for several years, was approved for use in the United States for the treatment of acute rejection. In the past decade, the manufacturers of OKT3 and daclizumab have discontinued production of each medication, and they are no longer available for clinical use.

In 1999, a class of new immunosuppressive medications, the mTOR inhibitors, was introduced. Initially, sirolimus was approved by the FDA; a similar drug, everolimus, was later introduced in Europe and gained FDA approval in 2010. The last major immunosuppressive medication to garner FDA approval for kidney transplantation was belatacept in 2011. The therapeutic armamentarium for transplant immunosuppression thus has continued to broaden and become more complex, as has the variety of potential drug combinations and protocols.

To address this complexity, this chapter is divided into five sections. Part I reviews the drugs in current clinical use, emphasizing cyclosporine, tacrolimus, MMF, sirolimus, and corticosteroids. Part II reviews the currently available biologic agents approved for use in transplantation. Part III discusses the clinical trial process used to develop new immunosuppressive agents and reviews available data on promising new agents at different stages of development. Part IV discusses combinations of these drugs in the form of clinically applied immunosuppressive protocols, both conventional and innovative. Part V discusses the treatment of the various forms of kidney transplant rejection.

Part I: Immunosuppressive Agents in Current Clinical Use

MECHANISM OF ACTION OF IMMUNOSUPPRESSIVE DRUGS: THE THREE-SIGNAL MODEL

The molecular mechanisms that are the target of immunosuppressive drugs are discussed in detail in Chapter 2. The three-signal model of T-cell activation and subsequent cellular proliferation, illustrated in Figure 6.1, is a valuable tool for understanding the sites of action of the agents discussed below. In brief, *signal 1* is an antigen-specific signal provided by the triggering of the T-cell receptors by antigen-presenting cells (APCs) and is transduced through the CD3 complex. *Signal 2* is a non–antigen-specific co-stimulatory signal provided by the engagement of B7 on the APC with CD28 on the T cell. These two signals activate the intracellular pathways that lead to the expression of interleukin-2 (IL-2) and other growth-promoting cytokines. Stimulation of the IL-2 receptor (CD25) leads to activation of mTOR (mammalian target of rapamycin) and provides *signal 3*, which triggers cell proliferation. As each of the immunosuppressive agents is discussed below, it is useful to refer to Figure 6.1 to review their relative sites of action.

Calcineurin Inhibitors: Cyclosporine and Tacrolimus

The term *calcineurin inhibitors* (CNI) is useful because it emphasizes the similarity in the mechanism of action of the two drugs, *cyclosporine* and *tacrolimus,* which have served as the backbone of solid-organ transplant immunosuppression for the past 30 years. Although they are biochemically distinct, they are remarkably similar, not only in their mechanism of action, but also in their clinical efficacy and side-effect profile. They are, therefore, considered together; discrete differences

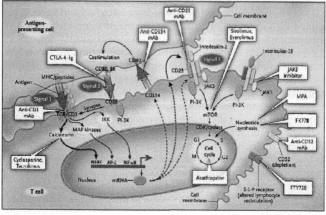

FIGURE 6.1 Anti-CD154 antibody, FTY720, and FK778 have been withdrawn from clinical trials. MPA, mycophenolic acid. (From Halloran PF. Immunosuppressive drugs for kidney transplantation. N Engl J Med 2004;351:2715–2729, with permission.)

between them are discussed in the text and summarized in Table 6.1. The choice of agent is discussed in Part IV.

Each agent will be discussed with regard to its pharmacodynamic and pharmacokinetic properties. *Pharmacodynamics* describes the effect a drug has on the body. This includes the agent's therapeutic activity (its mechanism of action) and any untoward effects it may cause (its adverse effect profile). *Pharmacokinetics* are the affect the body has on a drug (absorption, distribution, metabolism, elimination, therapeutic drug level monitoring, and drug–drug interactions).

Cyclosporine is a small cyclic polypeptide of fungal origin. It consists of 11 amino acids and has a molecular weight of 1,203g/mol. It is neutral and insoluble in water but soluble in organic solvents and lipids.

TABLE 6.1	Some Comparative Features of Cyclosporine and Tacrolimus	
Feature	**Cyclosporine**	**Tacrolimus**
Mode of action	Inhibition of calcineurin	Inhibition of calcineurin
Daily maintenance dose	About 3–5 mg/kg	About 0.15–0.3 mg/kg
Administration	PO and IV	PO, IV, and SL*
Absorption bile dependent	Sandimmune, yes; Neoral, no	No
Oral dose available (capsules)	100 mg; 25 mg	5 mg; 1 mg; 0.5 mg
Drug interactions	Similar	Similar
Capacity to prevent rejection	+	++?
Use with MPA	+	+[†]
Use with sirolimus, everolimus	+[‡]	+[‡]
Prolonged release formulations	−	+
Nephrotoxicity	+	+
Steroid sparing	+	++?
Hypertension and sodium retention	++	+
Pancreatic islet toxicity	+	++
Neurotoxicity	+	++
Hirsutism	+	−
Hair loss	−	+
Gum hypertrophy	+	−
Gastrointestinal side effects	−	+
Gastric motility	−	+
Hyperkalemia	+	+
Hypomagnesemia	+	+
Hypercholesterolemia	+	−
Hyperuricemia, gout	++	+

Data are based on available literature and clinical experience.
−, No or little effect; +, known effect; ++, effect more pronounced; ++?, probable greater effect; IV, intravenous; MPA, mycophenolic acid; PO, by mouth; SL, sublingual.
*IV rarely needed because sublingual absorption is good.
[†]Dose of MMF may be less when used with tacrolimus.
[‡]Nephrotoxicity may be exaggerated when used in full dose.

The amino acids at positions 11, 1, 2, and 3 form the active immuno-suppressive site, and the cyclic structure of the drug is necessary for its immunosuppressive effect. Tacrolimus, still often called by its nickname FK *(Eff-Kay)* from its laboratory designation *FK506,* is a macrolide antibiotic compound isolated from *Streptomyces tsukubaensis.* It is a 23-membered macrolide lactone with a molecular weight of 804 and is practically insoluble in water, freely soluble in ethanol, and very soluble in methanol and chloroform. Due to their molecular size and physical properties, these agents are not significantly dialyzed and both can be administered during dialysis treatment without dose adjustment.

Pharmacodynamics

Mechanism of Action. The CNIs differ from their predecessor immu-nosuppressive drugs by virtue of their selective inhibition of the im-mune response. They do not inhibit neutrophilic phagocytic activity as corticosteroids do, nor are they myelosuppressive. Cell surface events and antigen recognition also remain intact (see Chapter 2). Their im-munosuppressive effect depends on the formation of a complex with their cytoplasmic receptor proteins, cyclophilin for cyclosporine and tacrolimus-binding protein (FKBP) for tacrolimus (see Fig. 6.1). These complexes binds with calcineurin, whose normal function is to act as a phosphatase that dephosphorylates certain nuclear regulatory proteins (e.g., nuclear factor of activated T cells) and hence facilitates their passage through the nuclear membrane (see Chapter 2). Inhibi-tion of calcineurin thereby impairs the expression of several critical cytokine genes that promote T-cell activation, including those for IL-2, IL-4, interferon-gamma (IFN-γ), and tumor necrosis factor-alpha (TNF-α). The transcription of other genes, such as CD40 ligand and the proto-oncogenes H-ras and c-myc, is also impaired. The importance of these factors in T-cell activation is discussed in more detail in Chapter 2, but as a result of calcineurin inhibition, there is a quantitative limita-tion of cytokine production and downstream lymphocyte proliferation.

Cyclosporine enhances the expression of transforming growth factor-beta (TGF-β), which also inhibits IL-2 and the generation of cytotoxic T lymphocytes, and may be responsible for the development of interstitial fibrosis, an important feature of CNI nephrotoxicity. TGF-β has also been implicated as an important factor in the prolif-eration of tumor cells, which may be relevant to the course of certain post-transplantation neoplasms (see Chapter 11). The in vivo effects of cyclosporine are blocked by anti–TGF-β, indicating that TGF-β may be central to the mediation of both the beneficial and detrimental effects of CNIs.

Patients receiving successful CNI-based immunosuppression maintain a degree of immune responsiveness that is still sufficient to maintain host defenses. This relative immunosuppression may be a reflection of the fact that at therapeutic levels of these drugs, calcineurin activ-ity is reduced by only about 50%, permitting strong signals to trigger cytokine expression and generate an effective immune response. In stable patients receiving cyclosporine, CD4$^+$ T cells have reduced IL-2 production to a degree that is inversely correlated to drug levels. The degree of inhibition of calcineurin activity and IL-2 production may be at the fulcrum of the delicate balance that exists between too much and too little immunosuppression.

Adverse Effects

Nephrotoxicity.   Nephrotoxicity is the major "thorn in the side" of these remarkable drugs. Theories linking the mechanism of immunosuppression and nephrotoxicity are discussed later. The terms *cyclosporine* and *FK toxicity* are often used loosely, and it is important to note that these terms encompass several distinct, overlapping syndromes (Table 6.2).

Functional Decrease in Renal Blood Flow and Filtration Rate.   The CNIs produce a dose-related, reversible, renal vasoconstriction that particularly affects the afferent arteriole (Fig. 6.2). The glomerular capillary ultrafiltration coefficient (Kf) also decreases, possibly as a result of increased mesangial cell contractility. Most of the studies on the mechanism of this effect have used cyclosporine rather than tacrolimus.

TABLE 6.2	Syndromes of Calcineurin Inhibitor Nephrotoxicity

Exaggeration of early post-transplantation graft dysfunction
Acute reversible decrease in GFR
Acute microvascular disease
Chronic nonprogressive decrease in GFR
Chronic progressive decrease in GFR
Hypertension and electrolyte abnormalities
   Sodium retention and edema
   Hyperkalemia
   Hypomagnesemia
   Hyperchloremic acidosis
Hyperuricemia

GFR, glomerular filtration rate.

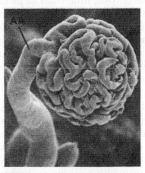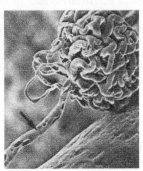

FIGURE 6.2 Cyclosporine-induced afferent arteriolar vasoconstriction. **A:** Control rat showing afferent arteriole (AA) and glomerular tuft. **B:** Constricted afferent arteriole *(arrow)* and glomerular tuft after 14 days of cyclosporine at 50 mg/kg/day. (From English J, Evan A, Houghton DC, et al. Cyclosporine-induced acute renal dysfunction in the rat: evidence of arteriolar vasoconstriction with preservation of tubular function. Transplantation 1987;44:135–141, with permission.)

The picture is reminiscent of "prerenal" dysfunction, and in the acute phase, tubular function is intact.

The normal regulation of the glomerular microcirculation depends on a complex, hormonally mediated balance between vasoconstriction and vasodilation. Cyclosporine-induced vasoconstriction is caused, at least in part, by alteration of arachidonic acid metabolism in favor of the vasoconstrictor thromboxane. Cyclosporine is also a potential inducer of the powerful vasoconstrictor endothelin, and circulating endothelin levels are elevated in its presence. Cyclosporine-induced changes in glomerular hemodynamics can be reversed by specific endothelin inhibitors and by anti-endothelin antibodies. The sympathetic nervous system is also activated.

Several *in vivo* and *in vitro* studies have suggested that alterations in the L-arginine nitric oxide (NO) pathway may be involved in CNI-induced renal vasoconstriction. NO causes relaxation of preglomerular arteries and improves renal blood flow. The constitutive enzyme endothelial nitric oxide synthase (NOS) is produced by renal endothelial cells and modulates vascular tone. Both acute and chronic cyclosporine toxicity can be enhanced by NOS inhibition with *N*-nitro-L-arginine-methyl ester and ameliorated by supplementation with L-arginine. Interestingly, sildenafil (Viagra) increases GFR in transplant patients, presumably by reversing this effect.

CNI-induced renal vasoconstriction may manifest clinically as delayed recovery of early malfunctioning grafts or as a transient, reversible, dose-dependent, blood-level–dependent elevation in serum creatinine concentration that may be difficult to distinguish from other causes of graft dysfunction. Vasoconstriction may be a reversible component of chronic CNI toxicity, which may amplify the functional severity of the chronic histologic changes seen with prolonged use. The vasoconstriction may be more pronounced with cyclosporine than with tacrolimus and also helps to account for the hypertension and the tendency for sodium retention that are commonly associated with cyclosporine use.

Chronic Interstitial Fibrosis. Interstitial fibrosis, which may be patchy or "striped" and associated with arteriolar lesions (see Chapter 15), is a common feature of long-term CNI use. This lesion may produce chronic renal failure in recipients of renal and nonrenal organ transplants; however, several long-term studies show that in the dose regimens currently employed, kidney function may remain stable, although often impaired, for many years. The mechanism of CNI-induced interstitial fibrosis remains poorly defined.

Evidence from experimental models suggests that chronic nephropathy involves an angiotensin-dependent upregulation of molecules that are important in the scarring process, such as TGF-β and osteopontin. Enhanced production of TGF-β in normal T cells may provide the link between the immunosuppressive effects of the CNIs and their nephrotoxicity, and variation in fibrogenic gene expression may help explain the varying consistency of this effect. CNI-induced hypomagnesemia may induce interstitial inflammation and enhance the production of TGF-β, thereby perpetuating chronic fibrotic lesions. Interstitial fibrosis may also be a reflection of intense and prolonged vasoconstriction of the renal microcirculation. Cyclosporine may also impair the regenerative capacity of microvascular endothelial cells and induce apoptosis. The resulting chronic renal ischemia may enhance the synthesis and accumulation of extracellular matrix proteins in the interstitium.

Acute Microvascular Disease. Thrombotic microangiopathy (TMA) (see Chapters 10 and 15) is a distinct form of CNI-induced vascular toxicity that may manifest as renal involvement alone or as a systemic illness. It produces a syndrome reminiscent of thrombotic thrombocytopenic purpura (TTP). In TTP, potentially pathogenic inhibitory antibodies against the von Willebrand factor (vWF)-cleaving protease ADAMTS13, a zinc metalloprotease, have been detected. A similar mechanism has been described in CNI-induced TMA.

Electrolyte Abnormalities and Hypertension. Impaired sodium excretion is a reflection of the renal vasoconstrictive effect of CNIs. Patients receiving long-term cyclosporine therapy tend to be hypertensive (see Chapter 11) and to retain fluid. Studies show activation of the renin–angiotensin–aldosterone system and sympathetic nervous system and suppression of atrial natriuretic factor, which results in attenuation of the natriuretic and diuretic response to an acute volume load. NO production is also impaired. Hypertension tends to be less marked (or the need for antihypertensive drugs may be less) for patients receiving tacrolimus, possibly because it produces less peripheral vasoconstriction than does cyclosporine.

Hyperkalemia is common and occasionally requires treatment, although it is rarely life-threatening as long as kidney function remains good. It is not uncommon for patients taking CNIs to have potassium levels in the mid-fives. Hyperkalemia is often associated with a mild *hyperchloremic acidosis* and an intact capacity to excrete acid urine. The clinical picture is thus reminiscent of type IV renal tubular acidosis. Patients receiving cyclosporine may have an impaired capacity to excrete an acute potassium load, and there is evidence to suggest impaired production of aldosterone, an acquired impaired renal response to its action, and inhibition of cortical collecting duct potassium secretory channels. Hyperkalemia may be exaggerated by concomitant administration of β blockers, angiotensin-converting enzyme inhibitors, and angiotensin receptor blockers. A defect of collecting tubule hydrogen ion secretion has been described with tacrolimus. Both drugs are magnesuric and hypercalciuric, and hypomagnesemia is commonly associated with their use. In liver transplantation, hypomagnesemia may predispose patients to seizures; this has been observed rarely in kidney recipients. The urinary loss of calcium and magnesium is due to downregulation of specific transport proteins. Magnesium supplements are often prescribed but may be ineffective because of a lowered renal magnesium threshold (see Chapter 20). Hyperuricemia, because of reduced renal uric acid clearance, is a common complication of CNI use, particularly when diuretics are also employed. While both cyclosporine and tacrolimus can produce hyperuricemia, only cyclosporine has been associated with gout, which has been reported in up to 7% of patients. This may resolve when cyclosporine is switched to tacrolimus. Treatment is discussed in Chapter 11.

Methods of Amelioration. The vexing issue of CNI nephrotoxicity has spawned a variety of clinical and experimental approaches designed to modify the renal effects of these drugs, particularly their capacity to produce vasoconstriction. Low-dose dopamine is used in some centers in the early postoperative period to "encourage" urine output. Calcium channel blockers given to both the donor (see Chapter 4) and the recipient (see Part IV) may reduce the incidence and severity of delayed graft function. Omega-3 fatty acids in the form of 6 g of fish oil each day were thought to increase renal blood flow and GFR by reversing the cyclosporine-induced imbalance between the synthesis of vasodilator and vasoconstrictor prostaglandins, but long-term studies have shown no such benefit. The prostaglandin agonist misoprostol and thromboxane synthetase inhibitors may have a similar effect. Various protocol adjustments, discussed later in this chapter, can also be employed to minimize CNI toxicity.

Nonrenal Calcineurin Inhibitor Toxicity

Gastrointestinal. Episodes of hepatic dysfunction typically manifesting as subclinical, mild, self-limited, dose-dependent elevations of serum aminotransferase levels with mild hyperbilirubinemia may occur in nearly half of all kidney transplant recipients taking cyclosporine and occur less frequently in those taking tacrolimus. No specific hepatic histologic lesion has been described in humans, and the hyperbilirubinemia is a reflection of disturbed bile secretion rather than hepatocellular damage. Cyclosporine does not itself produce progressive liver disease; other causes, most frequently one of the viral hepatitides, need to be considered. Cyclosporine therapy is associated with an increased incidence of cholelithiasis, presumably resulting from an increased lithogenicity of cyclosporine-containing bile. Varying degrees of anorexia, nausea, vomiting, diarrhea, and abdominal discomfort occur in up to 75% of patients receiving tacrolimus, and less frequently in patients receiving cyclosporine.

Cosmetic. The cosmetic complications of cyclosporine must be treated seriously, particularly in women and adolescents, because of the misery they can produce and the temptation to resolve them through noncompliant behavior. Cosmetic complications are often exaggerated by concomitant use of corticosteroids. They are less prominent for patients receiving tacrolimus.

Hypertrichosis in varying degrees occurs in nearly all patients receiving cyclosporine and is particularly obvious in dark-haired girls and women. A coarsening of facial features is observed in children and young adults, with thickening of the skin and prominence of the brow. Tacrolimus may produce hair loss and frank alopecia. Gingival hyperplasia, which can be severe, may develop in patients receiving cyclosporine and is exaggerated by poor dental hygiene and possibly by concomitant use of calcium channel blockers. Azithromycin, a macrolide antibiotic that typically does not affect cyclosporine metabolism, may reduce gingival hyperplasia. Gingivectomy may occasionally be indicated, and switching from cyclosporine to tacrolimus is usually effective. Cosmetic complications tend to become less prominent with time. Sympathetic cosmetic counseling is required. Cyclosporine may increase prolactin levels, occasionally producing gynecomastia in men and breast enlargement in women.

Hyperlipidemia. Cyclosporine has been implicated as one of the various factors responsible for the generation of post-transplantation hyper-cholesterolemia (see Chapter 11). The mechanism of this effect may be related to abnormal low-density lipoprotein feedback control by the liver, to altered bile acid synthesis, or to occupation of the low-density lipoprotein receptor by cyclosporine. Up to two-thirds of patients develop *de novo* hyperlipidemia in the first post-transplantation year. The effect is less marked with tacrolimus, and lipid levels may decrease when patients are switched from cyclosporine to tacrolimus.

Glucose Intolerance. Post-transplantation glucose intolerance and new-onset diabetes mellitus after transplantation (NODAT) are discussed in Chapter 11. CNIs are toxic to pancreatic islets, although tacrolimus is more so, possibly as a result of increased concentrations of FKBP relative to cyclophilin in islet cells. The effect is dose related and may be exaggerated by concomitant corticosteroid use. Morphologic changes in the islets include cytoplasmic swelling, vacuolization, and apoptosis, with abnormal immunostaining for insulin. Obesity, African-American or Hispanic ethnicity, family history of diabetes, and hepatitis C infection may predispose to NODAT. Figure 6.2 shows the incidence of diabetes before and after transplantation by type of CNI as reported to the United States Renal Data System.

Neurotoxicity. A spectrum of neurologic complications has been observed in patients receiving CNIs; they are generally more marked with tacrolimus. Coarse tremor, dysesthesias, headache, and insomnia are common and may be dose- and blood-level related. Patients may complain of discrete cognitive difficulties coinciding with peak drug levels. The use of the prolonged-release formulations of tacrolimus (see below) may reduce tacrolimus-induced neurotoxicity by virtue of its pharmacokinetic characteristics of having lower Cmax concentrations. Furthermore, with immediate-release tacrolimus, administering a higher evening dose than that given in the morning (i.e., 3 mg in the morning and 4 mg in the evening) may also lead to an improvement in neurologic symptoms owing to reduced morning peak levels (Fig. 6.3).

More severe complications are uncommon in kidney recipients, although isolated seizures may occasionally occur, and full-blown leukoencephalopathy has been described clinically and on brain imaging. Bone pain in long bones has also been described.

Infection and Malignancy. Infection and malignancy inevitably accompany immunosuppression and are discussed in detail in Chapters 10 and 11. Despite their immunosuppressive potency, the incidence of infections and common *de novo* neoplasms has not significantly increased since the introduction of the CNIs, although the course of malignancies may be accelerated.

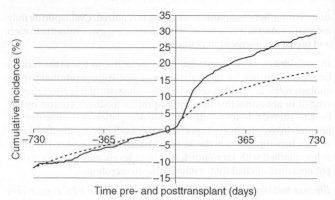

FIGURE 6.3 Incidence of diabetes before and after transplantation by type of calcineurin inhibitor (*solid line*, tacrolimus; *dashed line*, cyclosporine). Note that the incremental incidence of diabetes for cyclosporine was 9.4% at 1 year and 8.4% at 2 years. The incremental incidence of diabetes for tacrolimus use was 15.4% at 1 year and 17.7% at 2 years. (From Woodward RS, Schnitzler MA, Baty J, et al. Incidence and cost of new onset diabetes mellitus among U.S. wait-listed and transplanted renal allograft recipients. Am J Transplant 2003;3:590–598, with permission.)

Thromboembolism. *In vitro*, cyclosporine increases adenosine diphosphate–induced platelet aggregation, thromboplastin generation, and factor VII activity. It also reduces production of endothelial prostacyclin. These findings may be causally related to the somewhat increased incidence of thromboembolic events that have been observed in cyclosporine-treated kidney transplant recipients. The finding of glomerular microthrombi as part of CNI-induced microangiopathy was discussed previously.

Pharmacokinetics
Formulations
Cyclosporine. The original formulation of cyclosporine, the oil-based Sandimmune, has largely been replaced by the microemulsion formulation, Neoral. Both formulations are available in two forms: a 100-mg/mL solution that is drawn up by the patient into a graduated syringe and dispensed into orange juice or milk, and 25-mg and 100-mg soft-gelatin capsules. Patients usually prefer the convenience of the capsule that is typically administered twice daily. Due to the nature of the microemulsion formulation, these gelatin capsules should be kept in the original packaging as long as possible prior to administration. Gelatin capsules that have been exposed to heat or have been removed from the blister packaging for more than 14 days may exhibit decreased efficacy secondary to evaporative loss of emulsifiers.

The development of generic formulations of cyclosporine and other immunosuppressive agents is controversial because of the critical importance of these drugs to the success of transplantation and the corporate and financial implications of their introduction. If a generic formulation is used, an AB-rated product is mandatory. AB-rated drugs are molecular entities that meet the *bioequivalence* standards established by the Food and Drug Administration (FDA). Typically this is established in studies with healthy volunteers using a single dose to determine if key pharmacokinetic parameters are within 80% to 125% of the branded drug as determined by relatively simple statistical methods. If a generic formulation demonstrates pharmacokinetic properties within these parameters, it is assumed that the same molecular entity, at similar concentrations and with similar elimination characteristics, will exhibit a similar efficacy and adverse-effect profile as the branded drug. This assumption spares the generic drug maker from performing the same extensive clinical evaluations required of new drugs, and information on discrete differences in their pharmacokinetics in different ethnic groups is not always available. Because of the pharmacokinetic properties of cyclosporine exhibiting inherent variability and the difference between therapeutic and toxic or ineffective concentrations being very small, the drug is considered to have a *narrow therapeutic window*. While the standards for proving the bioequivalence of generic forms are more rigorous in some countries, in the United States this is not the case. Nonetheless, generic formulations of cyclosporine, such as the capsule *cyclosporine USP Modified* (Teva Labs) and the capsule *Gengraf,* are in widespread use in the United States; other generic formulations are available outside of the United States. The generic formulations are generally claimed to have an absorption profile that is very similar to that of Neoral. Because they are AB rated, in the United States they may be substituted for Neoral cyclosporine without the approval of the prescriber. Several small studies show a reduction in cyclosporine drug level by approximately 15% to 20% when using a 1:1 conversion between brand name and generic. If generic formulations are used, it is probably better to use them consistently and to avoid switching formulations. If conversions are made between the different formulations, it is wise to monitor drug levels and renal function (see Part IV). Patients should be counseled regarding the use of generic immunosuppressive medications to alleviate any potential anxiety regarding the use of nonbranded dosage forms and to enhance medication adherence. Extensive experience with generic formulations of cyclosporine has not demonstrated them to be inferior to the brand drug.

Tacrolimus. Tacrolimus (Prograf) is available in an intravenous formulation, and as 5-mg, 1-mg, and 0.5-mg immediate-release capsules. A suspension formula can be compounded, but is not commercially available. The immediate-release products are typically administered twice daily. Several generic brands are also commercially available. Like cyclosporine, conversion studies demonstrate an approximate 15% reduction in tacrolimus levels with a conversion from brand name to generic. These studies indicate that conversion is safe, but patients should be monitored closely during the process. Switching between formulations that can occur during inpatient hospital readmissions and discharges especially requires close monitoring.

Additionally, two long-acting once-daily formulations (Astagraf XL, Astellas, and Envarsus XR, Veloxis) are now also available. Astagraf XL comes as 0.5, 1, and 5 mg prolonged-release capsules and is approved for *de novo* use in kidney transplant recipients. Envarsus XR is available in 0.75, 1, and 4 mg prolonged-release tablets and has received FDA approval only for conversion from immediate-release tacrolimus in kidney transplant recipients. Importantly, these once-daily dosage forms are not bioequivalent to once-daily formulations or each other and inadvertent switching has the potential to be problematic (Fig. 6.3).

Absorption and Distribution

Cyclosporine. The bioavailability (F) of the microemulsion formulation is better than that of Sandimmune, and there is less variability in cyclosporine pharmacokinetics. Peak cyclosporine levels ($Cmax$) of Neoral cyclosporine are higher, and the trough concentration ($Cmin$) correlates better with the systemic exposure, as reflected by the *area under the curve* (AUC).

The improved gastrointestinal (GI) absorption of the microemulsion and lesser dependence on bile for absorption may reduce the necessity for intravenous cyclosporine administration. Compared with intravenous infusion, the bioavailability of the orally administered drug is in the range of 30% to 45%. Conversion between the oral and intravenous forms of the drug perioperatively requires a 3:1 dose ratio and is administered twice daily as 4-hour infusions. Bioavailability of oral cyclosporine increases with time, possibly as a result of P-gp inhibitory properties of the drug. As a result, the amount of cyclosporine required to achieve a given blood level tends to fall with time and typically reaches a steady level within 4 to 8 weeks. In general, food tends to decrease the absorption of cyclosporine, although some foods can lead to increased absorption (see "Metabolism" below and Chapter 20).

The microemulsion formula of cyclosporine reaches maximal blood concentrations in approximately 2 hours. The volume of distribution is 3 to 5 L/kg, with the majority of the drug found in erythrocytes. It also exhibits very high protein binding in the plasma, especially to lipoproteins. As such, whole blood is the preferred matrix for concentration determination. The half-life varies from 6 to 27 hours with a clearance of 5 to 7 mL/min/kg. In prepubertal patients, the clearance is approximately 25% greater. The drug is primarily eliminated in the bile with only 6% of the dose excreted in the urine, and with only 0.1% excreted unchanged. CYP3A4 is the primary enzyme system that metabolizes cyclosporine. While over 30 metabolites have been identified, three primary metabolites are found in the blood, urine, and bile. These metabolites can be pharmacologically active and the plasma levels of the most important cyclosporine metabolite, M17, may be similar to that of the parent compound. However, the clinical significance of this activity is not clear.

In the blood, one-third of absorbed and infused cyclosporine is found in plasma, bound primarily to lipoproteins. Most of the remaining drug is bound to erythrocytes. Whole-blood drug levels (see "Therapeutic Drug Level Monitoring" below) are thus typically three-fold higher than plasma levels. The binding of cyclosporine to lipoproteins may be important in the transfer of the drug through plasma membranes, and the toxic effects of cyclosporine may be exaggerated by low cholesterol levels and reduced by high cholesterol levels. The binding of cyclosporine to the low-density lipoprotein receptor may account for the hyperlipidemia associated with its use.

Tacrolimus. GI absorption is independent of bile salts. Despite its relatively poor bioavailability, it is rarely necessary to use the intravenous formulation. If necessary, the drug can be administered through a nasogastric tube or sublingually. Intravenous dosing is approximately one-third of the total daily dose required by the oral route and is administered via a 24-hour continuous infusion. Sublingual dosing is more variable, but is usually one-half that required by the oral route. This dosing is achieved either by opening a capsule and allowing the contents to dissolve under the tongue or by using a compounded suspension similarly held under the tongue. The latter may be better tolerated owing to flavoring additives in the specially compounded suspension.

With the immediate-release dosage forms, it is absorbed primarily from the small intestine, and its oral bioavailability is about 25%, with large interpatient and intrapatient variability, particularly for patients with GI disease. Maximal blood concentrations are reached in 1 to 3 hours. Gastric emptying of solids is faster in patients taking tacrolimus than in those receiving cyclosporine, a property that may be beneficial for patients with gastric motility disorders. Diarrhea may lead to increased absorption of tacrolimus from the lower GI tract with resultant toxic levels. Interestingly, immediate-release tacrolimus displays diurnal variation in its absorption profile. Cmax concentrations after morning dosing are typically greater than those found with the evening dose. This can have implications for utilizing dosing strategies as an adverse-effect management tool (see below).

The prolonged-release formulation, Astagraf XL, has a Cmax which occurs after approximately 2 hours, whereas that of Envarsus XR is approximately 6 hours. The AUC_{0-24} of both formulations is similar in stable renal transplant patient over 6 months postoperatively; following daily dosing of approximately 5 mg following 14 and 7 days of dosing, respectively, both formulations yield an AUC_{0-24} of about 220 ng·hr/mL. However, the 24-hour concentration time curves of the two formulations readily display the differences in the prolonged-release technologies that each employs (Fig. 6.4). The primary differences are the Cmax levels achieved; the Envarsus XR formulation provides a much more blunted and prolonged profile while the Astagraf XL achieves higher Cmax values. Food has a similar effect on absorption with both the immediate- and prolonged-release formulations as with cyclosporine; patients should be counseled to be consistent in how they take these medications with respect to meals.

Tacrolimus also has a high affinity for formed blood elements, but it differs from cyclosporine in that, although it is highly protein bound, it is not significantly associated with lipoproteins, and it has a less unfavorable effect on the cholesterol level than does cyclosporine. Approximately 95% of the agent is bound to erythrocytes secondary to the high concentration of FKBP found in these cells. Both agents cross the placenta and enter breast milk; breast-feeding is not recommended for female renal transplant recipients who have had successful pregnancies post-transplant.

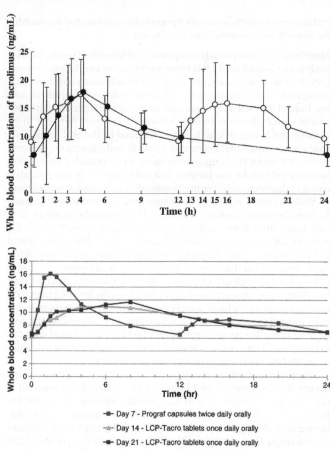

FIGURE 6.4 Pharmacokinetic profile of the two new prolonged-release formulations of tacrolimus, Astagraf XL and Envarsus XR versus immediate-release tacrolimus. **A:** White circles immediate-release data; black circles extended-release data. Whole-blood tacrolimus concentration–time curve in renal transplant patients taking Tac-BID (white circle, n = 47) and Tac-QD (black circle, n = 25). Each point and bar represents the mean +/–SD. Tac-BID, twice-daily tacrolimus; Tac-QD, once-daily tacrolimus. (From Niioka T, Satoh S, Kagaya H, et al. Comparison of pharmacokinetics and pharmacogenetics of once- and twice-daily tacrolimus in the early stage after renal transplantation. Transplantation 2012;94(10):1013–1019, with permission.) **B:** Mean whole-blood tacrolimus concentration in patients on days 7, 14, and 21 versus time. (From Gaber AO, Alloway RR, Bodziak K, et al. Conversion from twice-daily tacrolimus capsules to once-daily extended-release tacrolimus (LCPT): a phase 2 trial of stable renal transplant recipients. Transplantation 2013;96(2):191–197.

Metabolism and Excretion. Both cyclosporine and tacrolimus are metabolized extensively by the cytochrome P450 (CYP) 3A enzymes, specifically 3A4 and 3A5. This primarily occurs in the small intestine, liver, and to a certain extent in the kidney. Both agents and their metabolites are also substrates for P-glycoprotein (P-gp) efflux pumps.

P-gp is a member of the ABC (ATP binding cassette) transporter family that is encoded on the *ABCB1* gene. These ATP-dependent pumps are found in hepatocytes, distal and proximal renal tubular cells, intestinal epithelium, and the luminal surface of capillary endothelial cells in the brain. Patient-to-patient differences in the expression of CYP3A4/5 and *ABCB1* lead to large variations in absorption, metabolism, and distribution of the CNIs. Importantly, this may lead to differences in drug concentration at target sites which has the potential to influence efficacy and toxicity, as well as drug–drug interactions.

In the gut, the CNIs are repeatedly taken up and transported out of intestinal enterocytes by P-gp allowing for reuptake and repeated exposure to CYP3A4/5, leading to significant presystemic metabolism. Because of this, these agents can exhibit relatively poor bioavailability. Certain food items have CYP3A4/5 and/or P-gp inhibitory properties that can dramatically decrease this presystemic metabolism and lead to elevated levels of CNIs. Interestingly, both agents are P-gp substrates and inhibitors; however, only cyclosporine is a potent P-gp inhibitor in gut enterocytes. Similarly, only cyclosporine has inhibitory properties of organic anion transporter protein B1 (OATP1B1) in the liver. This property of cyclosporine has ramifications in its drug–drug interaction profile whereby cyclosporine has the ability to alter the metabolism of other pharmaceutical agents that are P-gp and/or OATP substrates; a property that is not found with tacrolimus.

CYP3A5 plays a larger role in tacrolimus metabolism than with cyclosporine; it has a two-fold higher intrinsic clearance than with CYP3A4. This produces four primary metabolites, some of which may have immunosuppressive and nephrotoxic potential, but at the concentrations achieved, this is not clinically significant. Genetic variations of CYP3A5 can result in changes to the activity of the CYP3A5 protein. Importantly, individuals homozygous for the G allele at the single nucleotide polymorphism (SNP) rs776746 (CYP3A5 *3/*3) have a nonfunctional CYP3A5 protein and have vastly reduced dosing requirements to achieve therapeutic concentrations compared to CYP3A5*1 allele carriers. Pharmacogenetic testing to determine the presence of CYP3A4/5 polymorphisms may play a future role in individualizing and optimizing CNI dosing.

Because both CNIs are excreted in the bile with minimal renal excretion, drug doses do not need to be modified in the presence of kidney dysfunction. The pharmacokinetic parameters of both drugs may vary among patient groups, and these variations may have clinical consequences. Pediatric and African-American transplant recipients may require relatively larger doses and short dosage intervals. Longer dosage intervals may be required in older patients and in the presence of liver disease.

Therapeutic Drug-Level Monitoring

The measurement of cyclosporine and tacrolimus levels is an intrinsic part of the management of transplant patients because of variation in interpatient and intrapatient metabolism. There is also a relationship, albeit an inconsistent one, between blood levels of the drug and episodes of rejection and toxicity. Drug-level monitoring is the source of much confusion because of the various assays available and the option of using different matrices (i.e., plasma or whole blood) for their measurement.

When Sandimmune was introduced, the trough level of cyclosporine (drawn immediately preceding the next dose, or Cmin), rather than the peak level, was measured because its timing was more consistent and appeared to correlate better with toxic complications. More sophisticated techniques of monitoring were suggested whereby a full, or abbreviated, pharmacokinetic profile is constructed to calculate the AUC, which reflects the bioavailability of the drug and may theoretically allow for more precise and individualized patient management. Although attractive, these techniques never proved popular because of their cost and inconvenience.

Evidence suggests that because of the more consistent absorption of Neoral cyclosporine, its peak level (typically 2 hours after dosing) may correlate better with drug exposure and clinical events than the trough level. So-called C_2 monitoring is applied routinely in some centers and clinical trials. For tacrolimus, the trough levels are usually used for monitoring, and this level is an adequate approximation of drug exposure: some programs use peak tacrolimus levels. Recommendations for target blood levels at different stages after transplantation are discussed in Part IV.

Cyclosporine concentrations can be measured in plasma or whole blood. Whole blood (ethylenediaminetetraacetic acid [EDTA] anticoagulated) is the recommended specimen type because the distribution of cyclosporine between plasma and erythrocytes is temperature dependent. The clinician cannot begin to assess the significance of a cyclosporine level without knowing what kind of assay is being used. Several methods are currently available to measure cyclosporine, and each differs in specificity for parent compound. *High-performance liquid chromatography* (HPLC) is the most specific method for measuring unmetabolized parent cyclosporine and is considered the reference method. HPLC, however, is expensive and labor intensive and is not available at all centers. Immunoassays, which use monoclonal antibodies against cyclosporine, are commonly used and have largely replaced HPLC because they can be performed on automated chemistry analyzers. The most commonly used immunoassay to measure cyclosporine in whole-blood samples is the Abbott (Chicago, IL) fluorescence polarization immunoassay (FPIA), which has significant cross-reactivity with cyclosporine metabolites and overestimates cyclosporine by as much as 45%. Samples for quantitation of peak cyclosporine levels should be clearly identified when sent to the laboratory and should be reported as such. These samples may exceed the linearity of the assay and will need to be diluted for accurate quantitation. For monitoring of tacrolimus concentrations, most laboratories use the Abbott monoclonal antibody-based *microparticle enzyme immunoassay* (MEIA) that can be performed on an automated instrument (IMx). This assay permits accurate estimation of tacrolimus levels as low as 2 ng/mL. Abbott has also developed a *chemiluminescent microparticle immunoassay* (CMIA) that is available on the ARCHITECT family of instruments with a reported detection limit of less than 1 ng/mL. New methodologies employ *electrochemiluminescence immunoassay* (ECLIA) techniques similar to CMIA with a reported detection limit of 0.5 ng/mL utilizing a 300-μL sample size. Importantly, reports of falsely elevated tacrolimus levels have illuminated a potential drawback to conjugated antibody magnetic immunoassay techniques and any clinical suspicion of aberrant lab values should be confirmed utilizing a different methodology.

Liquid chromatography/tandem mass spectrometry (LC-MS/MS) techniques have also been described that allow for the quantification of several immunosuppressant agents in a single analytical run; however, the highly technical nature of the methodology and the machinery required limit its application only to centers with highly developed clinical laboratories. Utilizing these powerful LC-MS/MS techniques, tacrolimus concentrations can be determined from a single dried spot of blood (i.e., a finger-prick sample), which may provide clinicians with a more patient-friendly monitoring strategy that may also aid in medication regimen compliance monitoring. Target cyclosporine (peak and trough) and tacrolimus (trough) levels are discussed in the section on immunosuppressive protocols.

Pharmacokinetic Drug–Drug Interactions

The interaction of CNIs with many commonly used drugs demands constant attention to drug regimens and cognizance of potential interactions. New drugs should be introduced with care, and patients should be warned to consult drug package inserts and physicians familiar with the use of cyclosporine and tacrolimus before considering new pharmacologic therapy. Some of the drug interactions discussed below are consistent and well established (and are emphasized in **bold** lettering); others have been described in small series and case reports or are anticipated based on the pharmacologic properties of the agents. Any drug that impacts on CYP3A4/5 or P-gp activity in the liver or intestinal tract, or that interacts with a drug that does, should be regarded as having a potential interaction with the CNIs. Some drugs affect CNI levels when administered orally, but not intravenously, because the drug interaction is taking place at the intestine. As discussed earlier, in addition to their effect on CYP3A4, CNIs inhibit P-gp and OATP1B1, and many of the interactions thought to be owing to CYP3A4 are, in fact, due to an effect on P-gp and or OATP1B1. The possibility that the CNI is affecting the blood level of the interacting drug should also be considered. Unless a comment is made to the contrary, the drug interactions noted below are common to both cyclosporine and tacrolimus, although more have been described with cyclosporine, which has been available longer. Drug interactions between CNIs and other immunosuppressive drugs are discussed in Part IV. Interactions with antibiotics are discussed below and in Chapter 21. Interactions with food are discussed in Chapter 20. Interactions with psychotropic drugs are discussed in more detail in Chapter 18. Drugs that cause impairment of graft function by virtue of their nephrotoxicity alone are not specifically discussed here. Table 6.3 lists agents with inducing and inhibiting properties at CYP3A by the expected magnitude of the interaction and Table 6.4 lists agents that have inhibitory activity at both CYP3A and P-gp. *It should be emphasized that the sections below are not intended to represent a complete listing of all reported and potential drug–drug interactions.*

TABLE 6.3	In Vivo CYP3A Inducers and Inhibitors and Their Relative Potency		

Strong Inducers (≥ 80% Decrease in AUC)	Moderate Inducers (50%–80% Decrease in AUC)	Weak Inducers (20%–50% Decrease in AUC)
Carbamazepine, phenytoin, rifampin, St. John wort*	Bosentan, efavirenz, etravirine, modafinil, nafcillin	Amprenavir, aprepitant, armodafinil, Echinacea*, pioglitazone, prednisone, rufinamide
Strong Inhibitors (≥ 5-fold Increase in AUC or > 80% Decrease in CL)	**Moderate Inhibitors (≥ 2 But < 5-fold Increase in AUC or 50%–80% Decrease in CL)**	**Weak Inhibitors (≥ 1.25 but < 2-fold Increase in AUC or 20–50% Decrease in CL)**
Boceprevir, clarithromycin, conivaptan, grapefruit juice†, indinavir, itraconazole, ketoconazole, lopinavir/ritonavir, nefazodone, nelfinavir, posaconazole, ritonavir, saquinavir, telaprevir, telithromycin, voriconazole	Amprenavir, aprepitant, atazanavir, ciprofloxacin, darunavir/ritonavir, diltiazem, erythromycin, fluconazole, fosamprenavir, grapefruit juice†, imatinib, verapamil	Alprazolam, amiodarone, amlodipine, atorvastatin, bicalutamide, cilostazol, cimetidine, cyclosporine, fluoxetine, fluvoxamine, ginkgo*, goldenseal*,isoniazid, nilotinib,oral contraceptives, ranitidine, ranolazine, tipranavir/ritonavir, zileuton

CL, Clearance.
*herbal product.
†The effect of grapefruit juice varies widely among brands and is concentration-, dose-, and preparation-dependent. Studies have shown that it can be classified as a "strong CYP3A inhibitor" when a certain preparation was used (e.g., high dose, double strength) or as a "moderate CYP3A inhibitor" when another preparation was used (e.g., low dose, single strength).

TABLE 6.4	Examples of In Vivo CYP3A and P-gp Inhibitors and Their Relative Potency	

CYP3A Inhibition	P-gp Inhibitor	Non–P-gp Inhibitor
Strong	Itraconazole, lopinavir/ritonavir, clarithromycin, ritonavir, ketoconazole, indinavir/ritonavir, conivaptan	Voriconazole, nefazodone
Moderate	Verapamil, erythromycin, diltiazem, dronedarone	None identified
Weak	Quinidine, ranolazine, amiodarone, felodipine, azithromycin	Cimetidine

Data updated 7/28/2011
(From http://www.fda.gov/Drugs/DevelopmentApprovalProcess/DevelopmentResources/DrugInteractionsLabeling/ucm093664.htm#potency; accessed 09/02/2015.)

Drugs that Decrease Calcineurin Inhibitor Concentration by Induction of CYP3A Activity

Antituberculous Drugs. **Rifampin** (and **rifabutin** to a lesser extent) markedly reduces cyclosporine and tacrolimus levels, and it may be difficult to achieve therapeutic levels for patients taking rifampin, the use of which should be avoided if at all possible. Pyrazinamide and ethambutol may reduce drug levels, and their use requires monitoring. Isoniazid (INH) can be used with careful drug-level monitoring and is the preferred drug for tuberculosis prophylaxis if this proves essential (see Chapter 12).

Anticonvulsants. Of the so-called first-generation antiepileptic drugs, **barbiturates** markedly reduce cyclosporine and tacrolimus levels. Dose requirements may double or triple, and thrice-daily administration may be required under careful supervision. **Phenytoin** and primidone reduce levels and should be used with great care. The average requirement for cyclosporine or tacrolimus is about doubled for patients receiving phenytoin. **Carbamazepine** may also decrease cyclosporine levels, but the effect is less pronounced. Benzodiazepines and valproic acid do not affect drug levels, but the latter drug has been associated with hepatotoxicity. Modafinil can cause an up to 50% reduction in CNI levels. Patients taking these anticonvulsants before transplantation should have a neurologic assessment with a view toward discontinuing them when possible or exchanging them for one of the new generation of anticonvulsants that do not interact with CNIs.

Of the second-generation antiepileptic drugs, oxcarbazepine (Trileptal) may decrease cyclosporine levels. Gabapentin (Neurontin) and levetiracetam (Keppra) and other drugs in this category do not appear to have significant interactions.

Other Drugs. There are isolated reports of several antibiotics, including nafcillin, intravenous trimethoprim, intravenous sulfadimidine, imipenem, cephalosporins, and terbinafine, reducing cyclosporine levels. An increased incidence of acute rejection episodes has been described after the introduction of ciprofloxacin. The antidepressant herbal preparation *Hypericum perforatum* (St. John wort) may reduce cyclosporine levels by enzyme induction. Ticlopidine may reduce cyclosporine levels. Cholestyramine, GoLYTELY, sevelamer (Renagel), and olestra may reduce levels by impairing GI absorption. Corticosteroids are inducers of CYP3A, an effect that needs to be considered if their administration is discontinued. Following cessation of concomitant corticosteroid therapy, tacrolimus levels may increase by up to 25%. The serum creatinine level may increase as a result and lead to a confusing clinical picture. Caspofungin can reduce CNI levels, but this does not appear to be mediated through either CYP3A or P-gp.

Prolonged Use. If prolonged use of a drug that induces CYP3A activity is required, addition of a drug that inhibits or competes with the CYP3A system (e.g., **diltiazem, ketoconazole**) may facilitate the achievement of therapeutic CNI levels. Administration of the CNI on a thrice-daily basis rather than the usual twice-daily basis may also be effective.

Drugs that Increase Calcineurin Inhibitor Levels by Inhibition of CYP3A or by Competition for Its Pathways

Calcium Channel Blockers. **Verapamil, diltiazem, amlodipine**, and **nicardipine** may significantly increase CNI levels. Diltiazem and verapamil are sometimes added routinely as adjuncts to the immunosuppressive regimen. Their use may safely permit up to a 40% reduction in the cyclosporine dose. Careful monitoring of drug levels is required when these calcium channel blockers are used for the management of hypertension or heart disease, and physicians and their patients should be specifically warned that changing the dosage of these drugs is equivalent to changing the dosage of the CNI. Brand-name and generic forms of these drugs (e.g., Cardizem, Dilacor, Tiazac, and Cartia are all forms of diltiazem) may have different effects on CNI levels. Furthermore, immediate-release and delayed-release formulations may provide differing effects. Nifedipine, isradipine, and felodipine have similar hemodynamic effects but have minimal effects on drug levels.

Antifungal Agents. **Ketoconazole, fluconazole, itraconazole, voriconazole, and isovuconazole** markedly elevate CNI levels. The interaction with ketoconazole is a particularly potent one, which may permit a safe reduction of up to 80% in the cyclosporine or tacrolimus dose. Great care must be taken when stopping and starting these antifungal agents. An important interaction between ketoconazole and histamine blockers has also been described. The effective reabsorption of ketoconazole from the GI tract requires acidic gastric contents, and the addition of a histamine-2 receptor antagonist may reduce its absorption, indirectly producing a clinically significant fall in CNI levels.

Antibiotics. **Erythromycin,** even in low doses, may increase CNI levels. Other macrolide antibiotics (e.g., clarithromycin, josamycin, ponsinomycin) may also increase levels. There are conflicting reports on the impact of azithromycin on drug levels; however, this drug can generally be given in short courses without monitoring. Because erythromycin is prescribed so ubiquitously, physicians, dentists, and patients should be warned about this interaction. Chloramphenicol, now rarely used, may increase tacrolimus levels.

Antiretroviral Therapy. With the advent of highly active antiretroviral therapy (HAART), selected HIV-positive patients may be deemed candidates for kidney transplantation (see Chapters 8 and 12). Some of the antiretroviral agents, particularly protease inhibitors, are potent inhibitors of P-450. **Ritonavir** is the most potent inhibitor of P-450 that is clinically available, and when used alone or in combination (kaletra-retonavir/lopinavir), very small doses of CNI (e.g., 1 mg/week of tacrolimus) may maintain adequate drug levels. Tenofovir (a component of Truvada and Atrypla) is potentially nephrotoxic; however, recent data indicate that it may be less nephrotoxic than originally believed. Introduction of this agent to CNI-containing regimens should be done cautiously. Because of multiple drug–drug interactions, immunosuppressive management of HIV-positive patients requires a close and ongoing collaboration and coordination between infectious disease consultants and the transplant team.

Histamine Blockers and Proton Pump Inhibitors. There are conflicting reports regarding the use of cimetidine, ranitidine, and omeprazole with CNIs. These drugs may increase creatinine levels without reducing the glomerular filtration rate (GFR) by suppressing proximal tubular creatinine secretion. There may be increased hepatotoxicity when ranitidine and cyclosporine are used in combination. Other agents that inhibit CYP2C19 (i.e., fluconazole or fluvoxamine) can shunt omeprazole metabolism to the CYP3A pathway causing further increase in CNI levels.

Hormones. Corticosteroids in high and low doses may decrease the clearance of cyclosporine metabolites. This effect may be particularly pronounced during "pulse" steroid therapy and may result in a confusing clinical picture if the drug levels are measured by a nonspecific assay. Oral contraceptives, anabolic steroids, testosterone, norethisterone, danazol, and somatostatin may also increase drug levels.

Other Drugs. Amiodarone, carvedilol, allopurinol, bromocriptine, and chloroquine are reported to increase cyclosporine levels. Metoclopramide and grapefruit juice increase the absorption of CNIs (see Chapter 20).

Pharmacodynamic Drug–Drug Interactions

Drugs that May Exaggerate Calcineurin Inhibitor Nephrotoxicity. Any potentially nephrotoxic drug should be used with caution in combination with the CNIs because the vasoconstrictive effect of the drug tends to potentiate other nephrotoxic mechanisms. Well-substantiated enhanced renal impairment has been described after the introduction of **amphotericin** and **aminoglycosides**, and renal impairment may occur earlier than anticipated. **Nonsteroidal anti-inflammatory drugs** should be avoided if possible but can be given for short periods under supervision. CNIs may potentiate the hemodynamic renal dysfunction seen with **angiotensin-converting enzyme inhibitors** and **angiotensin receptor antagonists**. Metoclopramide may increase CNI levels by increasing its intestinal reabsorption. A syndrome of diarrhea, hepatopathy, and renal dysfunction has been ascribed to the interaction between cyclosporine and colchicine, particularly when given to patients with Familial Mediterranean Fever.

Lipid-Lowering Agents. The β-hydroxy-β-methylglutaryl-coenzyme A (HMG-CoA) reductase inhibitors (HCRIs) are frequent accompaniments of the immunosuppressive protocol (see Part IV). **Lovastatin** has been implicated in several cases of acute renal failure. When used in full doses in combination with cyclosporine, lovastatin can cause rhabdomyolysis with elevated creatine phosphokinase levels and acute renal failure. Myopathy alone has been observed in up to 30% of recipients of the lovastatin–cyclosporine combination, with symptoms of muscle pain and tenderness developing 6 weeks to 16 months after commencement of therapy. The myopathic syndrome has not been observed when lovastatin is used in a daily dose of 20 mg or less. Even this dose should be used with caution, however, and patients should be made aware of the potential interaction. The coadministration of lovastatin with gemfibrozil further increases the likelihood of rhabdomyolysis. The newer HCRIs—pravastatin, fluvastatin, simvastatin, atorvastatin, rosuvastatin—should be introduced at low doses and maximal doses avoided secondary to the inhibitory CYP3A and P-gp effects of cyclosporine. While this effect is not seen with tacrolimus, other CYP3A or P-gp inhibiting agents commonly used with tacrolimus-containing regimens can have similar effects (i.e., diltiazem). Cyclosporine may increase the levels of ezetimibe, but ezetimibe has not been reported to affect the levels of cyclosporine. Cholestyramine may interfere with cyclosporine absorption from the GI tract. Interactions with the new PCSK9 inhibitors have not yet been described, but their use in transplant patients should be carefully monitored.

Immunomodulators. The thalidomide derivatives lenolidamide (Revlimid) and pomalidomide (Pomalyst) have been recently approved for the use in multiple myeloma and myelodysplastic syndromes. These agents stimulate both cytotoxic T-cell and NK-cell activity via the upregulation of INF γ, IL-2 and IL-10 and the downregulation of IL-6. These actions can directly antagonize the mechanism of action of CNIs and other immunosuppressive agents and can lead to severe rejection episodes. Nivolumab, a fully human monoclonal IgG4 antibody, and Pembrolizumab, a humanized monoclonal antibody, target the programmed cell death receptor PD-1. Some neoplasms such as melanoma and non–small-cell lung cancer utilize PD-1 as a way to avoid immune system detection and activation. The blockage of this receptor can lead to T-cell activation and upregulation which can lead to severe rejection episodes.

Mycophenolic Acid

Mycophenolate mofetil, also known as MMF and its trade-name, CellCept, was introduced into clinical transplantation in 1995 after a series of clinical trials (see Part III) showed that it was more effective than azathioprine for the prevention of acute rejection in recipients of deceased donor kidney transplants when used in combination with cyclosporine and prednisone. MMF is a prodrug, the active compound of which is mycophenolic acid (MPA), a fermentation product of several *Penicillium* species; the mofetil moiety serves to markedly improve its oral bioavailability. An enteric-coated form of MPA (ERL-080, Myfortic) became available in 2004. The role of MMF and MPA in clinical transplantation is discussed in Parts IV and V. Generic formulations of MPA derivatives are available and became available in the United States in 2009.

Pharmacodynamics
Mechanism of Action. MPA is a reversible inhibitor of the enzyme inosine monophosphate dehydrogenase (IMPDH). IMPDH is a critical, rate-limiting enzyme in the so-called *de novo* synthesis of purines and catalyzes the formation of guanosine nucleotides from inosine. Depletion of guanosine nucleotides by MPA has relatively selective antiproliferative effects on lymphocytes; lymphocytes appear to rely on *de novo* purine synthesis more than other cell types that have a "salvage" pathway for production of guanosine nucleotides from guanine (Fig. 6.5). In principle, MPA is a more selective antimetabolite. It differs radically in its mode of action from the calcineurin inhibitors and sirolimus in that it does

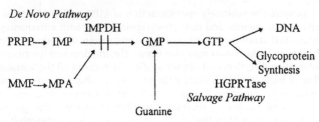

FIGURE 6.5 Mechanism of action of mycophenolate mofetil by inhibition of *de novo* purine synthesis. GMP, guanosine monophosphate; GTP, guanosine triphosphate; HGPRTase, hypoxanthine guanine phosphoribosyl transferase; IMP, inosine monophosphate; IMPDH, inosine monophosphate dehydrogenase; MPA, mycophenolic acid; PRPP, 5-phosphoribosyl-1-phosphate.

not affect cytokine production or the more proximal events following antigen recognition. It differs from azathioprine by virtue of its selective effect on lymphocytes. *In vitro*, MPA blocks the proliferation of T and B cells, inhibits antibody formation, and inhibits the generation of cytotoxic T cells. MPA also downregulates the expression of adhesion molecules on lymphocytes, thereby impairing their binding to vascular endothelial cells. The capacity of MMF to treat ongoing rejection (see Part IV) may be a reflection of its ability to inhibit the recruitment of mononuclear cells into rejection sites and the subsequent interaction of these cells with target cells. MMF may also exert a preventive effect on the development and progression of proliferative arteriolopathy, a critical pathologic lesion in chronic rejection (see Chapter 15). Retrospective analyses suggest that MMF reduces the rate of late allograft loss by an effect that is both dependent and independent of its effect on the incidence of acute rejection.

Adverse Side Effects
Extensive safety data are available from the clinical trials of MMF. Both MMF (CellCept) and enteric-coated MPA (Myfortic) are generally well tolerated and "user-friendly" compounds. The most common adverse events are related to the GI tract, with diarrhea occurring in up to one-third of patients, and varying degrees of nausea, bloating, dyspepsia, and vomiting occurring in up to 20% of patients. Frank esophagitis and gastritis with occasional GI hemorrhage occur in about 5% of patients and may be associated with cytomegalovirus (CMV) infection. The incidence of GI side effects may be higher if the dosage is greater than 1 g twice daily. Most of these symptoms respond promptly to transient reduction of drug dosage. The total daily dose can also be split into three or four doses. The GI side-affect profile of the enteric-coated formulation of MPA is not statistically significantly different from the original formulation, though practitioners frequently switch formulations when GI side effects develop. Persistent administration of MMF or MPA in the face of diarrhea is strongly discouraged and can lead to an inflammatory colitis. As with the CNIs, food decreases its absorption; however, coadministration with food may decrease the GI side effects.

Despite the relatively specific action of MPA on lymphocytes, leukopenia, anemia, and thrombocytopenia occur with a frequency similar to that seen with azathioprine and may require dose adjustment. Prolonged leukocytosis may also occur. The incidence of lymphoproliferative disorders and opportunistic infections in all the various clinical trials of MMF is marginally greater than that seen in control groups and is a nonspecific reflection of its greater immunosuppressive potency. Rare cases of progressive multifocal leukoencephalopathy (PML) have been described in patients receiving MMF, although it is difficult to definitively ascribe this catastrophic complication to the drug. Nephrotoxicity, neurotoxicity, and hepatotoxicity have not been observed with MMF.

Congenital malformations including ear malformations and spontaneous abortions have been reported in offspring of patients exposed to MPA during pregnancy, and MPA derivatives are regarded as being unsafe for use in pregnancy. To mitigate the pregnancy risks the FDA requires that a REMS (Risk Evaluation and Mitigation Strategy) program be instituted which requires additional patient education and the provision of a medication guide. Effective contraception should be employed and the drugs should be discontinued before planned pregnancy in females; immunosuppressive drug protocol adjustments may be required: azathioprine is often used to replace the MMF. No dose adjustment is required in males anticipating fatherhood.

Several studies have described a relationship between the AUC for MPA and its clinical efficacy and side-effect profile. The relationship to random trough levels is less consistent and limited sampling strategies are not clinically feasible. Therapeutic drug monitoring is generally not required for routine clinical management. In the event of side effects, the longer the period of drug-dose reduction or discontinuation, the greater is the subsequent incidence of episodes of acute rejection. Hence, the drug should be reintroduced as soon as possible and the clinical course carefully monitored.

Pharmacokinetics
Formulations. CellCept is the morpholinoethyl ester of MPA and is available for clinical use in immediate release 250-mg capsules and 500-mg tablets. A suspension formulation is also commercially available. The standard dose is 1 g twice daily. An intravenous preparation is available but is usually not required in kidney transplant recipients. Myfortic (ecMPA) is a delayed-release formulation of MPA as a sodium salt and is available in 180-mg and 360-mg tablets: the standard dose when used is 720 mg twice daily. The difference in mg strengths is owing to the molecular weight differences between the morpholinoethyl ester and sodium salt products. Both agents are also available as generics. It is unlikely that the generic formulations will undergo the same risk–benefit evaluation of the brand-name drugs. Because therapeutic drug monitoring is not routinely performed during administration of these drugs, it will be difficult to determine their relative clinical effectiveness, and they should be used with caution.

Absorption and Distribution

The pharmacokinetics of MPA is complex. Orally administered MMF is hydrolyzed to MPA presystemically and is rapidly absorbed, producing a peak level in approximately 1 hour. The bioavailability of MMF is roughly 90%, with 97% of the MPA protein bound to albumin. Orally administered ecMPA exhibits different absorption kinetics owing to the formulation; the tablets only dissolve under neutral pH conditions, and thus absorption only occurs in the intestine. It has a peak concentration after approximately 2 to 3 hours. For African-American patients, a higher dose may be required to produce the immunosuppressive benefit. Interestingly, the AUC of MPA increases with time; the same doses when used early postoperatively can produce much higher concentrations several months later. Patients should be continuously monitored for adverse side effects and periodically be evaluated for an MPA dose reduction, if clinically appropriate.

Metabolism and Excretion

MPA is glucuronidated via glucuronyl transferase enzymes in the liver to a pharmacologically inactive form (MPAG). Enterohepatic cycling of MPAG can occur via OATP transportation of MPAG from the liver into the bile. Gut bacteria can then enzymatically metabolize the MPAG to MPA. This produces a second absorption peak of MPA that occurs at 6 to 12 hours following administration and may account for some of its GI side effects. This property also makes therapeutic drug monitoring of MPA difficult owing to the affect this secondary peak has upon the AUC. MPA has a half-life of 6 to 18 hours that may be formulation-dependent. The primary route of excretion is via the kidneys as MPAG, with minimal amounts of MPA excreted unchanged in the urine, although a higher amount of MPA may be found in the urine with ecMPA use. The AUC of MPA is increased by renal impairment, although dose adjustments are not usually made. Neither MMF nor MPA is dialyzed.

Pharmacokinetic and Pharmacodynamic Drug–Drug Interactions

MPA is not metabolized through the CYP3A enzyme system, and the multiple drug interactions seen with the CNIs do not occur. MMF and azathioprine should not be administered concomitantly because of the potential for combined hematologic toxicity. Standard hematologic parameters must be carefully followed when MMF is used with sirolimus (see Part IV). Cyclosporine lowers MPA concentrations by decreasing its enterohepatic recycling via OATP1B1 inhibition. Trough levels of MPA increase when cyclosporine administration is discontinued. This interaction is not seen with everolimus, sirolimus, or tacrolimus, and the maintenance dosage of MMF, when used with standard doses and blood levels of these drugs, is typically 500 to 750 mg twice daily. MMF should not be administered simultaneously with antacids, cholestyramine, sevelamer, or oral ferrous sulfate, all of which decrease intestinal absorption. MMF, as opposed to azathioprine, can be administered with allopurinol without dose adjustment. Potential interactions may occur when MMF is administered concomitantly with acyclovir and ganciclovir, and it is wise to discontinue MMF when there is evidence of systemic herpes infection necessitating use of high dosages of the antiviral drugs.

mTOR Inhibitors: Everolimus and Sirolimus

The mTOR (mammalian target of rapamycin) is a key regulatory kinase in the process of cell division. The term *TOR* or *mTOR inhibitor* refers to two similar immunosuppressant drugs whose mode of action (see "Mechanism of Action," below) is closely linked to inhibition of this kinase. Sirolimus (Rapamune), also known as *rapamycin,* is a macrolide antibiotic compound that is structurally related to tacrolimus. Everolimus (Certican or Zortress) is a similar compound with a shorter half-life and is less hydrophobic. Everolimus is also marketed under the brand name Afinitor for nontransplant indications. Most of the clinical experience with this class of immunosuppressants is with sirolimus, everolimus was approved for use in the United States in 2010.

Sirolimus was introduced into clinical transplantation in the United States in 1999, after a series of clinical trials (see Part III) demonstrated that, when used in combination with cyclosporine and prednisone, it produced a significant reduction in the incidence of acute rejection episodes in the early post-transplantation period, compared with either azathioprine or placebo. These trials were similar in design to those that led to the introduction of MMF in that full doses of cyclosporine were administered and therapeutic drug monitoring was not routinely performed. In Europe, its introduction was delayed because of concerns regarding impairment of kidney function documented in similar trials. It was eventually approved for use in Europe in a protocol based on withdrawal of cyclosporine starting 3 months after transplantation (see "Side Effects"). Sirolimus has also been used with tacrolimus, with prednisone without a CNI, and with or without MMF. Sirolimus has not been rigorously compared with MMF; it is probably a more potent but also a more toxic immunosuppressant. Everolimus has been evaluated mainly in conjunction with cyclosporine and in a CNI-free regimen. The place of sirolimus and everolimus in clinical transplantation and dosing recommendations are discussed in Part IV.

Pharmacodynamics

Mechanism of Action. The immunosuppressive activity of the mTOR inhibitors appears to be mediated through a mechanism distinct from that of the CNIs. Like the CNIs, they bind to a cytoplasm-binding protein (the same one that binds tacrolimus, FKBP). The resultant sirolimus-FKBP ligand, however, does not block calcineurin (see Chapter 2, Fig. 6.1, and "Mechanism of Action" under "Calcineurin Inhibitors," above); instead, it engages a protein designated *target of rapamycin* (TOR) because its discovery was related to studies on the mechanism of action of rapamycin. TOR is a key regulatory kinase, and its inhibition reduces cytokine-dependent cellular proliferation at the G_1 to S phase of the cell-division cycle via the inhibition of Ca^{2+} dependent and independent events during the G_1 phase. Both hematopoietic and nonhematopoietic cells (i.e., endothelial cells, fibroblasts, hepatocytes, and smooth muscle cells) are affected. The result is a decrease in the production of IL-2, IL-3, IL-5, and IL-6. Additionally, in neutrophils, both agents prevent the release of vascular endothelial growth factor and IL-8, known pro-inflammatory mediators. Lastly, everolimus is unique in its ability to promote the release of IL-1 receptor antagonist, which has anti-inflammatory properties. Because rapamycin occupies the same binding protein as tacrolimus, it was originally presumed that it would impair the action of tacrolimus; the drug was thus developed in clinical trials as an adjunctive agent with cyclosporine. It now appears that the abundance of FKBP *in vivo* makes it unlikely that there would be inhibitive competition of tacrolimus and sirolimus for their receptor, and the drugs are often used in combination.

Adverse Effects

Nephrotoxicity. The TOR inhibitors, when administered alone, do not produce either the acute or chronic reductions in GFR that have been so consistently observed with CNIs. When administered with standard doses of CNIs, however, there appears to be a potentiation of nephrotoxicity that is not fully explained by their pharmacokinetic interaction and may be explained pharmacodynamically by potential antiproliferative effects of the agents on tubular epithelial cells. This phenomenon has been observed both in clinical trials and routine clinical use and is the basis for the recommendation that when the drugs are used in combination, the dose of the CNI should be an attenuated one (see Part IV). When cyclosporine is withdrawn from the cyclosporine–sirolimus combination 3 months after transplantation, there is a consistent and persistent improvement in renal function. This is manifested not only in lower serum creatinine levels and higher GFR but also in lower uric acid levels and blood pressure and less marked chronic histologic damage. The TOR inhibitor may be tubulotoxic and may produce hypokalemia and hypomagnesemia as a result of kaliuresis and magnesuria.

De novo proteinuria, nephrotic syndrome, and exaggeration of preexisting proteinuria have been observed with TOR inhibitor administration, possibly as a result of reduced tubular protein reabsorption and impaired podocyte integrity. Periodic quantitative monitoring of urinary protein excretion is recommended, and administration of TOR inhibitors in proteinuric patients should be avoided. TOR inhibitors have been associated with the development of localized limb edema and angioedema. Brawny limb edema may be owing to impaired lymphangiogenesis. Their concomitant use with other drugs known to cause angioedema, such as angiotensin-converting enzyme inhibitors, may increase this risk.

Impaired Healing. The TOR inhibitors block a critical step in cell division, and it is not surprising that their use would be associated with various manifestations of impaired healing and fibrogenesis. This property has been exploited in the coating of coronary artery stents with sirolimus to reduce the incidence of restenosis and may theoretically be of benefit in slowing tumor progression (see "Hematologic and Oncologic Effects," below). Sirolimus may delay recovery from post-transplantation delayed graft function by perpetuating acute tubular necrosis. The combination of sirolimus and tacrolimus has been reported to produce acute renal failure with a "cast nephropathy" as a consequence of tubular injury similar to that seen in myeloma. An increased incidence of lymphoceles and dehisced, poorly granulating wounds may occur when TOR inhibitors are used in the early postoperative period, particularly in obese patients. Painful mouth ulcers may also occur that resolve when the drug is discontinued.

For patients scheduled for certain elective surgical procedures (e.g., bowel anastomosis, hernia repair, skin flap) it may be wise to switch patients off mTORs a week prior to the procedure and recommence after wound healing; a CNI, MMF, or azathioprine can be used in the interim. For emergent surgery, the switch can take place immediately postoperatively.

Effects on Reproductive Health. In animal models, sirolimus is embryotoxic and fetotoxic. Its use is contraindicated in pregnancy, and effective contraception must be initiated before, during, and for 12 weeks after therapy has been stopped. Reversible oligospermia and reduced testosterone levels have been described during sirolimus administration, and male patients should be informed accordingly.

Hyperlipidemia and Hyperglycemia. Hyperlipidemia, hypercholesterolemia, and hypertriglyceridemia are common accompaniments of TOR inhibitor use and may occur in varying degrees in more than 50% of patients receiving these drugs. The effect has been ascribed to inhibition of lipoprotein lipase or to reduced catabolism of apoB100-containing lipoproteins. The hyperlipidemia is more pronounced for patients also receiving cyclosporine and tends to reach a peak 2 to 3 months after transplantation. In most patients, the elevation is manageable with treatment with statins, and based on the Framingham risk model, the associated coronary heart disease (CHD) risk is small. In an animal model of aortic atherosclerosis, sirolimus was described as having a protective effect despite the hyperlipidemia, presumably because of an anti-inflammatory effect. The overall impact of TOR inhibitors on clinical CHD has not been defined, but for most patients, the degree of hyperlipidemia does not contraindicate their use. TOR inhibitors may also be islet toxic and glucose metabolism does not improve when they are used in place of CNIs.

Pneumonia. In the early clinical trials of sirolimus, several cases of fatal *Pneumocystis* pneumonia were described in patients who did not receive prophylactic Bactrim. For this reason, it is recommended that Bactrim prophylaxis be continued for at least 1 year for patients receiving the drug (see Chapter 12). A noninfectious interstitial pneumonia has also been described, typically presenting as bilateral lower-lobe interstitial pneumonia. Pathologic features are similar to bronchiolitis obliterans organizing pneumonia with alveolar hemorrhage and lymphocytic infiltration. The diagnosis is one of exclusion, and the pneumonia typically resolves within 2 to 3 weeks of drug discontinuation.

Hematologic and Oncologic Effects. The TOR inhibitors can produce reversible "cytopenias," as do MMF and azathioprine, although the thrombocytopenia and anemia may be more pronounced. Hepatic artery thrombosis has been described in liver transplant recipients, but no increased thrombotic tendency has been described in kidney recipients. Thrombotic microangiopathy, well described with the CNIs (see "Acute Microvascular Disease" and Chapter 10), occurs with greater frequency when CNIs are used in combination with sirolimus, and cases have been described when sirolimus is used alone.

In the clinical trials and clinical experience of the TOR inhibitors, the incidence of malignancy and post-transplantation lymphoproliferative disease has been small. In animal models, sirolimus inhibits primary and metastatic tumors through antiangiogenesis and arrests malignant cell growth in the G_1/S phase. The potential of unlinking immunosuppression from tumor progression is clearly of critical importance in transplantation. Conversion from cyclosporine to sirolimus has been shown to be effective treatment for cases of Kaposi sarcoma, and in the CONVERT trial (see Part IV), the incidence of malignancy was lower in patients who were converted from cyclosporine-based to sirolimus-based immunosuppression. The ability to reduce malignancy has best been demonstrated for those patients who develop secondary skin cancer following kidney transplantation. In the TUMORAPA study, patients who developed cutaneous squamous cell cancer were randomized to receive sirolimus as a substitute for CNIs; the patients in the sirolimus arm had a 44% reduction in recurrence. The role of mTOR inhibitors in the management of post-transplant malignancy is discussed by Monaco in Selected Readings.

Pharmacokinetics

Formulations. Sirolimus is available as a 0.5-, 1-, or 5-mg tablet; an oral solution is also commercially available. While an intravenous preparation is not available, an intravenous preparation of *temsirolimus* could theoretically be used and has been described in kidney transplant recipients who have developed metastatic renal cell carcinoma. Everolimus (Zortres) is available as 0.25, 0.5, or 0.75 mg tablets and is the only formulation of everolimus approved for the prevention of rejection in transplant recipients. Everolimus as Afinitor is available in larger tablet sizes and a dispersible tablet designed to produce an oral solution; both of these are for once-daily dosing only. Importantly, these dosage forms of Afinitor have not been evaluated for maintenance therapy in solid-organ transplant.

Absorption and Distribution. Both agents are rapidly absorbed from the GI tract, reaching peak concentrations in 1 to 3 hours. Dosing with the oral solution of sirolimus has a lower F than that with the tablets and the two dosage forms should not be considered to be equivalent. Sirolimus is about 92% protein bound, mainly to albumin, while everolimus is less protein bound at approximately 74%. Excretion into breast milk is not known; nonetheless, breast-feeding while taking these agents is discouraged.

Metabolism and Excretion. Both drugs are largely metabolized by both CYP3A and *p*-glycoprotein in the gut and in the liver. They are also metabolized to a certain extent via CYP2C8. The native compounds are the major component in human blood and contributes most of the immunosuppressive activity. Concurrent use of cyclosporine greatly affects the metabolism of the TOR inhibitors via CYP3A and P-gp interactions. Sirolimus has a long half-life, averaging 62 hours, and a steady-state trough concentration can be achieved in most patients within 24 hours by administering a loading dose three times the size of the maintenance dose. Alterations of maintenance dosing can take 14 days before steady-state is re-achieved and has implications for therapeutic drug-level monitoring (see below). Everolimus has a half-life of approximately 30 hours and is usually not administered with a loading dose. Renal excretion is minimal, and dose adjustment is not required in renal dysfunction but is required in hepatic dysfunction. The majority of both agents are excreted in the feces via biliary elimination.

Therapeutic Drug-Level Monitoring. Therapeutic drug-level monitoring was not required in the initial labeling of sirolimus, but it has since become an essential component of its use. The target trough levels, using either chromatographic or immunoassay methodologies, vary between 5 and 15 ng/mL, depending on the concomitant use of a CNI and the clinical circumstances and are a good reflection of drug exposure. With the new CMIA methods, concentrations approximately 15% higher than those found with chromatographic methods are commonplace and should be considered when making dosing decisions. Because sirolimus has a long half-life, levels should be checked several days after a dosage adjustment is made, and once a steady-state has been reached, frequent monitoring may not be required. Everolimus has target trough whole-blood concentrations of 3 to 8 ng/mL in renal transplant recipients, also depending on the concomitant use of a CNI. The drug concentration is measured by LC-MS/MS, a methodology that is not available at all reference laboratories and can limit the turnaround time of results.

Drug Interactions. The TOR inhibitors and the CNIs are frequently administered together and are metabolized by the same enzyme CYP3A systems; therefore, the potential for interaction between them must be considered. In healthy volunteers, concomitant administration of sirolimus and the Neoral formulation of cyclosporine increased the AUC for sirolimus by 230%, when compared with administration of sirolimus alone; administration 4 hours after the cyclosporine dose increased the AUC by 80%. For this reason, it has been recommended that sirolimus be administered consistently 4 hours after the morning cyclosporine dose. In clinical practice, however, this recommendation is often ignored, which might account for some of the toxicity discussed earlier. The effect of sirolimus on cyclosporine metabolism is less marked, but over time, lower doses of cyclosporine are required to maintain target trough levels. Sirolimus and tacrolimus are typically administered simultaneously. Available information suggests, not surprisingly, that sirolimus interacts with calcium channel blockers, antifungal agents, anticonvulsants, and antituberculous agents in a manner similar to the CNIs (Tables 6.3 and 6.4).

Azathioprine

Azathioprine (Imuran) is an antimetabolite, an imidazole derivative of 6-mercaptopurine. It has been used in clinical transplantation for nearly 50 years. When cyclosporine was introduced, the role of azathioprine was largely relegated to that of an adjunctive agent, and with the introduction of MMF, its use has been discontinued in many programs. It can still be useful in certain circumstances and can be a valuable component of a low-cost immunosuppressive regimen (see Part IV).

Pharmacodynamics

Mechanism of Action. Azathioprine is a purine analogue that is incorporated into cellular deoxyribonucleic acid (DNA), where it inhibits purine nucleotide synthesis and interferes with the synthesis and metabolism of ribonucleic acid (RNA) (Fig. 6.1). Unlike cyclosporine, it does not prevent gene activation, but it inhibits gene replication and consequent T-cell activation. Azathioprine is a broad myelocyte suppressant. It inhibits the proliferation of promyelocytes in the bone marrow and, as a result, it decreases the number of circulatory monocytes capable of differentiating into macrophages. Thus, it is a powerful inhibitor of the primary immune response and is valuable in preventing the onset of acute rejection. It is ineffective in the therapy of rejection episodes.

Adverse Effects. The most important side effects of azathioprine are hematologic. Complete blood counts, including a platelet count, should be performed weekly during the first month of therapy, and less frequently thereafter. Delayed hematologic suppression may occur. In the event of significant thrombocytopenia or leukopenia, the drug can be discontinued for long periods if the patient is also taking a CNI, without great danger of inducing acute rejection. It is unnecessary to maintain a low white blood cell count for the drug to be an effective immunosuppressant.

The white blood cell count should be monitored with particular care when the corticosteroid dose is reduced or discontinued. Azathioprine may occasionally cause hepatitis and cholestasis, which usually present as reversible elevations in transaminase and bilirubin levels. The azathioprine dose is usually reduced or stopped during episodes of significant hepatic dysfunction. Pancreatitis is a rare complication. Azathioprine is converted to inactive 6-thiouric acid by xanthine oxidase. The inhibition of this enzyme by allopurinol demands that this drug combination be avoided or used with great care. When allopurinol is started, the azathioprine dose should be reduced to 25% to 50% of its initial level, and the white blood cell and platelet counts should be frequently monitored. Routine testing for thiopurine methyltransferase (TPMT) mutations is recommended in patients who are on azathioprine and in whom initiating allopurinol is considered. TPMT allows for degradation of 6-MP by an alternative biochemical pathway into the nontoxic 6-MMP. Patients with mutations in TPMT are at increased risk for bone marrow toxicity from the combination of azathioprine and allopurinol as there is no alternative metabolic pathway for 6-MP metabolism.

In the United States, the FDA has given azathioprine a pregnancy category D: there is positive evidence of human fetal risk based on adverse reaction data from investigational or marketing experience or studies in humans. Despite this, potential benefits may warrant use of the drug in pregnant transplant recipients and it has been used widely in pregnancy over a prolonged period of time without generating concern despite potential risks.

Dose and Administration

About half of orally administered azathioprine is absorbed; thus, the intravenous dose is equivalent to half the oral dose. Blood levels are not valuable clinically because its effectiveness is not blood-level dependent. The drug is not significantly dialyzed or excreted by the kidney. Dose reduction is often practiced during kidney dysfunction, although it may not be necessary. When used as the primary immunosuppressant, the daily oral dose is 2 to 3 mg/kg. When used as adjunctive therapy with a CNI, the dose is 1 to 2 mg/kg.

Corticosteroids

Corticosteroids have commanded a central position in clinical transplantation since they were first used to treat rejection in the 1960s. Despite this long experience, there remains only a general consensus on their best therapeutic use, and changing protocols often reflect both fear of prescribing them and fear of not prescribing them. The new generation of immunosuppressive drugs and protocols permit avoidance or withdrawal of corticosteroids for many patients, and in patients who continue to receive them, the dosage is typically quite small (see Part IV).

The diffuse effects of corticosteroids on the body reflect the fact that most mammalian tissues have glucocorticoid receptors within the cell cytoplasm and can serve as targets for the effects of corticosteroids. The immunosuppressive actions of corticosteroids can be somewhat simplistically divided into their specific actions on macrophages and T cells and their broad, nonspecific immunosuppressant and anti-inflammatory actions.

Pharmacodynamics
Mechanism of Action
Blockade of Cytokine Gene Expression. Corticosteroids exert their most critical immunosuppressive effect by blocking T-cell–derived and APC-derived cytokine and cytokine receptor expression. They inhibit the function of dendritic cells, which are the most important of the APCs (see Chapter 2). They are hydrophobic and can diffuse intracellularly, where they bind to cytoplasmic receptors found in association with the 90-kDa heat shock protein. As a result, the heat shock protein becomes dissociated, and the steroid–receptor complex translocates to the nucleus, where it binds to DNA sequences referred to as *glucocorticoid response elements* (GREs). GRE sequences have been found in the critical promoter regions of several cytokine genes, and it is presumed that the binding of the steroid–receptor complex to the GRE inhibits the transcription of cytokine genes. Corticosteroids also inhibit the translocation to the nucleus of nuclear factor-κB, a transcription factor that plays a major role in the induction of genes encoding a wide variety of cytokines. Corticosteroids inhibit the expression of IL-1, IL-2, IL-3, and IL-6, TNF-α, and IFN-γ. As a result, all stages of the T-cell activation process are inhibited. Cytokine release is responsible for the fever often associated with acute rejection. This fever typically resolves rapidly when high-dose corticosteroids are administered.

Nonspecific Immunosuppressive Effects. Glucocorticoids cause a lymphopenia that is a result of the redistribution of lymphocytes from the vascular compartment back to lymphoid tissue. The migration of monocytes to sites of inflammation is also inhibited. Steroids block the synthesis, release, and action of a series of chemokines, permeability-increasing agents, and vasodilators, although these anti-inflammatory effects are a relatively minor aspect of their efficacy in the prevention and treatment of acute rejection. The total white blood cell count may rise several-fold during high-dose steroid administration.

Adverse Effects. The ubiquitous complications of corticosteroids are familiar to medical practitioners and are not reviewed here in detail. They are a reflection of their profound immunosuppressive, anti-inflammatory, and hormonal action on numerous target tissues. The most important complications are cosmetic changes, growth impairment, osteonecrosis, osteoporosis, impaired wound healing and resistance to infection, cataracts, hyperlipidemia, glucose intolerance, and psychopathologic effects. There is marked variation in individual response to these drugs, presumably because of the varied concentration of tissue steroid receptors and individual variations in prednisone metabolism. In the dose regimens currently prescribed, untoward complications can be minimized, but not totally prevented.

Pharmacokinetics

Commonly Used Preparations. In clinical transplantation, steroids are used in three ways: as a high-dose intravenous or oral pulse given over 3 to 5 days; as a steroid cycle or taper with a gradually decreasing oral dose over days or weeks; or as a steady low-dose daily or every-other-day maintenance regimen. Corticosteroid dosage is discussed in Part IV.

Prednisolone, its 11-keto metabolite *prednisone,* and *methylprednisolone* (Solu-Medrol) are the corticosteroid preparations most commonly used in clinical transplantation. Prednisolone is the most active circulating immunosuppressive corticosteroid. Prednisone is the oral preparation usually used in the United States, whereas prednisolone is often preferred in Europe. Methylprednisolone is the most commonly used intravenous corticosteroid. These preparations have a half-life that is measured in hours, but their capacity to inhibit lymphokine production persists for 24 hours; therefore, once-daily administration is adequate.

Corticosteroids are metabolized by hepatic microsomal enzyme systems. Drugs such as phenytoin, barbiturates, and rifampin, which induce these enzymes, may lower plasma prednisolone levels, whereas oral contraceptives and ketoconazole increase levels. Unfortunately, there is no readily available plasma prednisolone assay for clinical use, although empirical adjustments in dose may be advisable when potentially interacting drugs are administered.

Part II: Biologic Immunosuppressive Agents

MONOCLONAL AND POLYCLONAL ANTIBODIES

The antilymphocyte polyclonal antibodies are produced by immunizing either horses or rabbits with human lymphoid tissue and then harvesting the resultant immune sera to obtain gammaglobulin fractions. Various polyclonal antibodies have been available for use in clinical transplantation since the 1970s. Currently, the primary polyclonal antibodies widely available for clinical use are preparations of rabbit anti-thymocyte globulin (rATG, Thymoglobulin). An equine anti-thymocyte globulin preparation is also available (eATG, Atgam), but not widely used. The intravenous immune globulins (IVIGs), which have been used in the treatment of antibody deficiency disorders for more than 30 years, are finding increasing relevance to current transplant therapeutics. They are made from pooled human plasma.

The monoclonal antibody muromonab-CD3 (Orthoclone OKT3) was the first monoclonal antibody approved by the FDA for use in humans. Largely because of frequent, potentially life-threatening, first-dose reactions, it is no longer used and its place in transplant therapy has been superseded by Thymoglobulin. The nomenclature used to name therapeutic monoclonal antibodies is unique and is governed by the World Health Organization. This is summarized in Tables 6.5 and 6.6. The humanized anti-CD25 monoclonal antibody preparations daclizumab (Zenapax) and basiliximab (Simulect) became available in 1998. In January 2009, Hoffman–La Roche removed daclizumab from the market, citing poor demand for the product. It is currently being studied in patients with multiple sclerosis. Rituximab (Rituxan) is an anti–B-cell monoclonal antibody developed for the treatment of hematologic malignancies that has proved useful in clinical transplantation.

Naming Conventions Used with Therapeutic Monoclonal Antibodies

Name = Prefix + Substem A + Substem B + Suffix

Substem A Abbreviations (Target)		Substem B Abbreviations (Source)	
-b(a)-	Bacterial	a	Rat
-c(i)-	Cardiovascular	axo	Rat/mouse
-f(u)-	Fungal	e	Hamster
-k(i)-	Interleukin	i	Primate
-l(i)-	Immunomodulating	o	Mouse
-n(e)-	Neural	u	Human
-s(o)-	Bone	xi	Chimeric
-tox(a)-	Toxin	xizu	Chimeric/humanized
t(u)	Tumor	zu	Humanized
-v(i)-	Viral		

Examples of Transplant-Related Monoclonal Antibodies

Medication	Naming Scheme			
	Prefix	Substem A	Substem B	Suffix
Alemtuzumab	Alem	Tu	Zu	Mab
Basiliximab	Basi	Li	Xi	Mab
Eculizumab	Ecu	Li	Zu	Mab
Rituximab	Ri	Tu	Xi	Mab

Alemtuzumab (Campath 1H) is an anti-CD52 humanized monoclonal antibody approved for use in B-cell chronic lymphocytic leukemia and now used in transplantation. While it was removed from commercial distribution in 2012, the manufacturer has a distribution program that still allows for its continued clinical use. Belatacept (Nulojix) is a fusion protein that contains a human IgG1 Fc fragment and the extracellular domain of CTL4-Ig. This molecule targets the CD80/86 receptor on antigen-presenting cells and subsequently blocks the CD28-mediated co-stimulation of T cells.

Biologic immunosuppressive agents can be used for induction immunosuppression and for the treatment of acute rejection; only belatacept is currently used for maintenance immunosuppression. The pharmacodynamic and pharmacokinetic properties of these large molecules are complex and not always fully elucidated. Due to their molecular size, they have very different pharmacokinetic profiles than the small-molecule immunosuppressive agents discussed previously. Their volume of distribution is usually relatively small and limited to the vascular compartment with slow diffusion into peripheral tissues and extracellular spaces. Metabolism to protein fragments and amino acids occurs in various organs and can be expected to be similar to that of endogenous IgG; uptake by the reticuloendothelial system is likely to be a key contributor to their elimination. Immune responses against the agent can occur, which can contribute to their elimination profile and may also affect their therapeutic efficacy. While hemodialysis will not remove these agents, plasmapheresis, a key therapy for antibody-mediated rejection, can be expected to rapidly clear them and dosing regimens should be carefully considered if the biologics will be used concurrently with that therapy. The biologic immunosuppressive agents will be discussed primarily based upon their pharmacodynamic properties. Table 6.7 reviews their major indications, which are discussed in detail in Part IV. The polyclonal antibodies (IVIG excluded) and alemtuzumab cause varying degrees of T-cell death and are sometimes referred to as *depleting antibodies*;

TABLE 6.7	Antibody Preparations for Renal Transplant Immunosuppression		
	Indication		
Treatment	**Induction**	**Rejection**	**Mechanism of Action**
Monoclonal			
Basiliximab	+*	—	Anti-CD25
Rituximab	(+)	(+)	Anti-CD20
Alemtuzumab	(+)		Anti-CD52
Eculizumab	—	—	Anti-C5
Polyclonal			
eATG (Atgam)	+	+	Lymphocyte depletion
rATG (Thymoglobulin)	(+)	+	Lymphocyte depletion
IVIg	(+)	(+)	Immune modulation

+, approved indication; (+) unapproved but commonly used indication.
*Concomitant administration of calcineurin inhibitor recommended.

the anti-CD25 monoclonal antibodies and belatacept cause T-cell dysfunction but are "nondepleting."

Rabbit Anti-Thymocyte Globulin

Rabbit anti-Thymocyte globulin (rATG) is a polyclonal antibody preparation made by immunization of rabbits with human lymphoid tissue; it has largely replaced eATG, which is less potent. In the case of Thymoglobulin (Genzyme), which is available in the United States, thymocytes are used for immunization; in the case of anti–T-lymphocyte immune globulin (ATG-Fresenius), which is available in Europe, an activated human T-cell line is used. The resultant gammaglobulin is then purified to remove irrelevant antibody material that may be responsible for some of the side effects.

Mechanism of Action

The precise mechanism of action of the polyclonal antibodies is not fully understood, but the immunosuppressive product contains cytotoxic antibodies directed against a variety of T-cell markers. After their administration, there is depletion of peripheral blood lymphocytes. The lymphocytes, T cells in particular, are either lysed or cleared by the reticuloendothelial system, and their surface antigens may be masked by the antibody. Of particular importance, Thymoglobulin causes sustained and rapid expansion of $CD4^+$, $CD25^+$, $FOXP3^+$ regulatory T cells that play an important part in maintaining immune homeostasis and limiting antigraft immunity (see Chapter 2). High levels of these cells improve the probability of reversal of acute rejection and lower the risk for graft loss after a rejection episode. Following the use of Thymoglobulin, a prolonged lymphopenia can ensue, and the CD4 subset may be suppressed for several years. The prolonged immunosuppressive effect may account for the relative infrequency of episodes of rejection recurrence.

Dose and Administration

The standard dose of rATG is 1.5 mg/kg given in a course lasting 4 to 10 days. Due to the commercially available single-use vial sizes, doses should be done in 25-mg increments. When rATG is used for induction, it may be more effective when started intraoperatively (rather than postoperatively) in reducing the incidence of delayed graft function. rATG may also be effectively dosed based on its impact on T-cell subsets. It is mixed in 500 mL of dextrose or saline and infused over 4 to 8 hours into a central vein or arteriovenous fistula. Use of a peripheral vein is sometimes followed by vein thrombosis or thrombophlebitis, although this may be prevented by adding hydrocortisone sodium succinate (Solu-Cortef), 20 mg, and heparin, 1,000U, to the infusion solution. To avoid allergic reactions, the patient should receive intravenous premedication consisting of methylprednisolone, 30 mg, and diphenhydramine hydrochloride (Benadryl), 50 mg given 30 minutes before injection. Acetaminophen should be given before and 4 hours after commencement of the infusion for fever control. Vital signs should be monitored every 15 minutes during the first hour of infusion and then hourly until the infusion is complete. The full course of thymoglobulin is typically given during a hospital admission, but patient can be discharged after the first two or three doses if appropriate outpatient facilities are available, particularly if the drug is administered via a peripheral vein.

Azathioprine, MMF, and sirolimus should generally be discontinued during the course of treatment to avoid exacerbating hematologic side effects. Cyclosporine or tacrolimus can be omitted during the course or given in a low dose, and oral prednisone is replaced by the methylprednisolone given in the premedication.

Adverse Effects

Most of the side effects of polyclonal antibodies relate to the fact that foreign protein is administered. Chills, fever, and arthralgias are common, although the severe first-dose reactions occur only rarely. There have been occasional cases of anaphylaxis. Serum sickness occurs rarely because the continued immunosuppression that follows the treatment course reduces the production of anti-idiotypic antibodies and the consequent immune complex deposition. Serum sickness typically presents with diffuse arthralgias, fever, malaise, and rash 1 to 2 weeks following infusion. It responds to an increase in prednisone dose to about 40 mg daily for several days.

Polyclonal antibody preparations can produce thrombocytopenia and leukopenia, necessitating reduction or curtailment of drug dosage. Leukopenia occurs in up to half of patients. The drug dose is usually halved for patients with either a platelet count of 50,000 to 75,000 cells/mL or a white blood cell count of less than 3,000 cells/mL. Administration should be stopped if the counts fall further. Occasionally, filgrastim (Neupogen) can be used to enhance white blood cell production of neutrophils so dosing can proceed. Therapeutic efficacy can be monitored by the differential on a complete blood count; an absolute lymphocyte count of 0.1% or less is targeted. Patients who do not respond may require a higher dosage or a prolonged treatment course.

Infection, most commonly with CMV, may be a late adverse sequela of depleting antibody use. The frequency of infection varies with the number of courses and the overall amount of immunosuppression given. Most programs routinely employ CMV prophylaxis before, during, and after a course of depleting antibody, with recipients of CMV-positive allografts representing a particularly high-risk population (see Chapter 12).

The development of lymphoma in transplant recipients is a well-recognized, although infrequent, consequence of effective immunosuppression. Use of repeat courses of depleting antibodies is associated with a particularly fulminant and typically rapidly fatal B-cell lymphoma that develops within the first few months after transplantation. Epstein–Barr virus (EBV) antibody-negative patients receiving a graft from an EBV-positive donor appear to be at greatest risk. The recognition, prevention, and management of post-transplant lymphoma are discussed in Chapters 11 and 12.

Alemtuzumab

Alemtuzumab (Campath 1H) is a recombinant DNA-derived humanized monoclonal antibody directed against the cell surface glycoprotein CD52 (Fig. 6.1). While initially approved for use in chronic lymphocytic leukemia, it is a depletional agent sometimes used in clinical transplantation, although it has not been formally approved for such use. Of note, the medication was withdrawn in 2012 and reintroduced as a treatment for multiple sclerosis with a higher cost. It has also been used as an induction agent and in the treatment of acute transplant rejection. When used at the time of transplantation as induction therapy (see Part IV), alemtuzumab induces a profound, rapid, and effective depletion of peripheral and central lymphoid cells that may take months to return to pretransplantation levels. Used as a single agent, it does not induce tolerance and episodes of acute rejection can occur even in the absence of T cells. Its use may facilitate minimization of maintenance immunosuppressive protocols and steroid sparing with monotherapy using sirolimus or low-dose calcineurin inhibitor. The terms *proper tolerance* and *near tolerance* have been used to describe the immunologic balance that results.

Alemtuzumab use in kidney transplantation is "off-label." Its ease of administration has made it an attractive alternative to Thymoglobulin. It is usually given as a single dose of 30 mg intraoperatively; a second dose is sometimes given. Because the drug is administered under general anesthesia, infusion-related events typically associated with the infusion of biologic agents are masked.

When used as an induction agent, alemtuzumab reduces the risk of rejection compared to basiliximab in unsensitized patients. However, when compared to rATG in randomized clinical trials, alemtuzumab has not been shown to be superior. In trials of patients undergoing steroid withdrawal, those receiving alemtuzumab have a greater risk of rejection.

Alemtuzumab induces profound lymphopenia, which may be prolonged requiring reduced doses of other myelosuppressive agents. There may be delayed incidence of cell-mediated acute rejection and possibly a higher incidence of antibody-mediated rejection that occurs as lymphocyte counts return to baseline. The hematologic, infection, and lymphoma risks are similar to those described for other depletional agents, and infection prophylaxis is mandatory.

Intravenous Immune Globulins

Pooled human gammaglobulin preparations, which were initially developed for the treatment of humoral immune deficiency disorders, are now used for a variety of autoimmune and inflammatory disorders. They are proving to be invaluable in certain defined situations in clinical transplantation when used alone or in combination with plasmapheresis (Table 6.8). Immune globulin preparations are made from pooled plasma from thousands of blood donors in a tightly regulated manufacturing process that essentially removes the risk for transmission of infectious disease. Immune globulins may be unselected, in which case they contain IgG molecules with a subclass distribution corresponding to that in normal human serum; they may also be selected because of the high titer of desired antibody in the donor plasma. CMV hyperimmune globulin (CMVIG, marketed in the United States as CytoGam), approved for CMV prophylaxis and treatment (see Chapter 12), is made from blood donors with a high titer of anti-CMV antibody.

TABLE 6.8	Clinical Uses of Immune Globulin Preparations in Transplantation

1. To reduce high levels of preformed anti-HLA antibodies in sensitized patients awaiting deceased donor transplants (see Chapters 3 and 7).
2. To facilitate living donor transplants in the face of a positive crossmatch or ABO incompatibility (see Chapters 3, 6, and 7).
3. To treat acute humoral rejection (see Part IV and Chapter 9).
4. To treat certain post-transplantation viral infection (see Chapter 11).

Mechanism of Action

The mode of action of IVIG is complex (Table 6.9), and the broad range of its activities is a reflection of the importance of immunoglobulins in immune homeostasis in health. In highly sensitized patients, IVIG inhibits anti-HLA antibody and produces long-term suppression or elimination of anti-HLA reactive T cells and B cells. The cytokine signaling, critical for IgG synthesis, is inhibited, and alloimmunization is inhibited through blockade of the T-cell receptor (see Chapter 2). Although discussed here in the context of immunosuppressant medications, IVIG is better regarded as immunomodulatory in its activity, and its use is not associated with the familiar complications of immunosuppression.

TABLE 6.9	Immunoregulatory Effects of Immune Globulin

Fc Receptors
Blockade of Fc receptors on macrophages and effector cells
Induction of antibody-dependent cellular cytotoxicity
Induction of inhibitory Fc γ receptor IIB

Inflammation
Attenuation of complement-mediated damage
Decrease in immune complex–mediated inflammation
Induction of anti-inflammatory cytokines
Inhibition of activation of endothelial cells
Neutralization of microbial toxins
Reduction in corticosteroid requirements

B Cells and Antibodies
Control of emergent bone marrow B-cell repertoires
Negative signaling through the Fc γ receptors
Selective downregulation and upregulation of antibody production
Neutralization of circulating autoantibodies by anti-idiotypes

T Cells
Regulation of the production of helper T-cell cytokines
Neutralization of T-cell superantigens

Cell Growth
Inhibition of lymphocyte proliferation
Regulation of apoptosis

(From Kazatchkine MD, Kaveri SV. Immunomodulation of autoimmune and inflammatory diseases with intravenous immune globulin. N Engl J Med 2001;345:747–755, with permission.)

Dosage, Administration, and Adverse Effects. The dose of IVIG is protocol dependent, and readers should consult the package insert and administration precautions of individual preparations before their use. All preparations are administered slowly over several hours. The standard dose is 2 g/kg up to a maximum of 140 g in a single administration given over 4 to 8 hours. The dose of CMVIG varies from 100 to 150 mg/kg and is often given following plasmapheresis, with one plasma volume exchange replaced by either 5% albumin or fresh-frozen plasma. Minor reactions, such as flushing, chills, headache, nausea, myalgia, and arthralgia, occur in about 5% of patients soon after commencement of IVIG infusions. These symptoms resolve when the infusion is temporarily discontinued or its rate reduced. Aseptic meningitis, which can be prevented by the administration of nonsteroidal anti-inflammatory agents, may occur in the first 72 hours following the infusion; it typically resolves spontaneously.

Thrombotic complications have been reported to follow IVIG infusion, including cases of myocardial infarction. Of particular importance to transplant recipients is the development of acute kidney injury. IVIG products differ in osmolality, pH, and sugar and sodium content. Most preparations of IVIG contain carbohydrate additives such as sucrose or sorbitol, which can induce osmotic injury (*osmotic nephrosis*) to the proximal tubular epithelium. Proximal tubular cells swell and are filled with isometric vacuoles. Patients with impaired baseline renal function may suffer further deterioration of function that may necessitate dialysis and may produce a confusing clinical picture. The tubular injury is self-limited and typically resolves within several days. Patients should be warned of the possibility of transient graft dysfunction, which may be prevented by administration while on dialysis. Practitioners must familiarize themselves with the IVIG preparation available at their institution and to the specific risk profile associated with them.

Anti-CD25 Monoclonal Antibodies
Mechanism of Action
The anti-CD25 monoclonal antibodies *basiliximab* (Simulect) and *daclizumab* (Zenapax) are targeted against the α chain (also referred to as CD25) of the IL-2 receptor (Fig. 6.1). The receptor is upregulated only on activated T cells (see Chapter 2), and as a result of the binding of the antibody, IL-2-mediated responses are blocked. The anti-CD25 monoclonal antibodies thus complement the effect of the CNIs, which reduce the production of IL-2. They are designed to prevent, but not treat, episodes of acute rejection. Zenapax is no longer available for clinical transplantation.

Basiliximab and daclizumab are two similar compounds that were introduced into clinical transplantation by virtue of their capacity to reduce the incidence of acute rejection episodes when used in combination with cyclosporine and corticosteroids (see Part III). They both originate as murine monoclonal antibodies, which are then genetically engineered so that large parts of the molecule are replaced by human IgG.

The resulting compounds have low *immunogenicity* because they do not induce production of significant amounts of human antimurine antibody. As a result, they have a prolonged half-life in the peripheral blood, and they do not induce a first-dose reaction. In the case of basiliximab, the entire variable region of the murine antibody remains intact, whereas the constant region originates from human IgG; the resulting compound is strictly deemed *chimeric* and is of 75% human and 25% murine origin.

Dose and Administration

The immunosuppressive potency of basiliximab is presumed to be related to its capacity to produce complete and consistent binding to the IL-2 receptor α sites on T cells. The drug has a half-life of longer than 7 days, which permits a long dosage interval. Two intravenous doses of 20 mg are given, the first dose preoperatively and the second dose on postoperative day 4; this regimen produces saturation of the IL-2α receptor sites for 30 to 45 days.

Adverse Effects

Other than occasional anaphylaxis or first-dose reactions described with basiliximab, there is a remarkable absence of significant adverse effects associated with its use. In the clinical trials leading to its introduction, the incidence of typical transplant-related side effects was not greater in the treatment groups than in the control group.

Rituximab

Rituximab (Rituxan) is a chimeric monoclonal antibody directed against the CD20 antigen on B lymphocytes. A rapid and sustained depletion of circulating and tissue-based B cells follows its intravenous administration. B-cell recovery begins about 6 months after completion of treatment. Rituximab is approved for use in the treatment of certain forms of non-Hodgkin lymphoma. It has also been used in a variety of presumed autoimmune diseases to suppress antibody formation. In clinical transplantation, it has been used off-label in a variety of ways: in an attempt to reduce high levels of preformed anti-HLA antigens; to facilitate living donor transplantation in the face of a positive crossmatch or ABO incompatibility; to treat acute humoral rejection; to treat recurrent post-transplantation focal and segmental glomerulosclerosis; and to treat post-transplantation lymphoproliferative disease, which is usually CD20$^+$ (see Chapter 11). The standard dosage is 375 mg/m^2. Infusion-related reactions such as hypotension, chills, fever, and rigors are fairly common and infusion rates should be started slowly and incrementally increased as tolerated. Premedication with methylprednisolone, acetaminophen, and diphenhydramine is advisable. Rare cases of PML have been associated with its use. Patients must be screened for hepatitis B as several fatalities have been reported in patients receiving rituximab who had active hepatitis B. The reader should refer to the package insert for precise dosing and administration guidelines.

Belatacept

Belatacept (Nulojix) is a second-generation co-stimulatory blocker that selectively blocks T-cell activation. The compound is not strictly a monoclonal antibody but is a human fusion protein containing cytotoxic T-lymphocyte–associated antigen 4 (CTLA-4) fused with the

Fc domain of human IgG1. Belatacept was approved as a prophylactic anti-rejection agent by the FDA in June 2011 following several clinical trials demonstrating comparable patient and allograft survival to cyclosporine. It is the most important new immunosuppressive agent for organ transplantation introduced in the last decade. It has the potential of replacing the standard CNI-based immunosuppressive protocols that have been in place for three decades.

Mechanism of Action

Belatacept has a similar structure to abatacept, with the exception of two amino acid substitutions. These substitutions permit for enhanced binding of CD80 (fourfold) and CD86 (twofold) on the antigen-presenting cell, with a 10-fold increase in T-cell inhibition *in vitro*. Blocking these ligands results in failure of "signal 2" activation in the three signal transplant model of T-cell activation. Normally, CD28 on the T cell will engage CD80 and CD86 on the antigen-presenting cell, resulting in the production of calcineurin and anti-apoptotic proteins. Blocking this pathway results in T-cell anergy and triggers apoptosis.

Adverse Effects

In three pivotal clinical trials, belatacept was demonstrated to be noninferior to cyclosporine in terms of graft and patient survival. In the initial phase II trial, there was no difference in acute rejection rates between the two regimens at 6 months. However, in two larger phase III trials, there was a higher risk of rejection (22% for low-dose belatacept vs. 17% for high-dose vs. 7% for cyclosporine). After 84 months of use, the less intensive belatacept cohort from the BENEFIT study experienced significantly better estimated GFR compared to cyclosporine (63.3 mL/min/1.73 m^2 vs. 36.6 mL/min/1.73 m^2, respectively: see Fig. 6.6). Furthermore, belatacept patients had a 43% reduced risk of graft loss or death after 7 years of use. While belatacept appears to be less effective than cyclosporine-based regimens at preventing early

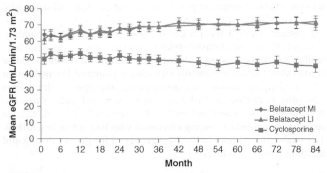

FIGURE 6.6 Glomerular filtration rate over the period from month 1 to month 84. The estimated glomerular filtration rate (eGFR) was determined by repeated-measures modeling, with time as a categorical variable. I bars indicate 95% confidence intervals. (From Vincenti F, Rostaing L, Grinyo J, et al. Belatacept and long term outcomes in kidney transplantation. N Engl J Med 2016;374(4):333–343, with permission.)

acute cellular rejection episodes, it is not less effective at preventing late cellular rejection. Additionally, donor-specific antibody development (DSA's, see Chapter 3) is less common in belatacept treated patients, a good prognostic marker for long-term function. Lastly, cardiovascular and metabolic risk factors can be expected to be reduced, providing further potential benefits to patients. Because of the design of the belatacept trials, no long-term direct comparisons to tacrolimus-based regimens are currently available.

Results from the belatacept trials demonstrated a significant increased incidence of post-transplant lympho-proliperative disease (PTLD, 1.4% in the belatacept group vs. 0.4% in the cyclosporine group). Progressive Multifocal Leukoencephalopathy (PML) was also observed. Many of the PTLD cases had central nervous system (CNS) involvement. This risk was especially true for EBV-seronegative individuals who received belatacept (7.3%). In the long-term follow-up results, PTLD cases mainly occurred in the initial 24 months of therapy. As such, belatacept should *only* be used in patients who have demonstrated EBV-seropositivity, typically to EBV viral-capsid antigen. Due to the risk of PTLD and PML, the FDA has designated belatacept as a REMS medication, requiring providers to discuss these potential adverse effects with patients and to review symptoms consistent with CNS PTLD or PML prior to drug infusions. The overall rate infection was similar between belatacept and cyclosporine. Infusion reactions were noted in 2% of patients but were generally mild.

Pharmacokinetics

Formulations. Belatacept is administered only as an intravenous infusion and comes in 250-mg vials that require reconstitution prior to use. Dosing is done in 12.5-mg increments owing to the reconstituted drug concentration. Further dilution up to 250 mL can be done with either normal saline or 5% dextrose. The standard dose is weight-based at 5 or 10 mg/kg delivered over 30 minutes through a peripheral line using an inline filter that is low protein binding. Belatacept can be administered in an outpatient environment.

Patients with *de novo* introduction of belatacept at the time of transplantation are given 10 mg/kg on postoperative days 1 and 5, followed by repeat dosing at weeks 2 and 4. After the fourth dose, two regimens are available, a high- and low-dose protocol. The high-dose protocol involves infusion of a dose of 10 mg/kg every 2 weeks until 3 months post-transplant, followed by a monthly dose of 10 mg/kg between months 4 to 6, and a maintenance dose of 5 mg/kg monthly. The low-dose protocol calls for 10 mg/kg monthly for months 2 and 3 post-transplant, followed by 5 mg/kg monthly thereafter.

For patients already on a CNI, conversion to belatacept may be warranted. Conversion requires an overlapping of immunosuppression such that the belatacept is slowly introduced at 5 mg/kg every 2 weeks for five doses before transitioning to a maintenance dose of 5 mg/kg monthly. CNI tapering is performed concurrently, with typical target drug levels at time of belatacept initiation. By the second infusion, the goal of CNI level is 40% to 60%, by the third week post initial infusion, the desired goal is 30% of the target CNI levels, and by the third infusion, 1 month following initiation of belatacept, the CNI can be discontinued.

Part III: Clinical Trials and New Immunosuppressive Agents

During the 1990s, a series of promising new immunosuppressive agents underwent laboratory and clinical evaluation in a successful attempt to broaden and improve the immunosuppressive therapeutic armamentarium; these included tacrolimus, MMF, sirolimus, and the anti-CD25 monoclonal antibodies. Other than the off-label use of the drugs noted above, belatacept has been the only major new molecular entity introduced into routine clinical transplantation practice. The race for the introduction of new drugs into clinical transplantation practice can be likened to an obstacle course. Many promising drugs (e.g., FTY720, FK778, efalizumab) have faltered and fallen from consideration usually because of unanticipated side effects manifesting in advanced clinical trials.

The great success of organ transplantation that was achieved in the 1990s with currently available agents is, paradoxically, making it exceedingly difficult (and enormously expensive) to prove the added benefit of new agents. In clinical trials of new agents, as discussed later, the use of the traditional marker of drug or protocol superiority—patient or graft survival—proved to be impractical and has largely been replaced by alternative end points.

Clinical Trials

Before any clinical trials can be performed with an investigational agent, an *investigational new drug* (IND) application has to be submitted to the FDA or to an equivalent regulatory body outside of the United States. Approval of the IND application is based on the evaluation of preclinical studies that suggest potential therapeutic benefits of a new agent and on the evaluation of studies in a variety of animals that suggest its safety. Phase 1 clinical studies are performed in healthy human volunteers or patients to evaluate human metabolism, pharmacokinetics, dosage, safety, and, if possible, effectiveness. Phase 2 includes controlled, open-label, clinical studies conducted to evaluate the effectiveness of the drug for a particular indication and to determine dose regimens, common side effects, and risks. Phase 3 studies are expanded trials based on preliminary evidence from the previous phases that suggest efficacy and safety. They are sometimes called *pivotal trials* because they are critical for FDA-approved licensing and registration. They typically involve large, usually *multicenter*, clinical trials that are *randomized* and, if possible, *double-blinded* using *placebo controls*. These studies serve to refine dosage, determine benefit, and further evaluate the overall risk-to-benefit ratio of the new drug. In organ transplantation, particular care has to be taken to ensure that any potential benefit of a new agent is not outweighed by the consequences of too much immunosuppression or by organ-specific toxicity. Successful completion of phase 3 should provide an adequate basis for product labeling and permit approval of the drug for its defined indications. Following introduction of a new drug into the clinical marketplace, phase 4 studies may be performed under the auspices of the manufacturer or of independent investigators or at the request of the FDA to further refine the role of the drug in clinical practice.

Any human use of an experimental drug is strictly governed by the predetermined rules of the experimental protocol under which the drug is administered. Patients must read, understand, and sign an informed consent form that clearly defines the nature of the experiment in which they are involved and its potential risks and benefits. They must also receive a copy of the *patient's bill of rights,* which clearly defines the nature of their commitment, and authorize the release of personal health information according to the provision of federal privacy laws (the Health Insurance Portability and Accountability Act [HIPAA]). The experimental protocol and consent form must have been approved by an *institutional review board* (IRB) or *human subjects protection committee* (HSPC), and the medical staff administering the protocol must feel totally comfortable with it. After a drug is licensed, it is often used off-label for indications, or in doses, different from those precisely defined. Such use does not require a formal consent procedure, although it is wise to inform the patient that the drug is being given for an unapproved use.

Clinical Trial Design in Transplantation

Immunosuppressive practitioners must understand the way in which new agents are introduced because clinical trials of new immunosuppressive agents not only have led to their clinical use but also have largely determined the way in which these agents are used. It is also particularly important to appreciate what primary *end points* were used to determine the efficacy of the new agents. The choice of primary end point, the frequency with which this end point occurs in the control population, and the anticipated capacity of the new agent to change the incidence of the end point (estimated from phase 2 studies) permit a statistical evaluation of the number of patients required to be enrolled in the study so that the study has sufficient statistical power to determine the effectiveness of the new agent. Secondary end points usually include side-effect comparisons, renal function estimations, and long-term effects on patient and graft survival. Studies may not have the *statistical power* to provide answers to the questions posed by the secondary end points.

When the clinical trials for cyclosporine use in kidney transplantation were designed in the late 1970s and early 1980s, the primary end point used was improvement of patient and graft survival, which cyclosporine indeed achieved. Tacrolimus was introduced based on its capacity to produce results equivalent to cyclosporine. OKT3 was introduced based on its superior capacity, when compared with corticosteroids, to reverse episodes of acute rejection, and Thymoglobulin was introduced for its superiority in reversing acute rejection when compared with Atgam. MMF, sirolimus, anti-CD25 monoclonal antibodies were introduced based on their capacity, when combined with cyclosporine and prednisone, to reduce the incidence of acute rejection episodes. Belatacept was introduced based on superior allograft function at 1 year post kidney transplantation.

End Point for Studies of New Immunosuppressive Drugs

The incidence of acute rejection episodes, typically biopsy proven (see Chapter 15), became the most frequently used marker of the effectiveness of new immunosuppressive drugs for the following reasons:

1. Because of the excellent results of kidney transplantation with currently available immunosuppressants, with 1-year graft survival

rates of greater than 90% in most centers and minimal mortality, it is statistically extremely difficult to prove the benefit of new agents or protocols in terms of patient or graft survival.

2. Acute rejection is a potent risk factor for the development of chronic allograft failure (see Chapter 10). In retrospective analyses, patients who have suffered episodes of acute rejection have a long-term graft survival rate that is 20% to 30% less than the graft survival rate of patients who have not suffered acute rejection.

3. Acute rejection episodes are morbid events in themselves, requiring intensification of immunosuppression and sometimes hospital admission.

4. Most acute rejection episodes take place within the first few months of transplantation, and their presence can be proved on biopsy. This permits a rapid evaluation of the effectiveness of a new agent or protocol (a luxury that is not available when immunosuppressive drug trials are performed in other clinical circumstances, such as systemic lupus erythematosus or rheumatoid arthritis).

A statistically significant reduction in the incidence of acute rejection episodes was achieved in the pivotal clinical trials leading to the introduction of MMF, the mTORs, and the anti-CD25 monoclonal antibodies. A significant effect on patient and graft survival was not achieved, probably because the studies did not have the statistical power to show such an effect.

As new immunosuppressive drugs and protocols are introduced and the incidence of acute rejection decreases, it is becoming increasingly difficult to prove the statistically significant benefit of newer drugs. In the pivotal trials leading to the introduction of MMF, sirolimus, and the anti-CD25 monoclonal antibodies, the incidence of acute rejection in the patients receiving the experimental drug protocol was compared with the incidence of acute rejection in patients receiving *standard therapy* with cyclosporine, prednisone, and azathioprine. The success of MMF in reducing the incidence of acute rejection led to it becoming part of an updated standard therapy protocol in many centers (see Part IV). As a result, for trials of newer agents, statistical proof of further reduction in the incidence of acute rejection will likely be more difficult to achieve. In current and future trials, end points may be based on functional parameters such as estimates of renal function (such as that seen in the belatacept studies), on histologic parameters such as scores for chronic allograft injury (see Chapter 15), on immune parameters (see Chapter 2), on the incidence of delayed graft function, or on a composite of multiple end points.

The phased evaluation of new drugs discussed above is designed primarily to lead to the introduction by pharmaceutical manufacturers of individual new agents that are safe and efficacious. These trials, however, may not address the clinical questions posed by practitioners who are more concerned with the safety and effectiveness of drug combinations. The comparison groups in formal registration trials are previously approved protocols that often do not represent "standard of practice" at the time the trials are completed—hence, their information may be of limited practical value to practitioners. Postregistration trials often describe single-center experience, and the clinical value of retrospective database analyses is intrinsically limited. Large, multicenter, randomized trials such as the CAESAR, ELITE-Symphony, and CONVERT trials attempted to evaluate immunosuppressive drug protocols in a manner that addresses these concerns.

New Immunosuppressive Drugs

Multiple new drugs and therapeutic concepts are at different stages of development. Those drugs that are in advanced clinical trials and show promise of introduction into the clinical arena are discussed below.

Other Monoclonal Antibodies

Efalizumab (Raptiva) is a humanized CD11a-specific IgG1 targeted against the lymphocyte-associated function-1 (LFA-1) molecule. LFA-1 binds to intercellular adhesion molecules, and the interaction is important in the recruitment of leukocytes to the sites of inflammation (see Chapter 2) and in stabilizing the interaction between T cells and APCs. Efalizumab has been approved for the treatment of severe psoriasis and was being developed for use in transplantation as a subcutaneously administered immunosuppressant in CNI-free protocols. Phase 1 and 2 studies show the drug to be effective, although in high doses, there was an increased incidence of PTLD. Cases of PML were reported in patients with psoriasis, and the FDA has halted its development for transplantation in the United States.

Alefacept (Amevive) is a humanized LFA-3–IgG1 fusion protein that binds to CD2 on T lymphocytes and blocks the interaction between LFA-3 and CD2 and interferes with T-cell activation. It has been approved for use in psoriasis. The phase 2 clinical trial in which it was paired with tacrolimus was never published, as an interim analysis did not provide sufficient evidence of benefit to convince the manufacturer to continue its development.

ASKP1240 is an anti-CD40 monoclonal antibody that consists of fully human IgG4. This biologic interrupts the co-stimulatory CD40–CD154 pathway by preventing the interaction between CD40 and CD154. The agent has shown promise in animal models and phase I trials.

Janus Kinase and Protein Kinase Inhibitors

Janus Kinases (JAKs) are a family of cytoplasmic tyrosine kinases involved in cell surface signaling. Tofacitinib (CP-690550) has been evaluated in clinical trials and appears to be an effective immunosuppressant, although high doses have been associated with an increased risk for infections. The phase 2 trials were conducted on unsensitized patients and demonstrated an equal rate of rejection compared to a cyclosporine-based regimen; however, BK nephritis and CMV infections were higher in some of the higher-dosing groups and hematologic toxicity was higher when used with MMF.

Sotrastaurin (AEB071) is a protein kinase inhibitor whose development for use in a CNI protocol was discontinued because of treatment failure but is been developed in Europe in combination with everolimus.

Bortezomib

Bortezomib (Velcade) is a proteosomal inhibitor that is FDA approved for the treatment of multiple myeloma. The immune-modulating effects of the drug are pleiotropic and result, in part, from its proapoptotic effects on plasma cells. Bortezomib also suppresses T-cell function, and the drug has potential for the treatment and prevention of both antibody-mediated and cell-mediated rejection. Preliminary studies suggest that the drug is effective and safe and that it reduces levels of donor-specific antibodies (DSAs; see Chapter 3). DSAs are increasingly thought to be an important cause of chronic rejection and graft loss, and if bortezomib is shown to be able to reduce or remove them over the long term, it may provide a valuable means to prolong graft function. Other proteosome-inhibiting agents are also available. These include carfilzomib and the newly FDA-approved ixazomib, the first orally active agent in this class, but published clinical transplant experience with these agents is lacking.

Eculizumab

Eculizumab (Soliris) is a humanized monoclonal antibody that targets complement protein C5. Binding inhibits the activity of C5 convertase, thus blocking the formation of C5a and C5b which are needed to form the membrane attack complex. It is currently approved by the FDA to treat paroxysmal nocturnal hemogloinuria or atypical hemolytic uremic syndrome. While the agent can be used to treat these disorders if they recur post-transplant (see Chapter 11), eculizumab has also been used in transplant recipients to prevent complement-mediated microvascular damage that is associated with ongoing antibody-mediated rejection. Several small studies have examined its usefulness in the transplant setting and its use appears promising. Cost concerns generally limit its off-label use to severe and refractory cases. Ongoing studies hope to establish its usefulness in the treatment of antibody mediated rejection, desensitization of preexisting donor specific antibodies, or for the prevention ischemia reperfusion injuries.

Immune Modulation and Tolerance Induction

Immune modulation is a somewhat vague term used to describe attempts to modify the immune response in a nonspecific fashion in order to facilitate allograft acceptance without impairing effector cells or mechanisms. Several techniques fall within this category. Infusion of *donor-specific bone marrow* or *stem cells,* or *total lymphoid irradiation,* in combination with short-term nonspecific immunosuppression, has produced long-term graft survival in the absence of immunosuppressive therapy in experimental and clinical organ allografts. The donor bone marrow provides an as yet unidentified signal for tolerance. *Blood transfusions* are known to exert beneficial effects on animal and human allograft survival through a variety of potential mechanisms. The tolerogenic effect of bone marrow and blood may also be a result of the development of a state of microchimerism (see Chapter 2). A randomized trial of perioperative donor-specific blood transfusions in live donor transplants showed no practical benefit. Although some success has been achieved with these innovative techniques, they all require heavy initial immunosuppression, and there is often evidence of residual immune response. Long-term follow-up studies of HLA incompatible transplants indicates a high rate of chronic allograft rejection. The data on two-haplotype pairs is encouraging. However, these protocols are not yet ready for broad clinical application, and require a living donor.

Part IV: Immunosuppressive Protocols

GENERAL PRINCIPLES OF PROTOCOL DESIGN

The variety of immunosuppressive drugs available for use in clinical transplantation permits permutations that make up immunosuppressive protocols. Transplant centers tend to be loyal to their own protocols, which have often been developed in response to local needs and experience. Financial considerations, both for patients and institutions, may determine the choice between similar agents. Protocols should be regarded as guides for therapy that need not necessarily be adhered to slavishly. They may require modification from patient to patient with new knowledge and experience. In an era in which short-term success rates for deceased donor transplantation of 95% are commonplace, it may take experience with hundreds of patients followed for prolonged periods to prove the benefit of a new or modified approach.

There are limited prospective data on the effects of different protocols on 5- and 10-year graft survival. Most of the data on long-term protocol design come from retrospective analysis and analysis of large databases. Although valuable, these analyses bring with them intrinsic design flaws. For instance, in a prospective blinded study, it is possible to ensure that the groups that are compared are demographically and clinically similar and that investigator bias in the choice of protocol is negated. In database analyses, such assurances are absent, and analyses are limited by the reliability of the data that are entered. Database analyses, however, permit evaluation of a very large number of patients over a prolonged period and may permit recognition of trends and associations not noted in short-term prospective studies on a limited number of patients. The relevance to individual patients of outcome studies based on database analysis must be considered with circumspection.

Table 6.10 lists the components of a conventional immunosuppressive protocol. These components are relevant to all recipients with the possible exception of two-haplotype–matched living related donors. The broad range of immunosuppressive drugs now available has also led to the development of a series of innovative protocols. In some programs, innovative protocols have become the local standard of therapy. For all protocols, because the risk for acute rejection is highest in the first weeks and months after transplantation (*induction phase*) and diminishes thereafter (*maintenance phase*), immunosuppression should be at its highest level in this early period and should be reduced for long-term therapy. The most feared side effects of immunosuppression—opportunistic infection and malignancy—tend to reflect the total

TABLE 6.10	Components of the Conventional Immunosuppressive Protocol	
Class of Agent	**Options**
Calcineurin inhibitor	Cyclosporine, tacrolimus
Corticosteroids	Dose and regimen
Adjunctive agent	Azathioprine, MMF, sirolimus
Antibody induction	Lymphocyte depleting or nondepleting
Supplementary agents	CCB, HCRI
Infection prophylaxis	Bactrim, antifungals, antivirals

CCB, calcium channel blocker; HCRI, HMG-CoA reductase inhibitor; MMF, mycophenolate mofetil.

amount of immunosuppression given rather than the dose of a single drug. The total quantity of immunosuppression should thus be monitored and considered in all stages of the post-transplantation course.

Conventional Immunosuppressive Protocols

Conventional immunosuppressive protocols consist of a CNI, an adjunctive agent, corticosteroids, and the possible addition of antibody induction. With conventional protocols, most programs are able to achieve 90% to 95% graft survival with an acute rejection rate of 10% to 20%.

Cyclosporine or Tacrolimus?

The two CNIs remain the backbone of transplant immunosuppression and are likely to remain so until such time as similarly effective but less toxic—in particular, nephrotoxic—agents are introduced into clinical practice. Although much has been made of discrete differences between cyclosporine and tacrolimus, the fact is that these drugs are remarkably similar, and both are highly effective. Table 6.1 summarizes their similarities and differences. These differences may guide the choice of agent in individual patients. For example, cyclosporine may be preferred in some centers for African-American patients because of the increased incidence of post-transplantation glucose intolerance in patients who receive tacrolimus; tacrolimus may be preferred in adolescents and other patients who are concerned about cosmetics because of the more marked cosmetic changes associated with cyclosporine; cyclosporine may be preferred in some patients because of the generally milder neurologic side effects; tacrolimus may be preferred in recipients of simultaneous kidney and pancreas transplants because of its somewhat greater immunosuppressive potency despite its greater islet toxicity (see Chapter 16); tacrolimus-induced hair loss in adult females may prompt conversion to cyclosporine.

Prospective data comparing the two drugs have tended to favor tacrolimus. These studies are often difficult to interpret, however, because of protocol design and the introduction of improved formulations and drug-level monitoring of cyclosporine. There has·been a steady trend during the past decade toward greater use of tacrolimus. In the United States, about 95% of patients receive tacrolimus at the time of discharge from hospital, and most of the remainder receive cyclosporine. A similar trend has been observed in Europe.

Which Adjunctive Agent?

In this discussion, the term *adjunctive agent* is used to describe the immunosuppressive drugs that are used in combination with a CNI in the early post-transplantation period to enhance the potency of the immunosuppressive protocol as reflected by a decreased incidence of acute rejection episodes. Most programs continue to use combination therapy over the long term. Azathioprine has been replaced by MMF or enteric-coated MPA (most commonly MMF) in most centers because of its superior capacity to reduce the incidence of acute rejection and evidence, that has been the subject of some controversy, that long-term outcomes are also improved. The MMF/MPA combination with tacrolimus is used in over 90% of patients in the United States.

Sirolimus became available for clinical use in late 1999. In its initial U.S. package insert, it was used in a manner similar to MMF with a full-dose of the CNI and a fixed sirolimus dose. It is now rarely used this way, and drug-level monitoring of sirolimus is regarded as mandatory for optimal use, typically with attenuated doses of CNI. Because of the side-effect profile of sirolimus and the failure to show superiority over MMF in most clinical circumstances (see discussion of Symphony trial, below), it is used as a primary agent in only 5% of cases in the United States. Sirolimus may be of particular value in patients deemed to be at high risk for post-transplantation malignancy or those who develop *de novo* malignancy, especially skin cancer, after transplantation (see Chapter 11). Everolimus has been shown to be a useful adjuvant agent and can even be used as a primary immunosuppressant when initiated a postoperatively, in a sequential manner.

Antibody Induction

Antibody induction is the term used to describe the use of the depleting antibodies (Thymoglobulin, alemtuzumab) or the nondepleting anti-CD25 monoclonal antibody (basiliximab) in the immediate postoperative period. Induction protocols with Thymoglobulin are an alternative to the use of a CNI in the early post-transplantation period (though the CNI is given at standard or attenuated doses at many programs) and are therefore different from induction using a nondepleting antibody, in which concomitant use of a CNI is mandatory. In *sequential* therapy, Thymoglobulin is administered and the CNI is introduced only when renal function has reached a predetermined level (e.g., a plasma creatinine level of 3 mg/dL). The antibody is discontinued as soon as adequate CNI levels are achieved. A patient with a well-functioning graft may thus receive only a few days of antibody treatment.

Table 6.11 lists the advantages and disadvantages of depletional antibody induction. The benefits of Thymoglobulin and alemtuzumab induction suggest a similar degree of effectiveness. There remains much discussion regarding the relative benefits of Thymoglobulin and the anti-CD25 monoclonal antibody. For low-risk patients, they are as effective as the depletional agents. A prospective trial of the two forms of induction in high-risk recipients (see "High-Risk and Low-Risk Groups," below) was discontinued because of an apparent benefit of Thymoglobulin. This benefit, however, was not recognized

T A B L E 6.11	Potential Advantages and Disadvantages of Depleting Antibody Induction

Potential Advantages
Improved graft survival for high-risk patients
Period of delayed graft function may be foreshortened
Onset of first rejection is delayed
Obviates early use of calcineurin inhibitor
May permit less aggressive maintenance regimen

Potential Disadvantages
Risk for first-dose reactions
May prolong hospital admission stay
Greater cost
Higher incidence of cytomegalovirus infection
Increased risk of post-transplant lymphoma
Increased short- and long-term mortality reported

in a retrospective analysis. Long-term retrospective studies have not shown significant benefit of routine induction therapy in terms of patient and graft survival.

In many programs, depletional antibody induction is reserved for immunologically high-risk recipients or for patients in whom delayed graft function is anticipated. Depletional antibody induction may also be indicated for patients requiring anticonvulsant drugs that may make it difficult to achieve therapeutic levels of the CNI in the early post-transplantation period. In the United States, about 90% of patients receive some form of antibody induction, most frequently with Thymoglobulin.

High-Risk and Low-Risk Groups
All patients are not equal with respect to the chances of rejection or graft loss, and protocols should be individualized to take this into account. Patients undergoing simultaneous kidney–pancreas transplantation and patients with high levels of preformed antibodies or previously failed transplants may require more intense therapy. Patients with delayed graft function have an increased susceptibility to episodes of acute rejection. In several clinical trials, African-American patients have required higher doses of immunosuppressive drugs to achieve the same immunosuppressive benefit, and some programs take this into account routinely in protocol design. Young patients tend to be immunologically aggressive; protocol design for children is discussed in Chapter 17. Older patients may not tolerate heavy immunosuppression, and kidneys from older donors may be less tolerant of immunologic and other insults. Recipients of transplants from well-matched deceased donors or from living related donors, particularly from two-haplotype–matched donors, may require less immunosuppression.

How Long to Continue Immunosuppression?
The immune system has a long memory! Immunosuppression is required for the functional life of the graft, even if it has lasted two decades or more. Discontinuation of immunosuppressive drugs, even many years after transplantation, may lead to late acute rejection or

accelerated chronic rejection. In stable patients, carefully monitored reduction or even discontinuation of individual components of the immunosuppressive protocol may be safe.

When to Stop Immunosuppression?

The minimal mortality that is now associated with kidney transplantation is to a large degree the result of an appreciation of when to minimize or stop immunosuppression and abandon a kidney. Discontinuation of immunosuppression may be necessary for patients with resistant opportunistic infection or malignancy (see Chapters 11 and 12). Patients with deteriorating graft function despite more than two or three appropriately treated rejections are better allowed to return to dialysis and seek another transplant. Withdrawal of immunosuppression can result in rejection and the development of HLA antibodies, resulting in a higher PRA (see Chapter 3). The decision to withdraw immunosuppression should take into account when one expects the recipient with a failed allograft to be retransplanted. In patients with an expected waiting time less than 2 years, or with a living donor, continuation of low intensity immunosuppression is recommended to avoid sensitization. Patients with failed transplants who continue to make significant amounts of urine while on dialysis may also benefit from continuation of a low-intensity immunosuppression. Patients who have received corticosteroids for prolonged period may be adrenally suppressed and the steroid dose should be discontinued very slowly. With the constant introduction of new immunosuppressive agents into clinical practice, great care and judgment are needed to avoid the temptation of excessively adding or exchanging new agents.

Specific Protocol Recommendations
Cyclosporine

Cyclosporine, 6 to 10 mg/kg/day orally, is given as a single dose or twice daily starting immediately before transplantation or on the first postoperative day. Cyclosporine can be administered by intravenous infusion over 4 hours or can be given as a constant infusion over 24 hours; the dose is one-third of the oral dose. For patients who receive depleting antibody induction, oral cyclosporine may be started several days before the completion of the course of therapy so that drug levels will be therapeutic at the time of the final antibody dose. Doses are then adjusted to maintain levels within the ranges given in Table 6.12. It is wise to continue to monitor levels of cyclosporine, although the degree of reliance on these levels and the frequency of their measurement vary from program to program. The desired dose and target levels are influenced by the concomitant use of adjunctive agents and history of rejections. By 3 months after transplantation, most patients are receiving cyclosporine in a dose of 3 to 5 mg/kg/day.

There is still no clear consensus regarding the best dose or drug level for long-term cyclosporine use, and it is unfortunate that prospective randomized trials comparing cyclosporine dose ranges are not available. Drug-level monitoring with 2-hour (C2) peak levels may be more effective than trough-level monitoring. Recommended peak levels have not been extensively validated with varied transplant populations and protocols, and the recommended levels noted in Table 6.10 should be

TABLE 6.12	Approximate Therapeutic Ranges for Calcineurin Inhibitors			
	Cyclosporine			Tacrolimus
Post-transplantation Month	HPLC and CMIA (ng/mL)	FPIA (ng/mL)	C2 levels* (µg/mL)	CMIA (ng/mL)
0–2†	150–350	250–450	1.2–1.5	10–15
2–6	100–250	175–350	0.8–1.2	6–10
>6	100	150	0.5–0.8	4–8

CMIA, chemiluminescent microparticle immunoassay; FPIA, fluorescent polarization immunoassay; HPLC, high-performance liquid chromatography.
*Drawn within 15 minutes of 2 hours postdose. For C2 levels, no change in target levels is required for different assay types.
†In the first few days after transplantation, the trough cyclosporine level should not fall below 300 ng/mL by HPLC.

considered accordingly. Fear of progressive nephrotoxicity has tempted many clinicians to permit low levels, yet such a policy may allow for the insidious development of chronic rejection. Retrospective studies show that continued use of cyclosporine is conducive to prolonged adequate graft function.

Tacrolimus

The recommended starting dose of oral tacrolimus is 0.15 to 0.30 mg/kg/day administered in a split dose every 12 hours, typically 2 to 4 mg twice daily. Intravenous tacrolimus is rarely required in kidney transplantation and sublingual administration should be considered first. Doses are adjusted to maintain tacrolimus drug levels at between 10 and 15 ng/dL during the first few post-transplantation weeks and somewhat lower thereafter (Table 6.12). There is marked inter- and intrapatient variation in the dose of tacrolimus required to achieve these levels, with some patients receiving as little as 2 mg daily and some patients receiving 10 times that dose. The relationship between drug levels and manifestations of toxicity varies considerably among patients.

Switching Calcineurin Inhibitors

If side effects develop with one of the CNIs, it is quite reasonable to switch to the other agent. Common reasons for switching are cosmetic (tacrolimus to cyclosporine for hair loss and the converse for hirsutism; cyclosporine to tacrolimus for gingival hypertrophy). In some patients, new-onset diabetes mellitus (see Chapter 11) may respond to conversion from tacrolimus to cyclosporine. The dose chosen at the time of switching must be individualized. There is no need to overlap the drugs, and steroid "coverage" is usually unnecessary. Patients should be monitored carefully after switching.

Corticosteroids

The use of corticosteroids in the peritransplantation period has been dramatically reduced with the availability of CNIs. A large dose of methylprednisolone is still typically given intraoperatively in a dose of up to 1 g. In standard protocols, the dose is then reduced rapidly from 150 mg on day 1 to 20 mg on day 14. Some programs avoid the steroid cycle altogether, modifying it or starting at 30 mg daily or even less.

The maximal oral dose of prednisone at one month should be 15 to 20 mg, and 5 to 10 mg at 3 months. The long-term maintenance dose is 5 mg in most programs. Rejection episodes may occasionally occur when even very small dose reductions are made in patients after 3 months. High maintenance dose protocols of steroids sometimes used for collagen vascular disease and vasculitides are unnecessary and contraindicated in kidney transplantation.

Adjunctive Agents

The standard dose of MMF in adults is 1,000 mg twice daily, although African-American patients may benefit from a higher dose (1,500 mg twice daily) in the early post-transplantation period. Patients on full-dose tacrolimus may require a lower dose. Some evidence suggests that measurement of mycophenolic acid AUC may be useful in predicting the effectiveness of MMF; however, the more convenient trough levels have not been convincingly shown to be useful and are generally not measured. If the dose of MMF is reduced or held for short periods in the event of side effects, the dose of CNI and prednisone should be maintained. The longer the MMF dose is reduced, the greater is the risk for subsequent rejection, and patients should be monitored accordingly. Most programs continue to administer MMF for prolonged periods; administration for at least 1 year has been shown, in retrospective studies, to produce measurable benefit in graft survival and to reduce the incidence of late acute rejections.

The maintenance dose of sirolimus is typically 2 to 5 mg once daily with target blood levels similar to those described for tacrolimus (see "Tacrolimus" above). If the accompanying CNI is totally discontinued, the dose requirements of sirolimus to maintain adequate levels may increase. The standard recommended dose of sirolimus is 2 mg administered once daily 4 hours after the morning dose of cyclosporine although many patients take the two drugs simultaneously. If sirolimus is to be the primary agent, a loading dose of 6 mg is given on the first day of treatment to accelerate the achievement of a stable trough level. African-American patients may require a higher dosage. Trough drug-level monitoring is now routine. If sirolimus is given with tacrolimus, a combined trough level of 10 to 15 ng/dL is typically adequate. Sirolimus administration should be accompanied by low-dose prophylaxis with sulfamethoxazole/trimethoprim for at least 1 year; some centers will use this indefinitely.

Everolimus is typically dosed at 0.75 to 1.5 mg twice daily and is also therapeutically monitored. A drawback to its use is the length of time required for concentration results to return from the laboratory and this can lead to subtherapeutic or extratherapeutic levels being

The inclusion of *calcium channel blockers,* usually either diltiazem or verapamil, in the standard immunosuppressive regimen has several potential advantages. In addition to their antihypertensive properties, both drugs may minimize CNI-induced vasoconstriction and protect against ischemic graft injury and nephrotoxicity. Both drugs compete with the CNIs for excretion by the CYP3A enzyme system, raising drug levels and permitting safe administration of lower doses. Calcium channel blockers may also possess some intrinsic immunomodulatory activity of their own related to the role of cytosolic calcium levels or gene activation. The routine inclusion of calcium channel blockers in the post-transplantation protocol may improve 1-year graft survival rates by 5% to 10%.

Protocols for Living Donor Transplants

Excellent results were achieved for two-haplotype–matched living-related transplants immunosuppressed with azathioprine and prednisone alone before the introduction of cyclosporine into routine clinical practice. Despite this experience, most transplantation programs now use CNI-based protocols for these patients because of the lesser incidence of acute rejection. Two-haplotype–matched transplant recipients receiving CNIs may be good candidates for steroid avoidance or withdrawal. MMF can potentially be used to replace the CNI. For all other living donor transplants, conventional protocols are CNI-based and are similar to those described for deceased donor transplants. Routine lymphocyte-depleting antibody induction is not required, and some programs dispense with antibody induction altogether.

Low-Cost Protocols

The immunosuppressive drugs and protocols described above are expensive to a degree that may preclude transplantation in the developing world, or for those without adequate health insurance and drug cost coverage in the developed world. In the developing world, most transplants are from living donors in unsensitized recipients. In these circumstances, excellent results can be achieved without using antibody induction and with the less expensive generic preparations of CNIs combined with azathioprine and low-dose steroids, both of which are inexpensive. The dose of azathioprine is 1 to 3 mg/kg. Drug levels are not measured, and the dose is usually fixed with adjustments made for hematologic toxicity. For patients who cannot afford long-term maintenance therapy with MMF or sirolimus, azathioprine is a far better alternative to no immunosuppression at all. The annual cost of azathioprine is about $900, compared with $12,000 for MMF.

Innovative Transplantation Protocols

The availability of multiple immunosuppressive agents has stimulated attempts to minimize or avoid the most toxic components of the standard protocol. The most obvious targets for such efforts are corticosteroids and the CNIs.

Steroid Withdrawal and Steroid Avoidance. *Steroid withdrawal,* the discontinuation of steroid administration days, weeks, or months after transplantation, needs to be differentiated from *steroid avoidance,* in which steroids are not administered at all. Steroid withdrawal may be rapid (within a week of transplantation) or delayed. The difference between the two techniques is more than semantic, and there is some evidence that rapid withdrawal may be safer than later steroid withdrawal. Rapid withdrawal may also be safer than total steroid avoidance. Because most of the side effects of steroids are a result of the high doses that are given in the early postoperative period and high-dose maintenance therapy, there is good reason to focus efforts on rapid withdrawal or the use of low-dose maintenance therapy.

Nearly one-third of all transplant recipients are discharged from the hospital in the United States without steroids, indicating that steroid avoidance is standard of practice in many programs. Most steroid-free protocols administer antibody induction with ATG followed by combinations of a CNI and sirolimus or MMF. Patients who are withdrawn from steroids may have an increased incidence of acute rejection episodes and some return to steroid use. African-American patients and presensitized patients may not be suitable candidates for withdrawal. A clear-cut benefit of withdrawal, in terms of certain steroid-related side effects (e.g., bone disease, hyperlipidemia), has been difficult to confirm, presumably because even those patients receiving steroids receive very low doses. Steroid withdrawal in selected patients may be associated with a lower incidence of cardiovascular events. Some evidence suggests that there may be long-term deterioration in graft function after steroid withdrawal. The risks and benefits of steroid withdrawal should be thoroughly reviewed with patients before protocol changes are made.

Calcineurin Inhibitor Avoidance, Withdrawal, and Dose Minimization. Avoidance, or at least minimization, of the nephrotoxic effects of the CNIs is indeed a worthy goal which has been tested in a number of large multicenter clinical trials. In low-risk patients, protocols avoiding or withdrawing CNIs by using combinations of anti-CD25 monoclonal antibodies, corticosteroids, and MMF, or by using sirolimus or everolimus alone, reportedly permit excellent graft survival but with an unacceptably high incidence of acute rejection episodes and side effects related to the TORs. Some protocols effectively combine sirolimus, MMF, and corticosteroids; dose adjustments resulting from hematologic toxicity are common. CNI avoidance or early withdrawal is not standard therapy.

The most promising protocol option for CNI withdrawal in the event of side effects, is switching to a belatacept-based protocol combined with MMF. Kidney function is better preserved. Recall that only EBV-immune patients can be offered this option.

ABO- and HLA-incompatible Kidney Transplantation

Transplantation across the traditional immunologic barriers of ABO blood type and HLA donor specific antibodies has become achievable in certain cases. In some cases patients with healthy living donors cannot undergo transplantation owing to ABO blood group incompatibility. This may be the only living donor available to the patient who would otherwise have deceased donor transplantation as the only other option available to them. In order for an ABO-incompatible pair to proceed, the recipient should have a baseline blood group isoaglutinin titer measured. The isoaglutinin titer is useful in predicting if therapy can permit ABO incompatible transplantation, and determining the number of pretransplant treatments required. There are programmatic differences but most employ a combination of plasmapheresis and IVIG until the isoaglutinin titer is $< 1:8$. Once this achieved the transplant can occur with careful monitoring of titers post-transplant. Post-transplant plasmapheresis may be indicated in patients in whole the titer rapidly rises post-transplant. In patients who are refractory to post-transplant plasmapheresis, splenectomy may be indicated. Recipients may receive rituximab, tacrolimus and mycophenolate prior to organ transplantation.

Patients with HLA donor-specific antibodies may also undergo treatment to permit transplantation with an HLA incompatible donor. This process can be done for incompatible living pairs, or for patients on the deceased donor transplant list who are highly sensitized. For living pairs the degree of HLA incompatibility should be assessed by the number of donor specific antibodies and their mean florescence intensity (MFI). There are two common protocols in use: (1) use of rituximab with high-dose IVIG (2 g/kg with maximum dose of 140 g) and (2) a combination of plasmapheresis with low-dose IVIG (100 mg/kg). HLA antibodies must be monitored post treatment to ensure that they are lowered. Other adjunctive therapies include rituximab and bortezomib.

Because of the inevitable complexity, cost, and risk, associated with desensitization protocols, kidney paired exchange may be a better approach for incompatible pairs. Kidney paired exchange is discussed in detail in Chapter 7, Part IV.

Part V: Treatment of Kidney Transplant Rejection

ACUTE CELLULAR REJECTION

First Rejection
Pulse Steroids

High intravenous doses of steroids, typically referred to as "pulses," reverse about 75% of first acute rejections. There are numerous ways to pulse a patient, and there is no good evidence that the higher-dose pulses (500 to 1,000 mg methylprednisolone for 3 days) are more effective than the lower-dose pulses (120 to 250 mg oral prednisone or methylprednisolone for 3 to 5 days). Most programs still prefer to use intravenous methyl-prednisolone, which is given over 30 to 60 minutes into a peripheral vein. Pulse therapy is suitable for outpatient use when clinically indicated. The dose of prednisone can be continued at its previous level when the pulse is completed, although some programs elect to *recycle* the prednisone dose after the pulse has been completed. High maintenance doses of prednisone are not indicated. It is wise to repeat antibiotic prophylaxis with sulfamethoxazole/trimethoprim after a steroid pulse.

Antibody Treatment

Thymoglobulin is highly effective therapy for the management of a first acute rejection, and about 90% of such rejections are reversed. Despite its effectiveness, most programs still prefer to use pulse steroids as their first-line acute rejection therapy because of convenience, lesser risks for side effects, and lower costs. Thymoglobulin may be a better first-line option for particularly severe or vascular rejections (Banff grade IIB or greater; see Chapter 15). The anti-CD25 monoclonal antibodies are not designed to be used in the treatment of established acute rejection. Antibiotic prophylaxis with antiviral, antifungal, and anti-pneumocystis agents should reinitiated.

Recurrent and Refractory Rejections

Repeated courses of pulse steroids may be effective in reversing acute rejections, but it is probably not wise to administer more than two courses of pulse therapy before resorting to antibody treatment. Many programs use antibody treatment for all second rejections unless the rejection is clinically mild or separated from the first by at least several weeks. Antibody treatment is particularly valuable for rejection episodes that are steroid resistant and may succeed in reversing a high percentage of such rejections.

Some programs commence antibody treatment if there is not an immediate response to pulse therapy, whereas others wait several days. If renal function is deteriorating rapidly in the face of pulse steroids, it is probably wise to start antibody treatment early. Switching from cyclosporine to tacrolimus, or adding MMF or sirolimus in patients who have not previously received it, may be indicated for recurrent rejections.

The term *refractory rejection* is not well defined. It usually refers to ongoing rejection despite treatment with pulse steroids and antibody. The management of these patients is problematic. Second courses of depletional antibodies can be given in selected patients, and long-term graft function can be achieved in 40% to 50% of such patients. When deciding whether to give a second course of an antibody preparation, the clinician should bear in mind the severity and potential reversibility of rejection on biopsy and the increased risk for infection and malignancy that ensues, particularly if two courses are given close together.

Late Rejections

The terms *early rejection* and *late rejection* are not well defined. The differentiation between early and late rejection is not just semantic; each may respond differently to therapy. Early rejections are easier to reverse likely because of the persistence of Foxp3 regulatory T Cells ([Tregs], see Chapter 2) in the early post-transplant period. For practical purposes, a late rejection is one that occurs more than 3 to 4 months after transplantation and may be a first, or more frequently, a recurrent rejection. Late rejections can also be divided into those that occur in the face of apparently adequate immunosuppression and those that occur as a result of inadequate immunosuppression, often in nonadherent patients. Late rejections are often a prelude to chronic rejection and accelerated graft loss, and the histologic findings are often mixed. The initial treatment of a late rejection is typically pulse steroids. There is evidence that late rejections associated with noncompliance are more likely to respond to therapy. Use of Thymoglobulin for late steroid-resistant rejection has not been systematically studied, and careful clinical judgment must accompany the decision to prescribe it; this decision should be made by a transplantation program. It may be wiser to accept graft dysfunction or loss rather than use repeated courses of high-dose immunosuppression in an already chronically immunosuppressed patient.

Antibody-Mediated Rejection

The clinical and pathologic recognition of antibody-mediated rejection are discussed in Chapters 10 and 15, with particular emphasis on the role of the C4D immunostain. Two related treatment protocols are effective: high-dose IVIG or low-dose IVIG combined with plasmapheresis.

A dose of 2 g/kg of IVIG is usually adequate; plasmapheresis plus IVIG is usually performed every other day until levels of donor-specific antibodies are brought under control and the serum creatinine has improved to within 30% of their previous baseline value. In severe cases, for patients with high-titer donor-specific antibodies, rituximab may reduce antibody burden and graft injury. Furthermore, the use of bortezomib is an attractive option due to its effects on active antibody secreting plasma cells and not just CD-20 + B lymphocytes seen with rituximab. Antibody-mediated rejection may recur and may be followed by episodes of acute cellular rejection. Patients must be monitored carefully in the weeks following treatment. Patients who have a reduction in DSA MFI by > 50% have improved outcomes compared to those individual who are unable to achieve such reductions.

Episodes of antibody-mediated rejection may occur months, years, or even decades after transplantation likely because of the unrecognized persistence of donor-specific antibodies often in a background of medication nonadherence. Treatment of these late episodes is problematic because of the concomitant presence of other forms of allograft injury. The therapeutic options are the same as for the treatment of early episodes though they have not been shown to be effective and should be applied, if at all, with careful consideration of risk and cost.

Immunosuppressive Management of Chronic Allograft Failure

The clinical course, pathology, and multifactorial etiology of chronic allograft failure are discussed in Chapters 11 and 15. Before making changes in the immunosuppressive protocol in a patient with a failing allograft, every effort must be made to rule out potentially reversible causes of graft dysfunction, and it must be appreciated that many of the histologic changes are irreversible. Table 6.13 lists the issues that must be considered in all patients with presumed chronic allograft failure before changes are made in the immunosuppressive protocol.

Several single-center studies and retrospective analyses have suggested that CNI dose reduction or discontinuation while maintaining adjunctive therapy is a safe and effective means of delaying the inevitable progression of chronic allograft failure. Switching to belatacept-based immunosuppression may also be an option. The aptly-termed Creeping Creatinine study (see Dudley et al in Selected Readings) was a multicenter, randomized, prospective study that evaluated the benefit of substitution of MMF for cyclosporine in patients with chronic allograft failure. An effective response to treatment was

 TABLE 6.13   Steps to Take Before Manipulating Immunosuppression for Patients with Chronic Allograft Failure

1. Have reversible causes of deteriorating graft function been ruled out?
2. Is the patient clinically euvolemic?
3. Is there evidence of recurrent disease?
4. Have drug formulations been recently changed?
5. Have interfering drugs been introduced?
6. Is the patient (and physician!) adherent to the immunosuppressive regimen?
7. Have "nonimmune" interventions been applied?

defined as a stabilization or reduction in the serum creatinine level, as evidenced by a flattening or positive slope of the 1/creatinine plot and no graft loss. The response rate was nearly 60% in the group whose cyclosporine was replaced by MMF, compared with 32% in the group whose cyclosporine dose was continued unchanged. This study and others support the following general principles that serve to guide immunosuppressive management of chronic allograft failure:

1. Intensification of CNI dosage is generally not beneficial and may lead to exaggeration of nephrotoxicity.
2. Consideration should be given to reduction or even discontinuation of CNI therapy. Such a therapeutic maneuver requires careful follow-up to screen for episodes of deteriorating graft function.
3. Reduction of CNI dosage is generally accompanied by addition of, or continuation of, a nonnephrotoxic immunosuppressant.
4. There is most experience and documented benefit with MMF in these circumstances, although sirolimus may be an appropriate alternative in the absence of proteinuria. Trials of belatacept in this situation in EBV-positive patients are in progress.
5. Patients with chronic allograft failure that have deposition of C4D as a marker of ongoing humoral injury may represent a separate category that may benefit from carefully considered intensification of immunosuppression or use of IVIG.
6. Introduction of a new immunosuppressive agent in previously immunosuppressed patients has potentially dangerous consequences. Patients should be monitored carefully and consideration given to prophylaxis to prevent development of infectious complications.
7. High baseline doses of corticosteroids are not indicated. Pulse steroid therapy may be valuable for episodes of deteriorating function, but repeated treatment should be avoided. Ideally, use of pulse steroids in these circumstances should follow histologic confirmation of an element of acute rejection.
8. Because repeated pulse steroid therapy should be avoided, it is rarely indicated to perform repeated biopsies in patients with established chronic allograft nephropathy.
9. If graft function continues to deteriorate despite the above measures, plans should be made to prepare for end-stage renal disease treatment options,
10. Once dialysis has started immunosuppression should be minimized. The decision regarding discontinuation of immunosuppression will be determined by a number of factors including presence of residual function and urine output and avoidance of sensitization in the event that a repeat transplant is anticipated.

Selected Readings

Part I

Barbarino JM, Staatz CE, Venkataramanan R, et al. PharmGKB summary: cyclosporine and tacrolimus pathways. Pharmacogenet Genomics 2013;23:563–585.

Budde K, Bunnapradist S, Grinyo JM, et al. Novel once-daily extended-release tacrolimus (LCPT) versus twice-daily tacrolimus in de novo kidney transplants: one year results of a phase III double-blind, randomized trial. Am J Transplant 2014;14:2796–2806.

Danovitch G. Mycophenolate mofetil: a decade of clinical experience. Transplantation 2005;80:S272–S274.

de Fijter J. Cancer and mTOR inhibitors in transplant recipients. Transplantation 2017;101:45–55.

Knops N, Levtchenko E, van den Heuval B, et al. From gut to kidney: transporting and metabolizing calcineurin-inhibitors in solid organ transplantation. Int J Pharm 2013;452:14–35.

Letavernier E, Bruneval P, Vandermeersch S, et al. Sirolimus interacts with pathways essential for podocyte integrity. Nephrol Dial Transplant 2009;24:630–638.

Naesens M, Kuypers D, Sarwal M. Calcineurin inhibitor nephrotoxicity. Clin J Am Soc Nephrol 2009;4:481–508.

Shaw L, Figurski M, Milone M, et al. Therapeutic drug monitoring of mycophenolic acid. Clin J Am Soc Nephrol 2007;2:1062–1072.

Staatz CE, Tett SE. Clinical Pharmacokinetics of once-daily tacrolimus in solid organ transplant patients. Clin Pharmacokinet 2015;54(10):993–1025.

Van Gelder T. What is the future of generics in transplantation? Transplantation 2015;99:2269–2273.

Vincenti F, Friman S, Scheuermann E. Results of an international, randomized trial comparing glucose metabolism disorders and outcome with cyclosporine versus tacrolimus. Am J Transplant 2007;7:1506–1514.

Werk AN, Cascorbi I. Functional gene variants of CYP3A4. Clin Pharmacol Ther 2014;96:340–348.

Wiseman A. Immunosuppressive medications. Clin J Am Soc Nephrol 2016;11:332.

Zalztman J. Is there a role for mTOR inhibitors in renal transplantation. Transplantation 2017;100:228–229.

Part II

Bollée B, Anglicheau D, Loupy A, et al. High-dosage intravenous immunoglobulin-associated macrovacuoles are associated with chronic tubulointerstitial lesion worsening in renal transplant recipients. Clin J Am Soc Nephrol 2008;3:1461–1468.

Cantarovich M, Durrbach A, Hiesse C, et al. 20-Year follow-up results of a randomized controlled trial comparing antilymphocyte globulin induction to no induction in renal transplant patients. Transplantation 2008;86:1732–1737.

Hellemans R, Bosmans J, Abramowicz D. Induction therapy for kidney transplant recipients: do we still need Anti-IL2 receptor monoclonal antibodies. Am J Transplant 2017;17:22–27.

Lopez M, Clarkson M, Albin M, et al. A novel mechanism for anti-thymocyte globulin: induction of CD4$^+$, CD25$^+$, Foxp3$^+$ regulatory cells. J Am Soc Nephrol 2006;17:2844–2853.

Malvezzi P, Jouve T, Rostaing L. Costimulation blockade in kidney transplantation: an update. Transplantation 2016;100:2315–2323.

Pestana JO, Grinyo JM, Vanrenterghem Y, et al. Three-year outcomes from BENEFIT-EXT: a phase III study of belatacept versus cyclosporine in recipients of extended criteria donor kidneys. Am J Transplant 2012;12(3):630–639.

Vincenti F, Rostaing L, Grinyo J, et al. Belatacept and long-term outcomes in kidney transplantation. N Engl J Med 2016;374:333–343.

Vo A, Cam V, Toyoda M, et al. Safety and adverse events profiles of intravenous gamma-globulin products used for immunomodulation: a single-center experience. Clin J Am Soc Nephrol 2006;1:844–855.

Vo A, Lukovsky M, Toyoda M, et al. Rituximab and intravenous immune globulin for desensitization during renal transplantation. N Engl J Med 2008;359:242–251.

Weaver T, Kirk A. Alemtuzumab. Transplantation 2007;84:1545–1547.

Part III

Everly M, Everly J, Susskind B, et al. Bortezomib provides effective therapy for antibody- and cell-mediated acute rejection. Transplantation 2008;86:1754–1758.

Fremeaux-Bacchi V, Legendre C. The emerging role of complement inhibitors in transplantation. Kidney Int 2015;88:967–973.

Hardinger KL, Brennan DC. Novel immunosuppressive agents in kidney transplantation. World J Transplant 2013;3:68–77.

Kawai T, Cosimi A, Spitzer T, et al. HLA-mismatched renal transplantation without maintenance immunosuppression. N Engl J Med 2008;358:353–361.

Krämer BK, Klinger M, Vitko S, et al. Tacrolimus-based, steroid free regimens in renal transplantation: 3-year follow-up of the ATLAS trial. Transplantation 2012;94:492–498.

Lachenbruch P, Rosenberg A, Bonvini E, et al. Biomarkers and surrogate end-points in renal transplantation: present status and considerations in clinical trial design. Am J Transplant 2004;4:451–457.

O'Leary JG, Samaniego M, Barrio MC, et al. The influence of immunosuppressive agents on the risk of de novo donor-specific HLA antibody production in solid organ transplant recipients. Transplantation 2016;100:39–53.

Starzl T. Immunosuppressive therapy and tolerance of organ allografts. N Engl J Med 2008;358:407–411.

Weir MR, Mulgaonkar S, Chan L, et al. Mycophenolate mofetil-based immunosuppression with sirolimus in renal transplantation: a randomized, controlled spare-the-nephron trial. Kidney Int 2011;79:897–907.

Vicenti F, Silva HT, Busque S, et al. Evaluation of Tofacitinib exposure on outcomes in kidney transplant patients. Am J Transplant 2015;15:1644–1653.

Parts IV and V

Abramowicz D, Hadaya K, Hazzan M, et al. Conversion to sirolimus for chronic renal allograft dysfunction: risk factors for graft loss and severe side effects. Nephrol Dial Transplant 2008;23:3727–3729.

Augustinne J, Hricik D. Steroid withdrawal: moving on to the next question. Am J Transplant 2009;9:3–4.

Axelrod D, Naik A, Schnitzler M, et al. National variation in use of immunosuppression for kidney transplantation: a call for evidence-based regimen selection. Am J Transplant 2016;16:2453–2462.

Craig J, Webster A, McDonald S. The case of azathioprine versus mycophenolate: do different drugs really cause different transplant outcomes? Transplantation 2009;87:803–804.

Danovitch GM. Immunosuppressive medications for renal transplantation: a multiple choice question. Kidney Int 2001;59:388.

Danovitch GM. Management of immunosuppression in patients with chronic allograft nephropathy. Kidney Int 2002;61:S80.

Dudley C, Pohanka E, Riad H, et al. Mycophenolate mofetil substitution for cyclosporine a in renal transplant recipients with chronic progressive allograft dysfunction: the Creeping Creatinine Study. Transplantation 2005;79:466–475.

Ekberg H, Tedesco-Silva H, Demirbas A, et al. Reduced exposure to calcineurin inhibitors in renal transplantation. N Engl J Med 2007;357:2562–2575.

Halloran P, Bromberg J, Kaplan B, et al. Tolerance versus immunosuppression: a perspective. Am J Transplant 2008;8:1365–1366.

Krämer B, Del Castillo D, Margreiter L, et al. Efficacy and safety of tacrolimus compared with ciclosporin A in renal transplantation: three-year observational results. Nephrol Dial Transplant 2008;23:2386–2392.

Leichtman A. Balancing efficacy and toxicity in kidney transplant immunosuppression. N Engl J Med 2007;357:2625–2627.

Le Meur Y, Aulagnon F, Bertrand D, et al. Effect of an early switch to belatacept among CNI-intolerant graft recipients of kidneys from extended criteria donors. Am J Transplant 2016;16(7):2181–2186.

Matas A, Gaston R. Moving beyond minimalization trials in kidney transplantation. J Am Soc Nephrol 2015;26:2898.

Schena F, Pascoe M, Albaru J, et al. conversion from calcineurin inhibitors to sirolimus maintenance therapy in renal allograft recipients: 24-month efficacy and safety results from the CONVERT trial. Transplantation 2009;87:233–242.

Vincenti F, Schena F, Paraskevas S, et al; for the FREEDOM Study Group. A randomized, multicenter study of steroid avoidance, early steroid withdrawal or standard steroid therapy in kidney transplant recipients. Am J Transplant 2008;8:307–316.

Wiseman A. Induction therapy in renal transplantation: Why? What agent? What dose? We may never know. Clin Am J Nephrol 2015;10:923.

Living Donor Kidney Transplantation

Anjay Rastogi, Mara Hersh-Rifkin,
H. Albin Gritsch, Jeffrey L. Veale,
Suzanne McGuire, and Amy Waterman

Advances in immunosuppressive therapy, refinement in surgical techniques, minimization of risk, in public awareness, altruism, and goodwill, have allowed living donor kidney transplantation to evolve from the first historic successful identical twin donor transplantation in 1954 to the current practice whereby virtually all biologically related and unrelated, medically and psychosocially suitable, individuals can be considered as donors. During the decade from 1994 to 2004, the number of living donor kidney transplantations in the United States almost doubled, reaching a peak level of 6,647 in 2004. Since then, numbers have fallen somewhat to 5,628 in 2015. The preference for living donation can be attributed to the superior patient and graft survival rates achieved with living compared to deceased donor transplantation, the advent of laparoscopic donor nephrectomy, improved patient and public awareness, and as a response to the long waiting lists for a deceased donor transplant. More specific and accurate information on the long-term risks of living donation are now available and will be discussed. Approximately 45% of all kidney transplants in the United States are from living donors.

Both within the United States and around the world, there are wide variations in the use of living kidney donors. These differences reflect varying medical and societal cultural values and varying realities in the availability of sophisticated care for patients with advanced kidney disease (see Chapters 1 and 22). Differences can also be driven by the availability of deceased donor organs relative to the number of patients waiting for transplants, attitudes of local physicians regarding the risk of living donation, and the degree of government oversight. European countries have lagged behind the United States in living donation, though by 2016, 20% of kidney transplants were from living donors. The United Kingdom is an exception among European countries and living donation accounted for close to 50% of all kidney transplants in 2016. In Japan, strong cultural and, until recently, legal barriers have limited deceased donor transplants, and living donation is the most common form of transplantation. Although illegal throughout the developed world (see Chapter 19) and proscribed by national and international professional transplantation organizations, commercial living donation, typically from vulnerable populations, remains a common practice in parts of the world. In 2006, the World Health Organization (WHO) estimated that up to 10% of organ transplantations were performed in this manner, though there is reason to believe that this number has fallen under the influence of the Declaration of

Istanbul on Organ Trafficking and Transplant Tourism (see Chapters 19, 22, and 23) whose mission is to put an end to exploitation of living donors while promoting healthy and robust transplantation practice.

Part I of this chapter provides medical guidelines for evaluating a potential living donor candidate; Part II discusses psychosocial evaluation and advocacy; Part III reviews the relevant surgical issues and techniques; Part IV discusses innovative and controversial aspects of living donation; and Part V discusses education for the promotion of living donation. Readers are referred to excellent resource material available on this topic, in particular the proceedings of the Amsterdam Forum, and the Consensus Conference on Best Practices in Live Kidney Donation (see Selected Readings).

It is fitting to commence this chapter by quoting a statement that cannot be overemphasized: "At all stages of the evaluation and transplant process, the donor is as legitimately considered to be a patient as the transplant recipient" (see Dew et al. in Selected Readings). The donor is entitled to a degree of advocacy and mutual trust that is no less than is offered to the recipient. A successful outcome to a living donor transplant requires a good outcome for both the donor and the recipient, with outcome being assessed in its broadest sense, medically and psychosocially, in the short- and the long term.

Part I: Medical Evaluation of Living Kidney Donors

INFORMED CONSENT

Informed consent is a core value in living kidney donation (Table 7.1). Living donor consent is also discussed in Chapter 19. Emphasis on the adequacy of the consent process is particularly important because, as opposed to standard medical procedures, living donation is not specifically designed to help the donor or advance the donor's health. Moreover, living donation has the potential for contravening that basic tenet of medical ethics, *primum non nocere*. The person who gives consent to donate an organ must be a competent adult (possessing decision-making capacity); willing to donate; free from coercion; medically and psychosocially suitable; fully informed of the risks and benefits of donation; and fully informed of alternative treatments available to the recipient (i.e., to understand that in the absence of their donation, the patient can, in most circumstances, continue dialysis). Under very specific and rare circumstances, an identical twin younger than age 18 (the established age for a consenting adult) might be allowed to donate to his or her identical twin sibling but only after thorough education on the risks of donation and alternatives for the intended recipient, and full understanding of the informed consent to proceed.

Two other principles of living donor consent have been endorsed: that of *equipoise*—the benefits to both the donor and recipient must outweigh the risks associated with the donation and the transplantation of the live donor organ; and that it is clear to the potential donor that his or her participation is completely voluntary and may be withdrawn

TABLE 7.1	Suggested Elements for Consent in the Living Donor Evaluation Process

The potential donor should understand the following:

- Undergoing evaluation is not a commitment to donate.
- I can stop at any time.
- The physicians may turn me down as a donor, and will inform me why.
- I will be evaluated by an independent donor evaluation doctor or team to protect my interests.
- The information obtained during the course of the evaluation is confidential.
- I will be tested for AIDS, hepatitis, and other infectious diseases.
- I may get unexpected information during the evaluation process that may have implications for my future health and insurability.
- There may be risks and discomfort associated with some of the testing (e.g., blood draws, intravenous contrast).
- There are potential financial costs to me related to time off work, travel expenses, and the like that might not be reimbursed.
- There are potential study uses to the information obtained during the evaluation. I may be asked to participate in a living-donor registry.
- It may be suggested to me that I have routine long-term medical follow-up after kidney donation.
- There are alternative treatments available to the recipient other than my donating a kidney to him or her.

Modified from a personal communication from D. Cohen, MD (February 2017)

at any time. To ensure that these principles are applied, it is recommended (and mandated in the United States and other countries) that all programs performing living donor transplantations have an independent donor advocate who is not part of the team caring for the recipient (see Part II). The availability of such an advocate (who may be the evaluating physician as long as he or she is not responsible for the care of the recipient) is now mandated in the United States.

A separate consent should be obtained for the donor evaluation itself. This helps ensure that, in addition to being informed of the risks of donation, the donor is informed about all aspects of organ donation and the implications of the evaluation process (Table 7.2).

THE EVALUATION PROCESS

The major components of the evaluation of potential living kidney donors are shown in Figure 7.1.

Preliminary Laboratory Evaluation: Donor Typing to Determine the Risk for Acute Transplant Failure

Mandatory preliminary laboratory evaluation of a potential living donor includes determination of ABO blood group compatibility, crossmatching against the potential recipient, and HLA tissue typing. To reduce cost, some programs delay the more sophisticated typing studies till the completion of the medical and psychosocial workup.

Which Donor to Choose?

In cases in which more than one donor is available, selection of the most appropriate donor depends on a variety of factors including the degree of

TABLE	
7.2	Consent for Medical Evaluation

The potential donor should be informed that he or she must undergo the following:
- A complete history and physical examination
- General laboratory testing
- Screening for HIV, hepatitis, and other infectious diseases
- Imaging studies requiring the use of intravenous contrast
- The potential donor should understand the following:
  - I may get unexpected information during the evaluation process that may have implications for my future health and insurability.
  - There may be risks and discomfort associated with some of the testing (e.g., blood drawn, intravenous contrast).
  - There may be potential short- and long-term risks associated with the surgical procedure.
  - I may need routine long-term follow-up after kidney donation.
  - The benefits to both the donor and recipient must outweigh the risks associated with the donation and the transplantation of the live organ.

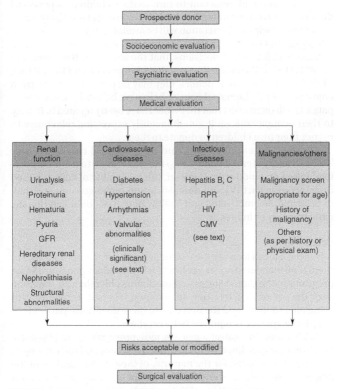

FIGURE 7.1 Major components of the evaluation of potential living kidney donors.

HLA matching and donor age. Biologically related donors are generally preferred over unrelated donors. When more than one family member is available, it is logical to commence evaluation of the best-matched relative (i.e., a two-haplotype match versus a one-haplotype match). If the donors have similar match grade (i.e., a one-haplotype–matched parent and a one-haplotype–matched sibling), it may be advisable to choose the older donor with the thought that the younger donor would still be available for donation if the first kidney eventually fails. When more than one one-haplotype–matched sibling is available, it may be worthwhile to check the tissue typing of one parent to determine which siblings shares the noninherited maternal antigens (see Chapter 3). Such sharing may improve long-term graft survival. There is some evidence that recipients of maternal kidneys may have a somewhat greater incidence of rejection and graft loss.

Patients and their loved ones often, understandably, pay much attention to "good matching." It should be noted, however, that other than for two-haplotype–matched siblings whose outcomes are superior, the outcomes for other degrees of matching of living donors are quite similar. Other factors, such as donor age and size, may be more important than the quality of the "match."

Parents often are reluctant to turn to their children as potential donors; yet as those parents age, it becomes less and less likely that a donor from their own generation will be available. It is useful to point out to parents that their grown children are adults who are capable of making independent decisions; that the welfare of the donor will be protected in the evaluation and donation period; and that, if they exclude their children as donors, they may be preventing them from enjoying the psychological gain of helping a beloved parent. Older patients will often insist that they would have been prepared to donate to their own parents while simultaneously expressing reluctance to permit their own children to donate to them.

Patients, potential donors, and their medical caregivers may "self-exclude" potential donors who they determine to be "incompatible" based on blood type. However, the availability of kidney paired exchange (see Part IV) and desensitization techniques means that, in principle, any motivated and healthy potential donor can donate, either directly or indirectly.

Donor Age

Advanced age can increase the risk for perioperative complications, but there is no mandated upper age limit for living kidney donation. Some programs in the United States exclude donors older than 70, donation after the age of 75 is relatively uncommon. There is a trend toward using older donors, and the outcome of these donations, particularly to older recipients, is reported to be excellent.

With respect to younger donor age, most programs regard 18 years to be a firm lower age limit. Donors in their late teens and early 20s must be carefully evaluated for the maturity of their understanding of the donation process and to ensure they are not being subjected to overt or covert pressure. The issue of the long anticipated life span of young donors and with it the exposure to the later risk for renal disease is discussed below. It is a fair generalization to say that there is a tendency to be more conservation regarding donation from the healthy young, particularly from ethnic minorities, and less conservative regarding donation from older individuals, even if they have isolated medical abnormalities, such that it is unlikely that their life span and renal function would be impacted by donation in the years that await them.

Counseling of Older Transplant Recipients

The treatment options faced by elderly patients with advance chronic kidney disease are discussed in Chapters 1 and 8. Approximately 10% of all living donations are to recipients who are older than 65 years. Transplantation of living donor kidneys into recipients in their 70s or older can be practically and ethically challenging. The elderly transplant candidates may be faced with a difficult dilemma: to wait for many years for a deceased donor kidney with the knowledge that their medical condition may continue to deteriorate, or to turn to a young family member for kidney donation while they are still medically suitable for the surgery and young and robust enough to enjoy the transplant.

When the potential donor is considerably younger than the recipient, the following questions should also be addressed: Is it reasonable to transplant a kidney from a very young donor into an elderly recipient who will only benefit from the kidney for a very limited number of years? Should the inevitable limit on extra years of life gained by the recipient place any limitations to the living donor transplantation? There are no formal guidelines that address the acceptable age disparity between living donors and recipients. In most cases, it is best to leave the decision in the hands of an educated and informed potential donor. Alternative approaches to the issue of age disparity are discussed in the section on paired-exchange living donation.

When an elderly transplant candidate does consider a living donor transplant, it is advisable that the transplant be performed as early as possible to maximize the benefit of the procedure. Furthermore, transplantation within a timely period has been shown to increase overall life expectancy, quality-adjusted life expectancy, and comorbidities for transplant recipients of all ages, whereas prolonged waiting time greatly decreased the clinical and economic benefit of transplantation.

General Assessment

The universal medical goals in the kidney donation evaluation process are to ensure that the potential donor has the following characteristics:

- Is sufficiently healthy from both the medical and psychosocial point of view to undergo the surgical procedure
- Has normal kidney function with minimal future risk for kidney disease
- Represents negligible risk to the recipient in terms of communicable disease or malignancy transmission
- Is not at increased risk for medical conditions that might require treatments that could endanger his or her residual renal function

Living donor evaluation requires a thorough history and physical examination supplemented by laboratory testing, age-appropriate

TABLE	
7.3	Living Donor Medical Evaluation

Laboratory Tests
- Blood group, HLA typing, crossmatch
- Urinalysis and urine culture
- Twenty-four-hour urine collection for protein and creatinine clearance or glomerular filtration rate determination by nuclear medicine test
- Complete blood count, prothrombin time, partial thromboplastin time
- Comprehensive metabolic panel (electrolytes, transaminase levels, albumin, bilirubin, calcium, phosphorus, alkaline phosphatase, fasting blood glucose, fasting lipid profile, cholesterol, triglycerides.)
- Viral serologies: HIV, hepatitis B and C viruses, Epstein–Barr virus, cytomegalovirus, herpes simplex virus, RPR
- Human chorionic gonadotropin quantitative pregnancy test in women younger than 55 years
- Serum protein electrophoresis in prospective donors older than 60 years

Other Tests
- Electrocardiogram
- Chest radiograph
- Papanicolaou test (for women)
- Mammogram for women 40 years and older
- Renal imaging: spiral computed tomography (CT), CT angiogram, or magnetic resonance angiogram

Further Testing Depending on Age, History, Abnormal Laboratory Findings, and Family History Screening
- Colonoscopy if 50 years or older
- Cardiac screening: echocardiograph, nuclear medicine stress test
- Twenty-four-hour ambulatory blood pressure monitoring
- Renal biopsy
- Cystoscopy
- PPD skin test
- Screening for hypercoagulability
- Glucose tolerance test with family history of diabetes mellitus or risk factors for development of diabetes (see text)
- Screening for APO L1 G1/G2 mutation in African Americans (see text)

medical screening, and renal imaging (Table 7.3). Donor history or characteristics known to confer significant risk to either the donor or recipient can automatically preclude donation. There must be detailed history of any drug the patient is taking to include prescribed and over-the-counter medications, and supplements including protein and creatine.

Obvious contraindications should be determined at the beginning of the donor assessment before subjecting unqualified donors to unnecessary tests (Table 7.4). Female patients should not be evaluated while pregnant or planning to become pregnant in the near future. The appropriate postpartum time when donor evaluation may be resumed has not been determined, but if the donor so desires, it is reasonable to evaluate for donation 6 months postpartum. Desire for future pregnancy does not in

| TABLE 7.4 | Contraindications to Living Kidney Donation |

Absolute Contraindications
- Evidence of renal disease (glomerular filtration rate < 80 mL/min, microalbuminuria or overt proteinuria)
- Significant renal or urologic abnormalities
- Transmissible infectious disease (HIV infection, hepatitis B, hepatitis C)
- Active malignancy
- Chronic illness that places patient at significant risk to undergo surgery
- Poorly controlled psychiatric illness or active substance use
- Cognitive deficit
- Current pregnancy
- Hypertension, uncontrolled or requiring multiple medications or history of hypertension with end-organ damage
- Diabetes mellitus
- Recurrent nephrolithiasis or bilateral stones
- History of thrombotic disorders with risk factors for future events or inherited hypercoagulable states
- Age <18 years and mental inability to make an informed decision
- Evidence of acute symptomatic infection (until resolved)
- High suspicion of donor coercion
- High suspicion of illegal financial exchange between donor and recipient

Relative Contraindications
- Age < 18 or >70 years
- Borderline or mild hypertension (see text)
- Borderline urinary abnormalities in the absence of renal function impairment
- Single prior episode of nephrolithiasis without evidence of secondary risk
- Obesity
- Young donor with risk factors for future development of diabetes mellitus (see text)
- Jehovah's Witness patient
- Metabolic syndrome
- African-American donor with two mutated alleles of APO L 1 G1/G2

general contraindicate donation. Unilateral donor nephrectomy does not increase obstetrical risks or complications or reduce birth weight or incidence of preterm delivery. There is, however, evidence to suggest that live kidney donation increases the risk of gestational hypertension and preeclampsia (11%) compared with experience among otherwise similar healthy women (5%). Women of childbearing age should be informed of this risk and the supporting evidence.

EVALUATION OF FUTURE DONOR RISK

The systematic evaluation of future donor risk focuses on life span, renal function, and covert renal disease. Cardiovascular disease risk factors include hypertension, diabetes, and obesity; risk for communicable disease or malignancy transmission to the recipient; and assessment of surgical risks. Estimation of donor risk can only be, at the very best, an approximation. Donors cannot be their own controls and the choice of control groups is difficult. Decades may pass between kidney donation and the development of complications, impairing the accuracy of projections based on short-term observations.

Assessment of Renal Function and Covert Renal Disease
Glomerular Filtration Rate

Measurement of creatinine clearance based on a 24-hour urine collection is generally adequate to assess the donor's renal function, although some centers prefer iothalamate or diethylenetriamine pentaacetic acid (DTPA) clearance. Many centers start with a 24-hour urine collection for creatinine clearance and only proceed to a renal nuclear scan study in cases with borderline renal function. It must be noted, however, that elderly donors, donors with low muscle mass, and vegetarians may have a low creatinine clearance without intrinsic renal disease. Creatinine-based prediction equations are not reliable in the donor population with relatively normal renal function and should not be used as the sole estimate of glomerular filtration rate (GFR). CKD-EPI and cystatin-based estimations are in general considered to be more accurate than MDRD-based estimation. A 24-hour urine collection is the preferred method to assess renal function because it also offers accurate data for proteinuria as well.

Although there is no absolute consensus on the level of renal function below which a person would not be deemed an acceptable donor, most centers use a cutoff GFR of 80 mL/min/1.73 m². The dietary intake of protein should be at least 1 g of protein per kg/body weight since a low-protein diet may decrease creatinine clearance by as much as 10 mL/min. Considerations for the lower limit of renal function allowable for kidney donation include a predicted fall in GFR to 75% of predonation level and the normal decline in GFR with aging at a rate of 4 to 5 mL/min/1.73 m² per decade of life starting at age 20 years. Other criteria used to preclude kidney donation include a projected GFR with removal of one kidney at 80 years of less than 40 mL/min/1.73 m². Healthy vegetarians in general tend to have a lower creatinine clearance than meat-eaters. A high animal protein meal prior to the test can have a significant impact on the outcome.

Abnormal Urinalysis

Proteinuria greater than 250 mg/day, in general, is a sign of renal disease and precludes donation. The collection should be repeated and its accuracy checked when the result is abnormal. An overestimate of proteinuria should be suspected if 24-hour urine creatinine–to–body weight ratios are greater than 25 mg/kg (>20 μmol/kg), especially in those with low muscle mass. An underestimate of proteinuria may have occurred if 24-hour urine creatinine–to–body weight ratios are less than 15 mg/kg (<132 μmol/kg). In those with borderline high proteinuria, it is especially important to rule out undercollections. The spot protein-to-creatinine ratio of a single early-morning urine specimen provides an accurate quantitative measurement. A ratio of <0.2 mg albumin/mg creatinine (<22 mg albumin/mmol creatinine) equates to urine albumin <0.2 g/24 hours. A 24-hour collection of urine for protein remains the "gold-standard" for quantitation of proteinuria.

Transient causes of proteinuria, including fever, urinary tract infection, or intense exercise, should be excluded. Orthostatic proteinuria, defined as elevated urine protein with assumption of the upright posture and normal protein excretion during recumbency should be ruled out. This benign phenomenon usually occurs in younger age groups and does not necessarily preclude donation. Borderline high proteinuria can be further evaluated for microalbuminuria. The presence of microalbuminuria in such cases should preclude kidney donation.

Isolated microscopic hematuria, based on repeat analysis, is not, in itself, a contraindication to kidney donation. A survey of transplant centers in the United States indicated that over one-third of centers were willing to accept donor candidates with isolated microscopic hematuria and a negative urologic evaluation and renal biopsy. Asymptomatic hematuria is a relatively common finding and only approximately 2% of those with hematuria were subsequently found to have serious disease. The sensitivity of urine dipstick is comparable to the evaluation of the urine sediment, and a negative result reliably excludes the presence of hematuria. However, the test is prone to false-positive results from contaminated samples, myoglobinuria, or hemoglobinuria, and should be confirmed by examination of the urine sediment. The differential diagnosis of hematuria is large. It includes benign conditions, such as exercise, menstruation, and benign prostate hypertrophy. It can also occur with intrinsic renal diseases or abnormalities within the urinary tract. The concurrent presence of urinary casts or dysmorphic red blood cells with or without proteinuria is indicative of underlying intrinsic renal disease. A family history of renal disease, urinary tract infections, stones, and tumors should also be excluded. Donor candidates with persistent isolated microscopic hematuria may require a complete urologic evaluation. A cystoscopy to exclude bladder pathology may be necessary. In the absence of any specific abnormalities, a kidney biopsy may be indicated to rule out glomerular pathology such as Alport syndrome, thin basement membrane disease, and immunoglobulin A (IgA) nephropathy. The risk and cost intrinsic to renal biopsies must be considered in the overall risk for donation. If a full evaluation for persistent isolated microscopic hematuria is negative, further evaluation for donation may be resumed because the risk for progressive renal disease is very small. Young patients with isolated urinary abnormalities should generally be excluded from donation.

Pyuria and/or bacteruria require further investigation. Common causes of pyuria should be ruled out. The urine test should be repeated after proper instructions. Urinary tract infections (UTI) and asymptomatic bacteruria are more common in women, with about one-third having a UTI at some time. In males it is uncommon, other than in the first year of life and over the age of 60 years owing to prostatic hypertrophy. Pyuria is the best determinant of bacteruria requiring therapy.

In the face of persistent sterile pyuria, renal tuberculosis should be ruled out with three morning urine acid-fast bacilli cultures. If no obvious infectious or inflammatory source can be found, a renal biopsy should be considered to rule out interstitial nephritis or chronic pyelonephritis. Evidence for renal tuberculosis, interstitial nephritis, or pyelonephritis is a contraindication to donation.

Uric Acid

An elevated blood level of uric acid has been shown to be a predictor of decline in kidney function. Potential donors should be screened for their blood uric acid levels. Uric acid levels can rise postdonation and this is something that should be discussed with the donors especially if they have a history of gout.

Inherited Renal Disease

When renal failure in the recipient is owing to an inherited disease or there is a family history of renal disease, the focus should be on excluding the disease in the genetically related donor. Knowledge of the etiology of the recipient's renal disease is a critical part of donor evaluation. For some hereditary renal diseases, a clear family history or unequivocal biopsy findings can provide valuable information; for others, in which biopsy documentation of the recipient's underlying renal disease is lacking, family information regarding extrarenal manifestations, such as ocular and hearing abnormalities in Alport syndrome, may provide information invaluable to the decision-making process of kidney donation. In some cases, the presence of these diseases precludes transplantation from related donors. Some more common genetic abnormalities are considered here.

Autosomal Dominant Polycystic Kidney Disease

The most commonly encountered hereditary renal disease is autosomal dominant polycystic kidney disease (ADPKD). The diagnosis of ADPKD in a person at risk is defined by specific age-dependent criteria. The newly updated, unified criteria can be used for diagnosis of both ADPKD 1 and ADPKD 2 genotypes. In families of unknown genotype, the presence of three or more (unilateral or bilateral) renal cysts is sufficient for establishing the diagnosis in individuals aged 15 to 39 years, two or more cysts in each kidney is sufficient for individuals aged 40 to 59 years, and four or more cysts in each kidney is required for individuals over 60 years old. Conversely, fewer than two renal cysts in at-risk individuals aged 40 to 59 years is sufficient to exclude the disease.

For potential donors older than 30 years, it is safe to proceed with donor nephrectomy if ultrasound or computed tomography (CT) reveals no evidence of cysts. Renal ultrasound is a sensitive, relatively inexpensive and noninvasive method of screening but can miss cysts smaller than 1 cm. For potential donors between the ages of 20 and 30 years, a negative ultrasound alone does not rule out ADPKD, and donation cannot be recommended without other evidence supporting the absence of the disease. It has been suggested that the greater sensitivity of heavily T2-weighted magnetic resonance imaging (MRI) in detecting smaller cysts may reliably exclude ADPKD at younger ages. However, the diagnostic criteria for ADPKD based on MRI have not been established. Genetic studies, such as linkage analysis and direct DNA sequencing, are gold-standard diagnostic tests. These tests, however, are often not feasible, routinely available, or 100% sensitive. Linkage analysis is rarely performed because of the requirement for testing of multiple affected and unaffected family members. Direct DNA sequencing may yield a definitive result in only 70% of cases. Nonetheless, it is generally considered safe to proceed with kidney donation if both imaging studies and genetic testing exclude the presence of ADPKD. For more information on ADPKD testing, readers are referred to http://www.athenadiagnostic.com.

Alport Syndrome
Most cases of Alport syndrome are transmitted as an X-linked recessive trait. In 15% of cases, the transmission is autosomal recessive. There are many different mutations that can lead to Alport syndrome, but they all cause a defect in the α_5 chain of type IV collagen in the basement membrane, which can lead to glomerulosclerosis and eventual renal failure. The mutation can be associated with basement membrane abnormalities in the eye and sensorineural part of the ear, causing ocular abnormalities such as lenticonus and deafness, respectively. Persons being evaluated as kidney donors with a family history of Alport syndrome need to be carefully screened for hematuria, hypertension, sensorineural hearing loss, and ocular abnormalities (anterior lenticonus, cataracts, retinal lesions). The absence of hematuria in an adult male 20 years of age or older essentially excludes the presence of the genetic defect. Adult female siblings with normal urinalysis have a low risk for being carriers and are acceptable as donors. However, female relatives with persistent hematuria are most likely carriers of the mutation and have a 10% to 15% risk for developing chronic kidney disease. Donation in the latter group is not advisable. Although genetic testing is possible, it is not readily available and generally not performed. Proteinuria is also associated with increased risk of renal failure in Alport families and should be considered exclusion criteria.

Fabry Disease
Fabry disease is an X-linked error of metabolism with systemic manifestations. It was considered an X-linked recessive disease, but now is has been shown that it can affect both males and females—heterozygote females are no longer considered carriers. Fabry disease usually lead to ESRD. Disease usually presents in early childhood in both male and female. However, heterozygote female patients with Fabry disease may present later in life and with vague symptoms. It has been shown that Fabry disease is underlying cause of renal failure in a significant percentage of ESRD patients with unknown cause. In assessing potential living donors, a thorough familial history with a focus on Fabry disease should be performed. In suspected cases, the donor must be screened for Fabry disease.

Thin Basement Membrane Disease
A biopsy diagnosis of thin basement membrane disease (TBMD) can result from an evaluation for persistent or strong family history of microscopic hematuria. Although TBMD generally has a benign prognosis, the impact of hyperfiltration after uninephrectomy may increase the risk for renal dysfunction. Donation from individuals with TBMD remains controversial. Prospective donors with TBMD may still be considered if they are older than 40 years of age and IgA nephropathy or Alport syndrome have been excluded. Early biopsy findings of female carriers of X-linked Alport syndrome and TBMD, however, may be difficult to differentiate histologically. Clinical characteristics that

T A B L E 7.5	Clinical Characteristics that Help Distinguish Thin Basement Membrane Disease from IgA Nephropathy and Alport Syndrome

Thin Basement Membrane Disease
- Gross hematuria uncommon
- Positive family history of hematuria
- Negative family history of renal failure

IgA Nephropathy
- Episodic gross hematuria common
- Family history of hematuria may occur in isolated cases
- May have family history of renal failure

Alport Syndrome
- May have episodic gross hematuria
- Typically with positive family history of renal failure
- Deafness may be present in families in which there is an X-linked mode of inheritance

help to distinguish TBMD from IgA nephropathy and Alport syndrome are shown in Table 7.5. The presence of hypertension, proteinuria, or both precludes donation. Prospective donors must be counseled that although TBMD typically has a benign outcome, slowly progressive renal insufficiency may occur. Potential donors should also be advised that long-term donor risk remains unknown and that any effect of TBMD on allograft function remains unclear. Development of glomerular diseases (most commonly IgA nephropathy) in the allograft organ may occur following transplantation from patients with TBMD.

Familial Primary Glomerulonephropathies
Familial forms of glomerulonephritis should be considered when more than one family member is affected with renal disease. Idiopathic steroid-resistant focal segmental glomerulosclerosis (FSGS), a glomerulopathy linked to mutations of various podocyte-associated proteins, is probably the best described familial primary glomerulonephritis. Other forms of familial glomerulonephritis such as IgA nephropathy, membranoproliferative glomerulonephritis, and familial membranous nephropathy have also been described. Genetic analyses for some of these conditions are available.

Systemic Lupus Erythematosus
Systemic lupus erythematosus (SLE) occurs in approximately 12% or more of first-degree relatives. Prospective living-related donors should be screened for antinuclear antibody (ANA), complement levels, and abnormal urinary findings. A history of deep vein thrombosis (DVT), stroke, pulmonary embolism, fetal loss, thrombocytopenia, hemolytic anemia, or livedo reticularis should lead to testing for antiphospholipid syndrome. A family member of a patient with SLE who has a positive ANA has an about 40-fold increased risk for developing lupus and generally should be excluded from donation. In unrelated potential donors, an isolated elevated ANA level is not considered a contra indication for donation.

Sickle Cell Trait
The literature on the potential risks to live kidney donors with sickle cell trait is sparse. Many programs do not routinely screen donors for sickle cell trait, but some do exclude donors with sickle cell trait when the diagnosis is made. There are currently no guidelines with respect to sickle trait screening, and center practice regarding exclusion of donors with sickle cell trait varies widely. Nonetheless, prospective donors with unexplained hematuria, women with recurrent bacteriuria or pyelonephritis, and those with a family history of sickle cell disease or sickle cell trait should be screened for sickle cell trait. It is probably prudent to exclude prospective donors with documented recurrent bacteriuria or pyelonephritis and those with evidence of papillary necrosis on imaging studies. Young prospective donors should be forewarned of the increased risk for medullary carcinoma, and regular postdonation follow-up is advised.

APOL 1 Gene Mutations
Individuals of African ancestry are known to be more predisposed to kidney disease. The observation that polymorphisms in the APOL1 gene, that confer increased risk of kidney disease, are disproportionately represented among African Americans thus has major implications for the evaluation of potential kidney donors of African ancestry. African-American kidney donors are at greater risk of developing ESRD than their European-American counterparts and it has been recommended that younger African-American potential donors and those with a significant family history of ESRD should be tested for the presence of two risks alleles—homozygosity or compound heterozygosity for APOL1 variants (G1 and G2). Two of these mutations (G1 and G2) which are found in 13% of African-American population are associated with increased risk of nondiabetic glomerosclerosis and FSGS and are associated with a steeper decline in GFR compared to non-Black population. Furthermore, renal allografts from these donors have an increased risk of rejection and transplant failure, including the renal allografts from deceased donors. The more prominent the African ancestry, the higher is the risk of renal failure in patients with two variants of these genes. Caution is advised regarding child to parent kidney donation in young African Americans since these potential donors may not display final kidney phenotypes until they are older.

Nephrolithiasis
The routine evaluation of donors should identify the presence of kidney stones. The obvious concern for kidney donation in a person with a prior history of kidney stones is the potential for stone recurrence in the remaining kidney with resultant obstruction. However, prospective donors with a distant history of stones (>10 years) but without metabolic abnormalities associated with stone formation (e.g., hypercalcemia, hyperuricemia, hyperoxaluria, hypocitraturia, or metabolic acidosis) are at low risk for stone recurrence and may be acceptable as living donors. An asymptomatic potential donor with a current single stone may be suitable for donation if the current stone size is less than 1.5 cm or potentially removable during transplantation. In addition, further

stone evaluation must reveal no evidence of metabolic abnormalities, urinary tract infection, nephrocalcinosis, and/or anatomic defects that may lead to infection struvite stones.

Prospective donors with a history of a kidney stone must be advised of increased risk for recurrence (50% in 5 to 7 years). The presence of underlying medical disorders associated with a high risk for recurrent stones such as cystinuria, primary or enteric hyperoxaluria, inflammatory bowel disease, and sarcoidosis contraindicates donation. A history of struvite stones contraindicates donation because these stones are associated with infection that are difficult to eradicate. A history of a single stone episode associated with treated primary hyperparathyroidism and normocalcemia does not necessarily preclude donation. The presence of nephrocalcinosis, bilateral stones, or history of stone recurrence despite preventive therapy contraindicates donation.

CT of the kidneys should be used to detect the current presence of stones or nephrocalcinosis in persons with a history of stone disease. Plain films cannot adequately assess radiolucent and small stones, whereas ultrasound can miss detection of the latter. Timed urine collections to assess metabolic abnormalities are not as predictive of the risk for recurrent stones as clinical parameters such as age and amount of time passed since an initial episode. Nevertheless, the data obtained may aid dietary counseling and selection of appropriate therapy. A stone initially detected in a person older than 50 is unlikely to recur. In contrast, the risk for stone recurrence is higher in individuals younger than 35 and must be considered during the donor evaluation process.

Hypertension
In general, screening for hypertension in a potential donor includes blood pressure measurement on three separate occasions. Elevated blood pressure, as defined by the Joint National Committee (JNC 7) for the diagnosis of hypertension, requires further evaluation with ambulatory blood pressure monitoring (ABPM) to exclude white-coat hypertension. The donor should have a mean awake blood pressure less than 135/85 mm Hg and sleep blood pressure less than 120/75 mm Hg. Most transplant program exclude prospective donors with blood pressures greater than 140/90 from donation. An echocardiogram may be considered to evaluate for cardiac hypertrophy in cases with borderline high blood pressure, or abnormalities suggesting cardiomegaly or left ventricular hypertrophy on chest radiograph or electrocardiogram, respectively. A history of mild hypertension may be acceptable for donation if the prospective donor is not African American and is older than 50 years without evidence of microalbuminuria or end-organ damage. In these circumstances, the risk for hypertension-induced chronic kidney disease within the prospective donor's lifetime is very small. The prospective donor with mild hypertension must have normal GFR for age and blood pressure controlled with lifestyle and behavioral modifications or use of no more than a single antihypertensive agent or a low dose of a combination agent. The donor should be counseled that the BP might go up slightly postdonation. Any secondary cause of hypertension should be ruled out and treated if identified before proceeding with the evaluation.

Diabetes

Diabetes mellitus is defined as having a fasting plasma glucose (FPG) level of at least 126 mg/dL ($\geq$7.0 mmol/L), or a plasma glucose level of at least 200 mg/dL (11.1 mmol/L) 2 hours after 75-g oral glucose challenge (oral glucose tolerance test), confirmed by repeat testing on a different day. FPG values between 100 and 125 mg/dL (5.6 to 6.9 mmol/L) define impaired fasting glucose (IFG), and 2-hour plasma glucose values between 140 and 199 mg/dL (7.8 mmol/L to 11.1 mmol/dL) define impaired glucose tolerance (IGT). Diabetes guidelines acknowledge that both IFG and IGT are important predictive factors for the progression to overt diabetes and well-established risk factors for microvascular and cardiovascular disease. Hb A1c, which estimates the glycemic control of the preceding 8 to 12 weeks, is a convenient measure since there is no need for serial samplings and there is no day-to-day fluctuation in its level. Hb A1c levels are now widely accepted as the best tool for screening diabetes and prediabetes.

All potential living donors should have FPG estimation. Prospective donors with an FPG between 100 and 125 mg/dL and those with risk factors for the development of diabetes in the absence of abnormal FPG should be evaluated with an oral glucose tolerance test (OGTT) and HbA1c. The latter include individuals with first-degree relative with type 2 diabetes, history of gestational diabetes or large birth weight (>9 pounds at delivery), obesity defined as having a body mass index (BMI) of more than 30, fasting hypertriglyceridemia of at least 250 mg/dL, high-density lipoprotein (HDL) level of no more than 35 mg/dL, or blood pressure higher than 140/90 mm Hg. Donors younger than 40 years with a second-degree relative with type 2 diabetes mellitus should also undergo OGTT and HbA1c.

Most transplant programs regard established diabetes mellitus as a contraindication to living donation, and many centers exclude individuals deemed high-risk. Absolute and relative contraindications to donation in the presence of glucose intolerance are shown in Table 7.6. Individuals with IFG and IGT should be counseled on lifestyle modifications, including weight control, diet, exercise, and tobacco avoidance. Prospective donors with IFG or IGT should be assessed on an individual basis, criteria for older patients may be liberalized. Donation is not recommended in individuals with mild or borderline IGT and additional risk factors. Individuals with blood glucose in the high range of IFG probably should not donate because of the greater tendency for deterioration. There should be particular concern for young donors of Hispanic, Native American, and Pacific Island ethnicity in the United States and of East Asian origin in the United Kingdom. Some programs will not consider prospective donors from these groups until their 30s. All prospective donors should be forewarned that both IFG and IGT are important predictive factors for progression to overt diabetes.

Women with a history of gestational diabetes have a high lifetime risk for developing type 2 diabetes—as high as 50% to 70% in some series—with the greatest increase in risk in the first 5 years after delivery, and a plateau in risk after 10 years. Therefore, acceptance for donation and counseling for future risk can be dictated by these time frames. An OGTT in conjunction with stimulated insulin levels may be

TABLE 7.6	Absolute and Relative Contraindications to Donation in Prospective Donors with Impaired Glucose Tolerance

Absolute Contraindications
- Known diabetes mellitus
- Fasting plasma glucose (FPG) level ≥ 126 mg/dL (7.0 mmol/L) on two or more occasions
- Plasma glucose level > 200 mg/dL (11.1 mmol/L) 2 hours after 75 g oral glucose challenge (oral glucose tolerance test) on two or more occasions

Relative Contraindications*
- Impaired fasting glucose (IFG), defined as FPG values between 110 and 125 mg/dL (6.1–6.9 mmol/L)
- Impaired glucose tolerance (IGT), defined as 2-hour plasma glucose values between 140 and 199 mg/dL (7.8 mmol/L to 11.1 mmol/dL)
- Individuals with IFG or IGT should be counseled on lifestyle modifications, including weight control, diet, exercise, and tobacco avoidance
- Prospective donors with IFG should be assessed on an individual basis
- Donation generally not recommended in:
  - Individuals with mild or borderline IGT and additional risk factors (first-degree relatives of patients with type 2 diabetes mellitus, obesity, gestational diabetes mellitus, dyslipidemia, belonging to an ethnic group with a high frequency of diabetes)
  - Individuals with blood glucose in the high range of impaired glucose tolerance (110–125 mg/dL, 6.1–6.9 mmol/L) should probably not donate because of the greater tendency for deterioration
- Prospective donors should be forewarned that both IFG and IGT are important predictive factors for the progression to overt diabetes

*Criteria may be liberalized for potential donors over the age of 50 in the absence of other abnormalities

more helpful in determining risk than an OGTT alone because some women with a history of gestational diabetes may have evidence of insulin resistance that may portend a higher risk for future development of overt diabetes.

Obesity
Obesity, defined as having a BMI greater than 30, is associated with increased risk for surgical complications as well as future medical problems including diabetes, hypertension, nephrolithiasis, glomerular disease with associated albuminuria or overt proteinuria, and end-stage renal disease (ESRD). Among obese individuals, an increased risk for proteinuria and renal insufficiency has been reported following unilateral nephrectomy. The relative risk for developing ESRD is three fold for a BMI between 30 and 35 and nearly five fold for a BMI of 35 to 40. The impact of other medical issues that may be present in this group, such as cardiovascular disease, sleep apnea, or fatty liver, should also be carefully assessed. Obese potential donors should be encouraged to lose weight before kidney donation. Donation is not advisable in the presence of other comorbid conditions. Approximately half of programs in the United States regard a BMI greater than 35 as a contraindication to donation, and some report excluding donors with a BMI over 30 (See Wong et al. in Selected Readings). BMI may be unreliable as a risk predictor and waist to hip ratio might be a better predictor, especially of cardiovascular outcomes.

Metabolic Syndrome and Fatty Liver

Metabolic syndrome is a common disorder which has various defini-tions. The American Heart Association and the National Heart, Lung and Blood Institute define metabolic syndrome as large waist size (40 inches or above in male and 35 inches or above in female) plus two of the following:

1. Hyperlidipemia, defined as TG $\geq$ 150 mg/dL or treatment with a lipid-lowering agent
2. HDL $\leq$ 40 mg/dL
3. Systolic blood pressure $\geq$ 135 mm Hg
4. Diastolic blood pressure $\geq$ 85 mm Hg
5. Fasting blood glucose $\geq$ 100 mg/dL.

Metabolic syndrome is a proven risk factor for cardiovascular disease. In addition, there are several concerns with regard to living donors with metabolic syndrome. Metabolic syndrome has been associated with decreased glomerular density, hyperfiltration, glomerulosclerosis, and a decline in GFR following uninephrectomy. Although metabolic syndrome is not, in itself, considered a contraindication for kidney donation in older donors, it is wise to consider it a contraindication in young donors, particularly if they are from at-risk ethnicities. All potential donors with metabolic syndrome should make appropriate lifestyle changes and show clinical improvement before donation.

Nonalcoholic fatty liver disease now affects 25% to 45% of population worldwide and approximately 30% in the United States. The prevalence is higher in patients with metabolic syndrome. Although it is generally considered a relatively benign process, approximately 4% progress to cirrhosis. Liver function should be assessed in all potential donors, especially if they tend to obesity or metabolic syndrome. Fatty liver should be evaluated to rule out any treatable cause besides lifestyle changes. Hepatitis in the setting of fatty liver should be considered a contraindication to donation unless it resolves or can be successfully treated. Alcohol consumption must be curtailed.

Smoking and Recreational Drugs

Current cigarette smokers in general are not considered as suitable donors. Smoking a risk factor for declining renal function in donors and studies have shown that there is significant risk of rejection and decreased function in kidney allografts taken from donors who have been smokers. Policies on marijuana use vary among programs but occasional recreational use should not necessarily exclude donation (see Chapter 18). Drug abuse including alcohol, cocaine, and meth are contraindications to donation and these patients should undergo a successful detoxification process before they are considered for do-nation. Potential donors requiring chronic narcotic use for pain relief must undergo psychiatric evaluation and are generally not suitable living organ donors.

Risk for Communicable Disease or Malignancy Transmission to the Recipient

The presence of chronic viral infections, such as HIV, hepatitis B, and hepatitis C, in the donor contraindicates donation because of the high risk for disease transmission to the recipient (see Chapter 12) and the risk for virus-induced renal disease in the donor. Transmission of human herpesvirus-8 (HHV-8) to the recipient has been associated with the development of T-cell leukemia and spastic paraparesis, and Kaposi sarcoma, respectively. The presence of active infection is a contraindication to living donation. International donors should be evaluated for diseases that might be endemic to their areas. It is recommended that potential donors who test positive for exposure to *Trypanosoma cruzi* (Chagas disease), which is endemic is Mexico, Central and South America, are excluded from donation as there is no cure for the disease which can be fatal in immunosuppressed transplant patients. However, some studies show that in the absence of acute or chronic symptoms of disease in seropositive donors, prophylaxis of recipients with benznidazole is been successful in preventing infection. Donors who test positive for antibody to Strongyloides can be treated with a single dose of ivermectin and are then able to proceed with donation with no additional risk to the recipient. The presence of active infection is a contraindication to living donation. Fully treated syphilis, tuberculosis, latent Epstein–Barr virus (EBV), West Nile Virus (WNV), and cytomegalovirus (CMV) do not preclude donation. Patients should be asked about high-risk sexual behavior.

Potential kidney donors should be screened for both personal and family history of cancer. They should undergo standard age-appropriate screening tests as recommended by the American Cancer Society and equivalent international organizations. Certain types of cancer have characteristics that would exclude any person with a prior history from donation. These cancers include those that are considered incurable, known to have a lengthy disease-free interval before possible recurrence, or reported to have the potential for increased virulence in the immunocompromised patient. A history of melanoma, renal cell carcinoma or urologic malignancy, choriocarcinoma, hematologic malignancies, gastric cancer, lung cancer, breast cancer, Kaposi sarcoma, or monoclonal gammopathy precludes living donation. Patients with certain local neoplasms, such as Stage 0 Ductal Carcinoma In Situ (DCIS) of the breast, encapsulated thyroid neoplasms, in situ squamous cell skin cancer or cervical carcinoma, may be acceptable as donors if the specific cancer is deemed cured and the potential for transmission is excluded. Oncology consultation is advisable. The effects of prior treatment of the malignancy on the prospective donor's renal reserve as well as potential nephrotoxicity from future treatment in case of recurrence are additional concerns. Patients at increased risk of skin cancer are advised to have a full skin survey to protect both the recipient and the donor.

Medical Clearance for Surgery

Certain characteristics and medical problems in prospective donors potentially increase the risks for postoperative complications and preclude donation. In general, underlying problems such as coronary artery disease (even if corrected), cerebrovascular disease, and significant chronic pulmonary disease increase the risk for having perioperative morbidity and contraindicate donation. Potential donors with multiple risk factors for coronary artery disease warrant noninvasive

T A B L E 7.7	Suggested Cardiovascular Evaluation of a Potential Living Donor

Exclusion Criteria as Donor
- Diabetes mellitus
- Untreated and/or symptomatic coronary artery disease
- Dilated cardiomyopathy
- Compensated or decompensated heart failure
- Untreated and/or clinically significant arrhythmias
- Untreated and/or symptomatic clinically significant valvular heart diseases

Indication for Cardiac Structural Evaluation with Two-Dimensional Echocardiogram
- Abnormal cardiac murmurs
- History of syncope, dizziness, palpitations, or short of breath
- Indications for Holter monitoring:
  - History of arrhythmias or possible arrhythmias
  - History of syncope, dizziness, or palpitations

Indications for Cardiac Stress Testing*
- Older age (>45 years in men or >55 years in women). May vary, depending on:
  - Donor's routine activity level
  - History of smoking
  - Family history of premature coronary artery disease
  - History of dyslipidemia (should be included in risk factor assessment; dyslipidemia alone is not an indication for cardiac stress testing)*
  - History of hypertension
  - Abnormal electrocardiogram (left ventricular hypertrophy, left bundle branch block, ST-T abnormalities)

*One or more of the indications listed or at the clinician's discretion.

screening. Suggested cardiovascular testing of potential living donors is outlined in Table 7.7.

Potential donors who smoke should be instructed to stop for at least 4 weeks before the surgical procedure to decrease pulmonary complications and strongly urged to quit permanently to decrease future health risks. Some transplantation centers will not accept a potential donor who continues to smoke. Pulmonary function testing for prospective donors is not routinely indicated unless the history or physical examination is suggestive of lung disease.

Coagulation Disorders

A history of hypercoagulability significantly increases the risk for perioperative thrombotic complications and may contraindicate donation. Persons with a family history of thrombotic disease or personal history of one episode of venous thrombosis or recurrent miscarriage should be screened for the presence of risk factors that would increase the risk for future events. Common factors to be considered include abnormal activated protein C resistance ratio associated with factor V Leiden mutation; lupus anticoagulant or anticardiolipin antibody; or prothrombin gene mutation (FII-20210). However, a person heterozygous for factor V Leiden mutation without previous thrombotic disease is not necessarily excluded from donation because the risk for complication is low. Individuals who have had a first confirmed episode of DVT and who are heterozygous or homozygous for the Leiden factor V mutation demonstrate, respectively, a 7-fold and an 80-fold increase in the relative risk for DVT. Appropriate perioperative prophylaxis to prevent thrombotic complications, as well as discussion of the significance of this abnormality, is advised. Disorders requiring chronic anticoagulation contraindicate donation.

LONG-TERM POSTNEPHRECTOMY ISSUES

Long-Term Risk for Chronic Kidney Disease and Life Expectancy

Within days to weeks after uninephrectomy, hyperfiltration in the remaining kidney increases the GFR to about 75% to 80% of predonation value: the amount of compensation is dictated by age-related renal reserve. Urine albumin excretion, attributable to single nephron hyperfiltration from reduced renal mass, may be elevated but is usually low grade and not associated with a higher risk for renal dysfunction. Similar to the nondonating population, an additional 5 mL per minute loss in GFR per decade occurred after donating. A systematic review, meta-analysis, and meta-regression study conducted by the Donor Nephrectomy Outcomes Research (DONOR) Network (see Garg and colleagues in Selected Readings) revealed that 7 years after donation, the average GFR was 86 mL per minute, and the average urine protein was about 150 mg/Postdonation studies that extend up to 12 years have shown rates of ESRD similar to those observed in the general population. However, comparison of ESRD risk between living kidney donors and the general population is not relevant since prospected donors are only accepted for donation if their risk of ESRD is determined to be minimal.

The risk for future development of chronic kidney disease and subsequent progression to ESRD in the remaining single kidney has always been a major concern for prospective donors and their advocates. A major review of the topic by Nguyen et al. in 2007 (see Selected Readings) quoted a mortality risk of 1/3,000 and an incidence of ESRD of 1/500 and claimed that the procedure was "reasonably safe". Since that time, however, several large studies have been reported that permit a much more refined consideration of donor risk.

Short-term donor mortality risk is small, less than that following a low-risk-level surgical procedure such as cholecystectomy. Long-term risk is much more difficult to assess because of the absence of a readily available control group and the decades of follow-up required, particularly in young donors. Certain pivotal studies are worthy of mention. In a Norwegian study by Mjoen et al. (see Selected Readings), kidney donors were found to be at increased long-term risk for ESRD, cardiovascular, and all-cause mortality compared with a control group of nondonors who would have been eligible for donation though the relative risk was small (see Fig. 7.2) and did not manifest for 10 to 15 years following donation. In a US study of nearly 100,000 kidney donors by Muzaale et al. (see Selected Readings), an increased risk of ESRD was found when the donors were compared to a matched group of healthy nondonors, though the magnitude of the absolute risk was small. Grams et al. (see Selected Readings) calculated that the 15-year observed risk of ESRD among kidney donors in the United States was

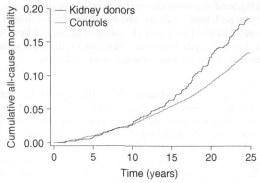

FIGURE 7.2 Cumulative mortality risk in kidney donors and controls, adjusted for year of donation. Controls are matched to donors for age, sex, systolic blood pressure, body mass index, and smoking status. (Reprinted from Mjoen G, Hallan S, Hartmann A, et al. Long-term risks for kidney donors. Kidney Int 2014;86:162–167, with permission from Elsevier.)

3.5 to 5.3 times as high as the projected risk in the absence of donation. The risk was highest in the youngest age groups, particularly among young African Americans. The authors of this study have developed an online risk tool to help evaluate, counsel, and accept living donor candidates (www.transplantmodels.com/esrdrisk): the value of this tool however, has not been definitively established.

These, and other, studies have led to some reevaluation and soul-searching in the living donor professional community. The studies also allow for a more granular assessment of risk, and along with it, better education of donors and their families. It has become clear that prediction of long-term risk is much more difficult in young donors than in older donors who have less time to be exposed to the impact of nephrectomy on GFR. Donors who are biologically related to recipients with immune-related kidney disease, African-American donors, and donors with ethnically associated risk factors of diabetes and hypertension are at increased risk, particularly if they are young. On the other hand, risk may have been previously overestimated in older donors with comorbidities that are highly unlikely to lead to ESRD in their remaining anticipated life span.

Hypertension

The incidence of hypertension requiring treatment increases with time following kidney donation, but most studies suggest a similar frequency compared with an age-matched population. A meta-analysis of more than 5,000 living kidney donors with an average follow-up of 7 years revealed that the donors may experience a 5-mm Hg increase in blood pressure (over that anticipated with normal aging) within 5 to 10 years after donation; this finding is clinically insignificant in most patients. Nonetheless, whether an increase in blood pressure from kidney donation increases cardiovascular disease risk remains to be defined. According to the Systolic Blood Pressure Intervention Trial (SPRINT), among patients at high risk for cardiovascular events but without diabetes, targeting a systolic blood pressure of less than 120 mm Hg, as compared to less than

140 mm Hg, results in lower rates of fatal and nonfatal major cardiovascular events and death from any cause. Healthy kidney donors would not typically fall into the "high risk" category as defined by this study. All in all, it would appear reasonable to target a systolic blood pressure of 130 mm Hg or less for long-term follow-up of donors.

Pregnancy

Concern about the impact of kidney donation on pregnancy and fertility is often an unspoken concern among female potential donors of childbearing age: the issue should be addressed proactively. Women of childbearing age should be told that unilateral donor nephrectomy should not have an effect on fertility, outcome of future pregnancies, incidence of preterm delivery, or low birth-weight. A greater incidence of preeclampsia, however, has been reported (11% in donors compared to 5% in matched non-donors). It is advisable to delay pregnancy for at least 6 months to allow for maximal compensatory hypertrophy of the single kidney and prudent to obtain early prenatal care with screening for hypertension, urinary abnormalities, and renal function. The desire for future pregnancy does not need to dictate the selection of which kidney to use for donation.

Long-Term Medical Care

In the United States, transplant centers are required to report follow-up donors at discharge (or 6 weeks postdonation, whichever comes first) 6 months, 1 year, and 2 years after donation. Donors can do these follow-ups with their local physicians and contact the transplant center for any recommendations. Recommendations for future medical care and risk modification for a kidney donor are not much different from those for the general population. Routine checkups, cancer screening appropriate for age, regular aerobic exercise, weight reduction, tobacco avoidance, and excessive alcohol abstinence should be emphasized. They should be advised to follow a healthy and balanced lifestyle. They should be provided with resources in case they are interested in learning more. Kidney donors with established medical issues before donation, such as mild hypertension, history of nephrolithiasis, or obesity, should have more frequent follow-up, and it could be argued that they should not be donors if they do not have access to such follow-up. Donors should be discouraged from using high-protein diets for weight loss or protein supplements for body building because they may contribute to hyper-filtration injury. They should be advised to avoid long-term regular use of nonsteroidal anti-inflammatory drugs. Registries for the long-term follow-up of donors are available. Donors should be warned that their serum creatinine values may rise by several decimal points, with a fall of estimated GFR, which can be a source of unnecessary anxiety.

Part II: Psychosocial Evaluation and Advocacy

The psychosocial evaluation is an important initial step in the evaluation of the potential donor (see also Chapters 18 and 21). It also presents a valuable forum for fulfilling the tenets of informed consent, exploring donor motivation, and excluding coercion. Significant psychiatric problems that would impair the person's ability to give informed consent or that might be negatively affected by the stress of surgery are considered contraindications to living donation (see Chapter 18, Table 18.2). The social support of the potential donor should be deemed adequate. The psychosocial evaluation of so-called nondirected or altruistic donors (see below) and donors who do not have a significant personal relationship with the recipient is particularly important because these donors may not enjoy the psychological gain of seeing the recipient benefit from their altruism (see Chapter 18). Most donors can look forward to stable or improved sense of psychological well-being and can be told of such. Depression is uncommon: donors may enjoy a so-called "halo" effect.

In the United States, the national Organ Procurement and Transplant Network (OPTN) mandates that a psychosocial assessment be performed on all potential living donors by a Master's degree prepared or licensed clinical social worker, psychologist or psychiatrist prior to donation, and it is often one of the first steps a potential donor takes during the initial evaluation process. This evaluation must include the documentation of:

- Potential issues that might complicate the living donor's recovery, including mental health issues that could be identified as a risk factors for a poor psychosocial outcome
- Evaluation for the presence of possible behaviors that may increase risk for disease transmission as defined by the US Public Health Guidelines
- If increased risk behaviors are identified, the potential donor is advised about disclosure of such behaviors to the recipient, and offered the option of withdrawing from the process without disclosure
- A review of the living donor's history of alcohol, smoking, and drug use
- The identification of factors that warrant either educational or therapeutic intervention prior to the final decision is made regarding donation
- Determination that the potential living donor understands both the short- and long-term medical and psychosocial risks for both the donor and the recipient
- An assessment of whether the decision to donate is free from any undue pressure or inducement by exploring the nature of the relationship, if any, between donor and recipient
- An assessment of the donor's ability to make an informed decision and ability to cope with the stress of major surgery and hospitalization. This includes an evaluation of the donor's plan for recovery with emotional, social, and financial support available as recommended
- A review of the potential donor's occupation, social support, health insurance/access to healthcare, and living situation
- Special consideration must be given to the psychosocial evaluation of young donors (under age 26) to include level of maturity, economic independence, level of education, and career or job stability

The initial psychosocial evaluation should be conducted in a private area with no other persons present. Involvement of family members or close friends (collateral interviews) can be included after the initial assessment, especially as it related to post donation care. When the psychosocial evaluation results in recommendations for any inter-vention prior to donation (e.g., alcohol or drug rehabilitation, mental health treatment) the potential donor should have the opportunity to return for a second evaluation with the provider who made the rec-ommendations to determine if the proposed recommendations have been met. It is often a good prognostic sign when the donor attends the recipient's pretransplantation evaluation appointments. The initial approach to the potential donor should ideally come from the patient and not the patient's nephrologist, transplant physician, or surgeon. In cases in which patients hesitate to approach family members, the nephrologist and transplant team should be prepared to facilitate the discussion of donation.

As the number of emotionally or biologically unrelated donors increases each year, the psychosocial evaluation of the nondirected or "Good Samaritan" donor has required a change in practice, necessitating a more in-depth evaluation regarding motivations for donating, and in the case of the nondirected donor, the issue of valuable consideration (see Chapter 19) must be addressed carefully.

Living donors may be reimbursed for legitimate expenses incurred as a result of donation and preparation for donation, such as travel and lodging. In the case of low income donors and recipients, finan-cial assistance may be available through the National Living Donor Assistance Center (NLDAC). In the United States, all medical costs directly associated with donation are covered by the recipient's health insurance. In 1999, the Organ Donor Leave Act was signed into law, al-lowing federal employees to take up to 30 days of paid leave as a result of organ donation. Many states have enacted donor leave laws that extend similar benefits to state and private sector employees, including tax credits or deductions. Some countries have more extensive forms of financial coverage. The topic of "financial neutrality" for living donors is discussed in Part IV.

The Role of the Independent Living Donor Advocate (ILDA)

The concept of a donor advocacy can be historically found in the earliest days of transplantation when a separate team was assembled to care for the living donor. Recommendations for donor care have since become more formalized, and in 2007 the Centers for Medicare and Medicaid Services (CMS) mandated that all transplant centers utilize an ILDA or team (IDAT) who serves to protect the rights of all living donors and potential living donors. The ILDA is defined as a skill set, not a profession, and can be a social worker, chaplain, nurse, psychologist, or physician.

The role of the ILDA is to be as an advocate for patient protection, and a safeguard for informed consent. The ILDA must be independent from recipient services and pressures often felt in high volume transplant centers, and at the same time knowledgeable regarding transplantation to promote donor understanding and informed consent.

The ILDA must:

- Be independent from the transplant recipient team
- Advocate for the rights of the living donor
- Have knowledge of living donation, transplantation, medical ethics, informed consent, and the potential impact of external pressures on the decision to donate
- Insure that the donor has received information on the informed consent process, evaluation process, surgical procedure, medical and psychosocial risks for donor and recipient, follow-up requirements
- Document that all of the above requirements have been met and that each of the topics has been reviewed

The role of the ILDA continues to evolve, and in some cases remains controversial, significantly in regard to possessing a narrowly defined "veto power" in circumstances when a potential donor is at high risk for coercion, uninformed about risk, or deemed unwilling.

Employment and Insurance

Most donors can return to their prior employment without limitation. In the United States, the federal government and many private employers provide employees with up to 30 paid working days after organ donation. Donors engaged in heavy physical labor may have some difficulty after open nephrectomy; this possibility should be discussed before the procedure and may be a particular problem in developing countries without laparoscopic donation potential (see Chapter 22). In general, kidney donors do not have insurability issues in terms of higher rates or an inability to obtain insurance. Any problems encountered are most likely attributable to the insurance company's incomplete knowledge regarding donor outcome and should prompt contact and education by the transplantation program. Most branches of the military will allow a person on active duty to donate a kidney and remain in the service, but it may affect the future ability to participate in all aspects of the military. A recent history of donation may preclude military recruitment. Future career plans should be discussed with prospective donors.

The Living Donor Protection Act (H.R. 4616) was introduced in the House of Representatives and the Senate on February 2016. The bill prohibits insurance companies from denying or limiting life, disability and long-term care insurance and from charging higher premiums to living organ donors. The bill also clarifies that living organ donors may use time granted through the Family and Medical Leave Act (FMLA) to recover from transplant surgery. The bill also directs the Department of Health and Human Services to add information on these new protections to its materials to encourage more Americans to consider living donation. Passage of the bill is anticipated.

Part III: Surgical Issues in Living Kidney Donation

In addition to the medical and psychosocial evaluation of the prospective donor detailed in Part I, the evaluation of the prospective donor by the donor surgical team is an intrinsic component of the kidney donor evaluation process. Generally, the surgical consultation represents the final medical visit for the donor candidate after the preliminary evaluation has been completed. It allows for appropriate patient selection, choice of the kidney for donation, and selection of the surgical technique to be employed and it ensures that the patient is fully informed of the risks of kidney donor surgery. The relative advantages and disadvantages of open and laparoscopic nephrectomy are summarized in Table 7.8. Laparoscopic nephrectomy has dramatically improved

TABLE 7.8	Relative Advantages and Disadvantages of Open Versus Laparoscopic Living-Donor Nephrectomy	
	Open	**Laparoscopic**
Safety record	Established international long-term record	Safety comparable to open nephrectomy with increasing surgical expertise; reoperation with or without conversion rates depends on surgeon expertise
Surgical complications	Retroperitoneal approach minimizes potential abdominal complications	Pneumoperitoneum may compromise blood flow
		Disadvantages: tendency to have shorter renal vessels and multiple arteries
		Advantages: magnified view of renal vessels
Scar formation	Long surgical scar with the potential for hernia and abdominal wall asymmetry	Minimal surgical scar: better cosmetic appearance
Operative time	2–3 hours	3–4 hours (increased warm ischemia time)
Postoperative pain	Occasionally persistent	Less postoperative pain (less analgesics required)
Hospital stay	4–5 days	1–2 days
Return to work	6–8 weeks	3–4 weeks
Recipient outcomes: graft function, rejection rate, urologic complications, patient and graft survival	Comparable	Comparable

the donation experience and has become "standard of practice" for living kidney donation.

HISTORY AND PHYSICAL EXAMINATION

The surgical evaluation provides an additional opportunity to identify issues that have not been revealed during prior visits as well as to focus on the details specific to donor surgery. The recipient's identity, the recipient's relationship to the donor, and the cause of the recipient's renal failure are reviewed. It is not uncommon for new issues to be raised at this visit, or for the social situation of the donor to have changed in a way that may affect the donor's candidacy or willingness to be a donor. Particular attention is focused on whether the patient has any urologic history, including as gross hematuria, nephrolithiasis, pyelonephritis, renal cysts, or renal tumors.

The physical examination includes measurement of vital signs and allows for confirmatory measurements of height and weight for the computation of the patient's BMI. Particular attention is paid to the abdominal examination to evaluate the patient's body habitus and to document any prior surgical scars relevant to the surgical approach. This simple evaluation is essential to identify patients appropriate for minimally invasive donor surgery. The relative size of the potential donor compared to the recipient may impact donor choice and if the donor is considerably smaller than the recipient the possibility of paired exchange donation may be considered (see Compatible Pairs in Part IV).

Review of Imaging

Donor imaging is also discussed in Chapter 14. CT-based imaging is routinely used to evaluate a potential donor's renal anatomy. The 64-slice multidetector (64-MDCT) urogram and angiogram phases generate high-quality images that allow for identification of intra-abdominal findings that may preclude donation; prompt further investigation; assess renal size; assess parenchymal and collecting system anatomy; and define the vascular anatomy. These images can be obtained using a less invasive approach than traditional arteriography and intravenous urography. GFR is closely related to kidney size, and CT scan is a better determinant of kidney size compared to ultrasound and is as precise as angiography in demonstrating kidney anatomy. Kidney size is a good predictor of allograft function.

Renal Nonvascular Anatomy and Abdominal Abnormalities

Incidental intra-abdominal pathology is often discovered at the time of the MDCT imaging. Adrenal nodules are detected in a small portion of patients and present a clinical challenge. If the adrenal lesions meets CT criteria for benign adenoma and a functional metabolic workup is negative, proceeding with donation is reasonable. Multiple phase MDCT images demonstrate the size of each kidney and the amount of renal parenchyma. Rapid symmetrical uptake of intravenous contrast, combined with prompt excretion and drainage, documents the relative renal function and can obviate the need for routine renal scans. Donors found to have disparities in renal size, contrast uptake or excretion, or renal scars may be further studied with an MAG3 renal scan to ensure adequate renal function (see Chapter 14). The affected kidney is then chosen to ensure the donor is left with the highest functioning renal unit. Delayed urogram phases also document the anatomy of the collecting system of each kidney and ureter. The identification of a calyceal diverticulum, asymptomatic hydronephrosis with ureteropelvic junction obstruction, or complete and partial ureteral duplication may alter the surgical approach.

Approximately 20% of kidneys evaluated using MDCT technology have incidental renal pathology such as low-density lesions considered "too small to characterize," renal cysts, and calyceal calcifications. This information does not necessarily preclude donation. Patients with a history of recurrent nephrolithiasis and those found to have bilateral, multiple unilateral, or large renal stones are not considered candidates for donor nephrectomy. Donor candidates found to have a single small asymptomatic calcification, particularly older donor candidates, undergo a thorough metabolic workup as detailed in Part I. If no abnormalities are detected, it is reasonable to proceed with donation, removing the affected kidney.

CT-based imaging can also supplement the patient selection process by elucidating the amount of perirenal fat and whether the kidney "rests" on the psoas muscle. This information can be used to select higher BMI donors that will still be amenable to a laparoscopic approach. This becomes particularly important in patients with complex vascular anatomy because the amount of perirenal fat can indicate significantly more and challenging dissection within the hilum. Figure 7.3 illustrates three patients with BMI values of 33 but varying amounts of perirenal fat.

Renal Vascular Anatomy

Vascular anatomy has become increasingly relevant to the surgical evaluation with the increasing adoption of laparoscopic approaches to kidney donor surgery, and 64-MDCT has demonstrated impressive sensitivity to identify small vascular structures. The increased resolution of 64-MDCT, along with three-dimensional reconstructions, will likely increase the operative safety as well identify small capsular and polar arteries such that attempts can be made to preserve these structures if indicated (Fig. 7.4). This imaging information can then be used to determine the appropriate kidney for donation. The left kidney is the preferred organ because of the longer length of the renal vein. It is routine to select the left kidney when one or two left renal arteries are identified. A right nephrectomy may be preferred when the left kidney is found to have more than two arteries. Arterial anatomy that is more complex is reviewed on an individual basis. Venous anatomy rarely precludes left-sided laparoscopic donor nephrectomy.

Risks of Surgery

Perhaps the most important aspect of the surgical visit for potential donors is a thorough review of the risks, benefits, and alternatives to kidney donation. It is critical for the patient to be fully informed of the risks of undergoing surgery and to have realistic expectations of the hospital and postoperative course. Occasionally, potential donors

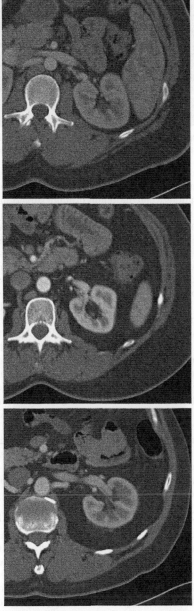

FIGURE 7.3 Three patients with a calculated body mass index of 33 and varying amounts of perirenal fat.

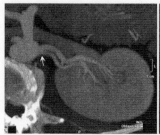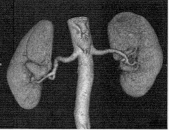

FIGURE 7.4 Example images from multidetector computed tomography illustrating an early bifurcation of a renal artery (*arrow*) and an example of three-dimensional renal reconstruction.

who have completed their medical and psychosocial evaluation will express reservations when the details of donor surgery are discussed. If necessary, a medical "alibi" can be provided to ensure that the potential donor does not feel undue pressure to proceed with the process that may have taken some time to complete and may be close to fruition.

When reviewing the risk for surgery, the risks common to the general anesthesia, including heart attack, stroke, blood clot, and pulmonary embolus, are discussed. The risk for death in healthy kidney donors is extremely low (estimated at 3 to 4 cases per 10,000 nephrectomies) but cannot be ignored. There may be bleeding, need for blood transfusion, wound infection, and postoperative pain. There is also a risk for injuring organs adjacent to the operative field. Specific to right donor nephrectomy, these structures include the liver, duodenum, colon, diaphragm, and pancreas. For a left-sided procedure, the structures at risk include the colon, small intestine, pancreas, spleen, and diaphragm. These injuries may require repair if identified at the time of surgery or may necessitate reoperation if identified after surgery. Cases of chylous ascites, intra-abdominal adhesions, and internal hernia formation have been reported. Minor risks include the development of wound infections, subcutaneous hematoma formation, and traumatic neuropathy, from either the incision or operative positioning. Risks particular to laparoscopic approaches include increased operative time and the occasional need to convert to an open procedure typically because of excessive bleeding.

SURGICAL TECHNIQUES FOR LIVING-DONOR NEPHRECTOMY

The introduction of laparoscopic living kidney donation has been a major advance in organ donation. First introduced with some trepidation in select centers in the mid-1990s, these procedures are now the preferred surgical approach in all transplant programs with the necessary surgical skill sets. The major benefits of laparoscopic techniques include significant reduction in surgical pain, postoperative convalescence, and recovery time. As a result, laparoscopic donor nephrectomy has been responsible for expanding the pool of living donors and may account for the increased popularity and frequency of living donation. Long-term renal function is not different between open nephrectomy and laparoscopic nephrectomy.

Laparoscopic Nephrectomy—Surgical Technique

Laparoscopic techniques require specially trained surgical staff. For laparoscopic donor nephrectomy, the donor is placed in the flank position, and a pneumoperitoneum is established with a Veress needle. A 5-mm visual trocar is placed three fingerbreadths below the xiphoid at the lateral border of the rectus muscle under direct vision. A 5-mm laparoscope is then inserted. Under direct vision, two additional 5-mm trocars are inserted along the lateral border of the rectus muscle. The surgery then proceeds as outlined next.

First, the white line of Toldt is incised down to the level of the iliac vessels in order to reflect the colon medially. The posterior peritoneum is then incised toward the crus of the diaphragm, mobilizing the spleen (for left-sided nephrectomy) or the liver (for right-sided nephrectomy) from the upper pole of the kidney. The colon is reflected medially to expose the gonadal vein. The vein is followed to the renal vein and the adrenal vein is identified. The adrenal gland is reflected medially to preserve the arterial supply to the upper pole. The gonadal vein is then dissected, clipped, and transected, a practice that does not increase the incidence of ureteral strictures in recipients. A plane lateral to the gonadal vein is then created, freeing the ureter down to the level of the iliac vessels. The renal hilum is elevated, and the renal artery and vein are carefully identified and circumferentially isolated. The remaining posterior and lateral attachments are then divided. Intraoperative mannitol is administered in two 12.5-g doses, with the first dose given at the start of surgery and the second dose delivered about 15 minutes before the ligation of the renal hilum. A horizontal midline incision, just large enough to accommodate the kidney, is made at the pubic hair line for an improved postoperative cosmetic result. The fascia is then incised vertically, and the midline is identified. A 15-mm trocar is placed through the superior portion of this incision to accommodate a vascular stapling device. The ureter is clipped at the level of the external iliac artery. The arteries and veins are divided with a vascular stapler, the ureter is cut, and the kidney is placed in an extraction sack. Heparin dosing, is unnecessary and protamine reversal can induce a hypercoagulable state. The two bellies of the rectus muscle are spread to allow for removal of the kidney and sack. After removal, the kidney is then placed in frozen saline slush, and the vascular staples are excised. The renal arteries are flushed with cold heparinized lactated Ringer solution.

The hand-assisted laparoscopic technique employs a relatively small abdominal incision to allow the introduction of the surgeon's hand to supplement the laparoscopic procedure and permit rapid, atraumatic removal of the kidney. Laparoscopic techniques can be rapidly converted to open nephrectomy in the event of uncontrolled bleeding or unforeseen anatomic abnormalities. Robotic techniques have been successfully used in some centers.

Open Nephrectomy

The traditional method for removing a kidney from a living donor has been an open surgical technique, using a modified flank incision. In select cases in which the donor has issues precluding laparoscopic access (e.g., significant prior abdominal surgery), or in some cases of complex vascular anatomy, an open surgical approach is preferred. The age of the recipient is not generally considered an indication for open renal procurement. Most donor surgeons use an extrapleural and extraperitoneal approach, just above or below the 12th rib. The kidney must be carefully dissected to preserve all renal arteries, renal veins, and the periureteral blood supply. Excessive traction on the renal artery is avoided to prevent vasospasm. After the renal vessels are securely ligated and divided, the kidney is removed and placed in a basin of frozen saline slush to decrease renal metabolism. The renal arteries are cannulated and flushed with heparinized solution as with laparoscopic donor nephrectomy.

Postoperative Management

In the operating room, donor nephrectomy patients may be given their first dose of ketorolac for effective pain control. Ketorolac is administered in 30 mg dosing every 6 hours for up to 48 hours. Its routine use decreases morbidity following donor nephrectomy without compromising renal function. For laparoscopic cases, the oral gastric tube is removed before extubation. The patient is transferred to the recovery room with a urethral catheter to gravity drainage. A mild bowel preparation is routinely employed before surgery. This allows the patient to be started on sips of clear liquids on the evening of the day of surgery. The diet is advanced to a full liquid diet on the morning of postoperative day 1, and to a regular diet thereafter as tolerated. Early ambulation is encouraged, as is aggressive pulmonary toilet. The combination of early mobilization and ketorolac-based analgesia during the first 48 hours facilitates early return of bowel function and shorter hospital stays. The average hospital stay after laparoscopic donor nephrectomy is 1½ days. Most donors can return to all but the most strenuous exercise or work by 3 to 4 weeks. Fatigue is a common complaint among donors during the recovery period and 2 or 3 months may pass before some donors report feeling energy and stamina levels have normalized. Laparoscopic procedures are associated with a faster recovery, less postoperative pain, and a full recovery in about 3 to 4 weeks. Complete recovery for open donor nephrectomy takes 6 to 8 weeks, although some donors complain of incisional pain for 2 to 3 months.

Part IV: Innovative Aspects of Living Kidney Donation

KIDNEY PAIRED DONATION

Approximately one in three potential living kidney donors will be ABO incompatible or crossmatch positive with their intended recipient. To circumvent this issue kidney paired donation (KPD) has been increasingly utilized over the past decade. Initially conceived in the 1980s and formally established in Korea in 1999, in its simplest form KPD can be used as a solution for donor–recipient pairs with ABO incompatibility. In this scheme, two or more incompatible donor–recipient pairs are matched to other pairs with complementary incompatibilities (i.e., donor swap). For example, a blood group A to B couple would be set up to exchange with a blood group B to A couple. Expansion of

The Evolution of Paired Exchange

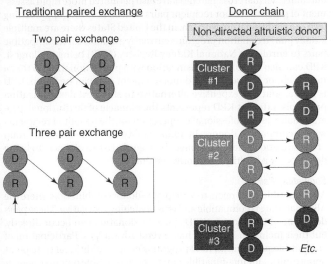

FIGURE 7.5 The evolution of paired exchange. (Courtesy of Garet Hill of the National Kidney Registry.)

this concept from ABO incompatible to immunologically (crossmatch) incompatible pairs can facilitate additional exchanges (Fig. 7.5).

Domino-Paired Kidney Donation/Donor Chain

Further evolution of the paired donation concept incorporates a nondirected donor (see below). To achieve optimal benefit from the nondirected donor, the donated kidney is matched to a recipient who has an intended, but incompatible, living donor. In turn, the recipient's incompatible living donor donates his or her kidney to the next incompatible pair, generating a domino effect which eventually terminates with a donor donating to a recipient on the deceased donor waiting list. If instead the final donor waits until a suitable match is found with a new incompatible pair, they become a "bridge" donor and can facilitate a nonsimultaneous extended altruistic donation (NEAD) (Fig. 7.5). In this way, nondirected donors can generate "clusters" or "chains" of living donor transplants with bridge donors perpetuating the chain. It is estimated that nondirected donors trigger an average of five transplants, and sometimes, many more.

Local and regional living donor exchange programs have been created, and some countries have developed national sharing programs. These programs use sophisticated computer algorithms to generate the best matches and even permit highly sensitized patients to be matched. The use of exchange programs is on the rise. In the United States in 2016 close to 15% of all living donor transplants were performed through a living donor exchange program. One of the "taboos" that has been broken in these programs is the "shipping" of living donor kidneys from one center to another, in a manner similar to the transportation of deceased donor kidneys. The short cold-ischemia times that such shipping entails does not appear to have an unfavorable effect on outcomes. Virtual crossmatches have also permitted more rapid assessment of potential donor recipient pairs with an accuracy approaching 99% of a traditional crossmatch. In the United States there are multiple kidney paired donation programs currently available for incompatible pairs to enroll, the National Kidney Registry (NKR) being the largest. KPD can also combine desensitization with paired donation so that a negatively, or less sensitized donor-recipient pair can be found. KPD is a safer and less expensive alternative to standard desensitization protocols. Efficient KPD represents the pinnacle of institutional, programmatic, and professional cooperation for the benefit of recipients with incompatible donors. Incompatability, by virtue of blood group or sensitization, should no longer be regarded as an obstacle to living donation by a healthy and motivated donor.

Compatible Pairs

A "compatible pair" refers to a recipient–donor combination where the ABO matching is compatible and crossmatching is negative. These pairs do not need to engage in KPD since the donation can occur directly, but their inclusion in chains has several advantages. Participation of compatible pairs within KPD programs creates additional transplant opportunities for incompatible pairs. The compatible pair may benefit by virtue of achieving a better match for themselves in terms of HLA matching, kidney size, or donor age, which may translate into better long-term transplant function.

ISOLATED MEDICAL ABNORMALITIES AND RISK ASSESSMENT

Donors have typically been accepted or rejected based on the evaluating physician's perception of safety for the donors. The most common reasons for declining an otherwise acceptable donor are mild hypertension, diabetes or prediabetes, and asymptomatic urinary abnormalities, because of the fear of increased risks for the development of ESRD. Indeed, no person can, or should, be told that the risk is nil. All risks are relative, and the risk for developing chronic renal failure in the face of mild hypertension or isolated microscopic hematuria appears to be low, with a reported incidence between 1 of 100 and 1 of 10,000 donations—an incidence that is considerably lower than for the general population. It has been suggested that rather than declining such borderline patients from the outset, an attempt should be made, based on available data on the demographics of renal disease, to give the potential donor an estimate of his or her risk and to permit the donor, within reasonable limits and after careful education, to decide on an acceptable degree of risk. Risk assessment is not absolute, however, and should be age adjusted: the finding of mild hypertension or a kidney stone in a 20-year-old will clearly be of much greater concern than similar findings in a 60-year-old. Young donors with isolated medical abnormalities are generally excluded from donation.

BIOLOGICALLY UNRELATED DONORS

The number of living unrelated donor transplantations performed in the United States is steadily increasing and as of 2016 constituted close to 50% of the living donors in the United States, a number about twice that of the previous decade. Most of these donors are "emotionally related" and have an apparent or easily documented close and long-standing relationship with the recipient (spouse, significant other, close friend, adopted sibling). An increasing number of prospective donors have much more casual relationship with the recipient (e.g., coworkers, acquaintances, members of faith community) or with little or no relationship to the recipient (e.g., solicited through the Internet, media appeals) are being performed in the United States, and about half of unrelated donors fall into this category. The survival benefit of transplants from unrelated donors exceeds that from remaining on dialysis even if the donors have some degree of HLA-incompatibility and sensitization (see Chapter 3 and Orandi et al. in Selected Readings).

Nondirected Donors

The biologically unrelated donors referred to above all donate to a specific individual who is known to them. A nondirected donor is one who comes forward to donate a kidney to someone unknown to them. The term *altruistic donor* (or *Good Samaritan donor*) is often used to describe these donors, but altruism is not a measurable factor and may certainly be present in all donors to a varying degree. Generally, the recipient of a kidney from a nondirected donor is a patient on the deceased donor waiting list with a compatible blood type, the most waiting time, and negative crossmatching (see Chapters 3 and 4). Nondirected donors may also play a critical role in living donor exchange programs as noted above. The nondirected donors do not know or select, and may never meet, the recipient and therefore may not observe or enjoy the recipient's gain of health following the kidney transplantation. The motives of altruistic donors are sometimes looked on with skepticism or suspicion. Public surveys in the United States report that up to 50% of the adult population would be willing, in principle, to anonymously donate a kidney to a stranger.

The evaluation of nondirected donors and of all donors whose relationship with the recipient is a tenuous one must emphasize a careful psychosocial examination to fully explore the motivation for donation and identify unrealistic expectations, misperceptions, covert depression, or anticipation of financial gain. Guidelines for the triage and evaluation of nondirected donors have been developed (see Chapter 18 and Adams et al. in Selected Readings). Less than 10% of persons who contact transplantation programs with a view to donating in a nondirected fashion actually become donors. Nonetheless, nondirected donors represented about 2% of all living donors in the United States as of 2016.

FINANCIAL INCENTIVES, DISINCENTIVES, AND NEUTRALITY

The shortage of organs for transplantation has engendered a lively and sometimes contentious debate as to the wisdom and ethical probity of payment for organs. Different forms of payment—*incentives*—have been suggested, including cash or cash equivalents such as grants for education, pensions, and the like. In the United States, the sales of human organs involving either direct monetary exchange or exchange of donor organ for valuable property violates the National Organ Transplant Act of 1984 (see Chapter 19). Similar legislation is in place internationally, and major professional transplantation organizations prohibit such payments. Donors however, often find themselves faced with expenses that may reach thousands of dollars. Reimbursement for expenses related to the donation process such as for traveling and lodging is not prohibited. A formal mechanism to make such reimbursements, in part or in full, is available in some countries, but is not available for most donors in the United States (see Chapter 21) and many other countries, a factor that could act as a *disincentive* to donation for some potential donors. Iran is currently the only country in which paid donation is officially sanctioned, almost all the donors are poor and uneducated and follow-up studies have shown that their lives are not improved, to the contrary, and that the payments have not "solved" their organ donor shortage.

The principle of "financial neutrality"—that organ donation should neither enrich donors nor impose financial burdens on them—is a basic precept of the policy statements on organ donation that has been promulgated by intergovernmental and professional organizations, and has received broad acceptance in the professional transplant community. The principles objectives are achieved through the legal prohibitions against the giving, receiving, or arranging of payments for organs. Together with these prohibitions, there exists a clear ethical and legal consensus that to remove the financial barriers that stand in the way of successful donation programs, all potential donors should be offered coverage of the actual amount of their lost earnings and actual expenses connected with the process of undergoing medical screening, organ removal, and recovery, including the costs of transportation, lodging, and replacement services for the care family members dependent on the donor. Costs of follow-up requirements and any postdonation complications should be covered. In those countries without universal health insurance, the provision of such insurance to donors is not consistent with financial neutrality since it represents a very considerable and potentially coercive financial incentive.

Despite the legal constraints on organ sales, commerce in kidney transplantation remains a common phenomenon in many parts of the world and, in some cases, has been linked to criminal activity. The donors are typically poor or under great financial stress, the recipients are often wealthy or come from other wealthier countries, and "middlemen" or "brokers" are often involved. The WHO has designated certain countries to be "hot-spots" of transplant tourism.

Arguments against paid donation express concern for the exploitation of the poor, commodification of the human body, and the documented negative impact on both living and deceased donation. Arguments made for allowing paid donation claim that the money paid to poor donors would have a significant positive impact on their quality of life, that paid donors are entitled to use their bodies as they see fit, that the risks of the procedure are small, and that there is no other way to address the organ donor shortage. Available data on the outcome of organ vending for the donors indicates that most of them have a poor psychosocial, and often poor medical, outcomes. Recipients of vended organs are subject to an increased risk for complications, particularly infection, likely as a result of a breakdown of trust and honesty that is a by-product of the commercialization of organ donation. Evidence from several countries has shown that commercialization of living organ donation, rather than addressing the organ shortage, comes at the expense of programs for related and unpaid living unrelated donation and of deceased donation.

An important distinction between legitimate "travel for transplantation" and "transplant tourism" is made in the Declaration of Istanbul (DOI, see Chapter 23). Physicians should discourage patients from engaging in transplant tourism and should inform them of its legal, ethical, and medical consequences. A pamphlet entitled "Thinking of Buying a Kidney: Stop" is available in multiple languages on the website of the DOI: www.declarationofistanbul.org. When faced with a patient who has returned to his or her country of origin after a paid donation, optimal care should be provided in a professional and nonjudgmental manner. Readers are also referred to the proceedings of the 2016 Madrid meeting on the prospective and retrospective aspects of transplant travel (see Dominguez Gil et al. in Suggested Readings).

Part V: Education for Living Donation

Education about living kidney donation is complex. It involves two or more learners including the potential recipient, the potential living donor, and any interested family members or friends. It requires communicating complex medical information about the risks and benefits of transplant and living donation to all of them. Many potential kidney transplant recipients feel uncomfortable asking others to donate and their concerns about future health problems for the living donor may lead them rule out the option of living donation even before they fully understand its advantages to their own health and the degree of risk to the donor. As a result family members and friends may never learn that they might be able to donate a kidney and have an opportunity to decide for themselves whether the risks of living donation are acceptable to them. Patients, potential donors, and medical professionals may have inaccurate or outdated information on "compatibility" and may self-exclude living donation (see Part I).

Living kidney donation is the optimal treatment option for most patients with advanced chronic kidney disease (CKD). Comprehensive education should be available to patients at all stages of CKD as well as to their potential living donors. Such education should occur multiple times for individuals across the stages of CKD progression, with distinct efforts being made to increase education for potential recipients and donors identifying as racial/ethnic minorities. Successful programs have been introduced at community nephrology clinics, dialysis centers, and transplant centers. Ideally, education should be tailored to an individual patient's level of readiness and other characteristics, so that they may develop skills to find and appropriately educate potential living donors from among their families and social support networks.

TAILORING EDUCATION TO READINESS LEVEL

Transplant education programs grounded in the so-called Transtheoretical Model (TTM) of Behavior Change (see Glanz et al. in Selected Readings) assess how ready an individual patient is to pursue living donation and deliver appropriate educational messages that are best tailored for each patient's stage of readiness. An assessment of a patient's readiness can be conducted by asking them which of the following statements is most true for them: "I am not considering taking actions in the next 6 months to pursue living donation" (Precontemplation); "I am considering taking actions in the next 6 months to pursue living donation" (Contemplation); "I am preparing to take actions in the next 30 days to pursue living donation" (Preparation); and "I am taking actions to pursue living donation" (Action). With access to educational materials and time to discuss the option of living donation with providers and other advocates, patients can progress forward in their stages of readiness, moving into planning or taking actions like talking with people they trust about whether to get a transplant, making a list of people who might become living donors, or asking someone to donate directly. However, if setbacks occur, patients can also move backwards to an earlier stage of readiness where they need additional support. Patients who first present for transplant evaluation in later stages of readiness (Action) have been shown to be more than 4 times more likely to receiving a living donor transplant years later. Readiness for living donation at the time of evaluation for transplantation (see chapter 8) is the single strongest predictor of ultimate living donation. An innovative "House Calls" program for African-American patients on the transplant waitlist found that well over a half were in early stages of readiness for living donation and that a single, 60 to 90 minute educational session in patients' homes substantially increased readiness, living donor inquiries and evaluations compared to standard print education (see Rodrigue et al. in Selected Readings).

Patients move from early to later stages of readiness for living donation when they perceive the advantages, or "pros," to taking a specific behavior to be greater than the disadvantages, or "cons," of taking it. Conversations about what is uniquely important to a kidney patient, including the possibilities of getting off dialysis, to feeling more "alive," to being able to eat restricted types of food, or being able to travel more, can help increase perceptions of the pros and cons, or fears and concerns, should also be addressed. Sometimes, patients are extremely concerned about something that has a low probability of actually happening, such as dying under anesthesia , fertility being affected, or the living donor having serious health problems. In these cases accurate information that communicates the low, but not absent risk of these negative outcomes should be provided.

Once a patient's level of readiness is known, providers can help the patient consider which small steps toward living donation are most appropriate, increasing the likelihood that the patient will move eventually into Action. Figure 7.6 demonstrates how best to orient discussions with patients in the four stages of readiness and suggests which steps may be most appropriate at each stage. Follow-up is critical, as repeated educational interactions are often more effective than

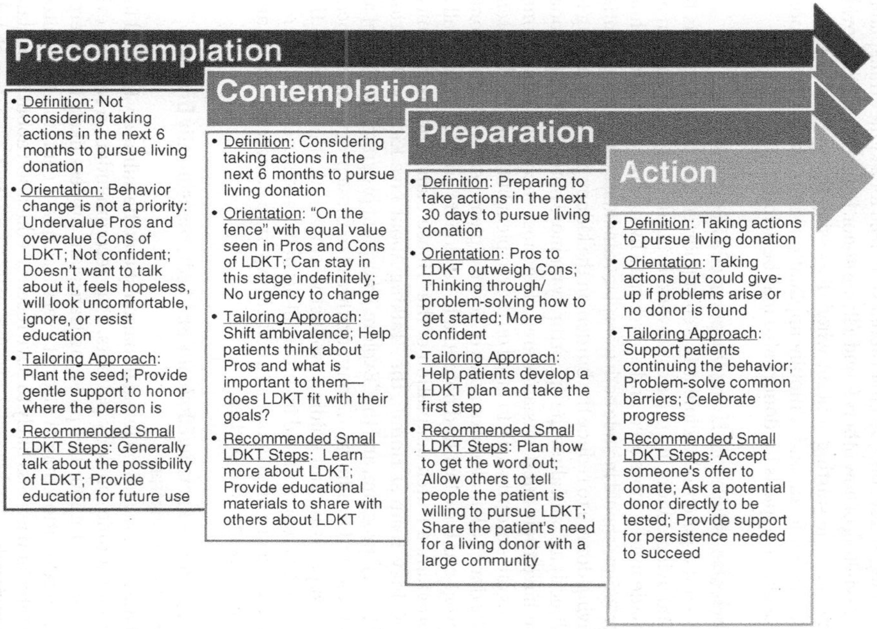

FIGURE 7.6 TTM tailored educational recommendations for increasing readiness to pursue living-donor kidney transplant. LDKT living-donor kidney transplant, TTM transtheoretical model of behavior change. (Reprinted from Waterman AD, Robbins ML, Peipert JD. Educating prospective kidney transplant recipients and living donors about living donation: practical and theoretical recommendations for increasing living donation rates. Curr Transplant Rep 2016;3(1):1–9, with permission of Springer.)

Precontemplation

- Definition: Not considering taking actions in the next 6 months to pursue living donation
- Orientation: Behavior change is not a priority; Undervalue Pros and overvalue Cons of LDKT; Not confident; Doesn't want to talk about it, feels hopeless, will look uncomfortable, ignore, or resist education
- Tailoring Approach: Plant the seed; Provide gentle support to honor where the person is
- Recommended Small LDKT Steps: Generally talk about the possibility of LDKT; Provide education for future use

Contemplation

- Definition: Considering taking actions in the next 6 months to pursue living donation
- Orientation: "On the fence" with equal value seen in Pros and Cons of LDKT; Can stay in this stage indefinitely; No urgency to change
- Tailoring Approach: Shift ambivalence: Help patients think about Pros and what is important to them— does LDKT fit with their goals?
- Recommended Small LDKT Steps: Learn more about LDKT; Provide educational materials to share with others about LDKT

Preparation

- Definition: Preparing to take actions in the next 30 days to pursue living donation
- Orientation: Pros to LDKT outweigh Cons; Thinking through/problem-solving how to get started; More confident
- Tailoring Approach: Help patients develop a LDKT plan and take the first step
- Recommended Small LDKT Steps: Plan how to get the word out; Allow others to tell people the patient is willing to pursue LDKT; Share the patient's need for a living donor with a large community

Action

- Definition: Taking actions to pursue living donation
- Orientation: Taking actions but could give-up if problems arise or no donor is found
- Tailoring Approach: Support patients continuing the behavior; Problem-solve common barriers; Celebrate progress
- Recommended Small LDKT Steps: Accept someone's offer to donate; Ask a potential donor directly to be tested; Provide support for persistence needed to succeed

203

single educational sessions. Video- and brochure-based education may improve effectiveness.

Knowledge about organ transplantation increases readiness to pursue living donation and racial/ethnic minority patients are more likely to be less knowledgeable. Helping patients learn more about the facts related to living donation will better prepare them for undergoing and completing evaluation, surgery, and successful recovery. Multiple interventions have been shown to increase knowledge, including the "House Calls" program, the "Explore Transplant" program (see Waterman et al. in Selected Readings).

Skill-Building to Help Identify Living Donors

Transplant centers should provide patients and their caregivers with training about how to successfully identify and approach potential living donors. Educational approaches that increase a patient's confidence reduce larger tasks like "finding a living donor" into smaller, more manageable pieces like, "making a list of your community" and "writing and sending an email about your need for a kidney transplant." Storytelling of how others found a living donor, letters or emails providing possible starting content when discussing the need for a kidney in written form, and a mobile application simplifying how to post Facebook appeals for donors also may be helpful.

Inclusion of Potential Living Donors in LDKT Education

Even if a potential recipient is well supported and taking actions to find living donors, no progress toward living donor transplant can be made until a motivated and appropriate living donor is found. Thus, programs should include both transplant candidates and their potential living donors to reduce the burden on the kidney patient of having to directly ask and allow the opportunity for more potential living donors to have their questions answered. The most successful educational programs are primarily focused on the recipient but also include potential donors. Four key examples of how recipient-centered educational programs have involved potential living donors are the "House Calls" program, a Dutch adaptation of the "House Calls" approach named "Kidney Team at Home", the "Talking About Live Kidney Donation (TALK)" program, and the "Explore Transplant program" (see Tan et al. in Selected Readings). A common thread to these programs is a focus on supporting and guiding productive communication between the potential recipient and members of his or her social network, often in the presence of a transplant medical expert to answer questions and concerns for both parties.

Educating a Racially/Ethnically and Socioeconomically Diverse Patient Population

Education regarding living donation should be culturally tailored for racial/ethnic minority patients. This recommendation reflects evidence that minorities pursuing transplant are less likely to undergo living donation than Whites at every transplant center in the United States and are less likely to have received education about transplant previously. Wherever possible, culturally-competent education should address the core causes of racial/ethnic disparities in living donation at all levels of the socioecologic model, which could include the patient, family and social network, medical providers, the healthcare system, and public policy.

Educational programs targeting Black and/or Hispanic kidney patients have aimed to increase knowledge or address fears by providing improved educational materials and longer educational conversations, supporting patients in completing small steps toward living donation, providing individually-guided navigation services, and assisting patients in obtaining financial resources to address socioeconomic barriers. These approaches have been successful in engaging kidney patients who are racial or ethnic minorities in education about living donation and in helping to identify potential living donors.

For living donor candidates facing large socioeconomic barriers to transplant of any racial/ethnic group, there is financial support available for some specific donation-related costs through the national living donor assistance program (https://www.livingdonorassistance .org). A financial toolkit for living donors has been designed to provide guidance and information on available resources to assist in mitigating donation-related costs with a goal of financial neutrality for donors (see Chapter 21).

Educational materials for both transplant candidates and potential donors are plentiful. Referrals to technology-based solutions including websites, videos, or mobile applications that help patients weigh the advantages and disadvantages of different renal replacement options, including living donation, may be helpful. There are also published recommendations for any program educating living donor candidates, particularly in covering the risks and benefits of donation (see Tan et al. in Selected Readings). Tailored educational resources for potential donors, including a website for altruistic donors to learn more (www .livingdonationcalifornia) and a website in Spanish have been made available (http://informate.org/english/).

Selected Readings

Adams P, Cohen DJ, Danovitch GM, et al. The nondirected live-kidney donor: ethical considerations and practice guidelines: a national conference report. Transplantation 2002;74:582–589.

Biancone L, Cozzi E, López-Fraga M, et al. Long-term outcome of living kidney donation: Position paper of the European Committee on Organ Transplantation (CD-P-TO), Council of Europe. Transpl Int 2016;29(1):129–131.

Cecka M. Transplantation: survival benefit of incompatible living donor kidney transplants. Nat Rev Nephrol 2016;12(6):321–323.

Chapman JR, Delmonico FL. Buyer beware transplantation. Kidney Int 2016;89(5):983–985.

Danovitch GM. The doctor–patient relationship in living donor kidney transplantation. Curr Opin Nephrol Hypertens 2007;16:503–505.

Danovitch GM. The high cost of organ transplant commercialism. Kidney Int 2014;85:248–250.

Danovitch GM, Chapman J, Capron A, et al. Organ trafficking and transplant tourism: the role of global professional ethical standards—the 2008 declaration of Istanbul. Transplantation 2013;95:1306–1312.

Davis C, Delmonico FL. Living-donor kidney transplantation: a review of the current practices for the live donor. J Am Soc Nephrol 2005;16:2098–2110.

Delmonico F, Council of the Transplantation Society. A report of the Amsterdam Forum on the Care of the Live Kidney Donor: data and medical guidelines. Transplantation 2005;79:S53–S66.

Dew MA, Jacobs CL, Jowsy SG, et al. Guidelines for the psychosocial evaluation of living unrelated kidney donors in the United States. Am J Transplant 2007;7:1047–1054.

Dominguez-Gil B, Muller E. Prospective and retrospective aspects of travel for transplant. Proceedings of the 2016 Madrid Conference [published online ahead of print 2017]. Transplantation.

Freedman B, Julian B. Should kidney donors be genotyped for APOL1 risk alleles. Kidney Int 2015;87:671–673.

Garg AX, Nevis I, McArthur E, et al. Gestational hypertension and preeclampsia in living kidney donors. N Engl J Med 2015;372:124–133.

Gaston R, Kumar V, Matas A. Reassessing medical risk in living kidney donors. J Am Soc Nephrol 2015;26:1017–1019.

Gill J, Dong J, Rose C, et al. The effect of race and income on living kidney donation in the United States. J Am Soc Nephrol 2013;24:1872–1879.

Glanz K, Rimer BK, Viswanath K. Theory, research, and practice in health behavior and health education. In: Glanz K, Rimer BK, Viswanath K, eds. Health Behavior and Health Education. 4th ed. San Francisco, CA: Jossey-Bass; 2008:23–38.

Grams M, Sang Y, Levey A, et al. Kidney-failure risk projection for the living kidney donor candidate. N Engl J Med 2016;374:411–421.

Ismael S, Duerinckx N, van der Knoop M, et al. Toward a conceptualization of the content of psychological screening in living organ donors: an ethical legal psychological aspects of transplantation consensus. Transplantation 2015;99:2413–2421.

Jacobs C, Gross C, Messersmith E, et al. Emotional and financial experiences of living kidney donors over the past 50 years: the RELIVE study. Clin J Am Soc Nephrol 2015;10:2221–2231.

Klarenbach S, Gill JS, Knoll G, et al. For the Donor Nephrectomy Outcomes Research (DONOR) Network. Economic consequences incurred by living kidney donors: a Canadian multicenter prospective study. Am J Transplant 2014;14:916–916.

LaPointe Rudow D, Hays R, Baliga P, et al. Consensus conference on best practices in live kidney donation: recommendations to optimize education, access, and care. Am J Transplant 2015;15:914–922.

Mjoen G, Hallan S, Hartmann A, et al. Long-term risks for kidney donors. Kidney Int 2014;86:162–167.

Muzaale A, Massie A, Wang M, et al. Risk of end stage renal disease following live kidney donation. JAMA 2014;311:579–586.

Nguyen T, Vazquez M, Toto R. Living kidney donation and hypertension risk. Lancet 2007;369:87–88.

Orandi B, Luo X, Massie J, et al. Survival benefit from HLA-incompatible live donors. N Engl J Med 2016;374:940–950.

Pei Y, Obaji J, Dupuis A, et al. Unified criteria for ultrasonographic diagnosis of ADPKD. J Am Soc Nephrol 2009;20:205–250.

Prasad GV, Ananth S, Palepu S, et al. Commercial kidney transplantation is an important risk factor in long-term kidney allograft survival. Kidney Int 2016;89(5):1119–1124.

Rodrigue JR, Cornell DL, Lin JK, et al. Increasing live donor kidney transplantation: a randomized controlled trial of a home-based educational intervention. Am J Transplant 2007;7(2):394–401.

Steiner RW. The risks of living kidney donation. N Engl J Med 2016;374:479–480.

Tan JC, Gordon EJ, Dew MA, et al. Living donor kidney transplantation: facilitating education about live kidney donation—recommendations from a consensus conference. Clin J Am Soc Nephrol 2015;10(9):1670–1677.

Waterman AD, McSorley AM, Peipert JD, et al. Explore Transplant at Home: a randomized control trial of an educational intervention to increase transplant knowledge for Black and White socioeconomically disadvantaged dialysis patients. BMC Nephrol 2015;16:150.

Wong G, Craig J, Chapman J. Setting the limit for living kidney donation-how big is too big? Kidney Int 2017;91:534–536.

8

Evaluation of Adult Kidney Transplant Candidates

Suphamai Bunnapradist, Basmah Abdalla, and Uttam Reddy

Kidney transplantation is the treatment of choice for most suitable end-stage kidney disease (ESKD) patients and must be discussed with patients with advancing chronic kidney disease (CKD) or prolonged irreversible acute kidney injury. The consideration of renal transplantation for patients with CKD should start from the time of its recognition, and preparation should occur in parallel with efforts to prevent and delay its progression. The improved life expectancy and quality-of-life benefits of transplantation over dialysis therapy have attracted an increasing number of patients to the transplantation option; ideally, patients are evaluated for, and undergo transplantation before the initiation of dialysis treatment.

Early referral to a transplant program is essential to optimizing transplant planning and outcomes. Transplant evaluation is aimed at not only assessing the chances of recovery from surgery, but also at maximizing short- and long-term survival, and assessing the likely impact of transplantation on quality of life. Evaluation of the suitability of kidney transplantation includes medical, surgical, immunologic, and psychosocial assessment. The patients' individual risks and benefits of transplantation are discussed so that they can make an informed decision about whether to proceed with transplantation. Various types of donors, their expected waiting time, and associated outcomes are also discussed with emphasis on living donation. After candidates are placed on the deceased donor list, a periodic reevaluation is necessary to address new issues that may affect transplant suitability and also to revisit potential living donor option. In this chapter, guidelines are provided for the evaluation of adult kidney transplant candidates. The evaluation should be tailored according to patient-specific conditions. Center expertise should be taken into account when determining which diagnostic studies should be performed.

The process of referral, evaluation, and preparation of patients for transplantation has been extensively reviewed in the professional literature. Several topics critical to the evaluation process are discussed in detail elsewhere in this book. The immunologic evaluation of transplant recipients is discussed in Chapter 3; recommendations for the screening of candidates for infectious disease are discussed in Chapter 12; evaluation of candidates with viral hepatitis and liver disease is discussed in Chapter 13; evaluation of diabetic candidates and the various options for pancreatic transplantation are discussed in Chapter 16; evaluation of children is discussed in Chapter 17; psychiatric evaluation is discussed in Chapter 18; psychosocial and financial issues and assessment of compliance are discussed in Chapters 18 and 21; evaluation of simultaneous liver and kidney transplantation is discussed in Chapter 13. Guidelines for the referral and management of patients eligible for solid-organ transplantation have been published under the umbrella of the American Society of Transplantation (available at www.myast.org). In 2014, the European Renal Best Practice Guideline on kidney donor and recipient evaluation and perioperative care was updated (see Abramowicz et al. in Selected Readings).

The evaluation of kidney transplant candidates should ensure that the process not be seen by the patient, the patient's family, or the transplant team as merely determining "thumbs up, or thumbs down" for transplantation. Rather, the process should be designed to determine the optimal mode of ESKD care after multiple considerations are taken into account. Patient advocacy must remain the guiding principle.

Part I: Evaluation of Transplant Candidates

BENEFITS OF EARLY REFERRAL

In ideal circumstances, preparation for transplantation begins as soon as progressive CKD is recognized. CKD care, care on dialysis, and transplant care are interdependent. Cardiovascular risk, which is a major determinant of post-transplantation morbidity and mortality, increases even in early CKD. The various aspects of the care of patients with CKD are beyond the scope of this text. Better-managed patients with CKD, both before and after commencement of chronic dialysis, make better transplant candidates. Patients without the major contraindications to transplantation listed in Table 8.1 should be referred to a transplant program when they approach stage 4 CKD or a glomerular filtration rate (GFR) less than 30 mL/min. Patients should understand that referral to a kidney transplantation program does not necessarily imply immediate transplantation. Patients who are likely not transplant candidates should still be given the option of a consultation with a transplant program so that they can better understand the option facing them.

TABLE 8.1	Major Contraindications to Kidney Transplantation

- Recent or metastatic malignancy*
- Untreated current infection
- Severe irreversible extrarenal disease
- Recalcitrant treatment nonadherence
- Psychiatric illness impairing consent and adherence
- Current recreational drug abuse
- Aggressive recurrent native kidney disease
- Limited, irreversible rehabilitative potential
- Primary oxalosis
- Uncorrectable chronic hypotension

*Excluding some low-grade localized malignacies

Early referral of patients to nephrologic care during the course of CKD permits better preparation for dialysis and transplantation. Patients who are referred to the care of a nephrologist at least 1 year before commencement of renal replacement therapy are documented to have decreased morbidity and mortality. Unfortunately, approximately 40% of incident ESKD patients receive little or no pre-ESKD care and many CKD patients are unaware of their problem until ESKD develops. Transplantation before the commencement of dialysis, called "preemptive transplantation," has been convincingly shown to improve post-transplantation graft and patient survival. Five- and ten-year graft survival rates are 20% to 30% better in patients who received either no dialysis or less than 6 months of dialysis than for those who received more than 2 years of dialysis before the transplant. The benefit of preemptive transplantation is likely largely a result of the avoidance of the cardiovascular consequences of long-term dialysis (see Chapter 1). A similar survival benefit is shown also in patients undergoing preemptive retransplantation.

In the United States, patients may begin to accrue points on the deceased donor transplant waiting list when the GFR is estimated to be 20 mL/min or less. However, less than 5% of patients added to the waiting list are predialysis. Because of the long wait anticipated for a deceased donor transplant, preemptive transplantation is infrequent in these patients, unless they are fortunate to be allocated a "zero-mismatch" kidney (see Chapter 5). The great advantage of early referral is that it permits recognition and evaluation of potential living donors and the elective timing of the transplantation so as to avoid dialysis and the necessity for placement of dialysis access. Avoidance of access placement is a great and tempting benefit, but it is one that must be considered carefully. If there is a reasonable doubt that a living donor is available, or that the workup of the donor can be completed expeditiously, it may be wiser to place a permanent access to avoid reliance on temporary access techniques that bring with them added morbidity.

Because of the varied course of advanced CKD, it is hard to provide a precise point when referral for transplantation should be made. Patients with diabetic nephropathy typically progress rapidly through the advanced stages of CKD, whereas patients with interstitial nephritis, for example, may progress slowly. Patients with a GFR in the 20s, and patients whose course suggests that they will become dialysis dependent in 1 to 2 years, should be referred.

Delays to Referral

All dialysis centers in the United States are mandated to be associated with kidney transplant centers, and all Medicare patients are legally entitled to referral for transplant evaluation. Unfortunately, there are wide variations in access to transplantation because of delays in the referral process that may tend to disadvantage ethnic minorities and other vulnerable population groups. The large size of the United States and its varied population density also introduce formidable geographic barriers to equality of access. It is the responsibility of nephrologists, dialysis unit staff, transplantation program staff, and the patients themselves to do their utmost to minimize delays and barriers to transplantation.

THE EVALUATION PROCESS

Patient Education and Consent

Patient education is at the core of the process. Transplant evaluation implies not only the medical assessment of the potential recipient by the transplant team but also the assessment by the patient of the transplant option and its relevance to their wellbeing. The evaluation process is an opportunity to counsel patients about their ESKD options and to advocate for their welfare. It should not be an obstacle course for patients to pass or fail!

Figure 8.1 illustrates the structure of the evaluation process. All potential transplant candidates should be encouraged to attend an information session, preferably accompanied by family members, caretakers, and friends. At the informational meeting, the risks of the operation and the side effects and risks of immunosuppression should be explained to the patient and family members. The surgical procedure and its potential complications should also be discussed. The relative benefits of living donor and deceased donor transplantations should be compared and contrasted in the context of the prolonged wait that is anticipated for a deceased donor transplant in the event that a living donor is not available. In the United States it is a requirement that graft survival statistics from the individual transplant program and from national data be shared with the patient and family members. Patients should be given to understand that statistics for graft survival for large cohorts of patients may not directly apply to their personal prognosis.

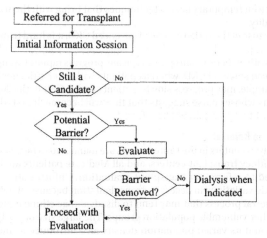

FIGURE 8.1 The renal transplant candidate evaluation process. (From Kasiske BL, Cangro CB, Hariharan S, et al. The evaluation of renal transplant candidates: clinical practice guidelines. Am J Transplant 2001;1(suppl 2):1–95, with permission.)

Patients are often understandably fearful of graft rejection. The nature of rejection should be explained to them in lay terms, and they should be informed that many incidences of rejection can be reversed without major consequence. Patients should be informed about the increased risk for infection, malignancy, and mortality together with donor risk factors; particularly those associated with deceased donation (see Chapter 4). Patients should be warned that even a successful transplantation may not last forever and that at some point they may be required to return to dialysis or undergo another transplant. The importance of adherence with dialysis and dietary prescription while waiting for transplantation and with immunosuppressive therapy after transplantation should be emphasized. The possibility of post-transplantation pregnancy should be discussed with women of child-bearing age and their partners (see Chapter 11).

In the United States, the Center for Medicare Services (CMS) requires that a formal consent process be made available to all patients seeking kidney transplantation. The transplant program, however, must ensure that the process is not merely a legalistic one and that patient consent truly represents an educated understanding of various options and expected outcomes.

Understanding the Allocation Algorithm

Allocation rules for kidneys from deceased donors vary from country to country, though the rules have much in common. Most uses a combination of donor and recipient factors including age, waiting time, presensitization, and HLA matching, together with logistic and geographic factors. No matter what the algorithm, it is important that it be clear and transparent and available to be presented in a manner than can understood by patients and their caregivers. The following section considers changes that have taken place in the allocation of deceased donor kidneys in the United States (see Chapter 5).

Until 2014, deceased donor kidneys in the United States were categorized as being standard criteria donor kidneys (SCD) and extended criteria donor kidneys (ECD) according to their expected post-transplant outcomes. In December 2014, Kidney Allocation System (KAS) was introduced to facilitate kidney allocation, minimize discard rates, and maximize the life years of kidney transplanted. The Kidney Donor Profile Index (KDPI, using ten attributes with index ranges from best outcomes 0% to worst outcomes 100%) is used as one of factors to allocate the kidneys. Regulations for the allocation of higher KDPI kidneys mandate that transplant candidates are informed about the benefits (shortening of waiting time) and risk (impaired long-term graft function) associated with their use. They are required to sign an informed consent document to opt in to receive kidneys from these donors. A cut-off of KDPI of 85% is usually used as the risk of subsequent graft loss increases significantly with KDPI higher than 85% although their outcomes are still better than those on dialysis. A useful guiding principle when counseling patients is to compare the additional risk of accepting kidney with a higher donor risk index with the risk of remaining on dialysis for a prolonged period while waiting for a kidney with a lower KDPI (see UNOS brochure at www.unos.org/wp-content /uploads/unos/Kidney_Brochure.pdf?e4f722).

Kidney transplant candidates each get an individual Estimated Post-Transplant Survival (EPTS) score, which ranges from 0% to 100%. The EPTS is a reflection of how long the candidate will need a functioning kidney transplant when compared with other candidates. Candidates with lower EPTS scores are likely to need a kidney longer than candidates with higher scores. Candidates with high EPTS score, therefore, should consider kidneys with higher KDPI kidneys. These usually include candidates 60 years of age or older (younger if they are diabetic or have coronary heart disease), have failing dialysis access, or are particularly intolerant of dialysis. Patients going on the transplant waiting list in their 60s may not survive long enough to enjoy an ideal kidney and would be well advised to accept an higher KDPI kidney if they are offered one. The waiting time for lower and higher KDPI kidneys varies geographically, and patients should be informed of the anticipated waiting time in their geographic area to facilitate an educated decision. Candidates should also be counseled about Public Health Service (PHS) increased risk donors and they must sign the informed consent to "opt in" to receive kidneys from these donors (For the 2013 definition of PHS increased risk donors, see https://optn.transplant .hrsa.gov/media/1163/2013_phs_guideline.pdf). These donor options should also be revisited while the candidates are on the waiting list.

Educational Resources

Potential transplant candidates and their family members should be encouraged to attend formal educational sessions and to obtain further information through available literature (see Chapter 21). They should also be familiar with the main features of deceased donor organ allocation policy as described above. Patient-orientated educational material is available in the United States in printed and electronic form from the American Society of Transplantation (AST) <www.myast.org>, the National Kidney Foundation (NKF) <www.kidney.org>, and the United Network for Organ Sharing (UNOS) <www.unos.org>. The UNOS website also provides detailed information on the performance of individual transplant programs, so-called "center-specific data," which can assist patients who have the opportunity to elect the program to which they wish to be referred. These data include both waiting list and transplant outcomes.

Who Is Not a Transplant Candidate?

The risks and benefits of transplantation should be explained during the initial session because some patients may decide that they do not want to proceed with the evaluation, thus avoiding the need for a costly and time-consuming evaluation. Table 8.1 lists the major contraindications to transplantation. Although some contraindications to transplantation are absolute, many are relative and determined by local policy and experience. For example, some programs exclude patients who are morbidly obese, or who continue to smoke despite being requested to stop. Attitudes vary about transplantation in the aged or the extent of cardiovascular disease deemed acceptable for transplant candidates. Of the over 400,000 patients on dialysis in the United States as of mid-2016, only about 25% are on the kidney transplant waiting list (see Chapter 1). Most of the unlisted patients are aged and have multiple medical morbidities, but many patients are potential candidates who have yet to be referred for transplantation or who have encountered delays in the process (see Kucirka et al. in Selected Readings). Patients should be presumed to be transplant candidates unless they have the major contraindication listed in the table. If there is any question regarding a transplant contraindication, the patient should be referred to the transplant program for consultation. Patients should be entitled to a second opinion if they find the recommendation of the transplantation program to be unreasonable or unacceptable to them.

The laws regarding the medicinal and recreational use of marijuana vary from country to country with a controversial global trend toward legalization. In the United States, there remains a contradiction between Federal law that regards marijuana use as illicit and the laws in over 20 states that are permissive in different degrees toward recreational and so-called "medicinal use." California passed a law in 2015 that bars medical officials from denying a patient a place on a transplant list solely upon a positive test for the use of medical marijuana unless the drug use is deemed clinically significant. Marijuana use, medicinally or otherwise, can and should be taken into account among the medical and social factors taken as a whole for any given patient (see also Chapter 18).

Conventional and Innovative Transplantation

Ideally, transplant candidates are unsensitized (see Chapter 3) and have motivated, healthy, ABO-compatible, crossmatch-negative, living donors available to donate to them. If no living donors are available, patients have no option but to wait for a deceased donor transplant, although some patients may elect to shorten their wait by agreeing to accept a lower-quality organ. Patients with hepatitis C in the absence of decompensated liver cirrhosis may elect to accept a kidney from a deceased donor with hepatitis C thereby foreshortening their waiting time. Treatment for hepatitis C can follow soon after the transplant (see Chapter 13). In the event that a potential living donor is available but is incompatible by virtue of ABO or histocompatibility differences, another living donor should be evaluated. If a living donor is available but apparently incompatible, innovative protocols may be available. ABO-incompatible transplantation and desensitization protocols for histo-incompatible donors are options, but paired exchange programs designed to facilitate ABO and histocompatible living donation are generally preferred (see Chapter 7) because of lower cost and greater safety.

ROUTINE EVALUATION

History and Physical Examination

A detailed medical history at the time of initial evaluation should be obtained, and efforts should be made to determine the cause of underlying renal disease. Medical records provided at the time of evaluation may be incomplete and "precooked" diagnoses should be regarded with healthy skepticism. This is particularly important in the era of the electronic medical record. As noted in Chapter 1, approximately 40% of patients present with CKD within a month of starting dialysis and may carry nonspecific or unsatisfactory diagnoses such as "CKD of unknown origin" or CKD owing to hypertension (very uncommon in non–African Americans). Defining a specific cause of CKD is particularly important in young people in whom the risk of recurrent disease or of covert urologic abnormalities is greater. Estimation of urine output is important because it may help to determine the significance of the urine output in the early postoperative period and helps to determine the necessity for further urologic evaluation. If a kidney biopsy has been performed, the report should be sought and reviewed. Family history is extremely important because it may provide information regarding the cause of the renal failure and may also allow the physician to initiate discussion regarding living-related donation. The evaluation of patients with potentially recurring renal diseases after transplantation is discussed later in the chapter and in Chapter 17.

A detailed cardiovascular history is mandatory for all candidates, and patients should be instructed to discuss significant cardiac symptoms with physicians while awaiting transplantation. Risk factors for coronary artery disease should be sought in the history, including a history of diabetes, smoking, family history of coronary artery disease, and previous cardiac events. Exercise tolerance should be assessed. A history of claudication warrants an evaluation for peripheral vascular disease and may also point toward a higher chance of ischemic heart disease. A full physical examination must be performed, including evaluation for evidence of congestive heart failure, carotid artery disease, and peripheral vascular disease. The presence of femoral bruits and poor peripheral pulses may warrant further evaluation of the pelvic vasculature with either a Doppler ultrasound or a magnetic resonance angiogram (see Chapter 14). The presence of strong femoral and peripheral pulses is a valuable indicator to the transplant surgeon that the pelvic vessels will likely be adequate for the transplant vascular anastomosis (see Chapter 9).

A detailed history of infectious disease should be obtained (see Chapter 12). This should include assessment for possible exposure to tuberculosis, such as history of residence or travel to endemic areas, prior exposure, any prior treatment, and duration of treatment. Evidence of other possible infections, including hepatitis and endemic fungal infections, should be sought.

A detailed history of malignancy should be obtained. The physical exam should include thorough examination of major lymph node groups and palpation of abdomen for organomegaly. Male prostate examination by rectal examination may reveal overt enlargement or mass which might affect transplant outcomes. The role of routine PSA testing is controversial and there is not enough evidence to recommend routine PSA screening for transplant purpose. The age-appropriate screenings for breast, cervical, and colon cancer should be part of CKD care and there are no recommendations for additional testing beyond what is recommended in CKD population.

Laboratory Testing

A complete blood count and a chemistry panel should be obtained along with a prothrombin time and partial prothrombin time. Blood should be sent for blood and tissue typing. Patients should be screened for evidence of hepatitis B and C, syphilis, HIV, and cytomegalovirus.

Screening for tuberculosis may be required for certain populations to assess for evidence of prior tuberculosis exposure or infection. A quantiferon TB test has gradually replaced purified protein derivative as a screening test owing to lower false-positive rate and chest radiography should be performed in those at high risk for granulomatous infectious disease. Those with risk factors for tuberculosis infection may require preventive therapy with isoniazid (see Chapter 12). A urinalysis and urine culture should be performed on all urinating patients. In the event of significant proteinuria, a 24-hour urine collection for protein should be obtained, which may reflect the cause of primary kidney disease and be a guide for further management. The ubiquitous urine protein/creatinine ratio is not a reliable marker of proteinuria in dialysis patients.

EVALUATION OF SPECIFIC TRANSPLANTATION RISK FACTORS RELATED TO ORGAN SYSTEM DISEASE

Cardiovascular Disease

The cardiovascular evaluation of diabetic transplant candidates is discussed in Chapter 16. Ideally, the transplant teams include a designated cardiologist to assist in the evaluation of the often-complex issues of assessing and managing cardiovascular disease (CVD) in the CKD population.

CVD is the leading cause of death after renal transplantation. Almost half of deaths in patients with functioning grafts occurring within 30 days after transplantation are owing to CVD, primarily acute myocardial infarction. CVD disease is the major cause of long-term mortality and death with graft function, and the major cause of late graft loss (see Chapter 11). All patients with CKD are at high cardiac risk, although for some, the risk is particularly high. Diabetic patients, older patients, patients on dialysis for prolonged periods, and patients with multiple Framingham Study risk factors for coronary artery disease are generally recommended to undergo noninvasive cardiac testing: routine testing of lower-risk asymptomatic patients may not be necessary. Because many dialysis patients are unable to exercise adequately, noninvasive testing usually takes the form of chemical stress echocardiography or scintography. Patients with a positive stress test should proceed to a coronary angiogram. A prior history of ischemic heart disease has been found to be a major risk factor for post-transplant ischemic events, so that all patients with a history of myocardial infarction or congestive heart failure should undergo cardiac stress testing or, possibly, angiography, even if the stress test is negative. Risk factors associated with post-transplant ischemic heart disease include age more than 50 years, diabetes, and an abnormal electrocardiogram. The American Heart Association and the American College of Cardiology Foundation have issued a scientific statement on cardiac disease evaluation and management among kidney and liver transplant candidates (see Lentine et al. in Selected Readings). Most transplant programs use noninvasive testing as their initial mode of screening for coronary artery disease, although some prefer to go directly to coronary angiogram. Data are not yet available to test the effectiveness of more expensive screening techniques such as using single photon emission computed tomography (SPECT), positron emission tomography (PET), or electron-beam computed tomography (CT). Both dobutamine stress echocardiogram and dipyridamole sestamibi have similar sensitivities in detecting coronary artery disease in the non-ESKD population. Specific sensitivities and sensitivities for the ESKD population are lacking and may be center dependent. Patients who have critical lesions should probably undergo correction with coronary artery bypass surgery, angioplasty, or stent placement before transplantation. Depending on the stent used, a finite period of antiplatelet therapy may be required which should be taken into account when timing a transplant. Severe uncorrectable coronary artery disease is a contraindication for kidney transplant.

Calcific aortic stenosis and valvular heart disease are common in transplant candidates. When they are suspected, it is important to perform an echocardiogram to elicit systolic or diastolic dysfunction because this may have important prognostic implications. Reversible myocardial dysfunction should be treated. Irreversible heart failure should probably preclude renal transplantation unless heart transplantation is also considered. However, many patients with mild-to-moderate cardiac dysfunction may respond to renal transplantation with an improvement in myocardial function. An improvement in the ejection fraction has been documented after transplantation. Figure 8.2 provides an algorithm that is acceptable to most transplantation programs. These recommendations, however, are made largely on the basis of evidence that is extrapolated from patients without CKD, and they are not based on the results of prospective clinical trials. It has been suggested that symptom-based evaluation may be as effective as routine cohort-based evaluation and, whereas cardiac testing may provide prognostic information useful for determining who should be accepted for transplantation, the benefits of such testing for treatment purposes are unproved.

Cerebrovascular and Peripheral Vascular Disease

Successful kidney transplantation has been shown to reduce the risk of vascular disease events involving the cerebral circulation by nearly 50%. Signs and symptoms of cerebrovascular disease in transplant candidates, particularly older candidates, must be evaluated. Dialysis patients experience significantly more ischemic and hemorrhagic strokes and transient ischemic attacks compared with transplanted patients. Risk factors identified for post-transplant cerebrovascular disease include a history of pretransplant cerebrovascular disease, age, smoking, diabetes, hypertension, and hyperlipidemia. There is no evidence, however, that routine screening of asymptomatic renal transplant candidates for cerebrovascular disease is beneficial. Patients who have suffered cerebral vascular events and have significant and fixed neurologic deficits may be poor candidates in terms of their perioperative risk and rehabilitative potential. The risk of recurrent stroke should be assessed by a neurologist for patients who have had recent transient ischemic attacks or other cerebrovascular events. Patients receiving anticonvulsant medications for a seizure disorder should

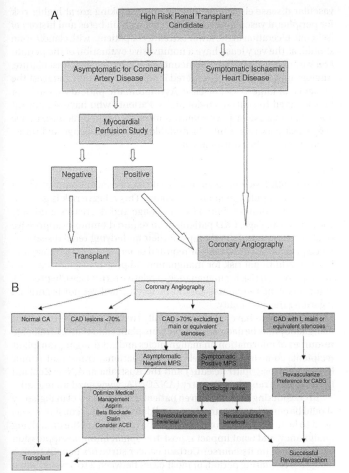

FIGURE 8.2 Proposed algorithm for cardiac evaluation for coronary artery disease in high-risk transplant candidates. (From Pilmore H. Cardiac assessment for renal transplantation. Am J Transplant 2006;6:659–665, with permission.)

undergo neurologic assessment to determine whether these medications can be safely discontinued. If anticonvulsants are required, it is preferable to use those that do not have a pharmacologic interaction with the calcineurin inhibitors (see Chapter 6).

Peripheral vascular disease is important both as a cause of allograft ischemia and lower-extremity amputation. There is a high incidence of peripheral vascular disease in diabetic recipients. Patients who have undergone lower-extremity amputations have a significantly higher mortality rate in the 2 years following transplant. Males, diabetics, patients with hypertension, lipid abnormalities, a history of vascular disease elsewhere, and cigarette smoking are at higher risk for peripheral vascular disease. Patients with diabetes and history of ischemic ulceration in the lower extremity or patients with claudication should, at the very least, have a noninvasive evaluation of the peripheral vasculature, preferably noncontrast CT of the pelvic vasculature. Angiography should be considered if noninvasive studies suggest the presence of large-vessel disease. Asymptomatic patients should not be subjected to routine angiography. Patients who have significant aortoiliac disease or have required intra-abdominal reconstructive arterial surgery represent a formidable surgical challenge and transplantation may be contraindicated.

Malignancy

Patients with ESKD have an increased risk of cancer compared with the general population at all age groups. This relative risk is greatest for patients younger than 35 years of age and decreases gradually with increasing age. CKD patients who required immunosuppressive treatment as part of the therapy of their underlying renal disease, or failed prior renal transplant, or required other solid-organ transplant, have an additional risk for malignancy. All post-transplant patients are at increased risk for malignancy in relative terms (see Chapter 11), and transplant candidates should be forewarned yet not frightened regarding this possibility.

Patients who have been successfully treated for a pretransplant malignancy may be deemed suitable transplant candidates. Invaluable resources of information on malignancies and solid-organ transplant recipients come from the Israel Penn International Transplant Tumor Registry (https://ipittr.uc.edu/) and the Australia and New Zealand Dialysis and Transplant Registry (ANZDATA, www.anzdata.org.au).

In considering whether a given patient with a history of malignancy should be considered a transplant candidate, two major considerations need to be taken into account: what is the prognosis of the underlying malignancy, and what impact is post-transplant immunosuppression likely to have on its course? Certain cancer survivors benefit from a disease-free waiting period, in most cases between 2 to 5 years. Some cancer types may not require any waiting period.

Previous editions of this text and other sources have provided recommended fixed period for transplant delay. A more nuanced and less proscriptive approach is based on an understanding of the course of a given malignancy, its pathology, staging, and response to therapy. There has been a trend to "downgrade" certain neoplastic lesions whose untreated prognosis is excellent. This includes ductal carcinoma in situ (DCIS) of the breast, and low-grade thyroid and prostate cancers. Routine prostate specific antigen (PSA) screening does not appear to confer a survival benefit. Small renal cell carcinomas may require no waiting period, whereas a delay of several years may be wise if the lesions are larger (more than 5 cm). Myeloma and plasma cell dyscrasias, once regarded as contraindications to transplant, are now often effectively treated and patients may be safely transplanted. The precise staging of melanoma is critical to recommendations regarding suitability; more advanced lesions require a wait of at least years, whereas superficial lesion may require no waiting period. In general, metastatic malignancies are contraindications to transplantation. Given the rapid progress being made in the management of multiple malignancies, oncologic consultation should be sought as part of the evaluation of transplant candidacy with a history of malignancy.

Infections

Pretransplant screening for infectious disease, together with recommendations for specific infections, is discussed in Chapter 12. Whenever possible, all treatable infections should be eradicated. The presence of chronic active infection precludes transplantation and the use of immunosuppressive therapy. Whenever possible, transplant candidates should receive immunization for infections that are prevalent, preferably before the development of ESKD. Osteomyelitis should be treated, and, if necessary, the infected parts should be removed surgically to prepare the patient for transplantation. Diabetic foot ulcers must be healed before transplantation.

An important change has taken place with respect to the candidacy of patients with HIV infection. Patients with HIV/AIDS are no longer regarded as inappropriate transplant candidates. The effective antiviral therapy has radically altered the prognosis of infected patients. Patients who are consistently receiving and tolerating an effective antiviral regimen (with an undetectable viral load and normal T-cell counts) can be considered candidates after completing their evaluation together with education with respect to their high-risk status. The availability and ongoing involvement of an infectious disease consultant familiar with the intricacies of highly active antiretroviral therapy (HAART) regimens is critical when HIV-positive patients undergo transplantation.

Gastrointestinal Disease

Diverticulitis. Diverticulitis is the most frequent cause of colonic perforation in renal transplant recipients. This may be related to the high prevalence of diverticulosis in patients on dialysis, especially patients with adult polycystic kidney disease. Mortality from colonic perforation is high, but the incidence of colonic perforation after renal transplantation has remained stable over many years. It seems reasonable that patients with a history of diverticulitis should be evaluated by a barium enema or a colonoscopy with consideration for resection of extensive disease if symptomatic diverticulitis persists.

Peptic Ulcer Disease. Peptic ulceration was once a frequent and sometimes lethal post-transplantation complication that required pretransplant screening in all patients and surgery in a selected few. With the use of histamine antagonists, antacids, and proton pump inhibitors (PPIs), the incidence of peptic ulcer disease has declined significantly. However, the evidence of an association of PPIs with the progression of CKD suggests that routine prophylaxis with these medications may be contraindicated. Transplantation is considered safe even in patients with a history of peptic ulcer disease, although active disease should be treated medically before transplantation. The role of *Helicobacter pylori* infection should be recognized, although routine screening for this organism is generally not recommended.

Cholelithiasis. Patients with a history of cholecystitis and cholelithiasis should undergo pretransplant evaluation with ultrasound to identify the presence of cholelithiasis and should be considered for cholecystectomy. Cholecystectomy may be wise for asymptomatic diabetic patients with cholelithiasis and is recommended for all symptomatic patients. Cholecystitis may be difficult to recognize after transplantation and can be a source of considerable morbidity.

Pancreatitis. A pretransplant history of pancreatitis increases the risk for post-transplant pancreatitis. Post-transplant pancreatitis has a high morbidity. Patients who have suffered episodes of pancreatitis may be more likely to develop post-transplant diabetes and should be forewarned. Both prednisone and azathioprine have been implicated in the etiology of pancreatitis. Hyperparathyroidism should be excluded as a possible factor. Other possible contributing factors, such as lipid disturbances, cholelithiasis, and alcohol, should be addressed before transplantation.

Pulmonary Disease

Surgical risks associated with severe lung disease include fluid overload, ventilator dependency, and infection. All patients should be screened with history, physical evaluation, and chest radiograph to identify lung disease that may increase the risk for major postoperative pulmonary complications. Formal pulmonary function testing may be required to assess surgical risk for patients with known lung disease, patients with signs and symptoms suggesting active lung disease, and patients with sleep apnea. Chronic lung disease may preclude safe general anesthesia, and patients who require supplemental oxygen are generally not transplant candidates. Patients with chronic obstructive lung disease and restrictive lung disease recipients have increased post-transplant infectious complications and mortality. Patients with evidence of chronic lung disease who continue to smoke must stop before transplantation. They should be directed to smoking cessation programs. Secondary pulmonary hypertension is more common due to long standing volume overload and diastolic dysfunction. Severe irreversible pulmonary hypertension is a contraindication to kidney transplantation. A careful assessment of its severity including repeated pressure measurement after dialysis to achieve a euvolumic state will help differentiate those with volume-related versus true pulmonary hypertension.

Urologic Evaluation

Ideally, the lower urinary tract should be sterile, continent, and compliant before transplantation. Urinalysis and urine culture should be performed on all urinating patients. Most patients will have undergone renal imaging studies as part of the evaluation of their underlying renal disease, and the studies themselves or reports thereof should be available at the time of the transplant evaluation. Dialysis patients who have not had an imaging study within the previous 3 years should have a renal ultrasound because of the risk for adenocarcinoma associated with acquired cystic disease.

A voiding cystourethrogram (VCUG) and other urologic procedures are generally not necessary unless there is a history of bladder dysfunction. Patients with a history of genitourinary abnormalities and individuals younger than 20 years may require a full evaluation including a VCUG, cystoscopy, and urodynamic studies. A history of nocturnal enuresis into late childhood is an important clue to the presence of bladder dysfunction and CKD in childhood (see Chapter 17).

Patients with bladder dysfunction secondary to neurogenic bladder and those who have chronic infection can often be managed without urinary diversion or bladder augmentation procedures. Self-catheterization may be an acceptable option for some patients, infection being a major complication. Graft implantation into the native bladder is always preferred. Diverted urinary tracts should be undiverted where possible to make the lower urinary tract functional before transplantation. Even a very small bladder may develop normal compliance and capacity after transplantation. Transplantation is possible for patients whose urinary tract has been diverted into an ileal conduit and cannot be undiverted. The rate of urologic complications is high, but the overall patient and graft survival is not different from patients with intact urinary tracts.

Older men frequently have prostatic enlargement and may develop outflow tract obstruction after transplantation. In general, if patients are still passing sufficient volumes of urine, the prostate should be resected preoperatively. Otherwise, the operation should be postponed until after the transplantation has been successfully performed. These patients may require an indwelling bladder catheter or be prepared to self-catheterize until the prostate has been resected. The possibility of chronic incontinence once a functioning transplant is in place should be considered, since this may have a major impact on quality of life.

Most patients with ESKD from adult polycystic kidney disease (PKD) do not require native kidney nephrectomy prior to transplant and there is adequate "room" to place the transplant. Some patients may benefit from unilateral or bilateral nephrectomy to reduce symptomatic bleeding or recurrent infection or for the discomfort suffered because of their massive size. Occasionally polycystic kidneys are so large that they reach deep into the lower abdominal quadrants and may need to be removed to make room for the transplant. For patients with PKD and CKD who are not yet on dialysis every attempt should be made to achieve preemptive transplantation. If necessary, the polycystic kidneys can be removed once transplant function is established.

Pretransplant nephrectomy may be indicated for patients with chronic renal infections or infected renal stones or obstructive uropathy complicated by chronic infections. Patients with uncomplicated recurrent urinary tract infection do not usually require pretransplant nephrectomy. Bilateral nephrectomy may be recommended in patients with congenital nephrotic syndrome and also in patients with persistent nephrotic syndrome and massive proteinuria despite optimal medical management. Adenocarcinoma of the native kidneys may manifest after transplantation and is associated with considerable morbidity and mortality. The major indications for pretransplant native kidney nephrectomy are listed in Table 8.2. If nephrectomy is required, it should be done 6 weeks to 3 months before transplantation, ideally by

TABLE 8.2	Indications for Pretransplantation Native Nephrectomy

Chronic renal parenchymal infection
Infected stones
Heavy proteinuria
Intractable hypertension
Polycystic kidney disease*
Acquired renal cystic disease†
Infected reflux‡

*Only when the kidneys are massive, recurrently infected, or bleeding.
†When there is suspicion of adenocarcinoma.
‡Uninfected reflux does not require nephrectomy.

laparoscopic technique. Occasionally, unilateral transplant nephrectomy is performed at the time of the transplant surgery, but this should be avoided if at all possible.

Renal Osteodystrophy and Metabolic Bone Disease

Patients with ESKD suffer from multiple bone disorders, including secondary hyperparathyroidism, osteomalacia, and dialysis-related amyloid bone disease (see Molnar et al. in Selected Readings and Chapter 1). Successful renal transplantation is the best treatment for most cases of osteomalacia and dialysis-related amyloid bone disease. Persistence of hyperparathyroidism after renal transplantation is common. Most renal transplant recipients have elevated parathyroid hormone (PTH) levels at the time of transplantation, and more than 30% of these patients continue to have elevated levels up to 3 years after transplantation. The duration of time on dialysis and the intensity of hyperparathyroidism before transplantation correlate with the severity of post-transplantation hyperparathyroidism (see Chapter 10). Hypercalcemia is the most common marker of hyperparathyroidism after transplantation. Every attempt should be made to minimize the effect of impaired calcium metabolism, metabolic acidosis, and secondary hyperparathyroidism in the pretransplantation period. Cinacalcet (Sensipar) is an approved and effective therapy, and it can be used safely after transplant to correct hypercalcemia. The data on cinacalcet on its long-term use especially when is PTH level is not markedly elevated is largely unknown. Patients with persistent hyperparathyroidism that is unresponsive to medical therapy or those with adenoma may need pretransplant parathyroidectomy. Older female and diabetic patients should be warned that they may be at an exaggerated risk for osteopenia and pathologic fractures after transplantation.

Hypercoagulable States

There appears to be an increased prevalence of several prothrombotic factors in renal transplant candidates, and thrombophilic patients are at a higher risk for early graft loss. All transplant candidates should have routine coagulation studies performed. Patients who have had a history of thrombosis, including recurrent thrombosis of arteriovenous grafts and fistulas, or spontaneous abortion, should have a more extensive coagulation profile performed. This should include screening for activated protein C (APC) resistance, factor V and prothrombin gene mutations, anticardiolipin antibody, lupus anticoagulant, protein C and S, antithrombin III, and homocystine levels. Approximately 6% of Caucasians have APC resistance, usually as a result of heterozygosity for the factor V Leiden mutation. They are prone to thrombotic complications and graft loss. All renal transplant candidates with systemic lupus erythematosus should have antiphospholipid antibodies measured.

Thrombophilia is rarely a contraindication to transplantation, although its recognition should initiate preventive strategies. Perioperative anticoagulation is discussed in Chapter 9. Therapeutic decisions for long-term anticoagulation need to be individualized with respect to the agent used and the length of treatment. Chronic anticoagulation of dialysis patients with recurrent access thrombosis but without an underlying coagulopathy is often ineffective and should be avoided. Long-standing warfarin administration has been associated with accelerated vascular calcification. The newer anticoagulation medications may not affect routine coagulation studies and there may be no readily available antidote, so that careful medication history is essential to avoid major bleeding complications

EVALUATION OF RISK FACTORS RELATED TO SPECIFIC PATIENT CHARACTERISTICS

Transplantation in Elderly Patients

The assessment of the transplant candidacy of elderly patients with advanced CKD is challenging. It requires both compassion for the unique predicament of the elderly patient and a dispassionate assessment of the complex issues that transplantation in elderly patients implies.

Patients over the age of 70 years are the fastest-growing segment of the ESKD population worldwide, though for reasons discussed below, the great majority not deemed kidney transplant candidates. There is no formal upper age limit at which patients may no longer be accepted for transplantation; successful outcomes have been described even in octogenarians (see Lonning et al. in Selected Readings). As of mid-2016, over 22% of all patients on the waiting list for renal transplantation in the United States are 65 years of age or older; over 5% are 70 years or older, and the "aging" trend is continuing. There has been a marked increase in the number of renal transplants performed in older patients in the past decade. Data from the United States shows that, as a group, patients 60 years or older, who are deemed appropriate transplant candidates and receive a renal transplant, survive longer than dialysis patients and have a better survival rate than patients who remain on the transplant waiting list. Similar data are also available for patients older than 70, and even for patients older than 75 years. This trend, however, has not been confirmed in older patients in the United Kingdom. Older transplant recipients have an increased risk for death owing to CVD in the few months after renal transplantation. They also tend to have longer initial hospitalizations but fewer acute rejection episodes because their immune system may be less aggressive. Older patients may be at increased risk for infection and malignancy related to immunosuppression. The metabolism of immunosuppressive drugs may be slowed by aging. The immunosuppressive management of elderly transplant recipients is discussed in Chapter 6.

The possibility of covert coronary artery disease should be routinely evaluated with stress testing, and the need for assessment of cerebrovascular and peripheral vascular disease should be considered on an individual basis. Older patients with significant vascular disease may not be appropriate transplant candidates. Standard malignancy screening recommendations should be applied compulsively in older patients. The assessment of older patients should also take into account their cognitive abilities and their capacity to ambulate and care for themselves in the post-transplantation period. Clearly, there are sprightly patients in their 70' s who are excellent transplant candidates, whereas many patients of this age group would do better to remain on dialysis. Of all the patients older than 65 years on chronic dialysis in the United States, only approximately 5% are on a transplant waiting list.

Most of the published data on transplantation in older patients relate to patients older than 60. Data on patients older than 70 are more limited. The available data also tend to relate to the "dry" statistics of patient and graft survival when compared to the standard center-based dialysis regimen. Comparisons to more innovative home-based dialysis techniques are awaited and home-based dialysis may represent an acceptable option to transplantation. Most older patients seek improved quality of life in their later years, which they may resent spending on dialysis. Older patients may have unrealistic expectations about their quality of life after transplantation—the transplant will not make them younger! They may also tend to underestimate or discount the risks associated with transplantation in their enthusiasm to be free from the constraints of chronic dialysis. The waiting time for a deceased donor transplant in the United States is such that older patients may not survive to be allocated a kidney by the standard algorithm, and to benefit from transplantation, and they should be encouraged to be prepared to accept a high KDPI or PHS higher-risk kidney (see Chapter 5), as noted previously.

Prolonged waiting times dramatically decrease the clinical benefits and economic attractiveness of transplantation, particularly among older transplant candidates. Older patients are often reluctant to accept living donor kidneys from their children, although these kidneys offer them the best and most realistic chance of meaningful improved survival and quality of life. Even devoted family members may have reservations about living donation for older family members with an intrinsically limited life span. These issues must be discussed with older patients and their families with particular care and compassion to optimize the chance of a satisfactory outcome. It should be made clear to older patients that data relating to relative post-transplant survival come from large database analyses and may not be relevant to individuals, many of whom may be anxious to hear apparently authoritative predictions about their anticipated expectancy.

Frailty

Chronologic age alone can be a misleading marker of transplant outcome and benefit. Frailty is a measure of physiologic reserve and augmented vulnerability described and validated in the geriatric population and is preferable to clinical "eyeballing" of transplant suitability in the aged.

TABLE 8.3	Components of Frailty*

1. Shrinking (self-report on unintentional weight loss of >10 lb in previous year based on dry weight)
2. Weakness (grip strength below an established cutoff based on sex and BMI)
3. Exhaustion (self-reported)
4. Low activity (kilocalories per week below an established cutoff)
5. Slowed walking speed (walking time of 15 ft below an established cutoff by sex and height)

*See Fried LP, Tangen CM, Walston J, et al. Frailty in older adults: evidence for a phenotype. J Gerontol A Biol Sci Med Sci 2001;56:M146–M156 and Dusseux et al in Selected Readings.

Higher severities of frailty are associated with greater mortality both on dialysis and after transplantation, prolonged post-transplant hospital admission, increased rates of delayed graft function, and readmission. Related and overlapping comorbidities, such as cognitive impairment, malnutrition, and functional status have a similar impact. Frailty estimation can be based on five components (see Table 8.3). Various tools are being developed and validated to identify elderly ESKD patients who are more likely to have acceptable long-term post-transplant outcomes. These tools will likely help identify elderly patients who will benefit most from transplant (see Dusseux et al. in Selected Readings) but have yet to be validated for this purpose in prospective clinical trials. Patients with low functional status that are deemed candidates by transplant centers and undergo kidney transplant may fare better compared to those waitlisted but still remaining on dialysis (see Reese et al. in Selected Readings)

Obesity

Malnutrition at the time of dialysis is a strong predictor of short-term and long-term mortality, whereas a high body mass index (BMI) has been associated with reduced mortality among hemodialysis patients, a phenomenon referred to as "reversed epidemiology." In contrast, morbid obesity is an important risk factor for renal transplant recipients (reversal of reversed epidemiology!) and has been considered by some transplant centers as an exclusion criteria. Approximately 20% of transplant recipients have a pretransplant BMI of greater than 30 kg/m^2, and this percentage is increasing. Obese renal transplant recipients have a higher risk for delayed graft function and suffer from more surgical complications, including more wound infections. Obesity is also associated with a prolonged post-transplant hospital stay, increased cost of transplantation, and a higher incidence of post-transplant diabetes and CVD (see Chapter 11).

Some programs exclude patients with a BMI greater than a fixed value (typically 35 or 40 kg/m^2) from transplantation, although the available patient and graft survival data in obese patients are not significantly worse than for nonobese patients. BMI alone can be a misleading predictor of risk, and fat distribution (estimated by waist /hip ratio) and muscle mass should also be considered. Abdominal obesity is a particular concern both in terms of surgical risk and as a marker for the metabolic syndrome. Patients with a large abdominal pannus are a special concern.

Special attention should be given to the cardiac evaluation of obese renal transplant candidates. Obese elderly patients and those with concomitant coronary heart disease may have a worse prognosis, and these patients may be better served by remaining on dialysis. It is tempting, and may seem intuitively appropriate, to recommend or even demand, weight loss in obese transplant candidates. Demands to lose weight, however, may put dialysis patients at risk and have not been proved to improve outcome. It is better to individualize transplant recommendations regarding weight loss rather than make broad exclusionary rules based on an arbitrary BMI or demands for BMI reduction. If weight loss is deemed necessary, it should be supervised by a trained dietitian (see Chapter 20). Studies evaluating bariatric surgery for transplant candidates are in progress and appear promising.

Hypotension

Whereas the great majority of CKD and ESKD patient are hypertensive, some tend to hypotension, either chronically or during dialysis treatments. Patients who have undergone native kidney nephrectomies are particularly prone to hypotension, as are long-standing diabetics as a result of autonomic neuropathy, and patients with a history of eating disorders and chronic interstitial nephritis. Chronically hypotensive patients should be evaluated for reversible causes, most frequently cardiac or adrenal in origin.

Chronically hypotensive patients, or those requiring midodrine or frequent saline infusions for symptomatic hypotension, represent a high-risk category for kidney transplantation. Delayed graft function, primary nonfunction, and repeated episodes of acute kidney injury (see Chapter 10) are more common. If uncorrectable, chronic hypotension may be a contraindication for kidney transplantation. If hypotensive patients are transplanted, every effort should be made to support the systolic blood pressure in the perioperative period.

Highly Sensitized Patients

The immunologic challenge faced by highly sensitized patients is discussed in Chapter 3. About 40% of patients awaiting deceased donor transplants in the United States have high levels of preformed cytotoxic antibodies that may prevent them from receiving a kidney or prolong their wait considerably. Cytotoxic antibodies result from failed prior transplants, multiple pregnancies, and multiple blood transfusions. Attempts have been made to reduce the antibody levels by infusion of intravenous immune globulin (IVIg), plasma exchange, and rituximab (see Chapter 6). Use of IVIg with rituximab in these circumstances appears to be the most promising (see Keith and Vranic in Selected Readings). Patients with high levels of antibodies should be warned of the probability of a prolonged wait for a kidney, though the additional points that the most highly sensitized patient are now given in the KAS has reduced the waiting time. The widespread use of erythropoietin in dialysis patients may serve to lower the level of preformed antibodies by

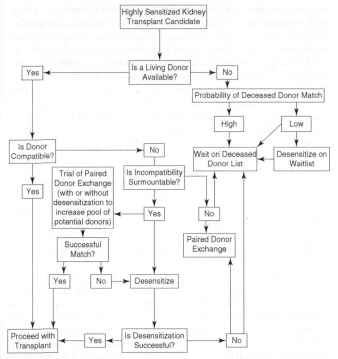

FIGURE 8.3 Algorithm for the management of the highly sensitized patient seeking kidney transplant.

There is no predefined level of incompatibility that is considered insurmountable and decision to pursue desensitization should be individualized for the potential recipient considering medical eligibility, degree of sensitization to the donor, and financial coverage. This decision making is highly center specific. The risks of early graft failure are significantly increased in those pairs with positive CDC crossmatch prior to desensitization and pursuing living donor transplantation in this setting should be attempted with caution. Paired donor exchange may offer candidates the opportunity to seek a more compatible donor, possibly obviating the risks and costs associated with desensitization. CDC, complement-dependent cytotoxicity. (Republished with permission of American Society of Nephrology, from Keith D, Vranic G. Approach to the highly sensitized kidney transplant candidate. Clin J Am Soc Nephrol 2016;11:684–693.)

minimizing blood transfusion requirements. Sensitized patients with potential living donors who are incompatible to them are best served by paired exchange transplantation (see Chapter 7, Part IV) so as to find a donor to whom they are unsensitized or less-sensitized. Paired exchange can be combined with desensitization (Fig. 8.3).

Previously Transplanted Candidates

The fate of second and multiple transplantations is dependent to a considerable extent on the timing and etiology of the prior transplant loss. Patients whose kidneys failed because of surgical complications or have kidneys that functioned for more than a year have a prognosis that is not significantly different from patients with primary transplants. If the primary transplant is lost to early rejection, the prognosis for another transplant is impaired and the patient will do best with a thorough immunologic workup to identify HLA and non-HLA antibodies and then undergo a well-matched deceased donor transplant if they are fortunate to be offered one, or compatible paired exchanged, or a two-haplotype-matched living-related transplant if a suitable donor is available. Patients must be made aware of their impaired prognosis. The prognosis of patients whose graft was lost owing to recurrent disease is generally poor, particularly if disease recurrence has been rapid and aggressive. In these circumstances, careful consideration needs to be given on when to consider retransplantation with a living donor. Patients with graft loss owing to BK nephropathy have been successfully retransplanted.

The process of evaluating a patient for a repeat transplant is the same as that for a primary transplant. Every effort must be made to understand the etiology of the loss of the previous transplant(s) and this is mandatory when the loss was rapid and nonsurgical in nature. If the transplant was lost owing to rejection, a careful assessment of medication adherence should be performed by the physician and social worker. For patients whose first transplant life was prolonged, special attention should be paid to the possibility of covert coronary artery disease or malignancy. Patients with a failing transplant should be referred early for retransplantation in the hope of avoiding the need to return to dialysis. Multiple transplanted patients are at an increased risk for immunosuppressant-related malignancy and infection and should be forewarned. Patients whose first deceased donor transplant was lost within the first 3 months, whether for technical or other reasons, are able to maintain their original waiting time on the UNOS waiting list (see Chapter 5).

Candidates with Other Solid-Organ Transplants

The topic of combined kidney and liver transplantation is discussed in Chapter 13. Experience with combined heart–kidney transplantation is more limited, but many of these procedures have been performed successfully. Approximately 20% of all nonrenal solid-organ transplant recipients eventually develop ESKD owing to a combination of preexisting acute and chronic kidney injury, calcineurin-inhibitor toxicity, post-transplant diabetes and other factors. These patients may become kidney transplant candidates and are similar in most respects to nontransplanted candidates except that they may have required months and years of immunosuppression. They may be more susceptible to the infectious and malignancy complication of immunosuppression and should be forewarned. Their candidacy will also depend on the function of the originally transplanted organ and on their anticipated life span and degree of rehabilitation. Living kidney donation is preferred so as to avoid or limit the need for dialysis.

RELEVANCE OF THE ETIOLOGY OF RENAL DISEASE TO THE TRANSPLANT EVALUATION

The cause of CKD is important for prognosticating transplant outcome. This information may also be critical in selecting a suitable living donor for transplantation. The risk for recurrence of the native kidney disease

TABLE 8.4	Risk for Recurrent Disease After Renal Transplantation

Recurrent Disease	Risk (%)
Focal and segmental glomerulosclerosis	20–40
Immunoglobulin A nephropathy	40–60
MPGN-I	30–50
MPGN-II	80–100
Membranous nephropathy	10–30
Diabetic nephropathy	80–100 (by histology)
HUS/TTP	50–75
Oxalosis	80–100
Granulomatosis with polyangitis	<20
Fabry disease	<5
Systemic lupus erythematosus	3–10

HUS, hemolytic uremic syndrome; MPGN, membranoproliferative glomerulonephritis; TTP, thrombotic thrombocytopenic purpura.

in the transplant is summarized in Table 8.4 which can be used as a guide to counsel patients. The effects of recurrent renal disease on the post-transplantation course are discussed in Chapter 11.

Diabetes Mellitus

The special considerations related to the evaluation of diabetic transplant candidates, who account for about 40% of the ESKD population in the United States, are considered in Chapter 16. Diabetic transplant recipients can develop histologic features of diabetic nephropathy as early as 3 years after transplantation, years earlier than in the native kidneys. However, patients should be informed that recurrent diabetic nephropathy is an uncommon isolated cause of graft failure, and its possibility should not be used as the sole reason to seek the more complex simultaneous kidney–pancreas transplantation. Optimal management of diabetes while on dialysis is a critical factor in the prevention of post-transplantation diabetic complications. Diabetic education should be reinforced at the time of transplant evaluation.

Many diabetic patients find that their insulin requirements, or requirements for oral agents, diminish with the development of ESKD and dialysis. These patients should be warned that they will likely become medication dependent again following a transplant. Non–insulin-dependent diabetics may become insulin dependent and this may impinge on their quality of life and that of their caregivers following a successful transplant (see Chapter 11). Insulin requirements increase owing to a combination of increased insulin clearance with improved renal function and the diabetogenic effects of immunosuppressive medications.

Focal and Segmental Glomerulosclerosis

This discussion relates to primary focal and segmental glomerulosclerosis (FSGS). FSGS that is secondary to reflux nephropathy, drug toxicity and obesity, for example, does not recur after transplantation. Evidence of focal sclerosis is often found on histologic evaluation of patients with hypertensive renal disease and other causes of CKD and should be differentiated from the primary disorder. Diffuse podocyte effacement on electron microscopy can differentiate primary FSGS from the secondary FSGS where the podocyte effacement is patchy. Presumably as a result of a yet to be identified serum factor that affects the permeability of the glomerular basement membrane (GBM), transplant candidates with primary FSGS have a high incidence of recurrence after transplantation, reported between 20% and 40%. The odds of recurrence are increased in patients who are younger (see Chapter 17), those with a history of heavy proteinuria and clinical nephrotic syndrome, those who had a rapid progression to ESKD, those with the collapsing variant, and those whose initial biopsy showed mesangial hypertrophy. The strongest predictor of recurrence is a history of recurrence in a previous transplant. Patients should be forewarned of the possibility of recurrence. If a living donor is being considered, both the transplant candidate and the potential donor should be aware of the risk for graft loss from recurrent FSGS. Plasma exchange before transplantation and in the early post-transplantation period has been suggested to reduce the risk for recurrent disease, but its effectiveness has been difficult to prove. Rituximab, abatacept, and Belatacept have been used as part of immunosuppression to prevent or treat FSGS but their results are less than satisfactory.

Some patients with FSGS continue to have heavy proteinuria (more than 10 g daily) while on dialysis. In these cases, native kidney nephrectomy may be indicated both for nutritional consideration and because persistent massive native kidney proteinuria makes the evaluation of post-transplant proteinuria very difficult. Post-transplant management and prevention of recurrent FSGS is a particular problem in children. Patients who have lost a prior transplant to recurrent FSGS are at a high risk for recurrence, and this is an important consideration in assessing their candidacy for a repeat transplantation. Some programs avoid living donor transplantation in these circumstances.

Recurrent Glomerulonephritis

The recurrence rates of the most common primary glomerulopathies are shown in Table 8.4 and are also discussed in Chapter 17. Recurrent disease estimates are imprecise because only about 20% of CKD patients have a specific histologic diagnosis at the time of presentation for transplant evaluation. The rate of recurrence of the glomerulopathies continues to increase with longer duration of follow-up after transplantation and may be more common in recipients of living related transplants. Evidence of histologic recurrence of immunoglobulin A (IgA) nephropathy is common, although graft loss due to recurrent IgA nephropathy is uncommon and has been reported in about 10% of patients. Recurrent IgA nephropathy in a prior transplant is generally not a contraindication for repeat transplantation, and re-recurrence is not inevitable. IgA nephropathy may be familial in some cases, and donors should be carefully screened. Membranous nephropathy, both primary and secondary can recur after kidney transplant. M-type phospholipase A2 receptor (PLA2R) has been identified as a major target antigen and autoantibodies against PLA2R were found in majority of patients with idiopathic but not secondary membranous nephropathy. Their detection may have a role in prognosis and responsive to treatment.

Atypical Hemolytic Uremic Syndrome

There is a high rate of recurrence of the nondiarrheal form of hemolytic uremic syndrome (aHUS) and before the introduction of eculizumab treatment, nearly 50% grafts failed from that recurrence (see also Chapter 17). Because the condition is rare, it may go undiagnosed. Patients with a history of renal failure and thrombotic microangiopathy (TMA) or rapid, nonsurgical, loss of a previous transplant with evidence of TMA should be evaluated for a diagnosis of aHUS. Older age at onset, a shorter interval between onset of ESKD and transplantation, the use of living donors, and the use of calcineurin inhibitors have all been associated with recurrence. Both the calcineurin inhibitor drugs may induce TMA (see Chapter 6), although its severity is typically less than in the recurrent form. Patients and living donors should be counseled regarding risks for recurrence in patients with a history of aHUS and consideration should be given to a calcineurin inhibitor-free regimens and the perioperative use of eculizumab. The great expense of eculizumab may be prohibitive in some circumstances and ideally, confirmation of its availability and insurance coverage should be made prior to transplantation.

Systemic Lupus Erythematosus and Vasculitis

Recurrence of SLE can occasionally lead to graft failure. Clinical activity of SLE should be quiescent before transplantation. The patient should not require cytotoxic agents, larger dose of mycophenolate or more than 10 mg of prednisone before transplantation to maintain quiescence. Clinically active SLE typically improves with the development of chronic renal failure, but may not do so in some patients, particularly African-American women. Some patients are clinically quiescent but maintain persistently abnormal levels of serologic markers of disease activity while on dialysis. It is the degree of clinical activity that should determine transplant candidacy.

Patients with antineutrophil cytoplasmic antibody (ANCA)-associated systemic vasculitis are at risk for recurrent disease; however, pretransplant ANCA levels are not predictive of recurrence in asymptomatic patients. Successful transplantation has been reported in active disease, but it is wise to wait until the disease is quiescent before transplantation.

Patients who have been immunosuppressed during the course of their native kidney disease may be at increased risk for post-transplant opportunistic infections and lymphoma. The risk for avascular necrosis is higher in patients with SLE, most of whom have received high doses of corticosteroids during the course of their illness. A subset of patients may also be at risk of thromboembolic events owing to their hypercoagulable state.

Oxalosis and Oxaluria

Primary oxalosis is a rare cause of renal failure. It is an autosomal recessive disorder owing to deficiency of the hepatic enzyme alanine glyoxylate aminotransferase. The presence of this enzyme leads to increased urinary secretion of calcium oxalate and nephrocalcinosis, which leads to CKD. Accumulation of oxalate occurs throughout the body. Failure of the graft usually occurs after transplantation with rapid deposition of oxalate in the graft, Failure of the graft usually occurs despite intensive therapy with perioperative intensive dialysis and oral phosphates, which are designed to minimize oxalate deposition. All reduce renal calcium oxalate deposition, whereas pyridoxine is a coenzyme that functions in conversion of glyoxylate to glycine. Combined liver and kidney transplantation is the best option for patients with primary oxalosis: the transplanted liver provides the absent enzyme (see Chapters 13 and 17). Because the usual parameters of hepatic function are normal in these patients, they may require a prolonged wait for a transplant in countries where the severity of hepatic dysfunction is the major determinant of liver allocation. It has been suggested that isolated kidney transplantation is a reasonable first option for patients with oxalosis as long as the precautions listed earlier are adhered to rigorously and patients are adequately warned of the recurrence risk.

Secondary hyperoxaluria is most commonly of intestinal origin and may also lead to recurrence in the allograft. Patients have usually suffered from inflammatory bowel disease or morbid obesity. If the underlying defect is reversible (e.g., intestinal bypass for obesity), consideration should be given to surgical reversal before transplantation. In urinating patients, the 24-hour excretion of oxalate should be checked to help assess the risk for recurrent oxalosis.

Fabry Disease

Fabry disease is owing to a deficiency of a-galactosidase enzyme, which results in accumulation of glycosphingolipid in the kidney and other organs. It was initially hoped that kidney transplantation would provide enough enzyme to prevent disease progression, but this has not proved to be the case and Fabry disease may recur and progress in the transplanted kidney. Recurrence is slow, and death is usually caused from sepsis and other systemic complications. Renal transplantation is the treatment of choice for patients with Fabry disease who do not have severe systemic disease. Fabrazyme is now available as a replacement recombinant form of the deficient human enzyme, which may have a major beneficial impact on the course of the disease.

Alport Syndrome

Patients with Alport syndrome have a genetic abnormality of type 4 collagen that is X-linked in 80% of patients. Autosomal recessive (15%) and autosomal dominant (5%) forms also occur. The introduction of normal collagen in the basal membrane of the transplanted kidney may induce antibody formation to donor kidney collagen found in the GBM. The precise incidence of anti-GBM antibody formation is unknown, although clinically significant anti-GBM nephritis is rare. Graft survival is not impaired in patients with Alport syndrome. Patients should be warned that there is a potential to develop clinically significant anti-GBM disease, which may occur in a subsequent transplant graft but usually without pulmonary involvement. The presence of inherited kidney disease always requires intensive family screening before consideration of living related donation.

Sickle Cell Disease

Sickle cell disease often leads to ESKD, probably by causing chronic intestinal fibrosis, but FSGS and nephrotic syndrome also do occur. Short-term patient and graft survival rates are not different from those in patients without sickle cell disease and long-term outcomes of patients with sickle cell disease have been shown to be comparable to matched control patients with diabetes. Occasionally, severe, and potentially lethal, sickling crises may occur after transplantation, presumably related to the improving hematocrit. Exchange transfusions may be an effective treatment. There is a trend toward improved survival for transplanted patients with sickle cell disease compared with sickle cell disease patients who remain on the waiting list. Renal transplantation appears to be the treatment of choice for patients without severe systemic complications.

Amyloidosis and Plasma Cell Dyscrasias

Patients with primary amyloidosis, multiple myeloma, and the plasma cell dyscrasias are high-risk transplant candidates. In the past, their mortality rate after transplantation was reported to be as high as 50% at 1 year, death being caused by infectious and cardiac complications. Patients were generally discouraged from renal transplantation. The prognosis of these diseases has been changed radically with the introduction of stem cell transplantation and the introduction on immunotherapy and protease inhibitors. Once therapy has been stabilized, kidney transplantation can be considered after hematologic consultation.

Patients with secondary amyloidosis may be acceptable candidates. The presence and extent of myocardial infiltration should be assessed. The subgroup of patients with amyloidosis complicating familial Mediterranean fever (FMF) may not tolerate the combination of colchicine and cyclosporine therapy as a consequence of systemic and gastrointestinal symptoms. Recurrence of amyloid deposition in the allograft is common.

The transplant evaluation of all patients older than 60 with an unexplained cause of renal failure should include plasma immuno-electrophoresis to screen for paraproteins. The rate of conversion from benign monoclonal gammopathy to frank multiple myeloma is about 1% per year and does not appear to be accelerated by solid-organ transplant. Patients should be informed of the higher morbidity risk in the post-transplantation period including infection risk and venous thromboembolic events (see Goebel et al. in Selected Readings).

Polycystic Kidney Disease

Patients with polycystic kidney disease are excellent potential transplant candidates. The graft and patient survival rates are not different from those in other low-risk groups. The necessity for pretransplant or post-transplant nephrectomy was discussed previously. There may be an increased risk for gastrointestinal complications after transplantation, usually related to diverticular disease. Patients with headaches or other symptoms of the central nervous system or with a family history of aneurysm should undergo noninvasive screening for cerebral aneurysm. The possibility of living-related donation and its workup in families with polycystic kidney is discussed in Chapter 7.

Part II: Management of the Waiting List for a Deceased Donor Kidney Transplant

As of early 2017, there were approximately 100,000 patients registered on the United Network for Organ Sharing (UNOS) kidney transplant waiting list in the United States. With close to 3,000 patients added to this list every month, this number will inevitably increase. The overall number of waitlisted patients includes candidates who have been placed on the list in an "inactive" status, typically because their evaluation is incomplete or new issues have developed which may be a contraindication to transplantation, presumably on a temporary basis. "Active" patients make up 60% of the overall transplant waiting list, and this number has been relatively stable with a more modest rise over the past 10 years. The rise of the listing of "inactive" patients was related in part to a UNOS policy change in 2003 wherein candidates could accrue waiting time while in inactive status. This resulted in a steady increase in the number of waitlisted patients who had inactive status. Some programs list all potential candidates "inactive" without formally evaluating them and only activate their candidacy when they are evaluated closer to the time they are likely to be offered a kidney. According to the revised UNOS national kidney allocation policy introduced in December 2014 (see Chapter 5), waiting time is now determined by first date of dialysis initiation or listing for transplantation when GFR is estimated to be less than 20 mL/min.

While the number of patients on the transplant waiting list has increased, the number of deceased donor transplants has trailed far behind the growing need, leading to longer waiting time and increased waitlist deaths. Some organ procurement organizations in the United States have waiting times on the order of 8 to 10 years for certain blood types. Approximately 30% of the candidates on the waiting list have been on dialysis for more than 6 years and 10% for more than 11 years. In addition, the population of kidney transplant candidates in the United States has grown older over the past 20 years. The proportion of candidates age 65 years or older is now over 20%. The mortality rate on the waiting list—both for active and inactive candidates—has been estimated at 5% per annum overall, and even higher for diabetic patients. Approximately half of the deaths on the waiting list occur in patients who are on inactive status. While waitlist times increase, patients face longer dialysis times at the time of transplant and tend to collect comorbidities which can impact post-transplant outcomes.

Waitlist management, therefore, has become one of the most significant issues facing transplant centers. Currently, no firm guidelines exist for frequency of pretransplant follow-up visits, storage sera for pretransplant crossmatch, cardiovascular workup, and screening for infection. Transplant programs vary in dealing with these items based on resources, staffing, and the length of the waitlist. As patients spend more time on dialysis awaiting transplantation, progression of their cardiac comorbidities, vascular disease and other complications makes transplantation more complicated. Cardiovascular health tends to deteriorate as patients remain on dialysis. The overall impression of the patient at time of initial evaluation may no longer apply during the patient's time on the waiting list. Proper waitlist management is essential to the functioning of a transplant program. It is critical that there be ongoing communication between dialysis units, patients, and transplant centers regarding health and psychosocial issues that may be relevant to the transplant candidacy. This could include any active infections, need for cardiac interventions, new malignancies, loss of insurance, and change in demographics and social support.

Many transplant programs attempt to reassess each patient's candidacy on an annual basis. In addition to updating a patient's medical status, this reassessment also provides an opportunity to review the availability of living donors and to reinforce transplant-related educational needs, and may serve to diminish a patient's sense of hopelessness. Specialized consents such as for PHS higher-risk kidneys, KDPI >85% kidneys (see Chapter 5), can be reconsidered. However, with the growing number of patients on the waiting list, annual follow up of all waitlisted patients can be difficult to achieve if the waitlist of a particular program is quite large. Devising an algorithm to update patient status remains an ongoing challenge for transplant centers that have lengthy waiting times. Some of the larger programs attempt to see the patients at the top of the waiting list (e.g., top 20 to 30 patients in each ABO blood group) as well as those patients who appear on a "match run" annually to re-assess their transplant candidacy and review the overall transplant process. For the other patients on the waiting list, these larger programs often send annual forms to the dialysis unit asking for up to date developments in a patient's clinical status. With the current allocation system which prioritizes HLA matching and highly sensitized patients, however, it is difficult to predict when a patient will be called with a kidney offer. Patients must be prepared at all times for the potential of transplantation, and a system must be in place to ensure their medical and psychosocial preparedness. The unpredictability has presented transplantation programs with a considerable challenge of attempting to ensure that large numbers of patients, most of whom are not under their direct care, are medically cleared for transplantation at all times. A consequence of their not being cleared is that transplantations may need to be cancelled; resulting in prolongation of ischemic injury to the allograft, or a decision may be made to proceed with the transplantation, placing the patient at unrecognized risk. "Unpredictability" has been implicated as a cause of death in the first post-transplantation year, particularly in older patients, diabetic patients, and patients with vascular disease.

As discussed above, cardiovascular screening is an essential part of the transplant evaluation process because of the high prevalence of cardiovascular disease in ESKD patients. The cardiovascular risk status of a transplant candidate is not static, and tends to deteriorate with time. Unrecognized progression of CAD may occur in the years that a patient remains on dialysis. Left ventricular function deteriorates particularly in the first year in patients on dialysis. Valvular disease, particularly aortic stenosis, may worsen over the years a patient is waiting on the list. As the waitlist ages, so does medical complexity of the patients that comprise it.

The primary goal of preoperative cardiac risk evaluation is to reduce morbidity and mortality of cardiovascular disease. A thorough history and physical examination are recommended to identify active cardiac conditions before transplantation remains paramount to any cardiac evaluation. Controversies regarding the best strategy for pretransplant assessment of cardiac disease are discussed above. Often times, the decision on cardiac assessment has to be individualized based on risk factors, residual renal function, functional status, and medical comorbidities. Once a patient has gained active status on the waiting list, the necessity of repeated cardiac risk assessment needs to be determined. One suggested approach is listed in Table 8.5. Annual cardiovascular screening or reassessment is typically recommended for asymptomatic

TABLE 8.5	Suggested Cardiac Surveillance for Waitlisted Transplant Candidates	
No Known CAD or Initial Evaluation		
Negative	**Frequency**	
1) Diabetic ESRD	Annually	
2) "High risk" Nondiabetic	Biannually	
≥2 traditional[*] or unconventional[†] risk factors		
or ≥1 CAD risk equivalents.[‡]		
3) Lower risk[§]	Every 2–3 years.	
Known CAD		
If not re-vascularized	Annually	
Medical management per ACC/AHA guidelines		
Successful Prior PCI	Annually	
Successful CABG	After 3 years, then annually	
Incomplete CABG	Annually	
Asymptomatic Aortic Stenosis[*]		
Mild	Echocardiography every 3–5 years	
Moderate[¶]	Echocardiography annually	

ESRD, end-stage renal disease; CAD, coronary artery disease; PCI, percutaneous coronary intervention; CABG, coronary artery bypass graft.

ESRD: end-stage renal disease; CAD: coronary artery disease; PCI: percutaneous coronary intervention; CABG: coronary artery bypass graft.

[*]Traditional risk factors: Age > 45 in men, >55 in women, diabetes mellitus, hypertension, dyslipidemia, obesity, history of angina pectoris, congestive heart failure, previous cardiac events, smoking, and family history.

[†]Unconventional risk factors: Left ventricular hypertrophy (LVH), coronary artery vascular calcification, dialysis duration ≥ 2 years.

[‡]CAD risk equivalent: Type 1 DM > Type 2 DM, Atherosclerosis in other vascular beds, history of stroke.

[§]Lower risk: defined as not meeting criteria (1) or (2).

[*]Clinical evaluation annually.

[¶]Cardiology consultation recommended.

patients who are at higher risk such as patients with known CAD or diabetes mellitus. It should be noted that there are no randomized trials that show that identification of CAD by screening the asymptomatic patient results in better outcomes, and the cost effectiveness of routine screening of transplant patients remains controversial. Currently, there is no strong evidence for or against routine cardiac screening of asymptomatic transplant candidates. More evidence is needed from randomized clinical trials, to guide strategies for pretransplantation cardiac risk assessment in potential kidney transplant candidates and to optimize risk factor management before transplantation.

Standard age-appropriate health maintenance is recommended for pretransplant patients that include age-appropriate cancer screening. It should be recalled that recommendation for routine screening that have been made for the general population may not be relevant for the ESKD population, whose life span is intrinsically limited. Optimal routine healthcare should be performed according to the best practices and published clinical practice guidelines. Routine updating of serologic and other blood test results that may be relevant to the transplant status is also suggested. When sera from waitlisted patients are collected at a predetermined interval and are available in the laboratory, a final crossmatch can usually be performed without obtaining a fresh sample from the patient. Typically, sera from nonsensitized transplant patients who are at the top of the waitlist are obtained quarterly, whereas for the remaining nonsensitized patients sera can be obtained semi-annually. This practice also depends on the size of a programs waitlist and their own preferences based on their immuno-genetics testing. For highly sensitized patients, screening tray sets should be prepared monthly.

The topic of "frailty" of transplant candidates has been discussed above. Waitlisted patients, frail or otherwise, benefit from ongoing physical activity and rehabilitation. They should be encouraged to lead an active life, physically, socially, intellectually, and professionally. The more active they are in these respects, the more likely they are to benefit from their long-awaited kidney transplant.

Selected Readings

Abramowicz D, Cochat P, Claas FH, et al. European Renal Best Practice Guideline on kidney donor and recipient evaluation and perioperative care. Nephrol Dial Transplant 2015;11:1790–1797.

Bunnapradist S, Danovitch GM. Kidney transplants for the elderly: hope or hype? Clin J Am Soc Nephrol 2010;11:1910–1911.

Casingal V, Glumac E, Tan M, et al. Death on the kidney transplant waiting list: good candidates or not? Am J Transplant 2006;6:1953–1956.

Danovitch GM, Hariharan S, Pirsch JD, et al. Management of the waiting list for cadaveric kidney transplants: a report of a survey and recommendations by the Clinical Practice Guidelines Committee of the American Society of Transplantation. J Am Soc Nephrol 2002;13:528–535.

Dusseux E, Albano L, Fafin C, et al. A simple clinical tool to inform the decision-making process to refer elderly incident dialysis patients for kidney transplant evaluation. Kidney Int 2015;88:121–129.

Exterkate L, Siegtenhorst BR, Kelm M, et al. Frailty and transplantation. Transplantation 2016;100:727–781.

Goebel T, Shiltz N, Woodside K, et al. Neoplastic and non-neoplastic complications of solid organ transplantation in patients with preexisting monoclonal gammopathy of undetermined significance. Clin Transplant 2015;29:851–857.

Grams ME, Massie AB, Schold JD, et al. Trends in the inactive kidney transplant wait-list and implications for candidate survival. Am J Transplant 2013;13:1012–1018.

Huang E, Bunnapradist S. Pre-transplant weight loss and survival after kidney transplantation. Am J Nephrol 2015;41:448–455.

Huang E, Poommipanit N, Sampaio MS, et al. Intermediate-term outcomes associated with kidney transplantation in recipients 80 years and older: an analysis of the OPTN/UNOS database. Transplantation 2010;90:974–979.

Kasiske BL, Cangro CB, Hariharan S, et al; American Society of Transplantation. The evaluation of renal transplantation candidates: clinical practice guidelines. Am J Transplant 2001;1(suppl 2):3–95.

Kattah A, Ayalon R, Beck LH Jr, et al. Atypical hemolytic uremic syndrome recurrence after kidney transplantation. Transplantation 2014;98:1205–1212.

Keith D, Vranic G. Approach to the highly sensitized kidney transplant candidate. Clin J Am Soc Nephrol 2016;11:684–693.

Kucirka L, Tanjala P, Segev D. Improving access to kidney transplantation: referral is not enough. JAMA 2015;314:565–567.

Lonning K, Midtvedt K, Leivestad T, et al. Are octogenarians with end stage renal disease candidares for renal transplantation[published online July 28, 2016]. Transplantation 2016.

McAdams-DeMarco MA, James N, Salter ML, et al. Trends in kidney transplant outcomes in older adults. J Am Geriatr Soc 2014;62:2235–2242.

McAdams-DeMarco MA, Law A, King E, et al. Frailty and mortality in kidney transplant recipients. Am J Transplant 2015;15:149–154.

Molnar MZ, Naser MS, Rhee CM, et al. Bone and mineral disorders after kidney transplantation: therapeutic strategies. Transplant Rev 2014;28(2):56–62.

Pilmore H, Chadban H. Cardiac screening for kidney transplantation: the clinical conundrum continues. Transplantation 2016;100:1396–1397.

Pruett T. Waiting for Godot: the plight of being on the kidney waiting list. Transplantation 2016;100:1402–1404.

Pruthi R, McClure M, Casula A, et al. Long-term outcomes and patient survival are lower posttransplant in patients with a primary renal diagnosis of glomerulonephritis. Kidney Int 2016;89:918–926.

Reese PP, Shults J, Bloom RD, et al. Functional status, time to transplantation, and survival benefit of kidney transplantation among wait-listed candidates. Am J Kidney Dis 2015;5:837–845.

Rossi A, Burris D, Lucas L, et al. Effects of a renal rehabilitation exercise program in patients with CKD: a randomized, controlled trial. Clin J Am Soc Nephrol 2014;9:2052–2058.

Sampaio M, Bunnapradist S. Posttransplant malignancy. In: Singh AK, Riella LV, eds. Scientific American Nephrology, Dialysis, and Transplantation [published online November 2016]. Hamilton, Canada: Decker Intellectual Properties; 2016.

Tong A, Hanson C, Chapman J, et al. 'Suspended in paradox'—patient attitudes to wait-listing for kidney transplantation: systemic review and thematic synthesis of qualitative studies. Transplant Int 2105;28:771–787.

The Transplant Operation and Its Surgical Complications

Nick G. Cowan, Jeffrey L. Veale, and H. Albin Gritsch

Kidney transplantation is an "elective" surgical procedure performed in patients who have undergone careful preoperative assessment and preparation. Chronic dialysis enables patients to be maintained in stable condition and provides time to address potentially complicating medical and surgical issues. In this respect, kidney transplantation differs from heart, lung, or liver transplantation, in which the condition of the patient is often deteriorating rapidly in the pretransplantation period.

THE TRANSPLANT OPERATION

Immediate Preoperative Preparations

If transplant candidates have been well prepared (see Chapter 8), it is rarely necessary to call off surgery because of last-minute findings. Occasionally, cancellation of surgery is required because of recent events, such as new onset of chest pain or electrocardiographic changes, diabetic foot ulcers, peritonitis, pneumonia, or new concerning imaging findings.

The decision to dialyze a patient before transplantation depends on the timing of the previous dialysis, clinical assessment of volume status, and serum electrolyte levels, particularly potassium. Prolonged periods without oral hydration and nutrition should be avoided to reduce hyperkalemia associated with hypoglycemia. Pretransplantation dialysis is associated with an increased incidence of delayed graft function. Because of the danger of intraoperative or postoperative hyperkalemia in oliguric patients, it is wise to dialyze patients with a serum potassium level of more than 5.5 mEq/L. In well-dialyzed patients, preoperative dialysis for fluid removal is usually unnecessary. If fluid is removed, it should be done with care to maintain the patient at or somewhat above dry weight to facilitate postoperative diuresis. If time constraints demand it, a brief preoperative dialysis lasting 1 to 2 hours may be all that is necessary to reduce potassium levels and to optimize the hemodynamic status.

Operative Technique

Because all kidney transplant recipients receive immunosuppressive drugs, and because many are anemic or malnourished at the time of surgery, wound healing is potentially compromised. Meticulous surgical technique, attention to detail, strict aseptic technique, and hemostasis are essential. Drains should be closed systems and should be removed as quickly as possible.

Incision

The patient is placed in a supine position and sequential compression devices are applied prior to induction of anesthesia. After the administration of prophylactic antibiotics, a lower abdominal *Gibson* incision is made (Fig. 9.1). It can be extended into the flank, or as high as the tip of the 12th rib, if more exposure is needed. In a first transplantation, the incision site may be in either lower quadrant. There are different approaches to the decision regarding which side to use. One approach is to always use the right side, regardless of the side of origin of the donor kidney, because the accessibility of the iliac vein makes the operation easier than on the left side. Another approach is to use the side contralateral to the side of the donor kidney; a right kidney is put on the left side, and vice versa. This technique was used when the hypogastric artery was routinely used for the anastomosis because the vessels lie in a convenient position and the renal pelvis is always anterior, making it accessible if ureteral repair is needed. The third approach is to use the side ipsilateral to the donor kidney; a right kidney is put on the right side, and vice versa. This choice is best when the external iliac artery is used for the arterial anastomosis. The

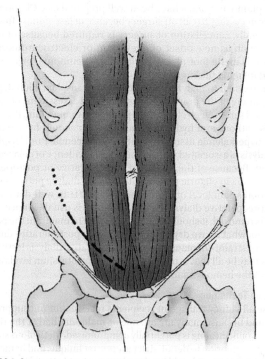

FIGURE 9.1 Standard incision for adult kidney transplantation. An oblique incision is made from the symphysis in the midline curving in a lateral and superior direction to the iliac crest.

vessels then lie without kinking when the kidney is placed in position. In repeat transplantations, the side opposite the original transplant is generally used. In repeat transplants, the decision regarding where to place the kidney is more complex; a transabdominal incision may be necessary, and more proximal vessels may be used. In patients with type 1 diabetes who may be eventual candidates for pancreas transplantation, the kidney is preferentially placed in the left iliac fossa to facilitate possible pancreas transplantation on the right side (see Chapter 16).

Venous Anastomosis

Using a 5-0 polypropylene suture, the donor renal vein is usually anastomosed end-to-side to the external iliac vein (Fig. 9.2). If there are multiple renal veins, the largest may be used; the others can be ligated safely because of internal collateralization of the renal venous drainage. If two veins are about the same size, they can be sewn together

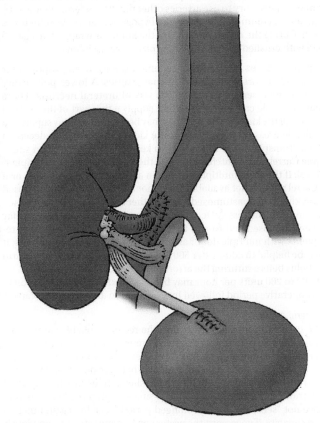

FIGURE 9.2 The standard hook-up. The donor renal artery is shown anastomosed end-to-side on a Carrel aortic patch to the recipient external iliac artery. The donor renal vein is anastomosed to the recipient external iliac vein. The donor ureter is anastomosed to the recipient bladder with an antireflux technique.

with the "pair of pants" technique, or individually anastomosed to the external iliac vein. With deceased donor renal transplants, the donor vena cava may be used as an extension graft for the short, right renal vein. The venous anastomosis is usually done first to minimize ischemia to the leg.

Arterial Anastomosis

The donor renal artery is usually sewn to the external iliac artery in an end-to-side manner using a 5-0 or 6-0 polypropylene suture (Fig. 9.2). In a deceased donor kidney transplantation, the donor renal artery or arteries are usually kept in continuity with a patch of donor aorta called a *Carrel aortic patch,* which makes the end-to-side anastomosis both easier and safer, and facilitates the anastomosis of multiple renal arteries. In living donor transplantation, a Carrel patch is not available, and the renal artery is sewn to the recipient artery. In small children and in patients undergoing repeat transplantation on the same side, it may be necessary to use arteries other than the external iliac artery. The aorta, common iliac artery, or hypogastric artery is sometimes used. During the anastomosis time, the kidney is wrapped in a gauze pad with crushed ice saline to minimize warm ischemia.

Multiple Arteries. A variety of techniques have been proposed for handling donors with multiple renal arteries. A lower-pole artery should be preserved to reduce the risk of ureteral necrosis. There may be visible capsular vessels that supply a tiny part of the cortical surface of the kidney. These vessels may be ligated, and tiny superficial ischemic areas on the surface of the kidney may result. In deceased donor transplantations, it is best to keep all the arteries on a single large Carrel aortic patch and to sew the Carrel patch to the recipient vessel. If there are multiple arteries in a living donor transplant, or if a Carrel patch is not available, the donor arteries can be anastomosed individually or anastomosed to each other before being anastomosed to the recipient vessel. Occasionally, a small lower-pole branch may be anastomosed end-to-end to the inferior epigastric artery. For recipients with multiple donor arteries or other risks for thrombosis, it may be helpful to administer 500 to 1,000 units of intravenous heparin by bolus before suturing the arterial anastomoses. A heparin infusion at 100 to 200 units per hour may be continued during the immediate postoperative period followed by transition to antiplatelet therapy.

Ureteric Anastomosis

The ureter can be anastomosed to the recipient bladder or into the ipsilateral native ureter as a uretero-ureterostomy. The native ureter may also be brought up to the allograft renal pelvis as a ureteropyelostomy. Most surgeons use the bladder whenever possible. Preferably, the recipient's bladder will have been shown to be functional before the transplantation; however, even small, contracted bladders that have not "seen" urine for prolonged periods usually regain function and capacity. If necessary, the ureter can be connected to a previously fashioned ileal or colonic conduit.

Reimplantation of the ureter into the bladder is aided by placement of a urethral catheter attached to a "Y-connector" which allows for inflow and bladder distention. There are several ways of reimplanting the ureter into the bladder. The most common approach is one in which the ureter is reimplanted extravesically, using the *Lich–Gregoir* technique. First, the bladder is distended with saline, and the extravesical tissues are dissected from the detrusor muscle. A muscular tunnel is then created by separating the detrusor muscle from the bladder mucosa for a length of about 2 to 4 cm. The ureter is prepared by removing redundant ureteral length, preserving adequate distal blood supply, and spatulating posteriorly. A mucosal opening is created and interrupted or running degradable fine suture, preferentially polydioxanone surgical suture, is used to approximate the ureteral and bladder mucosa. Finally, the detrusor muscle is closed exteriorly to create an antireflux mechanism (Fig. 9.3). Absorbable suture is used to prevent stone formation. Foley catheter drainage of the bladder is required for approximately 3 to 7 days, unless there are bladder abnormalities that may necessitate longer drainage.

Other, less common approaches include the *Barry* technique, the single-stitch *Taguchi* technique, and the intravesical *Leadbetter–Politano* technique. Whichever technique is used for the ureteral anastomosis, an indwelling stent should be placed in most cases. The practice of routine stenting is supported by randomized controlled trials in which ureteral stent placement reduced the risk of urine leak or urine obstruction. Although urinary tract infections (UTIs) were more common in stented patients, no difference in the incidence of UTIs

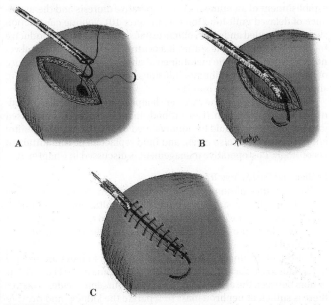

A

B

C

FIGURE 9.3 A Lich–Gregoir reimplantation. A single, small opening is made in the bladder **(A)**, and the ureter is sewn to the bladder mucosa over a ureteric stent **(B)**. The bladder muscle is used to create an antireflux mechanism **(C)**.

was seen when antibiotic prophylaxis was added. Routine stenting has also proved cost-effective because of the hospital costs associated with a single urinary complication. Additionally, stents are well tolerated by transplant recipients because the location of the ureter is high in the bladder dome and kidney denervation result in minimal trigonal irritation and reflux pain. Clear notation of stent placement and its subsequent removal must be made to prevent inadvertent stent retention because a retained stent may be difficult to remove intact and provides a nidus for recurrent urinary tract infections and stones. With the use of cotrimoxazole for prophylaxis against *Pneumocystis jirovecii*, and the removal of stents 3 to 4 weeks after transplantation, the incidence of urinary tract infections among stented recipients remains low.

Drains

Drains may be placed through a separate small incision into the perirenal space to drain blood, urine, or lymph. Some surgeons routinely place drains, whereas others do not. Closed drains, such as the Blake or Jackson–Pratt type, are preferred over the open Penrose-type drains because of a lower risk for wound infection. Placing a drain at the end of the procedure and leaving it for the initial postoperative course has been shown to reduce the incidence of lymphoceles. Drains should typically be removed once the output is less than 100 mL/day.

Intraoperative Fluid Management

Adequate perfusion of the newly transplanted kidney is critical for the establishment of an immediate postoperative diuresis and the avoidance of delayed graft function (see Chapter 10). Volume contraction should be avoided and mild volume expansion maintained, conducive to the recipient's cardiac status. If a central line is placed, central venous pressure should be maintained at about 12 mm Hg with the use of isotonic saline and albumin infusions, and mean arterial pressure should be kept above 80 mm Hg.

Before the release of the vascular clamps, a large dose of methylprednisolone is usually given. If an antibody induction agent is being used (see Chapter 6), it should be administered before this time. Mannitol and furosemide are also given, and fluid replacement is maintained accordingly. Postoperative management is discussed in Chapter 10.

En Bloc *and Dual Kidney Transplantation*

At the extremes of donor age, both donor kidneys are sometimes transplanted into a single recipient. The simultaneous use of both kidneys entails some additional technical risks to the recipient. Their use is a reflection of the donor shortage and reluctance to discard functional organs.

For donors younger than 2 years of age, both kidneys are usually transplanted *en bloc* with the donor aorta and vena cava (Fig. 9.4). For donors between the ages of 2 and 5 years, the surgeon decides whether there is sufficient nephron mass to separate the kidneys and provide allografts for two individuals. Separation can be considered when the allograft measures greater than 6 cm in length (the donor weight is usually $\geq$ 15 kg). For the *en bloc* procedure, the aorta and vena cava

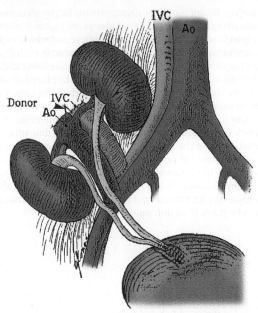

FIGURE 9.4 Pediatric *en bloc* kidney transplantation. The donor aorta (*Ao*) and inferior vena cava (*IVC*) are anastomosed to the external iliac vessels. The ureters are anastomosed to the bladder using pediatric stents. (From Bretan PN, Koyle M, Singh K, et al. Improved survival of en bloc renal allografts from pediatric donors. J Urol 1997;157:1592–1595, with permission.)

superior to the renal vessels are typically closed with 6-0 nonabsorbable monofilament suture. All the other branches of the great vessels are carefully ligated with 4-0 silk ties, the infrarenal aorta is then anastomosed to the external iliac artery, and the infrarenal vena cava is anastomosed to the external iliac vein.

The kidneys from pediatric *en bloc* donors must be carefully positioned to avoid kinking of the blood vessels or tension on the ureters. If the ureters are implanted into the bladder separately, and a complication occurs in one kidney, then the risk for compromising the other kidney is reduced. The rate of technical complications, most typically urine leaks and vascular thrombosis, varies between 10% and 20% with young donor kidneys transplanted individually or *en bloc*. The rate of thrombosis may be reduced by using a very low dose of an anticoagulant, such as intravenous heparin at 100 to 200 units per hour and converting to aspirin (81 mg) daily for 3 months.

Kidneys from older "marginal" donors are sometimes discarded for fear that they will not provide adequate renal function for their recipients. To avoid this waste, some centers now advocate the use of both kidneys (dual transplantation) from donors aged 60 years or older. Dual transplantation is appropriate if the calculated creatinine clearance is less than 90 mL/min at the time of admission, or if there is evidence of significant histologic damage on the biopsy specimen taken at the time of organ retrieval. These kidneys are typically placed into older recipients who are not significantly obese and whose metabolic requirements may be less. One kidney can be placed in each iliac fossa by using a preperitoneal midline incision or separate lower abdominal Gibson incisions. Alternatively, both kidneys can be placed on one side, preferably the right. For a unilateral incision, the right kidney is typically placed superolaterally, and the right renal vein with donor vena cava extension is anastomosed to the recipient vena cava. The right renal artery is then anastomosed to the common iliac artery. After revascularization of the right kidney, the left kidney is then placed in a more inferomedial position. The left renal vein and artery are anastomosed to the external iliac vessels (Fig. 9.5). The survival rate of dual kidneys is about 7% less than that for single kidneys, although when compared with the survival rate of single kidneys from donors older than 60 years, their outcome is similar.

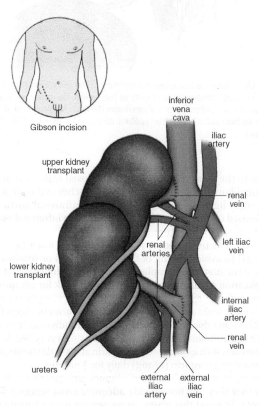

FIGURE 9.5 Dual transplantation of adult kidneys into a single recipient. (From Masson D, Hefty T. A technique for the transplantation of 2 adult cadaver kidney grafts into 1 recipient. J Urol 1998;160:1779–1780, with permission.)

SURGICAL COMPLICATIONS OF KIDNEY TRANSPLANTATION

The clinical presentation of surgical and nonsurgical complications of kidney transplantation may be similar. Graft dysfunction may reflect rejection or a urine leak; fever and graft tenderness may reflect wound infection or rejection. Post-transplantation events have a broad differential diagnosis that must include technical complications of surgery as well as immunologic and other causes.

The fundamental algorithm in the management of post-transplantation graft dysfunction requires that vascular and urologic causes of graft dysfunction be ruled out before concluding that an event is a result of a medical cause such as rejection or cyclosporine toxicity. The differential diagnosis of postoperative graft dysfunction is discussed in Chapter 10, and the radiologic diagnostic tools are discussed in Chapter 14. Doppler ultrasound is invaluable in the differentiation of medical and surgical postoperative complications.

Wound Infection

In the 1960s and 1970s, wound infection rates after kidney transplantation were as high as 25%. Wound infections now occur in less than 1% of cases. This improvement is a result of several factors: patients receiving transplants are healthier; lower steroid doses are used for both maintenance and treatment of rejection; and perioperative antibiotics are routinely used. Obviously, strict aseptic technique in the operating room is essential to prevent wound infection. If infections do occur, they should be treated with drainage and systemic antibiotics to avoid contamination of the vascular suture line and possible mycotic aneurysm formation. Patients who are obese or receiving the immunosuppressant agent sirolimus have a significantly higher incidence of wound infections.

Lymphocele

Lymphoceles are collections of lymph caused by leakage from severed lymphatics surrounding the iliac vessels or the renal hilum of the donor kidney. The incidence of lymphoceles reported in the literature varies widely. Some lymphoceles are small and asymptomatic. Usually, the larger the lymphocele, the more likely it is to cause pain, ureteral obstruction, or venous compression. Lymphoceles occasionally produce incontinence secondary to bladder compression, scrotal masses secondary to spontaneous drainage into the scrotum, or iliac vein obstruction that can result in deep vein thrombosis (DVT) or leg swelling. The incidence of lymphoceles can be reduced by minimizing the pelvic dissection, ligating lymphatics, and avoiding sirolimus in the early postoperative period. Additionally, placing an intraoperative drain and leaving it for the initial postoperative course has been shown to reduce lymphatic collections.

Lymphoceles are usually diagnosed by ultrasound (see Chapter 14). The characteristic ultrasound finding is a roundish, sonolucent, septated mass medial to the renal allograft. Hydronephrosis may be present, and the ureter may be seen adjacent to and compressed by the lymphocele. More complex internal echoes may signal an infected lymphocele. Usually, the clinical situation and ultrasound appearance distinguish a lymphocele from other types of peri-renal fluid collections, such as hematoma or urine leak. Simple needle aspiration of the fluid using sterile technique makes the diagnosis. The fluid obtained is clear and has high protein content, and the creatinine concentration approximates that of serum.

No therapy is necessary for the common, small, asymptomatic lymphocele. Percutaneous aspiration should be performed if there is suspicion of a ureteral leak, obstruction, or infection. The most common indication for treatment is ureteral obstruction. If the cause of the obstruction is simple compression caused by the mass effect of the lymphocele, drainage alone will resolve the problem. The ureter itself is often narrowed and may need to be reimplanted because of its involvement in the inflammatory reaction in the wall of the lymphocele. Repeated percutaneous aspirations are not advised because they seldom lead to dissolution of the lymphocele and often result in infection.

Infected or obstructing lymphoceles can be drained externally using a closed system. Sclerosing agents, such as povidone iodine (Betadine), tetracycline, or fibrin glue, can be instilled into the cavity and are moderately successful. Lymphoceles can also be drained internally by marsupialization into the peritoneal cavity, where the fluid is resorbed. Marsupialization can be accomplished through a laparoscopic or open surgical approach. It is important to ensure that the opening in the lymphocele is large enough to prevent peritoneal closure, which can produce recurrence or bowel entrapment and incarceration. Omentum is often interposed in the opening to prevent closure. Care must be taken to avoid injury to the ureter, which may lie in the wall of the lymphocele. On rare occasions, the actual site of lymph leak can be identified and ligated.

Bleeding

The risk for postoperative bleeding can be minimized by close attention to pretransplantation coagulation parameters, which should be considered during the pretransplantation workup (see Chapter 8). Aspirin and anticoagulant medications should be discontinued when possible before transplantation. Meticulous preparation of the allograft and hemostasis during the operation minimizes this risk for bleeding. If there is significant blood loss at the time of reperfusion, the vascular clamps should be reapplied and the graft carefully inspected. Anastomotic bleeding can usually be controlled with fine suture ligatures, and oozing will usually stop with gentle pressure and cellulose gauze. Early postoperative bleeding can occur from small vessels in the renal hilum, which may not have been apparent before closure because of vasospasm. After surgery, when perfusion improves, these hilar vessels can then bleed. Close observation of vital signs and serial hematocrits is necessary for the first several postoperative hours to recognize this type of bleeding. If postoperative bleeding occurs, coagulation parameters should be studied to ensure that there is no occult coagulopathy. Ultrasound can help to confirm and monitor a peri-allograft hematoma. If more than 4 units of blood are required within 48 hours, operative evacuation of the hematoma will usually accelerate graft function and patient comfort. Late profound hemorrhage can result from the rupture of a mycotic aneurysm. Nephrectomy and repair of the artery are usually required. Rarely, the external iliac artery may have to be ligated and blood supply to the ipsilateral leg provided by extra-anatomic bypass.

Thrombosis
Renal Artery Thrombosis

Renal artery thrombosis is most often seen in patients with thrombotic tendencies (see Chapter 8). It can also occur in kidneys with multiple arteries or when significant atherosclerosis is present in the donor or recipient vessels. Renal artery thrombosis occurs most often within the first 2 to 3 days after transplantation. The patient may experience a sudden cessation of urine flow without any discomfort. Thrombocytopenia and hyperkalemia may occur as platelets are consumed in the graft with a sudden elevation in creatinine. The diagnosis is made by Doppler ultrasonography or renal scan because no blood flow is seen to the allograft. Unfortunately, most grafts that develop arterial thrombosis are lost. Rarely, the diagnosis is made immediately, and the allograft is salvaged by rushing the patient to the operating room for emergent arteriotomy and thrombectomy. Recipients with significant risk factors for arterial thrombosis should be anticoagulated.

Renal Vein Thrombosis

Renal vein thrombosis typically occurs in the early postoperative period and may result from kinking of the renal vein, stenosis of the venous anastomoses, hypotension, hypercoagulable state, and acute rejection. With intraoperative venous thrombosis, the allograft appears swollen and cyanotic, and a clot may be palpable in the renal vein. Delayed renal vein thrombosis is usually diagnosed by Doppler ultrasonography because a clot may be visualized in the vein with decreased blood flow to the allograft. Although thrombolytic therapy may be helpful, when possible emergent thrombectomy with revision of the anastomosis should be attempted. Unfortunately, these grafts are usually lost because of the prolonged ischemia time and require allograft nephrectomy.

Deep Vein Thrombosis

DVTs can extend into the renal vein or cause life-threatening pulmonary embolism. Kidney transplant recipients are at a moderate risk for developing DVTs. Possible reasons for this includes stasis of the iliac vein from clamping during creation of the vascular anastomoses, endothelial injury, pelvic dissection, immobility, and perioperative dehydration. Ultrasonography is highly sensitive and specific in detecting proximal DVTs but far less satisfactory in detecting distal thrombi because of poor visualization of the calf veins. Patients with DVTs should receive anticoagulation therapy for at least 3 months. Heparin therapy is overlapped with initiation of warfarin and can be discontinued after 5 days provided the INR has been therapeutic (INR 2.0 to 3.0). The platelet count should be monitored for heparin-induced thrombocytopenia. Inferior vena cava filters should be inserted in patients with contraindications to anticoagulation. Prevention of venous thrombosis in transplant recipients should include intermittent pneumatic compression stockings as well as early ambulation. The addition of 5,000 U of unfractionated heparin subcutaneously is appropriate in those patients considered at increased risk for DVT; however, this risk must be balanced against an increased risk for hemorrhagic complications and caution is advised when considering dosage. Use of alternative agents such as low-molecular-weight heparin and new oral anticoagulants must be done with caution as they are dependent on renal function for clearance.

Renal Artery Stenosis

Transplant renal artery stenosis (TRAS) has been reported to occur in up to 10% of recipients. Soft bruits over the transplant incision are common are are usually of little significance. Loud prolonged bruits may suggest TRAS. Imaging with angiography remains the gold standard; however, it is often suspected on ultrasonography because administration of contrast is not recommended in patients with marginal renal function. A peak systolic velocity greater than 250 cm per second and a "tardus-parvus" arterial waveform are both suspicious for TRAS. Elevated peak systolic velocities in the renal transplant artery are common in the early postoperative period and frequently normalize with serial measurements. If stenosis is suspected in the first postoperative month, then surgical revision of the anastomoses is usually the best option. Graft loss after surgical repair has been reported in up to 30% of cases and is a reflection of the difficulty in directly approaching the vascular anastomosis in a noncollateralized kidney. Beyond 1 month, percutaneous transluminal angioplasty is usually favored. Table 9.1 lists potential causes of stenosis. The term *pseudorenal artery stenosis* has been used to describe the situation that can occur if an atherosclerotic plaque in the iliac vessels impairs blood flow to the transplant renal artery. The postulate that rejection can cause renal artery stenosis has not been conclusively proved. TRAS may be associated with difficult to treat hypertension and high hematocrit levels (see Chapter 11).

Urine Leaks

Urinary extravasation may be a result of distal ureteric ischemia because the allograft ureter receives blood supply solely from the renal artery. Therefore, preservation of all arterial branches (especially lower-pole arteries) is essential to ensure adequate blood supply to the distal

TABLE 9.1	Potential Causes of Renal Artery Stenosis

Rejection of the donor artery
Atherosclerosis of the recipient vessel
Clamp injury to the recipient or donor vascular endothelium
Perfusion pump cannulation injury of the donor vessel
Faulty suture technique: purse-string effect, lumen encroachment by the suture, improper suture material, fibrotic inflammatory reaction to polypropylene in the setting of abnormal hemodynamics
End-to-end anastomosis with abnormal fluid dynamics
Angulation as a consequence of disproportionate length between graft artery and iliac vessels
End-to-end anastomosis with vessel size disproportion
Pseudorenal artery stenosis by critical iliac atherosclerotic lesion
Kinking of the renal artery

ureter. Preserving peri-ureteral tissue during the donor nephrectomy and leaving the shortest length of ureter that allows for a tension-free bladder anastomosis in the recipient also helps to maximize distal ureteral blood supply. A stented Lich–Gregoir ureteric anastomosis to the bladder has been shown to have the lowest incidence of urinary leaks. A leak may also occur at the level of the renal pelvis or calyx and may result from obstruction. Leaks typically occur within the first few days after transplantation or at the onset of post-transplantation diuresis in patients with delayed graft function. The general presentation is increasing wound drainage, decreasing urine output and severe pain over the allograft. A leak may also cause the recipient to experience abdominal or scrotal pain and swelling. Agonizing pain over the allograft in the early post-operatve period should always raise the possibility of a urine leak. The diagnosis is made when the creatinine of the fluid drained from the incision or drain is elevated compared to plasma levels. The diagnosis is typically confirmed by cystogram, nuclear medicine scan, or antegrade nephrostogram.

A Foley catheter should be *immediately* placed if there is clinical suspicion of a leak. The catheter reduces intravesical pressure and occasionally may reduce or stop leakage altogether. Percutaneous antegrade nephrostomy may be used to diagnose the leak and control the flow of urine. Some leaks can be managed definitively with external drainage and stent placement alone. If the leak is caused by a ureteral necrosis, percutaneous treatment will never work and only delays definitive treatment. For these reasons, when leaks occur, early surgical exploration and repair are usually required.

The type of surgical repair depends on the level of leak and the viability of the tissues. If a ureteral leak is a simple anastomotic leak, resection of the distal ureter and reimplantation is the easiest solution. If the ureter is nonviable because of inadequate blood supply, ureteropyelostomy using the ipsilateral native ureter is a good option. Cystopyelostomy has also been done to replace a necrotic ureter. The bladder is mobilized and brought directly to the allograft renal pelvis without an intervening ureter. The bladder may need to be fixed superiorly by a *Psoas hitch* or extended by a *Boari flap*.

Urinary Obstruction

Common causes of urinary obstruction include catheter blockage, blood clots, extrinsic ureteric compression, ureteral stricture, stones, and prostatic hyperplasia. Low-grade obstruction in the early postoperative period may be a result of ureteral edema with vigorous diuresis and usually resolves. Obstruction is usually manifested by impairment of graft function and increasing hydronephrosis. It may be painless because of the absence of innervation to the transplanted kidney. Placement of an antegrade nephrostomy tube can rapidly reduce obstruction while serving as a conduit for an antegrade nephrostogram to help confirm the diagnosis.

The Foley catheter should be checked for blockage. Minor ureteric obstruction may resolve with proximal diversion and stenting. Ureteric strictures shorter than 2 cm can be treated endoscopically with a laser or cutting blade, balloon dilation, and stenting (Fig. 9.6). Ureteric strictures

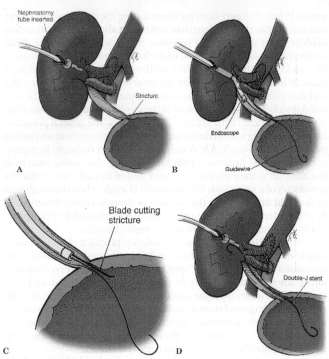

FIGURE 9.6 Stages in the endourologic treatment of ureteral structure.

longer than 2 cm require excision and reimplantation. If the length of the ureter is compromised, ureteropyelostomy using the ipsilateral native ureter or cystopyelostomy is a reasonable alternative. Extrinsic ureteric compression can often be successfully treated with external drainage of the lymphocele, hematoma, or urinoma.

Gastrointestinal Complications

Gastrointestinal complications are among the more common adverse events following renal transplantation and are often a result of immunosuppressive medications, infections, or bowel injury during surgery. Diarrhea, dyspepsia, and abdominal pain may result from mycophenolate and steroids may increase the risk of peptic ulcer disease. When managing gastrointestinal complications, it is important to note that sodium polystyrene sulfonate (Kayexalate)-sorbitol enemas should not be administered to uremic patients because they have been associated with colonic necrosis. Sodium phosphate (Fleet) enemas are to be avoided in patients with poor renal function because of the high phosphate load.

The incidence of colonic pseudo-obstruction (Ogilvie syndrome) is increased in renal transplant recipients. As the colon expands, the tissue strength is reduced. Immunosuppression with corticosteroids exacerbates this process, increasing the vulnerability to perforation by causing atrophy of the intestinal lymphatics and further thinning the bowel wall. When Ogilvie syndrome is recognized (pancolonic dilation $\geq$ 10 cm in the absence of an obstructive lesion), patients should receive nothing by mouth, and have opiates withdrawn and steroid doses tapered. If the renal allograft is functioning well, the addition of neostigmine usually proves efficacious; however, the drug is contraindicated in patients with renal insufficiency. Colonic decompression with a rectal tube or colonoscopy is indicated for patients who have failed to respond to conservative therapy after 24 to 48 hours. To prevent the catastrophic consequences of perforation, emergent laparotomy is indicated in patients who show signs of peritonitis or clinical deterioration.

ALLOGRAFT NEPHRECTOMY

Indications

Kidneys that have failed either for technical reasons or because of rejection may need to be removed. Indications for allograft nephrectomy are symptoms and signs that typically occur when immunosuppression is withdrawn but may be delayed by weeks or months. These can include low-grade fever, graft tenderness, abdominal pain, hematuria, and constitutional symptoms, and reflect "rejection of the rejected graft" after immunosuppression is withdrawn (see Chapter 11). It may be possible to lessen the symptoms and avoid nephrectomy by temporary reinstitution of steroids. Avoidance of nephrectomy is preferred because the procedure can result in significant morbidity and allosensitization affecting future transplantations. If the graft loss is acute and occurs within 1 year of transplantation, nephrectomy is necessary in most cases. Graft loss from chronic rejection after 1 year may not require nephrectomy. The rejected graft that remains *in situ* typically becomes a small, fibrotic mass.

Procedure

The removal of a failed allograft may result in increased perioperative morbidity compared with the transplantation itself because of the inflammatory response and scarring as a consequence of rejection. For this reason, the procedure should be performed at centers with appropriate experience. Usually, the old incision is reopened. Care must be taken to avoid the peritoneum, which may be draped across the anterior surface of the kidney. If the nephrectomy is performed soon after transplantation, the kidney can be removed entirely because it is not very adherent to surrounding structures. If there has been recurrent rejection, the kidney usually adheres to surrounding structures and most often needs to be removed using a subcapsular approach. It is almost always safe to leave a small amount of donor vessel in the recipient; this additional vessel length can help the surgeon achieve hemostasis with suture ligation.

Hemostasis should be meticulous. Some dead space is always left after nephrectomy. If this fills with blood, abscess formation is more likely. Although a closed drain may be used, it may inadequately drain the blood and create the potential for infection by its presence. Argon beam coagulation of the entire raw surface of the capsule should be considered.

Complications

Although there are few series in the literature, the reported morbidity for allograft nephrectomy is high. The potential complications include acute bleeding during surgery secondary to injury to the iliac artery or vein; injury to other surrounding structures, such as the bowel; infection; and lymph leaks. Leaving small segments of the allograft renal artery or vein does not usually cause long-term problems, although rupture can occur if the vessels become secondarily infected. Likewise, leaving a small amount of allograft ureter in place can result in some gross hematuria after the allograft nephrectomy; the hematuria is almost always limited and usually does not require reoperation.

NON–TRANSPLANT-RELATED SURGERY

Immunosuppressed transplant recipients may occasionally require significant surgical intervention not directly related to the transplantation, such as coronary artery bypass, cholecystectomy, hip replacement, or gynecologic procedures. Nephrologists or members of the transplantation team are often requested to aid in the perioperative management of such patients, and certain precautions are required (Table 9.2).

The renal function of many transplant recipients is impaired to varying degrees and the capacity to concentrate urine and lower urinary sodium concentration may be limited. Maintenance of euvolemia is, therefore, particularly important perioperatively to avoid further reduction in renal function. If a patient will be unable to take immunosuppressive medications orally for more than 24 hours, calcineurin inhibitors may be given sublingually or intravenously, but care should be taken to ensure proper dosing (see Chapter 6). In the event of an elective surgery requiring a skin flap, intestinal anastomosis, or hernia repair, patients on rapamycin should have the drug switched to an alternative a week prior to surgery until several days postoperative. Although functional adrenal suppression in patients taking 10 mg/day or less of prednisone is uncommon, a "stress dose" of 100 mg of hydrocortisone is typically given every 8 hours postoperatively until the patient can return to the preoperative oral prednisone dose. Additional agents, such as mycophenolate mofetil or rapamycin, can be safely withheld for 2 to 3 days.

TABLE 9.2	Precautions for Kidney Transplant Recipients Undergoing Post-transplantation Surgical Procedures

Maintain euvolemia.
Use nonnephrotoxic prophylactic antibiotics.
Give calcineurin inhibitor by mouth when possible and modify intravenous dose when necessary.
Ensure adequate imaging studies have been obtained to avoid injury to the allograft and ureter.
Provide perioperative steroid coverage.
Adjunctive immunosuppressants can be held for several days.
Avoid nephrotoxic antibiotics and analgesics.
Monitor graft function and plasma potassium and acid–base status.
Consider wound healing impairment.

Nonnephrotoxic antibiotics should be given prophylactically, and if intravenous contrast is required for radiologic studies, precontrast hydration with IV saline should be ensured. In patients with markedly impaired graft function, careful monitoring of postoperative plasma potassium levels and acid–base status is mandatory.

Surgical Considerations in Children

Urologic disease is the cause of renal failure in up to one-third of children with end-stage renal disease (see Chapter 17). It is therefore important to study bladder function in children with a history of urinary tract infections or voiding abnormalities. Reconstructive surgery must be coordinated with possible renal transplantation. The parents and child must be psychologically prepared to perform intermittent catheterization, which may be necessary postoperatively.

The transplantation procedure for children who weigh more than 20 to 25 kg is generally the same as the procedure for adults. There may be an increase in complexity of the surgical procedure in the setting of prior bladder procedures, including augmentation or prior Mitrofanoff creation. The placement of the allograft and method of ureteral reimplantation must be carefully planned to minimize postoperative complications. In children weighing less than 20 kg, comparatively large adult-size kidneys are implanted because kidneys from equivalently-sized infant donors are more prone to technical complications. In the smallest recipients, the venous anastomosis is often placed on the vena cava and the arterial anastomosis on the aorta in order to achieve the best position for the allograft in the right flank. In children who weigh more than 12 kg, an extraperitoneal approach can still be used. The right side is almost always preferable because of the easier exposure of the common iliac vessels. In children who weigh less than 12 kg, a midline transabdominal approach is generally necessary. The great vessels are approached by mobilizing the cecum, and the kidney is placed behind the cecum. To provide room for a large kidney in the right flank, a right native nephrectomy is sometimes necessary at the time of transplantation to create room for the allograft. Concomitant unilateral versus bilateral native nephrectomy should also be considered in recipients with a history of significant hydronephrosis, urinary obstruction, or urinary tract infection. In patients with severe hypertension refractory to multiple antihypertensive agents, bilateral native nephrectomy is generally performed before transplantation to avoid hypertension-related complications to the allograft. Before ureteroneocystostomy the transplanted ureter is often placed under the peritoneum, over the dome of the bladder, to avoid the potential for technical complications to the ureter should the child require exploratory laparotomy in the future.

Careful intraoperative fluid management is crucial to prevent thrombosis of large kidneys in small children. In general, generous fluid resuscitation with saline, colloid, and blood transfusions is necessary to provide adequate hemodynamic support before reperfusion. A constant dialogue with the anesthesia service is of paramount importance in this regard. In the smallest transplant recipients, reperfusion of a large kidney may consume a large portion of the circulating blood volume at reperfusion. In these patients, blood can be transfused in volumes of 10 mL/kg until the central venous and mean arterial pressures are adequate for reperfusion. This step serves to avoid early acute tubular necrosis that can be associated with hypotension and inadequate hemodynamic support before reperfusion. Furosemide (1 mg/kg) and mannitol (0.125 to 0.25 g/kg) are also administered at the time of reperfusion to generate a diuresis. In general, an intraoperative heparin infusion is also administered to reduce the risk for graft thrombosis, as this risk may be higher compared with adult transplant recipients. This is continued postoperatively with conversion to aspirin prior to discharge depending on the child's risk profile for graft thrombosis, as determined preoperatively (see Chapter 17).

Selected Readings

Alberts VP, Idu MM, Legemate DA, et al. Ureterovesical anastomotic techniques for kidney transplantation: a systematic review and meta-analysis. Transpl Int 2014;27(6):593–605.

Bunnapradist S, Gritsch HA, Peng A, et al. Dual kidneys from marginal adult donors as a source for cadaveric renal transplantation in the United States. J Am Soc Nephrol 2003;14:1031–1036.

Duty BD, Conlin MJ, Fuchs EF, et al. The current role of endourologic management of renal transplantation complications. Adv Urol 2013;2013:246520.

Gil-Vernet S, Amado A, Ortega F, et al. Gastrointestinal complications in renal transplant recipients: MITOS study. Transplant Proc 2007;39(7):2190–2193.

Knechtle S, Sudan D. Surgical technique in transplantation: how much does it matter? Am J Transplant 2015;15:2791–2792.

Marinaki S, Skalioti C, Boletis J. Patients after kidney allograft failure: immunologic and nonimmunologic considerations. Transplant Proc 2015;47:2677–2682.

Ngo AT, Markar SR, De Lijster, et al. A systematic review of outcomes following percutaneous transluminal angioplasty and stenting in the treatment of transplant renal artery stenosis. Cardiovasc Intervent Radiol 2015;38(6):1573–1588.

Pelletier SJ, Guidinger MK, Merion RM, et al. Recovery and utilization of deceased donor kidneys from small pediatric donors. Am J Transplant 2006;6:1646–1652.

Rouviere O, Berger P, Beziat C, et al. Acute thrombosis of renal transplant artery. Transplantation 2002;73:403–409.

Wilson CH, Rix DA, Manas DM, et al. Routine intraoperative ureteric stenting for kidney transplant recipients. Cochrane Database Syst Rev 2013;17(6):CD004925.

10

Post-transplant: The First 3 Months

Phuong-Thu T. Pham and
Gabriel M. Danovitch

It is convenient and practical to divide up the post-transplant period chronologically into the early post-transplant days, the first 3 months, and the later post-transplant period, which encompasses all that happens for the remainder of the life of the transplant. The period discussed in this chapter ends at the beginning of the fourth month. This division makes sense because many of the more acute events occur within the first 3 months, whereas thereafter, patients are more stable. Rejection is most common in the early period, as are some of the more significant infections. Relatively high levels of immunosuppressive medications are used at this time, and the side effects are more marked than they are later on. The later period is discussed in Chapter 11.

For most patients, this is one of the most exciting and yet anxious times in their lives, and it is important to recognize this as we engage in what for medical and transplant professionals have become quite routine tasks. The care of transplant recipients should ideally be a combined effort by medical and surgical teams that bring both their experience and expertise to the care of the patient. The best circumstance is for a single cooperative team to follow each patient together, making joint rounds and decisions about patient care. A relatively well-defined postoperative care pathway facilitates care, efficiency, and cost savings during this time of complex decision making. It is most useful to document all the events during the first admission in a manner that can be easily transmitted to the outpatient clinic. Some patients require readmission in this early period, and verbal and written communication between those caring for the patient in the clinic and the hospital is crucial to good care. The first 3 months are a time of relatively rapid change in management and also a time when surgical and immunologic complications are most common. It is sometimes tempting to focus most particularly on concerns related to graft function, immunosuppression, and rejection, but many of the medical issues discussed more completely in Chapter 11 are already present at this stage, and these too should be managed aggressively.

Early post-transplant factors including delayed graft function (DGF), acute rejection episodes, nephrotoxic agent–induced acute kidney injury (AKI), post-transplant hypertension, infections, and new onset diabetes after transplantation (NODAT) have been implicated in both short-term and long-term causes of morbidity and mortality. Routine postsurgical issues such as wound healing, ambulation, and bowel function must be addressed. Optimal management of the transplant recipient begins in the immediate postoperative period. This chapter provides a stepwise approach to the management of medical complications of the transplant recipient in the first 3 months after transplantation. Immunosuppressive therapy during this period is discussed in Chapter 6.

THE DAY OF THE OPERATION

Immediate Postoperative Assessment

The patient should be evaluated immediately upon arrival in the recovery room, preferably by a combined medical and surgical team who must be familiar with the pretransplant evaluation of the patient (see Chapter 8), the preoperative urine output, details of the source of the donor organ (see Chapters 4 and 7), and the intraoperative course (see Chapter 9). The initial assessment is similar to any major surgical procedure and attention should be paid to cardiovascular and respiratory stability. Most patients are successfully extubated and awake, and pain control should be administered. Intraoperative blood loss and volume replacement should be assessed and the operative report reviewed, paying particular attention to confirming that immunosuppression was given as ordered. Further evaluation should include a full metabolic panel, complete blood count, chest X-ray, and electrocardiography.

In general, it is possible to anticipate early graft function based on preoperative and postoperative characteristics of the donor and recipient as well as the intraoperative perfusion characteristics of the kidney allograft. In patients with minimal residual urine output, an immediate postoperative increase in urine output may serve as an indicator of early graft function. A brisk large volume diuresis following graft revascularization may be due to preoperative volume overload, osmotic diuresis in previously uremic patients, intraoperative use of mannitol or furosemide, or excessive intraoperative intravenous crystalloid or colloid administration. Total fluid intake and output should be monitored on an hourly basis. The intraoperative use of dopamine can be promptly discontinued in polyuric patients.

An abrupt cessation or significant reduction in urine output mandates immediate investigation. Irrigation of the Foley catheter to check for patency should be performed. Persistent oliguria or anuria, particularly in a recipient of a living donor kidney transplant, should prompt immediate evaluation with Doppler ultrasound to ensure ongoing blood flow to the allograft and to exclude surgical complications (see Chapter 14). The absence of blood flow to the allograft requires urgent evaluation by the surgical team for possible immediate reexploration. The length of time a patient remains in the recovery room may vary. A stable patient may typically be transferred to the general transplant care unit within 1 to 2 hours. Intensive care unit observation is usually not required except under special circumstances such as in patients with postoperative EKG changes or arrhythmias, hypotensive patients, or patients with known cardiomyopathy.

THE FIRST POSTOPERATIVE WEEK

It is important that both transplant physicians and nursing staff are experienced in the postoperative care of the transplant recipients and familiar with the importance of measuring urine output, establishing volume replacement, and maintaining hemodynamic stability. Strict control of blood glucose concentrations may not be necessary, and protocols should be in place, which maintain most blood glucose levels between 100 and 180 mg/dL while avoiding hypoglycemia. Patients who develop early post-transplant hyperglycemia or NODAT should be treated with insulin at the discretion of the clinicians. Transplant recipients with preexisting type 1 diabetes commonly require intravenous insulin infusion in the early postoperative period because of the exaggerated diabetogenic effects of high-dose steroid and calcineurin inhibitors (CNIs). Suggested postoperative orders on transfer to the transplant care unit are shown in Table 10.1. In general, stable patients should be encouraged to ambulate within 24 to 48 hours. Traditionally, a liquid diet

TABLE 10.1	Suggested Postoperative Orders on Transfer of Kidney Transplant Recipient from the Recovery Room

Postoperative Nursing Orders

1. Vital signs checked every hour for 12 hours, then every 2 hours for 8 hours, then every 4 hours for stable patients
2. Intake and output every hour for 24 hours, then every 4 hours
3. Intravenous fluid per physician
4. Daily weight
5. Turn, cough, deep breath every hour, encourage incentive spirometry every hour while awake
6. Out of bed on postoperative day 1, ambulate daily thereafter
7. Head of bed at 30 degrees
8. Dressing changes daily as needed
9. Check dialysis access for function every 4 hours
10. No blood pressure, venipuncture in extremity with fistula or shunt
11. Foley catheter to bedside drainage, irrigate gently with 30 mL normal saline as needed for clots
12. Catheter care every 8 hours
13. Notify physicians if urine output drops to less than 60 mL/h for 2 consecutive hours or greater than 300 mL/h for 4 hours or greater than 500 mL/h for 2 consecutive hours
14. Notify physicians if systolic blood pressure > 180 mm Hg or < 110 mm Hg
15. NPO until changed by surgical team
16. Chest radiograph immediately postoperatively

Postoperative Laboratory Orders

1. Complete blood count with platelets, electrolytes, creatinine, glucose, and blood urea nitrogen every 6 hours for 24 hours, then every morning
2. Calcineurin inhibitor level every morning
3. Chemistry panel including liver function tests, urine culture, and sensitivity twice weekly

With acknowledgment to Angela Phelps RN, Elizabeth Hands RN, and Maha Grissom RN.

is started when bowel function returns, but earlier feeding may safely stimulate bowel function (see Chapter 20). Intravenous fluid can usually be discontinued when the patient is able to tolerate solid food diet. Electrolyte abnormalities are not uncommon in the early postoperative period, and laboratory evaluation should initially be performed every 6 hours, and then daily. Wound care, management of Foley catheter and surgical drains, and close monitoring for early postoperative bleeding or urine leak are among other important aspects of early postoperative care of the transplant recipient. Attention should be paid to peripheral pulses and differences in the temperature of the feet, which could reflect impaired blood flow to the lower limb after vascular surgery on pelvic vessels. In a combined medical–surgical run transplant program, open communication between teams is critical for optimal patient outcomes. Surgical and urological complications are discussed in Chapter 9.

Hemodynamic Evaluation and Fluid Management

Frequent hemodynamic evaluation is important because hypotension and intravascular volume depletion may compromise allograft perfusion and graft function. The adequacy of urine output should be assessed in the context of these two parameters. This may require the use of central venous pressure or pulmonary wedge pressure measurements. However, for most stable patients, this is not necessary, and regular clinical assessment should be sufficient.

Patients who are dialyzed preoperatively are usually kept approximately 1 kg above their dry weight, and fluid replacement should be reduced in the face of persistent low urine output. In addition, it is useful to separate fluid replacement into "maintenance fluid" and "replacement fluid." Maintenance fluid is used to replace insensible loss, usually provided as 5% dextrose in water at 30 mL/hour. Urine output and any nasogastric fluid losses are replaced by replacement fluid using half-normal saline because the urine sodium concentration in the early postoperative period is usually 60 to 80 mEq/L. In general, specific management of patients in the first postoperative week depends on the immediate functional status of the graft, which may be categorized as immediate graft function, slow recovery of graft function (SGF), and DGF shown schematically in Figure 10.1. General guidelines for fluid management are summarized in Table 10.2. When necessary, potassium, bicarbonate, or calcium replacement should be given in a separate infusion. Mild hyperkalemia is more commonly encountered in kidney transplant recipients than hypokalemia, particularly in the early post-transplant period. The former is due in part to high-dose CNIs or other drug-induced hyperkalemia (discussed below under Common Laboratory Abnormalities). Serum electrolytes should be ordered at least every 6 hours as clinically indicated.

Patients with Immediate Graft Function

In patients with immediate graft function, urine output from the transplanted kidney generally exceeds 2 to 3 L/day and serum creatinine commonly decreases by 1.0 to 2.0 mg/dL daily. Patients with immediate graft function can usually be discharged on postoperative day (POD) 3 or 4 following successful Foley catheter removal and voiding trial. This is particularly important in older males who have been oliguric while on dialysis and may manifest acute prostatic symptoms when

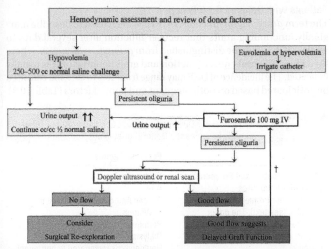

FIGURE 10.1 Suggested algorithmic approach to postoperative fluid management in an oliguric patient. *The volume challenge can be repeated after careful assessment of the volume status and fluid balance. †Repeated doses (or furosemide drips) may be effective in patients whose urine output fluctuates. Consider switching to IV bumetanide. Persistent oliguria will usually not respond to repeated doses.

TABLE 10.2	General Guidelines for Fluid Management

1. In the euvolemic patient, urine output should be replaced hourly with ½ NS cc per cc up to 200 cc. If the urine volume is greater than 200 cc/h, give 200 cc + ½ cc for each cc > 200.
2. Other fluid and electrolyte replacement will be determined appropriately for each individual patient after clinical assessment of volume status.
3. All fluids to be replaced by IV until oral fluids are reestablished by the surgeon.
4. Fluid management for diabetic transplant recipients:
   Replace insensible loss with ½ NS
   Replace other output with ½ NS

faced with a high urine output. In these circumstances, a longer period of Foley drainage may be required. Patients who receive basiliximab induction (see Chapter 6) therapy generally receive the second dose on POD 4, prior to hospital discharge.

Patients with Slow Recovery of Graft Function

Patients with SGF are generally nonoliguric and experience a slow decline in serum creatinine levels. These patients usually do not require dialysis support but require careful attention to fluid management. Volume depletion must be avoided to prevent precipitation of AKI. In contrast, overzealous fluid replacement in patients with slow graft function may result in overt pulmonary edema and the need for dialysis. The serum creatinine of patients with slow graft function generally does not normalize within the first postoperative week. Nonetheless, most patients can be discharged on postoperative day 5 to 7 with close outpatient follow-up.

Patients with Delayed Graft Function

The term *delayed graft function* (DGF) has been used to describe marginally functioning grafts that recover function after several days to weeks. DGF should be distinguished from *primary nonfunction*, where the kidney allografts never function and graft nephrectomy is usually indicated. The incidence of DGF may range from 10% to 50% and can often be anticipated based on both recipient and donor factors (Table 10.3).

 Risk Factors for Delayed Graft Function due to Acute Tubular Necrosis in Deceased Donor Kidney Transplantation[*]

Donor Factors	Recipient Factors
Premorbid Factors and Preoperative Donor Characteristics	**Premorbid Factors**
Kidney Donor Profile Index (KDPI) > 85% (see text). The donor characteristics used to calculate KDPI include the following:	Age
	African Americans (compared to Whites)
	Peripheral vascular disease
	Dialysis duration before transplant
• Age	Hemodialysis (compared to peritoneal dialysis)
• Height	
• Weight	Presensitization (PRA > 50%)
• Ethnicity	Reallograft transplant
• History of HTN	Obesity (body mass index > 30 kg/m²)
• History of diabetes	Hypercoagulability state[†]
• Cause of death (CVA/stroke, head trauma, anoxia, CNS tumor, other)	**Perioperative and Postoperative Factors**
• Serum creatinine	Hypotension, shock
• HCV status	Recipient volume contraction
• Donation after cardiac death status	Early high-dose calcineurin inhibitors
Donor macrovascular or microvascular disease	mTOR inhibitors[‡] (sirolimus and everolimus)
Brain-death stress	
Prolonged use of vasopressors	
Preprocurement ATN	
Nephrotoxic agent exposure	
Organ Procurement Surgery	
Hypotension prior to cross-clamping of aorta	
Traction on renal vasculatures	
Cold storage flushing solutions	
Kidney Preservation	
Prolonged warm ischemia time	
Prolonged cold ischemia time	
Cold storage vs. machine perfusion	
Intraoperative Factors	
Intraoperative hemodynamic instability	
Prolonged rewarmed time (anastomotic time)	

HTN, hypertension; CVA, cerebrovascular accident; CNS, central nervous system; ATN, acute tubular necrosis; PRA, panel reactive antibodies.
[*]The contributory role of certain risk factors may differ among studies.
[†]Such as the presence of factor V Leiden mutation or antiphospholipid antibodies.
[‡]May prolong the duration of DGF. Its use should be avoided in the early post-transplantation period.

Most patients with DGF are oliguric or anuric. Knowledge of the patient's native urine output is critical to assess the origin of the early urine output. When the transplant is from a living donor, postoperative oliguria is rare because of the short cold ischemia time. Nonetheless, if postoperative oliguria does occur, complications with vascular revascularization must be urgently considered. In contrast, when a patient receives a deceased donor kidney from a marginal donor kidney, DGF may be anticipated. The mate kidney from a deceased donor often behaves in a similar manner, and information on its function can be useful.

Anuria refers to negligible urine production. Oliguria in the peritransplant period typically refers to a urine output of less than 50 mL/hour. Before patients are subjected to a full evaluation for poor urine output, their volume status and fluid balance and patency of the Foley catheter must be assessed. If clots are present, the catheter should be removed and gentle suction applied in attempt to capture the offending clot. Thereafter, replacement with a large catheter may be required. If the Foley catheter is patent and the patient is clearly hypervolemic, 100 to 200 mg of furosemide may be given intravenously. If the patient is judged to be hypovolemic or if a confident clinical assessment cannot be made, a judicious trial of isotonic saline infusion may be given, with or without subsequent administration of furosemide as dictated by the patient's response to saline infusion alone. A suggested algorithmic approach to postoperative fluid management in an oliguric patient is shown in Figure 10.1.

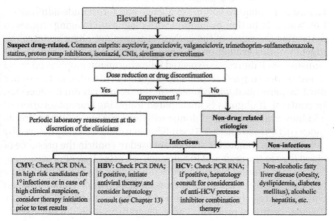

FIGURE 10.2 Algorithm for the management of elevated hepatic enzymes in kidney transplant recipients. CNIs, may cause transient, self-limited dose-dependent elevations of aminotransferase levels and mild hyperbilirubinemia secondary to defective bile secretion. (Modified from Pham PT, Danovitch GM, Pham PC. Medical management of the kidney transplant recipient: infections, malignant neoplasms, and gastrointestinal disorders. In: Johnson RJ, Feehally J, Floege J. Comprehensive Clinical Nephrology. 5th ed. Philadelphia, PA: Elsevier Saunders; 2015:1188–1201.)

Unless these patients have adequate residual urine output from the native kidneys, most patients with DGF will require temporary dialysis support for volume, hyperkalemia, or uremia. Indications for dialysis in the transplant recipient with postoperative allograft dysfunction are essentially the same as in any patient with postoperative AKI. Hyperkalemia should be treated aggressively. In anuric patients, it is wise to dialyze patient when potassium level is above 5.5 mg/dL. Other treatment modalities such as intravenous calcium and glucose with insulin are temporizing measures but do not obviate the need for dialysis. Sodium polystyrene sulfonate (Kayexalate) should not be administered in the early post-transplant period because it may induce colonic dilatation and predispose to perforation.

Patients with DGF often become volume overloaded in the early post-transplant period because they are frequently subjected to repeated volume challenges. It is not infrequent for such patients to gain several kilograms of fluid over their dry weight. Ultrafiltration with or without dialysis may be required. Care must be taken to avoid hypotension during dialysis because it may perpetuate graft dysfunction. In patients with established DGF, the dialysis requirement should be assessed daily until graft function improves.

Although peritoneal dialysis (PD) may be performed in patients with a functioning PD catheter in place, hemodialysis may be more effective in the early postoperative period when severe hyperkalemia is present or prolonged absence of bowel function is a problem. PD should be avoided when there is evidence of a peritoneal leak or infection.

Diagnostic Studies in Persistent Oliguria or Anuria

Failure to respond to volume challenge and furosemide administration warrants further evaluation with diagnostic imaging studies to determine the cause of the early post-transplant oliguric state. The urgency of this evaluation partially depends on specific clinical circumstances. If diuresis is expected following an uncomplicated living donor kidney transplantation and oliguria occurs, diagnostic studies must be performed *immediately*—in the recovery room if necessary. In contrast, if oliguria is anticipated following transplantation of a kidney from a deceased donor with a high Kidney Donor Profile Index ([KDPI] see Chapter 5), studies can usually be safely delayed by several hours. Diagnostic studies are used to confirm the presence of blood flow to the graft and the absence of a urine leak or obstruction. Doppler ultrasound has replaced scintigraphic studies of blood flow (see Chapter 14). If the study reveals no demonstrable blood flow, an emergent surgical reexploration is necessary to attempt to repair any vascular technical problem. These allografts may not be salvageable and are removed during the second surgery, sometimes they may recover function after a prolonged period of DGF. If adequate blood flow is demonstrated, the possibility of ureteral obstruction or urinary leak needs to be reconsidered and can be evaluated by the same imaging studies (see Chapter 14). In the first 24 hours after transplantation, as long as the Foley catheter has been providing good bladder drainage, the obstruction or leak is almost always at the ureterovesical junction and represents a technical problem that needs surgical correction. The differential diagnosis of DGF is shown in Table 10.4.

TABLE 10.4	Differential Diagnoses of Delayed Graft Function and Acute Kidney Injury in the Early Post-transplant Period

1. Prenatal (or Preglomerular Type)
   Volume contraction
   Nephrotoxic drugs causing preglomerular type AKI (e.g., cyclosporine and to a lesser extent tacrolimus, ACEI or ARBs, amphotericin B, intravenous radiocontrast dye)
2. Intrinsic Renal
   Acute tubular necrosis
   Early acute rejection
   Thrombotic microangioapthy (CNI- or mTOR inhibitor-induced, acute antibody-mediated rejection, atypical HUS, TMA associated with ADAMTS-13 deficiency or the presence of inhibitory antibodies, lupus anticoagulant or antiphospholipid antibody positivity, infection with CMV, parvovirus B19, or influenza A virus, the concomitant presence of hepatitis C and anticardiolipin antibody)
   Recurrence of primary glomerular disease (particularly FSGS)
3. Postrenal
   Catheter obstruction
   Perinephric fluid collection (lymphocele, urine leak, hematoma)
   Ureteral obstruction
      Intrinsic (blood clots, poor reimplantation, ureteral slough)
      Extrinsic (ureteral kinking)
4. Vascular Complications
   Arterial or venous thrombosis
   Transplant renal artery stenosis

Prerenal Causes of DGF

Intravascular Volume Depletion and Calcineurin Inhibitors. Severe intravascular volume depletion is usually suggested by a careful review of the patient's preoperative history and intraoperative report. If hemodialysis is performed preoperatively, it is preferable to keep the patients up to 1 kg above their dry weight to facilitate diuresis following graft revascularization. Both CNIs can cause a dose-related reversible afferent arteriolar vasoconstriction (see Fig. 6.2) that manifests clinically as delayed recovery of graft function. Intraoperative injection of the calcium channel blocker verapamil into the renal artery has been suggested to reduce capillary spasm and improve renal blood flow. Most centers advocate the use of nondihydropyridine calcium channel blockers (i.e., diltiazem) to counteract the vasoconstrictive effect of CNIs. Their use may permit a reduction in CNI dose up to 40% (see Chapter 6).

Intrinsic Renal Causes of DGF

Intrinsic causes of DGF typically include acute tubular necrosis (ATN), acute rejection, thrombotic microangiopathy (TMA), or recurrence of glomerular disease affecting the native kidneys.

Acute Tubular Necrosis. Acute tubular necrosis (ATN) is the most common cause of DGF. The two terms are often used interchangeably although not all causes of DGF are caused by ATN. Its incidence varies widely among centers and has been reported to occur in 20% to 25% of patients (range 6% to 50%). The difference in the incidence reported may be due in part to the differences in the criteria used to define DGF and/or the more liberal use of organs with high KDPI by some centers. The most common definition of DGF is based on the requirement for dialysis in the first post-transplant week; a definition that is convenient but is clearly inadequate because of varying levels of residual renal function that may obviate the necessity for dialysis. Unless an allograft biopsy is performed, post-transplant ATN should be a diagnosis of exclusion. In the absence of superimposed acute rejection or other pathologic findings, ATN typically resolves over several days and occasionally over several weeks, particularly in recipients of older donor kidneys. Recovery of ATN is usually heralded by a steady increase in urine output associated with a decrease in interdialytic increase in serum creatinine and eventual dialysis independence. Prolonged DGF should prompt a diagnostic allograft biopsy. Some centers perform serial biopsies in patients with prolonged DGF to exclude covert acute rejection or other intrinsic causes of allograft dysfunction. ATN is uncommon in living donor kidney transplants. Hence, early diagnostic allograft biopsy should be performed for unexplained DGF in living donor kidney transplants.

Risk Factors. Prolonged cold and warm ischemia times as well as an older donor age are well-established risk factors for DGF secondary to ATN. In addition to donor factors, recipient premorbid and peri- and postoperative factors may also predispose the kidney allograft to ATN. Table 10.3 summarizes potential risk factors for DGF due to ATN in deceased donor kidney transplants. A risk-prediction model, based on these factors, has been developed (see Irish et al. in Selected Readings) and may be valuable in clinical trials and the planning of perioperative immunosuppressive therapy. At the website www.transplantcalculator.com, an individual patient's predicted probability of developing DGF based on information available at the time of transplant can be estimated.

Potential Mechanisms of Post-transplant ATN. Post-transplant ATN is primarily a consequence of ischemia and reperfusion injury (IRI). Because of its importance and relevance to equivalent injury in other solid organs, it has been the subject of intensive study. Readers are referred to the references of Schroppel and Legendre and Cavaille Coll et al. in Selected Readings for a detailed consideration of the likely mechanisms at play. Organs from deceased donors are vulnerable to ischemic injury at various time points starting at the diagnosis of brain death, maintenance of circulatory and respiratory stability following brain death, procurement surgery and cold storage, and ending at the time of arterial anastomosis or rewarming time (see Chapter 4, Part I). Cell death, adaptive immunity, and innate immunity play important roles.

The use of kidneys with a high KDPI, and particularly kidneys recovered after circulatory death (donation after circulatory death [DCD], see Chapter 4), may increase the incidence of ATN. Patients receiving kidneys recovered after DCD have an incidence of DGF of over 40%, nearly twice the incidence of DGF compared with recipients of kidneys from heart-beating donors. Indeed, a DCD kidney is by definition susceptible to various degrees of warm ischemic damage and its use inevitably increases the incidence of post-transplant DGF.

To optimize the utilization of DCD kidneys, machine perfusion parameters and viability testing have been used by a number of centers to assess the extent of kidney damage and to predict graft function (see Chapter 4, Part I).

Following revascularization, the kidney allograft may be exposed to further IRI, particularly in donor organs with a long cold ischemia time. Clinically, patients may develop oliguria after having an initial good urine output. Renal blood flow is generally well preserved, leading to dissociation between flow and excretory function. Doppler ultrasound may show an elevated resistive index (RI) of greater than 80% (see Chapter 14).

In the presence of ATN, it is important to maintain adequate immunosuppression. Studies suggest that endothelial injury upregulates and exposes donor histocompatibility antigens, adhesion molecules, and costimulatory molecules, heightening the risk for acute rejection that occurs at a rate of approximately 50% greater than in kidneys that function immediately. Hence, efforts should be made to modify risk factors including minimization of cold ischemia time, avoidance of intraoperative and perioperative volume contraction, or use of CNI-sparing protocols to avoid their vasoconstrictive effect. Some centers advocate the use of sequential antibody induction therapy in the presence of anticipated or established DGF. In these cases, CNI is introduced when the serum creatinine reaches 2.5 to 2.9 mg/dL or less. The antibody can be discontinued once adequate CNI level has been achieved. Alternatively, a protocol consisting of induction therapy with anti-thymocyte globulin (Thymoglobulin) daily for 4 doses and delayed introduction of CNI until day 3 may be employed. As ATN may render the allograft more susceptible to immunologic injury, the use of anti-thymocyte globulin in this setting may also be beneficial because of its potent immunosuppressive effect. Intraoperative anti-thymocyte globulin administration has been reported to be associated with a significant decrease in DGF and better early allograft function compared to postoperative administration, presumably through modulation and attenuation of graft IRI. Mammalian target of rapamycin (mTOR) inhibitors should be avoided in the early transplant period because of their adverse effect on recovery of allograft function from ATN (see Chapter 6).

Prevention of ATN Using Drug Therapy. Low-dose dopamine infusions of 1 to 5 µg/kg/min are used routinely at some centers to promote renal blood flow and to counteract CNI-induced renal vasoconstriction. The benefits of dopamine have not been proved in randomized trials and its use is largely institution dependent.

Administration of calcium channel blockers (CCB) to the donor or recipient, or at the time of vasculature anastomosis, is routinely used in many transplant centers largely as a result of randomized clinical trials showing improved initial function with their use. The presumed mechanism of action is by virtue of a direct vasodilatory effect. The kidney may "pink up" when verapamil is injected into the renal artery during surgery. It is unknown whether the use of dopamine or CCBs confers a beneficial effect on long-term allograft function or graft survival beyond their vasodilatory effect and improvement in renal blood flow in the perioperative period. The requirement for perioperative dialysis may be reduced by these agents. Various pharmacologic approaches to the treatment of IRI have shown promising results in experimental animal models, but are yet to be proved successful in clinical settings (see Schroppel and Legendre in Selected Readings).

Long-Term Impact of DGF/ATN. Studies on the impact of DGF on long-term graft function have yielded conflicting results. This may be due in part to the lack of universally defined criteria for DGF, and differences in donor and recipient characteristics. In addition, in most studies, transplant biopsies were not performed and DGF was presumed to be due to ATN. Nonetheless, it does appear that prolonged delayed recovery of graft function and DGF concomitant with an increased incidence of acute rejection are associated with worse long-term outcomes. This emphasizes the importance of maintaining adequate immunosuppression and of repeating biopsies every 7 to 10 days to assess for covert acute rejection.

Regardless of the true impact of DGF (independent of other factors) on long-term graft survival, DGF has financial and programmatic significance. It is resource demanding and may affect the financial viability of transplant programs. Some programs may avoid accepting potentially viable organs for this reason.

Acute Rejection

Accelerated Acute Rejection. Accelerated acute rejection or delayed hyperacute rejection occurs within 24 hours to a few days after transplantation and may involve both antibody-mediated and cellular immune mechanisms. Repeat transplants, multiple pregnancies, or multiple blood transfusions are well-substantiated risk factors for hyperacute or accelerated acute rejection owing to preformed cytotoxic antibodies against human leukocyte antigens. However, with the currently sensitive cross-matching techniques and the availability of the single-antigen Luminex assays, hyperacute rejection has virtually been eliminated (see Chapter 3).

Early Acute Cell-Mediated Rejection. Acute rejections typically occur between the first week and the first few months after transplantation. In unsensitized patients with low levels of preformed antibodies, acute rejection rarely occurs in the first week. However, when the recipient has received recent blood transfusions, particularly if these were donor-derived blood, early acute cellular rejection may be more common. Over the last half decade, various desensitization protocols have allowed successful transplantation in highly sensitized kidney transplant candidates.

Acute Antibody-Mediated Rejection. Acute antibody-mediated rejection (AMR) can occur alone or in conjunction with cell-mediated rejection. It usually occurs early after transplantation and frequently, but not invariably, develops in the setting of preexisting sensitization. The advent of C4d staining and single-antigen Luminex assays to detect donor-specific anti-HLA antibodies has led to the recognition that AMR might have previously been diagnosed as hyperacute cellular rejection or rejection refractory to conventional therapy. Other alloreactive antibodies that have been shown to be associated with anti-HLA-negative AMR include antibodies against MHC-related chain A and B (MICA and MICB), anti-endothelial antibodies, and anti-angiotensin type 1 receptor antibodies. Although not yet widely available, high-resolution HLA typing for deceased donors permits detection of allele-specific, donor-specific antibodies with greater accuracy and assists clinicians in tailoring immunosuppression in highly sensitized transplant recipients, potentially preventing the development of AMR.

Clinical Manifestations of Acute Rejection. Acute rejection episodes most commonly present as asymptomatic rise in serum creatinine or failure of the serum creatinine to decrease below an elevated level. Since the introduction of CNIs and other potent immunosuppressive agents into clinical transplantation, the classic clinical signs and symptoms of acute rejection such as fever, malaise, graft tenderness, and oliguria are seen less frequently. A tender, swollen graft associated with a rising creatinine and fever can be due to acute rejection or pyelonephritis. Excruciating localized pain is usually a result of a urine leak (see Chapter 9). CNI toxicity and CMV (cytomegalovirus) or BK virus infection do not produce graft tenderness. Acute rejection and CNI toxicity can produce graft dysfunction in the absence of oliguria. Oliguria, however, can be seen in severe acute rejection, and its occurrence makes the diagnosis of drug toxicity less likely. In the presence of oliguria, the search for an anatomical cause is mandatory. The pathologic findings and treatment of acute rejection are discussed in Chapters 6 and 15.

Thrombotic Microangiopathy. Potential causative factors of post-transplant thrombotic microangiopathy (TMA) include acute antibody-mediated rejection (see Chapter 15); immunosuppressive drug-induced (CNI and mTOR inhibitors); recurrence of atypical HUS; TMA associated with ADAMTS-13 deficiency or the presence of inhibitory antibodies, and the presence of lupus anticoagulant or anticardiolipin; CMV infection, and less frequently systemic viral infection with parvovirus B 19 or influenza A virus. An increased incidence of TMA has also been described in a subset of transplant recipients with concurrent hepatitis C infection and anticardiolipin antibody positivity. Treatment should be directed against the underlying cause. Belatacept is a therapeutic option in patients with immunosuppression-associated TMA (see Chapter 6).

Recurrence of Glomerular Disease of the Native Kidneys. Recurrence of glomerular disease of the native kidneys is discussed in Chapter 11.

Postrenal Causes of DGF

Postrenal DGF is generally due to obstruction and may occur anywhere from the intrarenal collecting system to the level of the bladder-catheter drainage. The latter is generally due to blood clots and can often be managed by flushing the catheter with saline solution. Nursing care orders should routinely include irrigation of the Foley catheter as needed for clots or no urine flow. Other causes of early acute obstruction include technically poor reimplant and ureteral sloughing. Ureteral fibrosis secondary to either ischemia or rejection can cause intrinsic obstruction. The distal ureter close to the ureterovesical junction is particularly vulnerable to ischemic damage because of its remote location from the renal artery, and hence compromised blood supply. Ureteral kinking, lymphocele, and pelvic hematoma are potential causes of extrinsic compression in the early post-transplant period. Although uncommon, ureteral fibrosis associated with polyoma BK virus in the setting of kidney transplantation has been well described.

Potential etiologic factors of postrenal causes of DGF are summarized in Table 10.4. Surgical and urological causes of obstructive uropathy are discussed in Chapter 9.

Vascular Causes of DGF

Renal Artery Stenosis. Transplant renal artery stenosis (RAS) may occur as early as the first week, but it is usually a later complication. RAS may amplify the effect of CNI toxicity, volume depletion and angiotensin converting enzyme inhibitor (ACEI) and angiotensin receptor blocker (ARB) use. Acute deterioration of graft function or severe hypotension associated with the use of ACEI or ARB should raise the suspicion of RAS. Other clinical manifestations may include accelerated or refractory hypertension and peripheral edema in the absence of proteinuria. The latter is a clinical example of so-called Goldblatt II type hypertension produced in animal models by partially clamping the renal artery when the contralateral kidney is removed (single-kidney RAS). Although invasive, renal angiogram remains the gold standard for establishing the diagnosis of RAS. Color Doppler ultrasound is highly sensitive and can serve as an initial noninvasive imaging study to assess transplant vessels (see Chapter 14). In patients with preexisting diffuse vascular disease, the possibility of stenosis of the iliac artery proximal to the transplanted renal artery should be excluded. Such lesions may limit flow to the transplanted kidney causing signs and symptoms similar to those of transplant RAS, a phenomenon referred to as pseudo-RAS. Vascular clamp injury to the iliac vessels proximal to the transplanted renal artery may also cause RAS and may be associated with claudication to the ipsilateral buttock or leg.

Graft Thrombosis. Arterial or venous thrombosis generally occurs within the first 2 to 3 postoperative days but may occur as long as 2 months post-transplant. Thrombosis occurring early after transplantation is most often due to technical surgical complications, whereas the later onset is generally due to acute rejection. In patients with initial good allograft function, thrombosis is generally heralded by the acute onset of oliguria or anuria associated with deterioration of allograft function. Clinically, the patient may present with graft swelling and tenderness or gross hematuria. In patients with DGF and good residual urine output from the native kidneys, there may be no overt signs or symptoms and the diagnosis rests on clinical suspicion and prompt imaging studies. The diagnosis is usually made by Doppler ultrasound or isotope flow scan. Suggested risk factors for vascular thrombosis include arteriosclerotic involvement of the donor or recipient vessels; intimal injury of graft vessels; kidney with multiple arteries; history of recurrent thrombosis; thrombocytosis; younger recipients or donor age; and the presence of antiphospholipid antibody (anticardiolipin antibody or lupus anticoagulant). Some studies suggest that DCD kidneys are risk factors for graft thrombosis.

There is no consensus on the optimal management of recipients with an abnormal hypercoagulability profile, such as abnormal activated protein C resistance ratio or factor V Leiden mutation, antiphospholipid antibody positivity, protein C or protein S deficiency, or antithrombin III deficiency. However, unless contraindicated, perioperative or postoperative prophylactic anticoagulation should be considered, particularly in patients with prior history of recurrent thrombotic events. Transplant of pediatric en bloc kidneys into adult recipient with a history of thrombosis should probably be avoided.

Postoperative Bleeding. Any combination of the triad of hypotension, precipitous drop in hemoglobin/hematocrit levels, and pain should raise the suspicion of significant postoperative bleeding. The perinephric drain may fill with blood, and there may be a visible or palpable hematoma. If the hematoma is contained, the buildup of pressure will usually be sufficient to stop further bleeding. However, if the hematoma appears to be placing pressure on the ureter or surrounding vasculature, surgical evacuation may be necessary to prevent ureteric or vascular necrosis. Persistent bleeding refractory to blood resuscitation often requires surgical exploration. Retroperitoneal bleeding can be a source of significant blood loss and may be associated with significant pain. In patients with coronary artery disease and in diabetic and older recipients, it is advisable to maintain hemoglobin level above 10 g/dL.

MEDICAL MANAGEMENT IN THE FIRST WEEK

Hypertension and Hypotension

Many patients are hypertensive after surgery and this may resolve spontaneously or with adequate pain control. Although persistent severe hypertension requires treatment, aggressive lowering of blood pressure may increase the risk for ATN and DGF. In the acute setting, a systolic blood pressure of <180 mm Hg is acceptable because blood flow to the newly transplanted organ is dependent on an adequate mean systemic blood pressure. Intravenous labetalol or hydralazine can be used, or if the patient is able to take oral medications, clonidine or nifedipine can effectively lower blood pressure. However, it should be noted that there is a lack of conclusive evidence that one class of antihypertensive agent is superior to another in the transplant setting and treatment should be individualized. β blockers are generally used in the perioperative period because they have been shown to reduce cardiovascular events in high-risk candidates. Diuretics are used in nonoliguric patients who are volume expanded. ACEIs and ARBs can cause acute changes in kidney function as well as hyperkalemia and hence should be avoided until allograft function stabilizes. Nondihydropyridine calcium channel blockers such as diltiazem may permit CNI dose reduction. The concomitant use of β-blocker and nondihydropyridine CCB can occasionally cause symptomatic bradycardia and the potential for such drug interactions should not be overlooked. Long-term management of post-transplant hypertension is discussed in Chapter 11.

Though most dialysis patients are hypertensive, some tend to hypotension and their management on dialysis is difficult. In the event that these patients become transplant candidates (see Chapter 8), their perioperative management is challenging. It is essential to maintain adequate perfusion to the newly transplanted kidney and systolic blood pressure should be kept over 100 mm Hg and mean arterial pressure over 70 mm Hg with the aid of liberal fluid replacement, blood transfusion, use of vasoactive drugs both orally (midodrine) and intravenously, and fludrocortisone. Patients are best served by monitoring in an ICU environment and an arterial line may facilitate accurate measurement of blood pressure.

Hyperglycemia

Transplant recipients with preexisting diabetes or those who develop post-transplant hyperglycemia may require a more prolonged hospital stay for glycemic control. In the immediate postoperative period, hyperglycemia should be controlled with an intravenous infusion of insulin. In patients at risk for developing NODAT, and in those with type 2 diabetes who are not on insulin, consideration should be given to using cyclosporine-based immunosuppression because it is less diabetogenic than tacrolimus (see Chapter 6). In addition, steroid exposure should be minimized, with possible discontinuation of prednisone within the first few days in patients considered to be at low immunologic risk. The diabetogenic effects of various immunosuppressive agents are discussed in Chapter 6. Once patients are able to tolerate oral intake, they should be transitioned from intravenous insulin to a subcutaneous regimen. Those who were on insulin pump before transplant can resume their insulin pump therapy. However, they should be informed that their new insulin requirements will be higher particularly in the first postoperative week because of high dose of steroid. Patients with new onset post-transplant hyperglycemia should be started on a sliding-scale, rapid-acting insulin such as NovoLog if it is expected that their hyperglycemia will improve concomitant with reduction in steroid dosage. For diabetic patients on a regimen that includes a long-acting basal insulin and preprandial short-acting insulin, a correction scale using rapid-acting insulin should be used. During the first post-transplantation week, all hyperglycemic patients, including those with preexisting diabetes, should receive teaching from a diabetic educator, emphasizing the effects of immunosuppression, of missing meals, and of exercise on the use of insulin. Endocrinology consultation should be obtained at the discretion of the transplant physician. A structured diabetes education and discharge planning may reduce hyperglycemia-related hospital readmission rates.

Surgical Incision, Drains, and Stents

Improved surgical techniques and prophylactic antibiotics have made wound infections and dehiscence of the incision uncommon. Obese transplant recipients are at greater risk and should be evaluated frequently. Sirolimus may delay wound healing and increase the incidence of lymphocele formation and its use should be avoided in the early post-transplant period. The bladder catheter is usually removed on postoperative day 3 or 4, and the perinephric drain, if present, is usually removed on the following unless it continues to drain more than 100 mL/day. It is not uncommon for serosanguineous fluid to drain through the incision in the first few days. However, increasing wound drainage, particularly if associated with increasing graft tenderness and decreasing urine output, should raise the suspicion of a urine leak. The fluid drained should be sent for creatinine. In the presence of a urine leak, the fluid creatinine concentration is significantly elevated compared with that of the plasma. The diagnosis is confirmed by a voiding cystogram, nuclear medicine scan, or antegrade nephrostogram. Management of urine leaks is discussed in Chapter 9.

Surgical staples or sutures are generally removed 2 weeks after surgery. If a double-J stent was placed in the ureter at the time of transplant, patients should be advised of its presence and cystoscopic removal should be scheduled 3 to 4 weeks after transplant.

THE DAY OF DISCHARGE

It is imperative that all patients (together with family members or caregivers) attend the patient education session given by transplant coordinators in anticipation of discharge. The necessity of frequent outpatient visits in the first 3 months post-transplantation must be emphasized. Patients should receive clear instructions, easy-to-understand medication lists, and a log to record vital signs, and if applicable, blood glucose measurements along with insulin dosages and perinephric drain output. They must be taught to recognize the signs and symptoms of infection, allograft rejection, and potential adverse effects of immunosuppressive agents and drug–drug interactions. Women of childbearing age may regain fertility soon after a successful transplant and should be counseled about contraception and drug-induced teratogenesis. If available, patients are seen by a transplant pharmacist prior to their discharge. Patients should also be encouraged to engage in regular physical activities or exercise program. In addition, nutritional education should be provided to all patients irrespective of their diabetic status. The transplantation team should understand this enormous new burden on patients and provide them with psychosocial support if necessary (see Chapter 21). Although uncommon, patients may develop changes in mental status in the early post-transplant period, which warrant psychiatric intervention (see Chapter 18).

FROM DISCHARGE TO THE END OF THE FIRST 3 MONTHS

The first post-transplant month involves the transition from inpatient to outpatient care. Patients with immediate graft function are generally discharged on the third or fourth POD, whereas those with slow graft function are usually discharged on a day or two later. Patients who develop DGF and biopsy-documented ATN can usually be discharged on POD 8 to 10 after arrangements for outpatient dialysis have been made. The frequency of clinic visits may vary among centers. However, patients should be seen twice a week for the first 4 weeks, weekly for the next month, and biweekly after the first 2 months (or more frequently at the discretion of the clinicians depending on the complexity of their early postoperative course). Laboratory assessment during the first 2 to 3 months should include a comprehensive metabolic panel, a complete blood count with platelets, urinalysis, and immunosuppressive drug levels. Patient's log book should be reviewed and medications should be adjusted at the time of their clinic visit. Physical examination should focus on their volume status and the allograft surgical incision site. The importance of medical adherence, proper nutrition, and physical activity should be emphasized. Most patients with stable graft function and an uneventful postoperative course can return to work or their regular daily activities 2 to 3 months post-transplant. These patients are typically repatriated to their primary nephrologists 3 months after transplant. Those with DGF requiring dialysis support should be reassessed at each clinic visit. Prolonged DGF warrants surveillance biopsies to exclude covert acute rejection.

Acute Kidney Injury

An increase of 10% to 20% in serum creatinine from baseline commonly represents laboratory variability and can be rechecked within 48 to 72 hours at the clinician's discretion. However, a greater increase in serum creatinine should prompt further evaluation, particularly in high immunologic risk patients. Prerenal AKI is usually evident through obtaining a medical history and physical exam that should include serial assessment of body weight and postural change in blood pressure. In the era of potent immunosuppression, fever and graft tenderness are usually absent during acute allograft rejection episodes. Accurate diagnosis necessitates an allograft biopsy. All medications must be reviewed to exclude any drug-induced nephrotoxicity. A rise in serum creatinine associated with markedly elevated CNI concentrations may be managed expectantly by dose reduction. Acute CNI toxicity typically improves within 24 to 48 hours after dosage adjustment. Hence, a persistently elevated serum creatinine warrants further evaluation. In contrast, acute kidney allograft injury in the face of persistently low CNI concentrations or in high immunologic risk transplant recipients (e.g., high pretransplant panel reactive antibodies, reallograft transplant, and historical donor specific antigens [DSA]) raises the possibility of acute rejection and requires more aggressive diagnostic and therapeutic intervention. Initial evaluation with Doppler ultrasound to exclude vascular complications and to rule out hydronephrosis or perinephric fluid collection (because of lymphocele, hematoma, or urine leak) is appropriate. If perinephric drains are still in place or if there is copious drainage through the incision, the fluid should be sent urgently for measurement of creatinine. Elevated fluid creatinine concentration to more than one and a half times over that of plasma suggests urine leak and appropriate steps should be taken. Diagnostic imaging studies and management of surgical and urological complications are discussed in Chapter 9. A diagnostic allograft biopsy can be performed after vascular and urologic causes of graft function have been excluded. In patients with high risk for complications (those who are anticoagulated or those in whom allograft biopsy may be difficult due to overlying bowels or obesity), it may be appropriate to proceed with pulse steroid without biopsy confirmation, particularly when there is a high clinical suspicion for acute rejection. The potential etiologic factors of AKI in the early post-transplant period are shown in Table 10.4. AKI in the early transplant period may predict impaired function at 1 year post-transplant.

Cyclosporine and Tacrolimus Concentrations

CNI therapeutic drug monitoring is an integral part of patient management because of inter- and intrapatient variability in pharmacokinetics and pharmacodynamics. Guidelines for drug monitoring are discussed in Chapter 6. There is a significant overlap between therapeutic range and toxicity. Acute rejection can occur in patients with high CNI concentrations and toxicity can be seen at seemingly low CNI concentrations. In contrast, low CNI levels in the first post-transplant year may be associated with subsequent biopsy-proven acute rejection. Acute CNI toxicity is due to intense afferent arteriolar vasoconstriction and reduction of glomerular capillary pressure (see Fig. 6.2). It is generally dose-related and reversible within 48 hours after dosage adjustment. Unexplained persistently elevated serum creatinine warrants a diagnostic allograft biopsy to exclude other causes of AKI such as TMA, acute antibody-mediated rejection, BK nephropathy, pyelonephritis, or recurrent primary glomerular disease, particularly focal segmental glomerulosclerosis (FSGS), or anti-GBM disease in patients with Alport syndrome (see Chapter 11).

BK Virus Infection

In kidney transplant recipients, BK virus infection is associated with a range of clinical syndromes, including asymptomatic viruria with or without viremia, ureteral stenosis and obstruction, BK nephropathy (BKN), and interstitial nephritis. BKN is an important cause of both acute and chronic allograft injury and may occur as early as the first week to as late as several years after transplantation. The prevention, recognition, and treatment of BK virus infection are discussed in Chapter 12 and its pathologic features in Chapter 15. Screening for BK viremia monthly for the first 3 to 6 months after transplantation then every 3 months until month 12 allows early detection of most cases of BK viral replication in kidney transplant recipients.

Fever

Isolated low-grade fever is common. Persistent low-grade fever should be evaluated to exclude an underlying infectious process. Potential sources include urine, lungs, and incisional site. The most common viral infection, CMV, may present with fever with or without gastrointestinal symptoms, unexplained fatigue, leukopenia, thrombocytopenia, or various signs and symptoms related to the specific affected organ. All febrile patients should be examined thoroughly, with close attention to the incision. Chest radiographs and urine culture should be done as clinically indicated. Potential infectious sources such as arteriovenous dialysis access, sinuses, dental hygiene, or perineum should not be overlooked. If the peritoneal or hemodialysis catheter is still present, peritoneal fluid or blood should be sent for cultures. The diagnosis and management of CMV infection and other post-transplant infectious complications is discussed in Chapter 12.

Graft Tenderness

In the early post-transplant period, the site of the surgical incision may be tender but incisional pain generally resolves within 1 to 2 weeks unless there is a hematoma or infection. The presence of fever, graft tenderness, and pyuria suggests pyelonephritis. In the CNI era, fever and graft tenderness are usually absent during acute rejection episodes. Persistent graft tenderness (with or without graft enlargement) and rising creatinine mandate a thorough evaluation to exclude infection, obstruction, bleeding, or acute rejection. Diagnostic work-up should include an allograft ultrasound to exclude a structural cause and urine culture to rule out pyelonephritis. An allograft biopsy should be performed for unexplained AKI and graft tenderness. Viral infections and CNI toxicity are not associated with graft enlargement or tenderness.

COMMON LABORATORY ABNORMALITIES IN EARLY POST-TRANSPLANT

Urinalysis

A routine urinalysis should be part of every clinic visit. Pyuria and microhematuria are common laboratory findings in the early post-transplant period. Pyuria usually indicates bacterial infection. However, sterile pyuria is not uncommon and can be due to the presence of an indwelling double-J stent, contamination from vaginal secretions, treated urinary tract infections, and although uncommon, pyuria has also been found to be associated with rejection.

If persistent, other causes of sterile pyuria such as fungal and tuberculosis should also be excluded. Microhematuria or transient mild gross hematuria is generally due to the presence of an indwelling ureteral stent or continued trivial bleeding at the ureteric anastomosis or from blood clots that are slowly dissolved in the bladder. Patients should be warned that their urine may clear and then appears blood-tinged again as the clots are lysed. Hematuria usually resolves following stent removal, but low levels of microscopic hematuria may persist in some patients. The native kidneys must be considered as a source. When there is bleeding into the urine, protein is also invariably present. Proteinuria from native kidneys generally resolves within the first month after transplantation. Persistent or worsening proteinuria is usually indicative of graft pathology. Primary FSGS may recur early after transplant and urine protein-to-creatinine ratio should be followed closely to monitor for disease recurrence. Allograft biopsy should be performed in patients with significant or worsening proteinuria.

Hyperkalemia

Mild hyperkalemia is commonly encountered in the early post-transplant period when relatively high-dose CNI is given. It is often associated with mild hyperchloremic acidosis, a clinical presentation reminiscent of type 4 renal tubular acidosis. Suggested mechanisms of CNI-induced hyperkalemia include hyporeninemic hypoaldosteronism, aldosterone resistance, and inhibition of cortical collecting duct Na^+K^+ ATPase or potassium secretory channels. In patients receiving a CNI, a potassium level in the range of 5.2 to 5.5 mmol/L is typically seen. At higher potassium concentrations, the use of drugs that may exacerbate hyperkalemia including ACEIs, ARBs, potassium-sparing diuretics, β blockers, and potassium-containing phosphate supplements should be avoided. Although both high- and standard-dose trimethoprim can cause hyperkalemia via an amiloride effect, the routine use of low-dose trimethoprim-sulfamethoxazole prophylactic therapy is rarely the cause of refractory hyperkalemia in kidney transplant recipients. Oral (but not rectal) sodium polystyrene sulfonate (Kayexalate), furosemide, or fludrocortisone may be used to treat hyperkalemia. Fludrocortisone may cause fluid retention and worsen blood pressure control and should not be overused. The concomitant presence of a metabolic acidosis may exacerbate hyperkalemia, and this may be corrected with bicarbonate replacement. All patients should be counseled on the dietary sources potassium.

Hypokalemia is less commonly seen than hyperkalemia. Potential etiologic factors include diuretic use, overzealous dietary potassium restriction, hypomagnesemia, and mTOR inhibitor use.

Parathyroid Hormone, Calcium, Phosphate, and Magnesium

Secondary hyperparathyroidism of some degree occurs in most post-transplant patients and tends to be more pronounced and persistent in those patients who have been on dialysis for long periods before their transplant. High post-transplant PTH levels may be accompanied by increased serum calcium and decreased serum phosphate levels.

Hypercalcemia due to hyperparathyroidism is common after transplantation typically reaching a peak at week 8. The concomitant presence of severe hypophosphatemia, particularly in patients with excellent graft function, may exacerbate hypercalcemia through stimulation of renal proximal tubular 1α-hydroxylase. Mild hypercalcemia induced by persistent hyperparathyroidism may be controlled by phosphate supplements. In patients with severe hypercalcemic hyperparathyroidism, treatment with the calcimimetic, cinacalcet, can reduce serum calcium and PTH levels and improve hypophosphatemia. Persistent severe hypercalcemia associated with hyperparathyroidism warrants further investigation. Parathyroidectomy should be considered in patients with tertiary hyperparathyroidism, persistent severe hypercalcemia (>11.5 to 12 mg/dL) for >6 to 12 months, or in those with symptomatic or progressive hypercalcemia (nephrolithiasis, persistent metabolic bone disease, calcium-related allograft dysfunction, progressive vascular calcification, or calciphylaxis).

Hypophosphatemia is frequently encountered in the first weeks after transplantation and can be multifactorial in etiology. Concomitant hypercalcemia suggests post-transplantation hyperparathyroidism. Early after transplantation, hypophosphatemia has been attributed to a massive initial diuresis in patients with good allograft function, defective renal phosphate reabsorption due to ischemic injury, glucosuria (due to hyperglycemia-induced osmotic diuresis), magnesium depletion, and corticosteroid use (by inhibiting proximal tubular reabsorption of phosphate). Fibroblast growth factor-23 (FGF23) with accompanying 1,25-dihydroxvitamin D deficiency may play a major contributory role in the development of early post-transplantation hypophosphatemia independent of PTH level. FGF23 levels fall rapidly after transplant. Phosphate supplement is usually given in the form of potassium phosphate and the presence of hyperkalemia may limit its use. Patients are often habituated to a low-phosphate diet and need encouragement to include phosphate-rich foods in their diet. Dairy products are one such source (see Chapter 20). Calcium-containing phosphate binders should be avoided, and if calcium supplements are prescribed, these should be separated from meals by at least 2 hours.

CNIs and sirolimus can cause hypomagnesemia by inducing urinary magnesium wasting. In the first 3 months after transplantation, a magnesium level below 1.5 mg/dL is common. Dietary magnesium intake is usually insufficient, and high-dose oral magnesium supplementation (i.e., 400 to 800 mg magnesium oxide 3 times a day) may be required. Intravenous magnesium should be considered in patients with severe hypomagnesemia (<1.0 mg/dL), particularly those with a prior history of coronary artery disease or cardiac arrhythmias. Magnesium supplement may be ineffective because of persistent urinary losses.

Hematologic Abnormalities
Anemia
In the immediate post-transplant period, aggressive perioperative volume expansion may result in dilutional anemia. Refractory or severe anemia (particularly in patients with a rapid fall in hemoglobin and hematocrit levels) mandates aggressive evaluation to exclude the possibility of surgical postoperative bleeding or bleeding of the gastrointestinal tract. Blood transfusions should be considered at the discretion of the clinicians.

Mild anemia is common in the early post-transplant period when erythropoietin is typically discontinued, but usually improves within several weeks to months. Assessment of baseline iron stores at the time of transplantation is advisable because iron deficiency is not uncommon in the dialysis population. Profound iron deficiency should be treated with intravenous iron as tolerated. In iron-replete patients, erythropoietin therapy is effective in correcting anemia in the majority of patients, though it is ineffective in the immediate postoperative period. Other potential etiologic factors of post-transplant anemia include impaired graft function, acute rejection episodes, recent infection, and medications (such as ACEI and ARBs, sirolimus, everolimus, azathioprine, and mycophenolate mofetil [MMF]). Parvovirus B19 infection can cause refractory anemia and should be excluded. Although uncommon, drug-induced hemolysis such as dapsone should also be considered. Glucose 6-phosphate dehydrogenase (G6PD) level should be checked prior to initiation of dapsone therapy.

Leukopenia and Thrombocytopenia
Leukopenia and thrombocytopenia are most commonly related to adverse drug effects from agents such as antilymphocyte antibodies, mycophenolic acid, sirolimus, everolimus, azathioprine, ganciclovir or valganciclovir, acyclovir, and trimethoprim-sulfamethoxazole, among others. The antiproliferative agents sirolimus, azathioprine, and MMF may cause anemia, pancytopenia, or isolated thrombocytopenia or neutropenia. The latter is more common in patients on prednisone-free protocols. Withholding of the offending agent or dose reduction generally corrects these hematologic abnormalities. Treatment with subcutaneous

granulocyte stimulating factors should be considered in patients with severe neutropenia, particularly when the absolute neutrophil count is below 500×10 E3/μL. Potential infectious causes of neutropenia or thrombocytopenia or both include CMV and parvovirus B19 infections. CNI-induced TMA can cause anemia, thrombocytopenia, and AKI without systemic signs or symptoms of hemolytic anemia.

Erythrocytosis

Post-transplant erythrocytosis (PTE) may develop within the first 2 years post-transplant and generally affects those with good allograft function. The incidence of PTE appears to have decreased to less than 10% concomitant with the more frequent use of ACEI and ARBs (see Chapter 11). Suggested risk factors for PTE include the presence of native kidneys, male gender, excellent graft function, the absence of rejection episodes, high baseline hemoglobin before transplant, and polycystic kidney disease as the cause of ESKD. Although transplant RAS has not been consistently shown to be a risk factor for PTE, imaging studies to evaluate the iliac and renal arteries should be considered in patients with refractory PTE. In addition, the possibilities of renal cell carcinoma in the native and transplanted kidneys should be excluded. Treatment is generally recommended for a hemoglobin level exceeding 17 to 18 g/dL or a hematocrit level greater than 51% to 52% because of the associated risk of thromboembolic complications, hypertension, and headaches. In the absence of baseline hyperkalemia, treatment with ACEIs or ARBs is often sufficient, although phlebotomy may occasionally be necessary.

Abnormal Hepatic Biochemical Tests

Mild elevation in the liver enzymes such as alanine transaminase and aspartate transaminase—"transaminitis"—is common in the early post-transplantation period and is generally caused by drug-related toxicity. Cyclosporine and less commonly tacrolimus may cause transient, self-limited, dose-dependent elevations of transaminase levels and mild hyperbilirubinemia owing to defective bile secretion. Elevated liver enzymes caused by drug-related adverse effects generally improve or resolve after drug discontinuation or dose reduction. Persistent or profound elevation in hepatic liver enzymes should prompt further evaluation to exclude infectious causes including CMV, hepatitis B, and hepatitis C. A suggested algorithm for the management of elevated hepatic enzymes is shown in Figure 10.2.

REFERRAL BACK TO COMMUNITY CARE

In the United States, patients are commonly repatriated to their primary nephrologists 3 months after transplant. Transition of care involves clear communication between the transplant physicians and the community nephrologists. Medical records related to the patient's post-transplant course should be transferred in a timely fashion. Any issues of special concern should be discussed. In the current era, electronic medical record transfer facilitates a smooth transition of patient care. Patients should be seen by their primary care provider monthly at this stage. Follow-up visits at the transplantation center every 3 months until the end of the first year, and annually thereafter are typically recommended.

However, patients should return to the transplantation center for assessment of any significant change in kidney function and of any new comorbidity. If an allograft biopsy is required, it is preferable that this should be performed at the transplant center because of the proximity of pathology expertise and a broad range of therapeutic options. Community physicians vary with respect to their degree of comfort in assuming the care of a kidney transplant recipient. Some transplant centers maintain control of the immunosuppression dosing for the life span of the allograft. However, the community physicians should be contacted to discuss any changes made, and both patients and their primary care providers should be made aware of any potential drug–drug interactions. Patients should always have access to their "mother" transplant center at a time of need.

Selected Readings

Cavaillé-Coll M, Bala S, Velidedeoglu E, et al. Summary of FDA workshop on ischemia reperfusion injury in kidney transplantation. Am J Transplant 2013;13:1134–1148.

Gaynor JJ, Cianco G, Guerra G, et al. Lower tacrolimus trough levels are associated with subsequently higher acute rejection risk during the first 12 months after kidney transplantation. Transplant Int 2016;29:216–226.

Gill J, Dong J, Rose, et al. The risk of allograft failure and the survival benefit of kidney transplantation are complicated by delayed graft function. Kidney Int 2016;89(6):1331–1336.

Hamed MO, Chen Y, Pasea L, et al. Early graft loss after kidney transplantation: risk factors and consequences. Am J Transplant 2015;17(4):362–367.

Kiberd BA. Posttransplant erythrocytosis: a disappearing phenomenon? Clin Transplant 2009;23(6):800–806.

Noris M, Remuzzi G. Thrombotic microangiopathy after kidney transplantation. Am J Transplant 2010;10(7):517–523.

Panek R, Tennankore KK, Kiberd BA. Incidence, etiology, and significance of acute kidney injury in the early post kidney transplant period. Clin Transplant 2016;30:66–70.

Pham PT, Danovitch GM, Pham PC. Medical management of the kidney transplant recipient: infections, malignant neoplasms, and gastrointestinal disorders. In: Johnson RJ, Feehally J, Floege J. Comprehensive Clinical Nephrology. 5th ed. Philadelphia, PA: Elsevier Saunders; 2015:1188–1201.

Schold J, Elfadawy N, Buccini L, et al. Emergency department visits after kidney transplantation. Clin J Am Soc Nephrol 2016;11:674–683.

Schroppel B, Legendre C. Delayed kidney graft function: from mechanism to translation. Kidney Int 2014;86:251–258.

Wolf M, Weir MR, Kopyt N, et al. A prospective cohort study of mineral metabolism after kidney transplantation. Transplantation 2016;100:184–193.

Wu WK, Famure O, Li Y, et al. Delayed graft function and the risk of acute rejection in the modern era of kidney transplantation. Kidney Int 2015;88:851–858.

11

Post-transplant Long-term Management and Complications

Edmund Huang and Bertram L. Kasiske

The previous chapter described the care of the patient during the first three post-transplant months. By the end of that period, as patients commence the period of long-term management, the risk for surgical complications, acute rejection, and major infections is diminishing, although these issues continue to be of concern for the rest of the first year, and to a lesser extent for the life of the transplant. By the end of the third month, most patients have had their immunosuppressive doses reduced to the levels that will continue for many years, and the treatment of their hypertension, diabetes mellitus, hyperlipidemia, and other medical issues should be under stable control. Fewer patients now lose their allografts within the first year, and most centers report a 1-year graft survival rate of close to 95%. There has been a gradual improvement in the time it takes for 50% of the grafts to fail—the graft half-life—and because of the thousands of transplants performed, there are many patients whose grafts have been in place for more than 10 years, and indeed for more than 20 years. The half-life of two-haplotype living donor transplants has been estimated to be more than 20 years, and that of deceased donor grafts more than 11 years. Many of the factors that affect the longevity of the graft are determined by the features of the graft itself and by the early post-transplant course. A major cause of graft loss is patient death (Fig. 11.1), predominantly from cardio-vascular disease (CVD, see Strategy 5 below). To promote longevity of the graft, the intensive treatment of the medical complications from which transplant patients suffer, particularly those that increase the risk for CVD, are therefore as important as the long-term modification of immunosuppression.

There is now a greater understanding of the role of chronic antibody-mediated rejection (AMR) on graft loss, and alloantigen-dependent factors are now thought to be important mediators of graft failure in many more cases than previously recognized. This new paradigm challenges older strategies of immunosuppression minimization in the late post-transplant period, which has now evolved to a more contemporary strategy of individualizing immunosuppression through the use of immune monitoring and immunologic risk stratification.

This chapter is divided into two sections. Part I describes the management of medical complications and considers strategies to improve patient and graft outcomes. Part II describes the factors thought to cause chronic allograft injury and strategies to reduce the rate of loss of kidney function. Part II also describes other causes of late graft loss apart from death after transplantation. Long-term immunosuppressive therapy and the immunosuppressive management of chronic allograft failure are discussed in

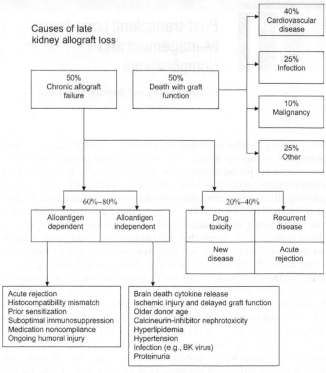

Causes of late
kidney allograft loss

| 50%
Chronic allograft failure | 50%
Death with graft function |

→ 40% Cardiovascular disease
→ 25% Infection
→ 10% Malignancy
→ 25% Other

60%–80%

| Alloantigen dependent | Alloantigen independent |

20%–40%

| Drug toxicity | Recurrent disease |
| New disease | Acute rejection |

Acute rejection
Histocompatibility mismatch
Prior sensitization
Suboptimal immunosuppression
Medication noncompliance
Ongoing humoral injury

Brain death cytokine release
Ischemic injury and delayed graft function
Older donor age
Calcineurin-inhibitor nephrotoxicity
Hyperlipidemia
Hypertension
Infection (e.g., BK virus)
Proteinuria

FIGURE 11.1 Causes of late kidney allograft loss.

Chapter 6, Part V; post-transplantation infectious disease is discussed in Chapter 12; post-transplantation liver disease is discussed in Chapter 13; and medication nonadherence is discussed in Chapter 21. Readers are also referred to the KDIGO (Kidney Disease Improving Global Outcomes) clinical practice guideline for the care of kidney transplant recipients (http://kdigo.org/home/guidelines/care-of-the-kidney-transplant-recipient).

Part I: Management of Post-transplant Medical Complications

Renal transplant recipients should be considered a subset of patients with chronic kidney disease (CKD-T). A minority of these patients have normal glomerular filtration rate (GFR). Whereas there are factors particular to transplant recipients that may increase the risk for certain diseases and of their complications, in general, guidelines for the management of patients with CKD and those recommended for the general population are applicable to the management of these patients. A continuous intensive and coordinated approach to the chronic conditions from which they suffer is an important part of their care. The transplant center, community physicians, and the patient are all part of the team that has to work to obtain optimal health for these patients and their transplants.

The great disparity between the demand for organs and their supply means that fewer patients than in the past will have multiple transplants, and after the first transplant fails, most will return to dialysis for a considerable period of time, perhaps for the rest of their lives. Both physicians and their patients need to understand this. It should make the prevention of risk factors and adherence to the medication schedules a priority for all these stakeholders. The treatment of chronic conditions can be frustrating and arduous, but the rewards obtained from realizing the benefits of persistence are great. We know from studies in the general population (e.g., in the treatment of hypertension, an established risk factor for stroke and CVD) that even when the evidence is overwhelming that treatment is beneficial, a minority of patients at risk are treated, and a minority of these achieve the targets set in management guidelines. Transplant patients, however, are already well connected to a system that should provide their care, and this should enable more successful prevention strategies. We know the major causes of morbidity and mortality in the late post-transplant period and in some cases have evidence to suggest effective measures to prevent post-transplantation complications. When evidence is not available from transplant studies, the data from the CKD and general population should be used, if available.

The success of treatment of chronic conditions is enhanced by frequent contact with the patient's physicians. The intensity of care provided to transplant recipients should be tailored to their needs, but in general, it is recommended that after a gradual reduction in the frequency of visits from twice monthly during the fourth month to monthly at 6 months, this monthly schedule should be maintained until the end of the first year. For the next year, the visits should be every 1 to 2 months and thereafter every 3 to 4 months as long as the transplant is functioning. Follow-up can occur at the clinic of the transplant center, with the community nephrologist, or with a community internist or family practitioner with experience in the care of transplant recipients. There should be frequent and open communication between the community physicians and the transplantation center. The transplant center should remain a source of care and expertise and patients and their caregivers should always have access to it.

The following strategies address the most important management issues in the late transplant period.

STRATEGY 1: AVOID REJECTION, BUT REDUCE IMMUNOSUPPRESSION WHENEVER POSSIBLE

Death is a common cause of renal allograft failure in the late post-transplantation period. The ultimate goal is to have all our patients die with a functioning graft, but not prematurely, as is now too often the case. CVD, cancer, and infection are the leading causes of death in the late post-transplantation period, and immunosuppression plays a major role in the pathogenesis of each of these complications. Each immunosuppressive agent has both immune and nonimmune toxicity. Immune toxicity is usually nonspecific: the result of the total amount of all immunosuppression over a given period of time. Immune toxicity can only be avoided if patients became tolerant to their transplanted kidney. Unfortunately, most patients will reject their kidney if immunosuppression is completely withdrawn, and the best we can do is to select the minimal amount of immunosuppression that prevents rejection. This minimal amount should ideally be tailored to the needs of specific patients, but we are currently able to do that only in a crude way.

Physicians and patients must choose among the most effective, but least toxic, of several different agents. In general, it is prudent to tailor the choice of agents to the risk profile or adverse effects that are most troubling to the individual while also considering the patient's risk for rejection. Switching a patient from cyclosporine or sirolimus to tacrolimus, for example, may reduce low-density lipoprotein cholesterol by the same amount as therapy with an HMG-CoA reductase inhibitor. Similarly, reducing cyclosporine or prednisone dose may help to control blood pressure. Patients with impaired baseline function in the absence of rejection may benefit from calcineurin-inhibitor (CNI) dose minimization or introduction of belatacept. Patients with severe tremor will be especially eager to reduce CNI dose in the late post-transplant period if this is possible. A significant number of patients receiving cyclosporine develop gum overgrowth. This is made worse by poor dental hygiene and by the concomitant use of calcium channel antagonists. This reverses if patients are switched to tacrolimus. Similarly, patients with difficult-to-control diabetes may be good candidates for minimizing doses of prednisone. New-onset diabetes in a patient receiving tacrolimus may respond to switching to cyclosporine or newer agents, such as belatacept. Bone marrow suppression may be an indication for reducing doses of mycophenolic acid or sirolimus. Tacrolimus may be the better CNI for patients with gout. Finally, many patients cannot afford to pay the high cost of immunosuppression. The use of expensive medications for patients who cannot afford them increases the risk for nonadherence and graft failure.

Patients should be risk-stratified to characterize their likelihood of losing their graft to alloantigen-dependent processes. A multivariate model incorporating recipient factors at 1 year post-transplant, including age, gender, ethnicity, renal function, presence of proteinuria, and prior acute rejection is highly predictive of 5-year graft survival (see Gonzales et al. in Selected Readings). Adding the presence of glomerulitis, which is indicative of microcirculatory inflammation related to AMR (see Chapter 15), and chronic interstitial fibrosis found on biopsies performed at 1 year improves the predictive discrimination further.

Donor-Specific Antibodies

The presence of donor-specific antibody ([DSA], see Chapter 3) is known to be associated with poorer allograft survival. The incidence of *de novo* DSA in the first year after transplant is reported to be around 2%, but increases to 10% at 5 years and approximately 20% at 10 years. Its development has prognostic significance, especially if it is associated with graft dysfunction or proteinuria. Although many patients with DSA will suffer from AMR, not all DSA is considered "equal" and some patients with DSA do not have graft dysfunction or signs of antibody-mediated injury on biopsy (see Fig. 11.2). Patients who have

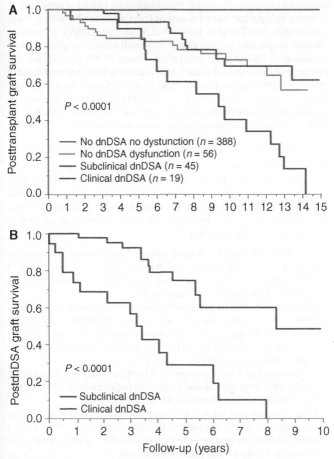

FIGURE 11.2 Death-censored graft survival. **A:** Kaplan–Meier plot of renal allograft survival by clinical phenotype. **B:** Kaplan–Meier survival plot of post-dnDSA graft survival by clinical phenotype at the time of dnDSA detection. dnDSA, *de novo* donor-specific antibody. (Reprinted from Wiebe C, Gibson IW, Blydt-Hansen TD, et al. Rates and determinants of progression to graft failure in kidney allograft recipients with *de novo* donor-specific antibody. Am J Transplant 2015;15(11):2921–2930, with permission.)

complement-binding DSA, as detected by a C1q-binding assay, are more likely to have lesions of AMR on protocol biopsy. DSA IgG subclass may discriminate between those who have an acute or subclinical AMR with the presence of IgG3 and IgG4 DSA subclasses having a positive predictive value of 100% to identify antibody-mediated injury.

Ideally, no DSA should be detectable at the time of transplant (see Chapters 3 and 8). A consensus recommendation has been made that all patients should be screened for DSA at least once in the first year after transplantation, with frequency of monitoring dictated by whether the patient had a preexisting DSA at transplant, prior history of sensitization to donor antigen but none present at transplant, or absence of donor sensitization (see Tait et al. in Selected Readings). If DSA is present, an allograft biopsy may be considered. Although many transplant centers do screen for DSA at some point after transplant, the practice has not yet become the standard of care, as it is unclear whether treatment of subclinical DSA (patients with DSA but no evidence of graft dysfunction), is effective or leads to an improvement in graft survival. However, it is generally regarded that patients who have known circulating DSA should not undergo immunosuppression minimization.

STRATEGY 2: ADOPT STRATEGIES TO PREVENT NONADHERENCE

There are few randomized, controlled trials to suggest how to prevent nonadherence with immunosuppressive medications. On the other hand, a number of observational studies have demonstrated that nonadherence is an important, preventable cause of allograft failure. These same studies have provided clues to preventive measures that are most likely to be effective.

- Minimize the number of daily doses of medication, discontinue nonessential medications, and whenever possible, use medications that can be taken once daily. The latter recommendation is particularly important in young adults.
- Educate patients. In particular, dispel the common misconception that the immunosuppressive effects of medications extend beyond the dosing interval. Patients need to be reminded at every follow-up visit that failure to take medications regularly will eventually result in graft failure.
- Educate and update physicians and medical staff regarding immunosuppressive protocols and individual regimens and the potential for drug interactions (see Chapter 6).
- Help patients to establish a system to remind them to take their medications. Enlist the help of friends, family, and public health aides. Mobile applications are widely available and may be used to remind patients to take their medications.
- Maintain close contact with patients throughout the late post-transplantation period. Insist that patients have routine follow-up with the transplant center and make every effort to locate patients who are lost to follow-up. Clinic visits and laboratory checks are a valuable reminder to patients of the importance of taking medications. When negotiating contracts with providers, insist that patients be allowed to follow-up with the transplantation center at regular intervals.
- Know whether your patients have trouble paying for their medications. If this is the case, assign someone to help them. Most transplant programs have found that it is often necessary to have a dedicated social worker or pharmacist available to help patients (see Chapter 21). Be prepared to offer less-expensive alternatives (see Chapter 6).
- Identify patients who are at high risk for nonadherence. Adolescent patients are at increased risk, often because they are fearful

of the cosmetic effects of prednisone and cyclosporine. Patients who are poorly educated are also at increased risk for nonadherence. Similarly, low family income is associated with nonadherence. Socioeconomic factors place members of racial minorities at increased risk for nonadherence. Studies show that patients who were nonadherent with medication, diet, and dialysis therapy before transplantation are more likely to be nonadherent after renal transplantation.

▪ Patients who are at high risk for nonadherence should be targeted with risk factor intervention in much the same way that we target patients who are at high risk for CVD with intensive risk factor management. In both instances, the benefit is likely to be the greatest when the risk is the highest.

STRATEGY 3: MONITOR KIDNEY FUNCTION CLOSELY

Frequent monitoring of kidney function in the late post-transplantation period helps to enforce adherence with immunosuppressive medications and provides the only reliable means to detect acute rejection at a time when it may still respond to treatment. A program requiring patients to make certain that serum creatinine is measured regularly and reported to the transplant center also provides an indirect means for the center to monitor compliance. Patients should also keep a record of their own creatinine values and thereby learn to self-monitor for significant change. Most electronic medical records have patient access portals that permit patients to follow their own lab tests: they should be encouraged to do so. Patients who fail to have their serum creatinine level checked regularly should be contacted and reminded of the importance of close, ongoing follow-up to prevent graft failure. Patients and caregivers should be constantly reminded that acute rejection rarely presents with signs and symptoms. Although immune monitoring holds promise as a more sophisticated way of recognizing acute rejection before it manifests clinically, the serum creatinine level is currently the only practical tool that can be used to screen for acute rejection in the late post-transplantation period. It is not too much to ask patients to have their serum creatinine level measured regularly in the late post-transplantation period. Measurement of cystatin C in conjunction with creatinine may provide a more accurate estimate of GFR in transplant patients than creatinine-only based estimations, and may be useful when patients have unusually low or high creatinine levels owing to extremes of body habitus or loss or gain of muscle mass.

At least once a year, and preferably more often, urine should be checked for albumin excretion. Persistent albuminuria (i.e., more than 1 g in 24 hours for at least 6 months) is associated with an increased risk for graft failure. Albuminuria can be most reliably detected by either a timed urine collection (which is cumbersome) or an albumin-to-creatinine ratio (ACR) measured in a random "spot" urine sample (which is convenient). Dipstick screening is less reliable because the protein concentration is also dependent on the state of diuresis.

STRATEGY 4: MAKE AN ACCURATE PATHOLOGIC DIAGNOSIS OF THE CAUSE OF GRAFT DYSFUNCTION

It is important to establish an accurate pathologic diagnosis in patients with deteriorating graft function. There is evidence to suggest that even low-grade tubulitis, or so-called borderline acute rejection, may increase the risk for allograft failure (see Chapter 15). The evidence supporting the clinical value of routine protocol biopsies, however, is mixed, and most programs do not perform them unless the patient is engaged in a research protocol. In general, the lower the risk for acute rejection, the less helpful a protocol biopsy is and vice versa. An increased serum creatinine level remains the prompt for biopsy and treatment. However, the message is clear: It is important to have a high level of suspicion for acute rejection and a low threshold for obtaining a renal allograft biopsy. An acute, sustained rise in serum creatinine should prompt immediate evaluation. The strategy of routinely monitoring serum creatinine levels will only be successful if biopsies are obtained quickly and acute rejection is treated. Such a strategy will also avoid unnecessary intensification of immunosuppression when rejection is not present. Unexpected diagnoses, such as recurrent disease, CNI toxicity, polyomavirus infection, and post-transplantation lymphoma, may require radically different therapeutic approaches. If a cause of chronic allograft dysfunction is established, repeated biopsies may be unnecessary because repeated treatment may be unwise (see Chapter 6).

STRATEGY 5: TREAT CARDIOVASCULAR RISK FACTORS AGGRESSIVELY

All patients with kidney disease have an elevated risk of CVD. Although the prevalence of CVD, including stroke, in kidney transplant recipients is lower than those who are maintained on dialysis, the prevalence remains quite high. It is estimated that one-third of transplant recipients have some form of CVD.

Statin use is associated with a 20% to 30% reduction in the risk of major cardiovascular events across a number of clinical trials. The risk reduction is independent of baseline low-density lipoprotein (LDL) cholesterol levels and treating to a specific target LDL is no longer recommended. The 10-year risk for major cardiovascular events should be estimated, and KDIGO suggests that statins should be started in patients with nondialysis CKD, if the 10-year risk is greater than 10%. The evidence is less clear in kidney transplantation, in which the 10-year risk for major cardiovascular events is generally less than 10% for most patients. The best available evidence comes from the Assessment of LEscol (fluvastatin) in Renal Transplantation (ALERT) trial, published in 2003, which observed a 17% nonsignificant reduction in major cardiovascular events, including cardiac death, nonfatal MI, or coronary revascularization procedure, over a 5- to 6-year follow-up period. Because the vast majority of participants were of low risk without prior CVD, there was a lower-than-expected event rate, which raised the possibility of inadequate statistical power. The trial was followed by a 2-year extension study, where all patients in the original study were offered open-label fluvastatin and compared to patients who consented to be a part of the extension study but did not wish to take fluvastatin. The extension study observed a 21% reduction in major cardiovascular events that was statistically significant. On this basis, KDIGO has suggested that all kidney transplant recipients be treated with a statin (level 2a recommendation). It is important to note that plasma levels of HMG-CoA reductase inhibitors are increased in cyclosporine-treated renal transplant recipients, and it is generally prudent to use about half the usually prescribed dose. Tacrolimus, on the other hand, has no effect on plasma levels of HMG-CoA reductase inhibitors, and dose adjustments of statins are not necessary when a patient is maintained on tacrolimus-based immunosuppression.

The use of aspirin in the general population is associated with an approximately 20% reduction in the rate of nonfatal myocardial infarction over 10 years, but limited benefit on mortality and stroke. The benefit of aspirin for primary prevention is offset by an increase in bleeding complications. In the CKD population, aspirin use is associated with a reduction in major cardiovascular events, with the greatest benefit observed in patients with lower GFR. However, similar to the general population, there is an increased risk of bleeding associated with chronic aspirin use, and the potential benefit of aspirin for primary prevention of cardiovascular events needs to be weighed against the potential risks of bleeding.

The use of aspirin for secondary prevention of cardiovascular events is well-established and should be used in those with a prior history of vascular disease, including prior myocardial infarction or known coronary artery disease, stroke or transient ischemic attack, angina, and peripheral arterial disease.

STRATEGY 6: TREAT HYPERTENSION AGGRESSIVELY

Hypertension occurs in 60% to 80% of renal transplant recipients. It is associated with an increased risk for graft failure. Studies in the general population show that treatment with antihypertensive agents reduces the risk for CVD; these findings parallel observational data in the kidney transplant population, where lower systolic blood pressure control is associated with improved graft survival, lower all-cause mortality, and lower cardiovascular mortality. Although optimal blood pressure targets have not been established through randomized, controlled trials in kidney transplantation, there is good reason to believe that treating blood pressure elevations would be beneficial in renal transplant recipients.

The Systolic Blood Pressure Intervention Trial (SPRINT) was designed to test the hypothesis that a systolic blood pressure of less than 120 mm Hg among patients at elevated risk of cardiovascular events (see Group et al. in Selected Readings). The study was stopped early once it became apparent that fewer patients with a lower systolic blood pressure target of <120 mm Hg would meet the primary endpoint compared to patients randomized to a higher systolic blood pressure target of <140 mm Hg. Although this trial was strictly a hypertension trial and not a trial of blood pressure management in CKD or post-transplant, 28% of the study population consisted of patients with CKD. In the absence of trials conducted specifically in kidney transplant patients, the evidence for an optimal blood pressure target in kidney transplantation is necessarily indirect. However, it is not unreasonable to extrapolate the findings of the SPRINT trial to kidney transplant recipients and to target a systolic blood pressure of close to 120 mm Hg.

All classes of antihypertensive agents can be used to lower blood pressure in renal transplant recipients. Although there are limited data on the effects of reduced dietary sodium chloride intake on blood pressure in renal transplant recipients, this is a reasonable first step. A low dose of thiazide diuretic is also reasonable for patients with creatinine clearance estimated to be greater than 25 to 30 mL/min. Low doses of thiazides (e.g., 12.5 to 25 mg/day) are effective, inexpensive, and do not generally perturb lipid or glucose metabolism. Both a low-salt diet and thiazide diuretics may help with edema, which is a common problem after transplantation. A thiazide diuretic may also help in the management of the hyperkalemia that is common in CNI-treated transplant recipients. Transplant recipients may be sensitive to volume contraction; therefore, diuretics may cause a reversible increase in serum creatinine levels. Thiazides often potentiate the antihypertensive effects of other agents, especially angiotensin converting enzyme inhibitors (ACEIs). β-blockers are also relatively inexpensive and are especially attractive for patients with ischemic heart disease, which is common after renal transplantation. Relative contraindications to β-blockers (e.g., peripheral vascular disease, reactive airways disease, and hypoglycemic reactions) are rarely a reason to forego the use of this important class of medication.

Physicians are sometimes reluctant to use ACEIs and angiotensin II antagonists (ARBs) in transplant patients for fear of inducing hemodynamic impairment of allograft function. Several studies, however, show that these drugs are generally safe, effective, and well tolerated. They may reduce proteinuria and stabilize the deterioration in renal function in patients with chronic allograft dysfunction, possibly reducing the production of transforming growth factor-β (TGF-β). They may also have additional benefit in reducing the incidence of cardiovascular events in high-risk patients, and may also reduce the degree of insulin resistance. Occasionally, ACEIs may increase serum creatinine, but this is usually a transient and reversible effect. Hyperkalemia can often be managed by adding a thiazide diuretic or a loop diuretic to the treatment regimen. The role of the newly FDA-approved patiromer (Veltassa) in the treatment of hyperkalemia is yet to be determined. ACEIs may cause anemia in transplant recipients; this side effect can be exploited for the treatment of post-transplantation erythrocytosis. Cough occurs in about 15% of patients taking ACEIs but is much less frequent with ARBs. Otherwise, ARBs appear to have all of the advantages and disadvantages of ACEIs.

Calcium antagonists are also effective in renal transplant recipients. They can contribute to edema, which is already prevalent among transplant patients. Non–dihydropyridine calcium antagonists (e.g., diltiazem and verapamil) increase CNI blood levels and can be used to help reduce the immunosuppressive drug cost. Dihydropyridine calcium antagonists have less effect on blood levels (see Chapter 6,

Part I). Calcium antagonists may cause gum overgrowth, particularly when used with cyclosporine. Vasodilators and α-blockers are also effective in treating hypertension, although they can cause reflex tachycardia and may need to be used in combination with β-blockers. Excess hair growth with minoxidil, the most potent vasodilator, limits its long-term usefulness in women. Other agents that are useful include sympatholytics, central and peripheral α-antagonists, and combined α- and β-blockers.

The possibility of renal allograft artery stenosis should be considered when hypertension cannot be controlled, particularly if attempts to reduce blood pressure result in decreased graft function (see Chapter 9). In addition, the presence of diuretic-resistant peripheral edema, a loud allograft bruit, renal dysfunction after administration of ACEIs or ARBs, and polycythemia should engender consideration of this diagnosis. Color-flow Doppler examination of the renal artery may aid the diagnosis (see Chapter 14), but interpretation of this test is difficult, and false-positive results are common. Radionuclide scanning is usually not helpful. Magnetic resonance angiography or renal arteriography should be used for diagnosis when suspicion of renal allograft artery stenosis is high, paying attention to the risk for iodine-containing dyes worsening renal function, and that of gadolinium causing nephrogenic fibrosing dermopathy in patients with a reduced GFR. The studies to exclude renal artery stenosis should also include studies of the proximal iliac artery because stenosis of this is not uncommon, and the effects may mimic those of renal artery stenosis ("pseudo-renal artery stenosis"). Percutaneous transluminal angioplasty may improve renal function and reduce the need for antihypertensive medications in 60% to 85% of cases. Restenosis may occur in up to 30%. Surgery should probably be reserved for critical stenosis that threatens the integrity of the graft.

The native kidneys often contribute to hypertension after renal transplantation. Studies to determine the role of the native kidneys in causing hypertension, however, are probably not useful. In particular, renal vein renin levels do not reliably predict blood pressure reduction after native kidney nephrectomy. Therefore, in difficult-to-control hypertension, consideration should be given to empirical removal of the native kidneys. Laparoscopic surgery may reduce the morbidity of post-transplantation native kidney nephrectomy.

STRATEGY 7: TREAT DIABETES MELLITUS AGGRESSIVELY

Transplant recipients with diabetes are at increased risk for developing CVD and other diabetic complications, including diabetic nephropathy. This is also true for those who develop new-onset diabetes after transplantation (NODAT). Abnormalities in glucose tolerance also occur in up to 30% of post-transplantation patients in the absence of a pretransplant or post-transplant diagnosis of diabetes; such abnormalities are less common in patients receiving cyclosporine compared with tacrolimus. Patients receiving belatacept are less likely to develop NODAT than those receiving cyclosporine. The risk of NODAT with mechanistic target of rapamycin (mTOR) inhibitors (see Chapter 6) is similar to that with tacrolimus, which may be owing to increased insulin resistance, β-cell toxicity, or impaired suppression of hepatic glucose production. The targets of treatment are the same as for all diabetic patients, and sufficiently intensive treatment should be given, even if this means the permanent use of insulin. Patients benefit from referral to a dietitian and an endocrinologist and should have the usual regular surveillance for vascular, ophthalmic, and neurologic disease. Their feet should be examined at every visit, particularly if they have a neuropathy. Caution should be exercised to not excessively lower the blood sugar. Aggressive treatment has been shown to reduce the risk for developing microvascular diabetic complications, including CKD and retinopathy. Patients should be treated with an ACEI or ARB, especially if they have any microalbuminuria. The immunosuppressive regimen should be evaluated to ensure that an excessive steroid dose is not being administered and to consider switching the CNI or using belatacept (see Chapter 6).

STRATEGY 8: ENCOURAGE A HEALTHY LIFESTYLE

Regular aerobic exercise should be part of the therapeutic regimen of all patients at high CVD risk and may be particularly beneficial in counteracting the effects of corticosteroids on muscle and bone. Near-normal levels of physical functioning are possible after transplantation, particularly for those patients who engage in regular physical activity. Patients should be encouraged to train for and participate in the Transplant Games (www.transplantgamesofamerica.org). Exercise may help to minimize post-transplantation weight gain and may be particularly important for patients with the metabolic syndrome. Readers are referred to Chapter 20 for detailed dietary recommendations for transplant patients.

Cigarette smoking appears to be just as prevalent among renal transplant recipients as it is in the general population. Cigarette smoking contributes to CVD and increases the already high risk for cancer after kidney transplantation. Studies in nontransplant populations also show smoking to be detrimental to kidney function. Thus, every effort should be made to encourage transplant recipients to quit smoking. Smoking cessation programs that make use of nicotine-replacement therapies have been shown, in clinical trials, to be effective. The American and Psychiatric Society and the Agency for Health Care Policy and Research have developed guidelines for smoking cessation.

STRATEGY 9: SCREEN FOR CANCER

After transplantation, there is a substantially increased incidence of a wide variety of cancers, most of which have known or suspected viral etiology (see Engels et al. in Selected Readings). Knowledge that many post-transplant cancers are caused by viruses has not yet produced effective prophylactic strategies. Successful treatment of cancer after renal transplantation relies on surveillance and early detection. Typically, guidelines for cancer screening developed for the general population are presumed to be effective for kidney transplant recipients. However, because the life expectancy of most transplant patients is less than that of the general population, the presumptions underlying recommendations for cancer screening may not be relevant to them. Decisions regarding routine screening for breast, colon, lung, and prostate cancers should be made on an individual basis, because their incidence does not appear to differ significantly in the kidney transplant population from the general population. Women who are older than 18 years should have an annual pelvic examination and Papanicolaou test to screen for cervical cancer. Anogenital carcinoma is common after renal transplantation. Yearly physical examination and pelvic examination in women are useful in screening for anogenital lesions. Skin cancer and kidney cancer surveillance are discussed below.

The management of immunosuppression in patients who have developed cancer is difficult, and each case should be considered individually. Transplant recipients are at elevated risk for cancer because of their use of chronic immunosuppression. When patients develop a malignancy that is related to immunosuppression, it is wise to minimize the immunosuppressive protocol, and in some cases, discontinuation of immunosuppression may be appropriate. The potential for graft loss needs to be weighed against the natural history and the staging of the malignancy. It is the patient who must ultimately decide on his or her priorities after receiving consultation from oncologic and transplant physicians.

There is a large body of clinical data that suggests that mTOR inhibitors (sirolimus and everolimus) are associated with a reduced risk for malignancy after transplantation (see Chapter 6, Part I). There are also theoretical reasons for basing immunosuppression on these drugs in patients with *de novo* post-transplantation malignancies. The benefit of this approach, however, has not been definitively established, but a useful algorithm to guide conversion from CNI to mTOR inhibitors has been proposed (Fig 11.3) and is discussed in Causes of Allograft Failure below. Post-transplantation lymphoproliferative disease (PTLD) is discussed later.

STRATEGY 10: PREVENT INFECTION

Infections in the late post-transplantation period are discussed in Chapter 12 together with recommendations for routine immunization (Table 12.4). Routine prophylaxis for *Pneumocystis jiroveci* infections with trimethoprim-sulfamethoxazole is probably not warranted late after transplantation. The exception may be for patients who are receiving high doses of immunosuppression to treat rejection or for patients receiving sirolimus (see Chapter 6, Part I). The same is true for cytomegalovirus (CMV) infection prophylaxis.

Influenza types A and B are likely to be at least as common, and probably more severe, in renal transplant patients as in the general population. Therefore, transplant recipients should receive annual influenza vaccination. Although vaccines are safe, they may be somewhat less effective in transplant recipients than in the general population because of the limitation in antibody response by immunosuppressant drugs. Nevertheless, the response to vaccination is high enough (50% to 100%) to warrant their use.

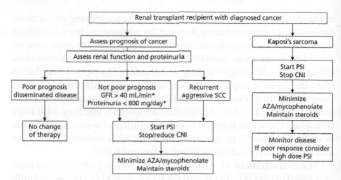

FIGURE 11.3 Recommendations to guide conversion from calcineurin inhibitors to proliferation signal inhibitors in renal transplant recipients. *Some clinicians may decide to convert patients with impaired renal function (e.g., GFR < 40 mL/min, proteinuria > 800 mg/day) if they feel that the benefits of PSIs* are warranted; this should be evaluated on an individual-patient basis. AZA, azathioprine; CNI, calcineurin inhibitor; PSI, proliferation signal inhibitor; SCC, squamous cell carcinoma. (From Campistol J, Albanell J, Arns W. Use of proliferation signal inhibitors in the management of post-transplant malignancies: clinical guidance. Nephrol Dial Transplant 2007;22(Suppl 1):i36–i41, by permission of Oxford University Press.)
*PSI is alternative term for mTOR inhibitor)

STRATEGY 11: PROTECT THE BONES

Renal osteodystrophy has traditionally been used as a broad term to describe a spectrum of bone disorders arising from hormonal and metabolic alterations that occur with CKD, including hyperparathyroidism, vitamin D deficiency, hyperphosphatemia, and hypocalcemia. The nomenclature has since been revised and replaced with the syndrome of chronic kidney disease–mineral and bone disorder (CKD–MBD), and the term *renal osteodystrophy* now specifically refers to bone pathology associated with CKD and requires a bone biopsy for definitive diagnosis. Regardless of the terminology used, the nomenclature highlights the notion that bone disorders can occur through a variety of different mechanisms in CKD. The net result is that patients with end-stage kidney disease (ESKD) are especially vulnerable to fractures, and this risk is carried over to the kidney transplant population.

In addition to disorders of mineral metabolism occurring in patients with ESKD, post-transplant bone disease is also influenced by the use of chronic immunosuppression. Kidney recipients are at increased risk for fractures compared to their waitlisted counterparts, although refinement in immunosuppression protocols is believed to have mitigated the risk considerably.

Bone mineral density (BMD) decreases within the first year after transplant when steroid doses are relatively high, but tends to increase and then stabilize thereafter, particularly at the lumbar spine and hip. The applicability of BMD measurement to the transplant population is unclear, as it is generally a poor predictor of subsequent fractures in transplant recipients, especially in those with advanced renal dysfunction (GFR < 30 mL/min/1.73 m^2). Corticosteroids are well-known to cause decreased BMD and to contribute to post-transplant osteoporosis, but withdrawal of corticosteroids at 7 days post-transplant compared to chronic corticosteroid maintenance has not been shown to reduce the fracture rate. Studies of BMD followed longitudinally in patients maintained on corticosteroid-free immunosuppression show stable BMD after transplant at the spine and hip, but decreased bone density peripherally at the forearm (see Iyer et al. in Selected Readings).

Hypophosphatemia is common early after kidney transplantation (see Chapter 10) and may result from vitamin D deficiency and elevated parathyroid hormone (PTH) concentrations and fibroblast growth factor (FGF)-23 levels, both of which induce phosphaturia. PTH levels generally fall over the first 6 to 12 months after transplant, but may remain elevated in approximately 20% to 30% of patients at 12 months post-transplant. FGF-23 levels begin to fall as early as the first week after transplantation and eventually approximate levels of eGFR-matched CKD patients.

Although the evidence supporting BMD screening in kidney transplant recipients is lacking, KDIGO clinical practice guidelines suggest that a screening bone density exam in the first 3 months after kidney transplant in patients who have a GFR $\geq$ 30 mL/min/1.73 m^2 is reasonable. Measurement of 25-OH vitamin D levels and calcitriol supplementation has been associated with improved post-transplant PTH levels with variable effect on BMD. Bisphosphonates are widely used in the general population for treatment of osteoporosis, but their utility in the renal transplant population is uncertain. Their use has been associated with preservation of BMD after transplantation, but has not been shown to decrease fracture risk. They are not recommended for use in patients with GFR < 30 mL/min/1.73 m^2 and may increase the risk for adynamic bone disease.

Hypercalcemia is common after transplantation, particularly in the first few months when PTH levels are elevated. The use of cinacalcet may be an effective means of achieving normocalcemia but may not result in normalization of PTH concentrations or improvement in BMD. Parathyroidectomy may achieve normocalcemia and improvement in femoral neck bone mineral density, but its effect on fracture risk is unclear. Indications for parathyroidectomy include severe hypercalcemia, nephrolithiasis or nephrocalcinosis, progressive renal dysfunction, and osteoporosis or asymptomatic vertebral fractures.

Newer agents, such as teriparatide (recombinant human PTH) and denosumab (inhibits osteoclast formation, decreases bone resorption) may be considered for treatment of post-transplant bone disease, but their use has not been evaluated systematically in the kidney transplant population.

STRATEGY 12: REGARD PERSISTENTLY IMPAIRED POST-TRANSPLANTATION FUNCTION AS A FORM OF CHRONIC KIDNEY DISEASE

Even well-functioning kidney transplants may have a GFR that falls within the definition of CKD and most allografts will eventually progress to ESKD. Patients should understand that "leading a normal life," the aim of transplantation, includes following quite precise recommendations for health maintenance. A balance needs to be struck by patients and their doctors between burdensome instructions and living the good life. It is clear, however, that patients with impaired baseline renal function are not normal, and their care should encompass the same principles that have become standard of care for other causes of CKD. Control of hypertension, use of ACEIs, control of mineral metabolism, treatment of anemia, and eventually preparation for ESKD options and timely dialysis access placement are fundamental to optimal long-term post-transplantation care. The immunosuppressive management of the failing graft is discussed in Chapter 6, Part V.

SPECIFIC MANAGEMENT ISSUES

Post-transplantation Lymphoproliferative Disease

The reported incidence of PTLD in the recipients of solid-organ transplants ranges from 0.8% to 15% and varies with the type of transplantation, the patient's age, and the immunosuppressive regimen employed. The incidence is about 12-fold higher than in the nontransplant population. There is a bimodal incidence, with most early cases recognized within the first post-transplant year. The incidence declines thereafter and then increases again approximately 4 years after transplantation. For kidney transplant recipients, the incidence is typically 1% to 2%. Despite the widespread use of potent immunosuppressive protocols, the incidence of PTLD in kidney transplant recipients does not appear to be increasing.

PTLDs have several unusual features that distinguish them from lymphomas found in the general population:

1. Most are non-Hodgkin lymphomas (Hodgkin disease is the most common lymphoma in age-matched controls), are of B-cell origin, and are CD20^{+}.
2. PTLD often presents as dysfunction of the transplanted organ and may be confused histologically with severe rejection. Disease is often localized in or near the allograft.
3. There is a high rate of association with Epstein–Barr virus (EBV) infection. Seronegative recipients of an organ from a seropositive donor are at highest risk for PTLD.
4. Extranodal involvement (central nervous system, liver, lungs, kidneys, and intestines) is common, and multiple sites are often involved.
5. The mortality rate is much greater with PTLD than with lymphomas in the general population. The course may be extremely fulminant, with progression to death within a few months of transplantation.
6. The prolonged or repeated administration of lymphocyte-depleting antibody preparations is a significant risk factor for the development of PTLD.
7. PTLD may respond to withdrawal or drastic reduction of immunosuppressive therapy. Standard chemotherapy may often be required.
8. Viral infection, particularly with CMV infection (see Chapter 12), may serendipitously reduce EBV replication and the incidence of PTLD.

9. Although typically considered to result from EBV infection of recipient B cells, PTLD may be of donor origin in some patients.

Role of Epstein–Barr Virus

EBV is a human DNA-transforming herpesvirus that primarily targets B lymphocytes. It is associated with an array of disorders ranging from infectious mononucleosis to nasopharyngeal carcinoma, Burkitt lymphoma, and B-cell lymphomas in immunocompromised patients.

About 10% of adults do not have serologic evidence of previous EBV infection. These patients are at higher risk for PTLD. EBV-seronegative recipients of a seropositive donor are at the highest risk, but even EBV-seronegative recipients of a seronegative donor are at elevated risk for PTLD compared to seropositive recipients. Transmission of EBV in transplant recipients is most commonly through the transplanted organ, but may also be transmitted through alternate sources, such as from bodily fluids, including saliva, blood, and semen. Most EBV-seronegative recipients will ultimately seroconvert after transplant, even if they receive a kidney from a seronegative donor. After transplant, the presence of EBV viremia may be associated with subsequent development of PTLD. Although its positive predictive value is low, the extent that this is influenced by reduction of maintenance immunosuppression upon detection of EBV viremia is unclear.

EBV undergoes lytic replication because of inadequate EBV immune surveillance. The resultant increased burden of EBV in the naive recipient then infects the recipient's B cells. EBV has the innate capability of transforming and immortalizing host B lymphocytes, producing *lymphoblastoid cells*. An extrachromosomal particle of EBV genome can be found within the B-cell nucleus. In an immunocompetent host, a latent carrier state is established when the proliferation of the transformed B cells is contained by a normal immune response with intact cell-mediated immunity. The presence of reactive T lymphocytes inhibits infected cell proliferation in a process called *regression*. Immunosuppressive agents, particularly the antilymphocytic antibody preparations (see Chapter 6), prevent regression, and EBV-transformed cells may proliferate uncontrollably.

EBV-associated PTLD appears to progress through stages of transformation to a malignant state. The first stage resembles an infectious mononucleosis syndrome, with the development of polymorphic diffuse B-cell hyperplasias without cytogenetic abnormalities or gene rearrangements. The second stage produces a subpopulation of cells with cellular and nuclear atypia and cytogenetic abnormalities. In the third stage, a malignant monoclonal B-cell lymphoma develops. A form of fulminant PTLD has been described, often following multiple courses of lymphocytic depletional agents. The disease may initially resemble a severe infectious mononucleosis-like illness but may progress rapidly, with death occurring within a few months of transplantation. At a later stage, the patient may present with localized lymphoproliferative tumor masses in the brain, lung, or gastrointestinal tract. Predictors of poor survival from PTLD include increased age, elevated lactic acid dehydrogenase values, severe organ dysfunction, multiorgan involvement, and constitutional symptoms (fever, night sweats, and weight loss).

Treatment of PTLD

Restoration of host immunity is probably the most important therapy for the control of lymphoid proliferation. Patients with evidence of polyclonality are most likely to respond to reduction of immunosuppression. For patients with monoclonal tumors, immunosuppression should be drastically reduced or discontinued altogether.

Single-agent rituximab, administered at a dose of 375 mg/m^2 weekly for four treatments, in conjunction with immunosuppression reduction has become the preferred treatment for PTLD, particularly for those with EBV detected on tumor histology. B cells, together with their EBV viral load, disappear from the blood after its administration. Overall response rates may approach 70%. This regimen appears to be most appropriate for lower-risk patients. A multivariate risk stratification model has been derived to predict response to single-agent rituximab for the treatment of PTLD (see Trappe et al. in Selected Readings) using patient age, performance status, and serum LDH concentration. This categorization clearly differentiated 1-year survival after single-agent rituximab therapy (100% for low-risk, 79% for intermediate-risk, and 36% for high-risk). It has been proposed that single-agent rituximab is a reasonable first-line therapy after reduction of immunosuppression for low-risk patients, but may not be appropriate for higher-risk patients. In these cases, combined cytotoxic chemotherapy may be employed, either administered together with rituximab or given sequentially.

The mammalian target of rapamycin inhibitors (mTOR; sirolimus and everolimus) are often used in patients with malignancy, as they inhibit signaling pathways that impede cell proliferation. *In vitro*, they inhibit the growth of EBV-positive lymphoblastoid B-cell lines. The literature supporting their use in the clinical management of PTLD is scant and limited to case reports. Despite the limited evidence, however, mTOR inhibitors are widely used in the setting of post-transplant malignancies, and it is not unreasonable to consider mTOR-based immunosuppression in patients who have developed PTLD.

Skin Cancer

The skin is the most frequent site of post-transplant malignancy accounting for nearly 40% of all post-transplant malignancies. Almost all the increased incidence of skin cancer is in White patients, approximately 50% of whom will develop skin cancer. The frequency may be more than a 100-fold greater than in the nontransplant population and varies with the intensity and duration of immunosuppression; sun exposure (forearms, bald scalp); light-colored skin type; geographic location (skin cancer is particularly common in Australia); ethnicity; and presence of prior skin cancer or precancerous lesions. Squamous cell carcinoma (SCC) and basal cell carcinoma (BCC) account for over 90% of post-transplant skin malignancies, but melanoma, Merkel cell carcinoma (MCC), and Kaposi sarcoma are also more common than in the nontransplant population. In the general population, the frequency of BCCs is greater than SCCs, whereas the ratio of SCC/BCC may be as high as 5 in transplant recipients. In addition to the impact of specific immunosuppressive agents (azathioprine, CNIs, see Chapter 6), oncogenic viruses play an important etiologic role, and the location of SCCs on the lips, oral cavity, and genitalia is a reflection of the causative role of human papillomavirus.

The key to the management of post-transplant dermatologic malignancies is prevention by education, awareness, and observation. Annual self-examination and examination by a physician are warranted to screen for squamous cell carcinoma and malignant melanoma. Suspicious lesions should undergo biopsy. Patients should be instructed to avoid excessive sun exposure and to use sunblock, although the effectiveness of this strategy in adults is uncertain. Patients with multiple lesions should undergo formal dermatologic surveillance on a regular basis. Treatment of specific dermatologic malignancies is beyond the purview of this text. Readers are referred to the International Transplant Skin Cancer Collaborative (ITSCC, www.itscc.org). Sirolimus has been shown to decrease the development of new nonmelanoma skin cancers and even regression of preexisting skin malignancies (see Chapter 6, Part I).

Cancer of the Native Kidneys

The incidence of cancer in the native kidneys is close to sixfold higher in kidney transplant recipients than in the nontransplant population because of the frequency of typically low-grade adenocarcinoma occurring in acquired cystic diseased kidneys. The role of routine ultrasound screening for such malignancies, however, remains controversial. The problem with routine screening is that it is likely to increase detection of low-grade tumors and lead to invasive treatments, which may not necessarily benefit the patient and could be harmful. On the other hand, certain higher-risk recipients with better-than-average life expectancy could potentially benefit from screening. This would include patients with diseases that carry an increased risk for renal malignancies, such as analgesic nephropathy, tuberous sclerosis, and known acquired cystic kidney disease. In evaluating hematuria post-transplant, the native kidneys should always be considered as a source.

Hematologic Disorders
Anemia

Anemia is common after renal transplantation. The presumption that the newly transplanted kidney will produce enough erythropoietin to lead to resolution of pretransplant and early post-transplant anemia is incompletely realized in many patients. It has been estimated that 25% of patients are anemic and 13% are iron deficient 12 months after transplantation. In addition to its clinical symptoms, anemia has been associated with worse patient and graft survival and higher rates of acute rejection compared with nonanemic transplant recipients. Anemia may further exaggerate left ventricular hypertrophy. Unrecognized iron deficiency is a frequent cause, and gastrointestinal bleeding should be excluded. Anemia from folate or vitamin B_{12} deficiency is unusual. Hemolysis is rare. In the late post-transplantation period, anemia is most commonly caused by immunosuppression or decreased kidney function. Azathioprine, mycophenolic acid, and sirolimus can cause anemia, thrombocytopenia, and leukopenia, and the doses of these medications may need to be reduced. Anemia has been reported in as many as 60% of patients receiving sirolimus. ACEIs and ARBs may also cause anemia. Parvovirus infection may be a cause of refractory anemia, and treatment with intravenous immune globulin might be effective. When no underlying cause can be found, renal function is impaired, and iron stores are adequate, erythropoietin or darbepoetin alfa (Aranesp) may be indicated. Anemia in patients with chronic allograft failure should be treated in a similar fashion as the anemia accompanying other causes of CKD. The guidelines for the use of erythropoietin have come under scrutiny because of concerns relating to an increase in CVD if the targeted hemoglobin is too high and because of possible effects on cancer growth. Current recommendations for the use of this erythropoietin in CKD should be used in treating transplant patients.

Erythrocytosis

Some degree of erythrocytosis has been reported to occur in up to 20% of patients after transplantation, most commonly during the first 2 years. It rarely occurs in patients who have undergone native kidney nephrectomy, suggesting that it is the native kidneys, rather than the transplant, that is the source of the problem, although stenosis of the transplant renal artery may be a factor. The cause of erythrocytosis appears to be related to defective feedback regulation of erythropoietin metabolism. Although increased erythropoietin production has been reported after transplantation, erythrocytosis is not directly related to erythropoietin levels, which may be low or undetectable in some cases. Elevated levels of insulin-like growth factor-1 (IGF-1) have been found, which may increase the sensitivity of erythroid precursors to erythropoietin. Erythrocytosis may also be a manifestation of transplant renal artery stenosis, and this diagnosis should be considered in any patient with the combination of hypertension, edema, allograft bruit, and erythrocytosis.

Hematocrit levels higher than 60% are associated with increased viscosity and thrombosis, and treatment should commence at a hematocrit level of greater than 55%. Low doses of ACEIs and ARBs are generally effective in reducing elevated hematocrit levels. Their mechanism of action may be related to the induction of apoptosis in erythroid precursors and to reduction of IGF-1 levels. Renal dysfunction after introduction of ACEIs should raise the possibility of transplant renal artery stenosis. Theophylline is a potential alternative to the use of ACEIs or ARBs, although it is less-well tolerated. Phlebotomy may be required in resistant cases.

POST-TRANSPLANTATION REPRODUCTIVE FUNCTIONS

Men

After successful transplantation, about two-thirds of male patients observe improved libido and a return of sexual function to predialysis levels. In some patients, there is no improvement, and occasionally sexual function deteriorates. Fertility, as assessed by sperm counts, improves in half of patients. The sex hormone profile tends to normalize; plasma testosterone and follicle-stimulating hormone levels increase; and luteinizing hormone levels, which may be high in dialysis patients, decrease to normal or low levels. CNIs may impair testosterone biosynthesis through direct damage to Leydig cells and germinal cells, and a direct impairment of the hypothalamic–pituitary–gonadal axis has been suggested. Chronic glucocorticoid use may also lead to reduction in testosterone levels. Mycophenolate has not been reported to have an effect on spermatogenesis or male fertility. Sirolimus, on the other hand, is associated with lower testosterone levels, sperm counts, and fathered pregnancy rates compared to that of transplant recipients maintained on sirolimus-free regimens. There is no increased incidence of neonatal malformations in pregnancies fathered by transplant recipients.

Additional factors may account for failure of male sexual function to improve after transplantation. Antihypertensive medications may be responsible in some patients, autonomic neuropathy may impair erectile function, and interruption of both hypogastric arteries may occasionally impair vascular supply. Male patients should be asked about their sexual function and referred for urologic evaluation when necessary. There is no specific contraindication to the use of sildenafil (Viagra) or similar agents in transplant recipients as long as standard precautions are taken regarding concomitant coronary artery disease (CAD).

Women

Women with CKD demonstrate loss of libido, anovulatory vaginal bleeding or amenorrhea, and high prolactin levels. Maintenance dialysis therapy results in improvement in sexual function in only a small percentage of women, and pregnancy is rare. After successful transplantation, fertility may be restored rapidly; menstrual function and ovulation typically return, and prolactin levels fall to normal in most women by the end of the first year.

Family Planning

All women of childbearing age should be counseled concerning both the possibility and the associated risks of pregnancy after kidney transplantation. Psychosocial issues should be discussed, genetic counseling should be provided for those with hereditary kidney disease, and consideration should be given to the long-term prognosis of the patient and the graft. Patients can be assured that birth defects are not increased with the use of azathioprine, or CNIs during pregnancy, although some degree of intrauterine growth retardation and prematurity are common. Data regarding the stability of graft function during and after pregnancy should be discussed. All pregnancies should be planned and prepared for. It is generally recommended that conception be delayed for a year after kidney transplantation and contraception practiced until then, though data to support this recommendation are scant.

Contraceptive counseling should begin immediately after transplantation because ovulatory cycles may begin within 1 to 2 months of transplantation in women with well-functioning grafts. Low-dose estrogen-progesterone preparations are effective and available in an oral formulation, transdermal patch, or vaginal ring. Any of these formulations may be used in kidney transplant recipients, although they should be used with caution because they may cause or aggravate hypertension or precipitate thromboembolism. In such patients, progestin-only preparations, available as pills, subcutaneous or intramuscular injections, or a subdermal implant may be used. CNI levels should also be monitored soon after the contraceptive is started.

Barrier contraception is the safest modality but depends on user compliance for efficacy. Intrauterine devices (IUD), both copper and levonorgestrel, represent another safe and effective option for contraception for kidney transplant recipients. Although there is only limited data on their use in the transplant population, their use in the HIV-infected population shows them to be highly efficacious without any increase in the rate of pelvic infection, and it is inferred that they may be safely and effectively used in kidney transplant recipients.

Pregnancy

Women with ESKD sometimes seek transplantation with the knowledge that a well-functioning graft will give them the only real chance for natural motherhood. It has been estimated that 3% of women of childbearing age conceive after transplantation. The incidence of spontaneous abortion is reported to be approximately 15%, and that of ectopic pregnancy less than 1%, (see Wyld et al. in Selected Readings) rates that are similar to those seen in the general population. Kidney transplant recipients, however, are at a much higher risk for preeclampsia and preterm birth than the general population. About one-third of pregnant transplant recipients seek therapeutic abortion, a number that likely reflects inadequate family planning in women who have not previously considered themselves to be fertile. More than 90% of conceptions that continue beyond the first trimester end successfully.

Table 11.1 lists the criteria that should ideally be met before conception. A 90% incidence of successful pregnancies has been reported for women with a baseline serum creatinine of 1.5 mg/dL or less. A higher serum creatinine level increases the risk for graft loss, which consistently occurs within 2 years of pregnancy in women whose baseline creatinine is greater than 2 mg/dL. Failure to meet all the listed criteria places the patient in a higher risk category but is not necessarily an absolute contraindication to pregnancy. Because female transplant recipients will generally be stopping their use of an anti-metabolite (mycophenolate or mTOR inhibitor), the patient's risk of rejection and prior rejection history should be taken into consideration before attempts at conception. The US National Transplantation Pregnancy Registry has been developed to provide current information concerning transplant recipient pregnancy for the benefit of patients and their physicians (http://www.ntpr.giftoflifeinstitute.org/).

TABLE 11.1	Criteria for the Reduction of Post-transplantation Pregnancy Risk

At least 1 year after transplantation
Serum creatinine < 2.0 mg/dL, preferably < 1.5 mg/dL
No recent episodes of acute rejection
Normotensive or minimal antihypertensive regimen
Minimal or no proteinuria
Normal allograft ultrasound
Pregnancy-safe drug regimen (see text)

Antenatal Care

Pregnancy in a patient with a kidney transplant should be considered a high-risk condition and should be monitored in a tertiary care center with consultation by a transplant nephrologist, obstetrician, and pediatrician. The pregnancy should be diagnosed as early as possible and accurate dating obtained by fetal ultrasound. For patients with good allograft function before conception, the GFR remains stable or increases, as it does during a normal pregnancy. The GFR may decline to prepregnancy values during the third trimester. Most studies suggest that pregnancy does not have an unfavorable effect on long-term graft function as long as baseline function is excellent. Proteinuria may increase to abnormal levels in the third trimester but usually resolves postpartum and is not of poor prognostic significance unless it is associated with hypertension. Approximately 30% of pregnant patients with kidney transplants develop pregnancy-induced hypertension, a figure that is fourfold greater than in uncomplicated pregnancies. The use of cyclosporine in pregnancy tends to increase the incidence of hypertension. If complications (usually hypertension, renal deterioration, and rejection) occur before 28 weeks' gestation, successful obstetric outcome is reduced by 20%. Prematurity (60%), growth restriction (52%), and the need for hospitalization in a neonatal intensive care unit (35%) are reported to be more common in transplant recipients than in patients with renal diseases who are not on immunosuppression.

Urinary tract infections are the most common bacterial infections and occur in up to 40% of pregnant transplant recipients. Pyelonephritis may develop despite adequate antibiotic treatment. Urinary tract infections are particularly common in patients who develop ESKD as a consequence of pyelonephritis.

Immunosuppression in Pregnancy

Prednisone. Prednisone crosses the placenta, but a large proportion is converted to prednisolone, which allegedly does not suppress fetal corticotropin. Adrenal insufficiency in the neonate has been reported with maternal prednisone ingestion. Very large doses of corticosteroids administered to animals have resulted in congenital anomalies (cleft lip and palate), but no consistent abnormalities have been noted in the offspring of women treated with corticosteroids during pregnancy for rheumatologic disease or kidney transplantation. Overall, low-dose prednisone is considered to be safe for use in pregnancy.

Azathioprine. At doses of 2 mg/kg or less, no anomalies attributable to azathioprine have been noted in human offspring. There are minimal data, however, on the long-term effects of azathioprine on first- or second-generation offspring. Azathioprine can cause transient gaps or breaks in lymphocyte chromosomes. Germ cells and other tissues have not been studied. It is not known whether the eventual sequelae could be the development of malignancies in affected offspring or other abnormalities in the next generation, although no such malignancies have been observed in several decades of use.

Calcineurin Inhibitors. There are no animal or human data showing teratogenicity or mutagenicity of cyclosporine or tacrolimus which appear to be safe during pregnancy. Intrauterine growth retardation and small-for-gestational-age neonates have been reported with cyclosporine use and may reflect chronic vasoconstriction. Cyclosporine is present in the fetal circulation at the same concentration found in the mother. The increased volume of distribution may produce low maternal blood levels, and dose elevations may be required. CNIs may enter breast milk and lactation is generally not recommended in transplant recipients, though adverse consequences for infants have not been reported.

Mycophenolic Acid. The US Food and Drug Administration (FDA) has added a "black box" warning to the product insert for mycophenolic acid preparations following a number of reports of first trimester pregnancy loss and congenital fetal abnormalities in children born to women taking these drugs at the time of and after conception. These include abnormalities of the face and ear. Women should be advised to discontinue these drugs for some months before attempting conception. Prescribers are recommended to complete the Mycophenolate Risk Evaluation and Mitigation Strategy (REMS), which was put in place by the FDA to educate healthcare providers about the pregnancy risks associated with the use of mycophenolate and the need to counsel women of childbearing age of the risks and the importance of pregnancy prevention and planning when taking mycophenolate. Pregnancies that are conceived while on mycophenolate should be reported to the Mycophenolate Pregnancy Registry (https://www.mycophenolaterems.com/).

Other Immunosuppressive Agents. The FDA categorizes the potential fetal risks of drugs used in pregnancy. Most immunosuppressive drugs fall into category C, which implies that "risks cannot be ruled out." Limited data are available concerning the safety of pregnancy for patients receiving newer immunosuppressive agents, such as belatacept (see Chapter 6); for the present, they should be avoided during pregnancy. Sirolimus should be discontinued 6 weeks before conception is attempted. At present, there is insufficient information about the biologic effect of even small amounts of immunosuppressive agents on the neonate, and breast-feeding should be discouraged.

Hypertension Control
Many transplant patients require antihypertensive drugs in pregnancy. Drugs that have been consistently shown to be safe should be used; these include methyldopa, hydralazine, and labetalol. ACEIs and ARBs are generally contraindicated in pregnancy, but it is probably safe to continue a pregnancy if their administration is discontinued as soon as pregnancy is diagnosed.

Labor and Delivery
Vaginal delivery is recommended because the transplanted kidney is placed in the false pelvis, and there is little risk for obstruction of the birth canal or mechanical injury to the allograft. Cesarean section is usually performed only for standard obstetric reasons. Great care should be taken to identify and protect the transplanted ureter. Preterm delivery occurs in about half of pregnancies in transplant recipients because of

the frequent occurrence of declining kidney function, pregnancy-induced hypertension, fetal distress, premature rupture of membranes, and premature labor. The incidence of small-for-gestational-age neonates is 20%. There is no increase in fetal abnormalities.

In the perinatal period, the steroid dose should be augmented to cover the stress of labor and to prevent postpartum rejection. Hydrocortisone, 100 mg every 6 hours, should be given during labor and delivery. Maternal hypertension and fluid balance should be monitored carefully. Graft function and the immunosuppressive regimen should be monitored with particular care in the first 3 months postpartum. Occasional cases of postpartum acute renal failure resembling hemolytic uremic syndrome have been described.

Part II: Causes of Late Allograft Failure

It is more difficult to define the cause of allograft failure than it may seem. Allograft failure is usually defined either by the patient's death or the patient's need to undertake new treatment for ESKD (i.e., chronic dialysis or retransplantation). Making a distinction between these two categories of allograft failure may have important implications for understanding how to prevent allograft failure. However, making the distinction may sometimes be difficult. For example, a patient with severe acute rejection may require dialysis support and may die of complications of immunosuppression before the rejection can be reversed. Did this patient die with a functioning graft, or was the graft loss because of acute rejection? Studies show, however, that most patients who die with a functioning graft have good allograft function (so-called "death with graft function"). In these cases, attempts to understand the pathogenesis of allograft failure should focus on understanding the cause of death and its pathogenesis. In the United States, death with graft function accounts for 40% to 50% of all graft losses (Fig. 11.1).

The goal of renal transplantation should be to have every patient who dies do so with a kidney that functions well. Unfortunately, most deaths that now occur with a functioning allograft are premature and are potentially preventable. Most of the premature deaths that occur in the late post-transplant period can be directly or indirectly attributed to the morbid events that initially led to CKD and the consequences thereof (see Chapter 1) and to allograft dysfunction or the immunosuppression used to prevent or treat allograft rejection. The three most commonly defined causes of death in the late post-transplant period are CVD, infection, and malignancy.

CAUSE OF DEATH AFTER TRANSPLANTATION

Cardiovascular Disease

Atherosclerotic CVD kills patients by causing myocardial infarction, congestive heart failure, stroke, ischemic colitis, and peripheral vascular disease. In the case of ischemic colitis and peripheral vascular disease, the terminal event may be infection (e.g., sepsis from a perforated bowel or cellulitis). To understand how to prevent post-transplantation

TABLE 11.2	Risk Factors for Post-transplantation Cardiovascular Disease
Risk Factor	**Strength of Evidence**
Pretransplantation cardiovascular disease	++++
Diabetes (including post-transplantation diabetes)	++++
Cigarette smoking	+++
Hyperlipidemia	+++
Hypertension	++
Platelet and coagulation abnormalities	++
Allograft dysfunction or rejection	++
Hypoalbuminemia	++
Erythrocytosis	+
Oxygen free radicals	+
Infections	+
Increased homocysteine	+

CVD deaths and complications, it is crucial to define the etiologic risk factors (Table 11.2). Some risk factors can be modified, and for some of these, there is strong evidence from studies in the general population that intervention improves survival. It is also important, however, to identify risk factors that cannot be modified because these risk factors help to identify high-risk patients who can be targeted for screening and possibly intervention as well as for treatment of other modifiable risk factors.

Patients with pretransplant CVD are at increased risk for post-transplantation CVD complications. Such patients should be targeted for aggressive management of modifiable CVD risk factors. Because atherosclerosis is a systemic illness, it should not be surprising that patients with a history of cerebral vascular disease (e.g., ischemic strokes) are at increased risk for ischemic heart disease. Although pretransplant CVD greatly increases the risk for post-transplant CVD complications, much of the risk for CVD in the late post-transplant period is acquired after transplantation. Identifying and aggressively managing high-risk patients is important. A decline in renal function has been identified as an important risk factor for CVD, and to the extent that the transplanted kidney is functioning well, this reduces the risk for CVD in transplant recipients. As renal function declines, this again becomes an additive risk factor for CVD.

Diabetes is the most common cause of ESKD leading to transplantation, and diabetes is the most important risk factor for post-transplantation CVD. Both type 1 and type 2 diabetes greatly increase the risk for ischemic heart disease, cerebral vascular disease, peripheral vascular disease, and death. Diabetic control may become difficult after transplantation and patients with type 2 diabetes often become insulin dependent.

About 20% of nondiabetic patients develop hyperglycemia after transplantation, and 5% to 10% require therapy with oral hypoglycemic agents or insulin. Older patients, obese patients, Blacks and ethnic minorities, and patients with a strong family history of diabetes are at higher risk for post-transplant diabetes. The effect of diabetes developed after transplantation on morbidity and graft survival is intermediate between that of patients without diabetes and those who have pre-transplantation diabetes. Corticosteroids, mTOR inhibitors, and the CNIs (tacrolimus more so than cyclosporine) all contribute in varying degrees to glucose intolerance (see Chapter 6).

Numerous epidemiologic studies of the general population show that cigarette smoking is an important modifiable risk factor for CVD. Smoking is as prevalent in renal transplant recipients as it is in the general population and is linked to CVD in the late post-transplant period.

Countless epidemiologic studies and numerous large, randomized, controlled trials in the general population show that hyperlipidemia causes CVD. The evidence is strongest that elevations in LDL cholesterol contribute to the pathogenesis of atherosclerosis; however, evidence is also strong that low levels of high-density lipoprotein (HDL) cholesterol also contribute to CVD risk. Several studies have found the same associations between lipoprotein elevations and CVD in renal transplant patients. The most important cause of hyperlipidemia after renal transplantation is immunosuppressive medication. Sirolimus, cyclosporine, and tacrolimus (in order of severity) all cause elevations in lipid levels to varying degrees (see Chapter 6). Other causes include corticosteroid dose, diet, genetic predisposition, proteinuria, and possibly decreased renal function.

Data from several epidemiologic and interventional studies show that hypertension contributes to CVD in the general population, although it has proved difficult to demonstrate that hypertension specifically causes CVD in renal transplant recipients. This may be because most transplant physicians treat blood pressure aggressively. Corticosteroids and the CNIs (cyclosporine more so than tacrolimus) can elevate blood pressure after renal transplantation. Graft dysfunction also contributes to hypertension. The presence of the native kidneys is associated with increased blood pressure after renal transplantation.

Allograft dysfunction is also associated with subsequent CVD complications. Decreased renal function and proteinuria can contribute to other risk factors, such as hyperlipidemia and hypertension. Allograft dysfunction is also more common in patients who have had acute rejection and have been treated with higher doses of immunosuppressive medications known to affect several CVD risk factors adversely. Allograft dysfunction may be an independent risk factor for CVD. It is speculated that allograft rejection may be associated with a systemic inflammatory response that may contribute to the pathogenesis of CVD. Hypoalbuminemia may also be an independent risk factor for post-transplantation CVD, and chronic inflammation may reduce serum albumin levels.

Atherosclerosis could be both a cause and an effect of chronic inflammation. Although epidemiologic studies have often reported an association between antioxidant vitamin use and CVD, more convincing clinical data supporting a role for oxygen free radicals in the pathogenesis of CVD have been elusive. In particular, most large, randomized, controlled trials in the general population have failed to show that antioxidant vitamins protect against CVD events. A number of epidemiologic studies implicate various infections, including CMV infection, in the pathogenesis of CVD. In addition, some studies have found evidence for the presence of infectious agents in atherosclerotic lesions. It is certainly plausible, however, that individuals with CVD may be more susceptible to infection and that infectious agents may play an innocent-bystander role in systemic atherosclerosis. Heart transplant recipients treated with CMV prophylaxis have been reported to have less CAD. On the other hand, an association between CMV or other infections and CVD in renal transplant recipients has been difficult to document despite the fact that the prevalence of such infections is high. Periodontal disease is common in patients with CKD and may cause a systemic inflammatory response that may contribute to cardiovascular risk. Post-transplant patients should maintain dental hygiene and have access to dental care.

Infection

Specific post-transplantation infections are discussed in Chapter 12. Infection is an inevitable companion of immunosuppression and is attributable to the overall level of immunosuppression. Certain infections occur more frequently at certain times after transplantation (see Chapter 12). CMV is arguably the most common infection after renal transplantation. Infection occurs most often in the early post-transplantation period when patients are most immunosuppressed. Fortunately, the availability of effective antiviral therapy has greatly reduced its lethal potential. BK virus is a human polyomavirus that has emerged as a serious infection that can cause graft dysfunction and, ultimately, graft failure (see Chapters 10 and 12). It is critical to identify BK virus because its morphologic characteristics can be confused with acute rejection and the therapeutic response is based on minimization of immunosuppression. Chronic liver disease, usually caused by viral hepatitis, is an important cause of post-transplantation mortality (see Chapter 13). Hepatitis C virus is the most common cause of hepatitis after renal transplantation. Influenza is an important cause of preventable morbidity and mortality after transplantation. Viral infections are associated with malignancy in the late post-transplantation period.

Bacterial infections are common in the late post-transplant period because of underlying risk factors and immunosuppression. As previously discussed, the high prevalence of peripheral vascular disease among diabetic patients and other transplant recipients greatly increases the risk for cellulitis and life-threatening bacterial sepsis. Ischemic bowel disease can also lead to septic shock and death. Bladder dysfunction, caused by diabetes and other anatomic urologic abnormalities, combine with immunosuppression to increase the risk for urinary tract infections and gram-negative bacterial sepsis. Tuberculosis is common among high-risk populations.

Several other, potentially life-threatening, opportunistic infections occur sporadically but are nevertheless relatively common in the late post-transplantation period. Examples include infection with *P. jiroveci*, *Toxoplasma gondii*, *Nocardia* species, *Aspergillus* species, *Listeria monocytogenes*, *Candida* species, *Cryptococcus neoformans*, *Histoplasma capsulatum*, *Coccidioides immitis*, and *Blastomyces dermatitidis*. Infection with opportunistic organisms can present as pneumonia, meningitis, cellulitis, osteomyelitis, or generalized sepsis. Diagnosis requires a high index of suspicion and an aggressive diagnostic approach.

Malignancy

Malignancies are common after renal transplantation; they are also more common in chronic dialysis patients. The risk for transmission of malignancies from the donor is extremely low, and almost all malignancies arise *de novo* in the recipient. Much of our knowledge of the malignancy and transplantation association comes from large registries, such as the Transplant Cancer Match Study (www.transplant-match.cancer.gov), the Israel Penn Transplant Tumor Registry (www.ipittr.uc.edu), and the Australia-New Zealand Dialysis and Transplant Registry (www.anzdata.org.au) (see also Engels et al. and Yanik et al. in Selected Readings). These data indicate that the incidence of non-cutaneous malignancies in renal transplant recipients is as much as 3.5-fold higher than that of age-matched controls. This increase can be attributed to an increased incidence of most tumors. However, the observed-to-expected incidence (the standardized incidence ratio) is not uniform among different types of tumors. Some tumors, such as breast cancer in women and prostate cancer in men, do not appear to be more common among renal transplant recipients than among the general population. Renal cell carcinoma is discussed above and may be no more common than in the dialysis population. The differences in the observed-to-expected incidence of different malignancies are consistent with the notion that more than one mechanism may explain the increased incidence of cancer after renal transplantation.

Some malignancies are undoubtedly caused by viral infections. Viruses that may otherwise reside in the host without untoward complications may cause potentially lethal malignant transformations in immunocompromised renal transplant recipients. Some of the tumors that occur with the highest incidence, compared with the general population, have possible viral causes. For example, PTLD has been linked to infection caused by EBV. Human herpesvirus-8 has been implicated in the development of Kaposi sarcoma after renal transplantation. Human papillomavirus has been implicated in the pathogenesis of squamous cell cancer of the skin, vulva, vagina, and possibly uterine cervix. Liver cancer may be caused by chronic infection with hepatitis B and C viruses.

Urinary malignancies may occur more frequently among renal transplant recipients because renal disease may sometimes be associated with malignant and premalignant conditions such as acquired cystic disease of the native kidneys. Similarly, an increased risk for the rarely occurring parathyroid cancer may be attributable to long-standing renal disease and events occurring before transplantation.

Other mechanisms are undoubtedly at play. Immunosuppressive agents may damage DNA and lead to malignant transformation of cells and may also inhibit normal immune surveillance and thereby allow cells that have undergone malignant transformation to grow and divide unchecked. In an animal model, cyclosporine has been shown to promote cancer progression by a direct TGF-β–related cellular effect that is independent of the host's immune cells. The antiproliferative effect of sirolimus may theoretically protect against tumor development and progression; epidemiologic studies have shown decreased incidence of cancers with its use.

Malignancies may occur at any time after transplantation. However, some are more likely than others to occur early after transplantation. These include PTLD (relatively common) and Kaposi sarcoma (relatively rare). Most other tumors tend to occur later. Moreover, the incidence of malignant tumors continues to increase throughout the late post-transplant period. The cumulative incidence of noncutaneous malignancies is about 33% by 30 years after transplantation. The cumulative incidence of skin cancer is much higher, but few patients die of skin cancer after renal transplantation.

It is the cumulative effects of immunosuppression *per se*, rather than any particular agent or agents, that is principally responsible for the increased incidence of noncutaneous malignancies after renal transplantation. Age increases the risk for post-transplant tumors, and it may be wise to minimize the amount of immunosuppression used in transplant recipients older than 60 or 65 years of age. Cigarette smoking is also associated with a higher risk for post-transplantation malignancies.

Tumor markers, carcinoembryonic antigen (CEA), cancer antigen 125 (CA125), and CA15-3 have a low specificity and sensitivity as screeners for malignancies in renal transplant recipients. The value of routine screening of the transplant population for common cancers (breast, colorectal, and prostate) has been questioned; the risk-to-benefit ratio of such screening may be less favorable in the transplant population than in the general population because the life expectancy of transplant patients is intrinsically limited. Decisions regarding cancer screening should be made on an individual basis.

Late Allograft Failure

The highest rate of allograft failure is in the first year after transplant, with 1-year graft survival reported at approximately 92% (http://optn.transplant/hrsa.gov). Graft survival is better with living donor transplant than deceased donor transplant (at 1 year, 95% versus 89%, respectively). Beyond the first year, the rate of all-cause graft loss is relatively constant and is estimated at approximately 3% to 5% per year. Fifty percent of deceased donor kidney transplants will have failed by approximately 9 years after transplant; half-life of a living donor transplant is estimated to be approximately 12 years. As described earlier, death with a functioning allograft is the most common cause of late allograft failure. Allograft half-life estimates increase to 14 years for a deceased donor transplant and 17 years for a living donor transplant after censoring for death with a functioning graft.

Factors that influence late allograft failure include either immune, or alloantigen dependent, and nonimmune, or alloantigen independent (Table 11.3). The distinction between alloantigen-dependent and alloantigen-independent factors is a convenient one, but multiple factors often coexist, and early events may program later events. For example, ischemic injury may make the graft more susceptible to acute rejection, and graft survival is impaired in the presence of

TABLE 11.3	Tailoring the Amount of Immunosuppression to the Individual	

Risk Factor	Patients Who May Need More Immunosuppression	Patients Who May Need Less Immunosuppression
Donor source	Deceased	Living
Major histocompatibility	>0 mismatches	0 mismatches
Prior transplant experience	>1, rejected quickly	0 or 1, prolonged survival
Age	<18 years old	>60 years old
Race	African American	White
Timing of acute rejection	Late	Early
Severity of acute rejection	Severe, vascular	Mild, cellular
Number of acute rejections	>1	0 or 1

hypertension. The pathologic features of late allograft failure are described in Chapter 15.

Clinically, late allograft failure presents as declining allograft function, often with proteinuria and hypertension. The clinical course may be unpredictable, and the biopsy findings are often poor predictors of the subsequent clinical course, particularly if the histologic findings are mild. Functional studies tend to underestimate the extent of morphologic injury. Patients with transplant glomerulopathy or severe arterial lesions on biopsy often have progressive declines in renal function.

Alloantigen-Dependent Risk Factors

The most convincing evidence that alloantigen-dependent factors are an important cause of graft loss comes from epidemiologic studies demonstrating associations between allosensitization, episodes of acute rejection, presence of donor-specific antibodies, and allograft failure. Nevertheless, not all rejection episodes should be considered equivalent, and the pathologic processes underlying the rejection episode, the severity, and the response to therapy predict the long-term outcome. T-cell–mediated rejection is an important cause of early allograft failure, but is a less common cause of late allograft failure except in circumstances of medication nonadherence. Acute rejections that occur late (after the first 3 months) appear to be more predictive of chronic allograft failure than those that occur during the first 3 months; rejections that occur very early and are reversed may have little or no effect on outcome. Rejections that are more severe, either by histology or by increase in serum creatinine, are more likely than less acute, severe rejections to herald late allograft failure. Multiple acute rejections also appear to be more predictive of late allograft failure.

The number of major histocompatibility complex (MHC) antigens that are mismatched between the recipient and donor is associated with late allograft failure (see Chapter 3). Among deceased donor kidney transplants, those that have zero MHC mismatches have the best long-term allograft survival. Less marked are differences in late allograft survival between kidneys that have one to six MHC mismatches. Haploindentical living-related transplants are associated with the longest long-term survival and are often managed with reduced-dose immunosuppression and transplants donated by an identical twin may be managed with no immunosuppression at all. The effect of MHC mismatches on graft half-life is further evidence that alloantigen-dependent factors are important in the pathogenesis of late allograft failure.

There is an association between detection of preformed antibodies (see Chapter 3) at the time of transplantation or development of *de novo* donor-specific antibodies and subsequent late allograft failure. As discussed in Part I, the presence of donor-specific antibodies and evidence of antibody-mediated injury on biopsy portend a poorer long-term prognosis. In some studies, up to 60% of patients with late allograft failure show evidence of antibody-mediated injury. The therapeutic implications of this finding are discussed in Chapter 6, Part V.

Alloantigen-Independent Risk Factors

Patients with delayed, or "slow," graft function have a higher rate of late allograft failure. One theory holds that ischemic injury and delayed graft function result in a reduced number of functioning nephrons and that inadequate "nephron dosing" causes late allograft failure. However, delayed graft function is also associated with an increased incidence of acute rejection that could also explain its adverse effects on late graft survival. Close surveillance of patients for acute rejection during and after periods of delayed graft function may reduce the rate of late allograft failure.

Donor age is clearly associated with a higher rate of late allograft failure. The inadequate number of nephrons may create a physiologic response that sets in motion mechanisms ultimately leading to graft failure. The accelerated senescence theory proposes that the intrinsic age of the kidney (genetically determined in every cell and expressed in telomere length) limits its longevity in the recipient; the aging process is further accelerated by the repeated injury and stress represented by the alloantigen-dependent and alloantigen-independent factors discussed previously. By whatever mechanisms, the use of older kidneys appears to be a major cause of late allograft failure. Nevertheless, older kidneys are still a valuable source of organs and are best used when directed to older recipients. There is little difference in patient survival when older recipients receive a kidney from a younger donor compared to an older donor. The use of older donor kidneys in the appropriate context can be an effective way to increase the donor supply to an ever-increasing population of patients needing a kidney transplant.

CNI nephrotoxicity is also an important cause of late allograft failure in kidney transplant recipients: Its prevalence may have been overstated in earlier publications. The histologic changes of chronic CNI toxicity are described in Chapter 15, and are characterized by arteriolar hyalinosis or striped cortical fibrosis. These lesions occur in more than 90% of patients treated with a CNI, but have been described to occur in two-thirds of patients not exposed to a CNI likely related to diabetes and hypertension.

Registry data show that elevated blood pressure is also associated with graft failure. Of course, it is plausible that graft dysfunction causes hypertension, rather than hypertension causing graft dysfunction. Unfortunately, there are no randomized trial results to determine whether aggressive blood pressure lowering will reduce the rate of late graft failure. Cigarette smoking is another risk factor that could have a negative effect on graft vasculopathy and contribute to chronic allograft injury. The incidence of persistent proteinuria after transplantation (more than 1 to 2 g per 24 hours for longer than 6 months) has been estimated to be about 20% and tends to be greater with longer duration of follow-up. Proteinuria is an important risk factor for graft loss. Proteinuria causes interstitial nephritis in experimental animals, and studies in humans with renal disease have consistently reported that the amount of urine protein excretion predicts renal disease progression. Thus, it is possible that proteinuria could cause tubulointerstitial damage and contribute to late allograft failure.

Renal Function Predicts Renal Function

Whatever the mechanisms underlying chronic allograft injury, the bottom line remains the same: The better and more stable the graft function, the better the long-term outcome. The serum creatinine measured at varying stages after transplantation (at discharge from hospital; 6 months; 1 year) is a valuable predictor of long-term outcome, and events occurring in the first year are critical for long-term survival. Renal function is a better predictor of graft survival than the incidence of acute rejection, delayed graft function, HLA mismatch, and other risk factors. Patients with a 1-year creatinine of less than 1.5 mg/dL and a change of creatinine of less than 0.3 mg/dL can look forward to excellent long-term graft outcome. Higher values are accompanied by a steadily increasing risk of graft loss.

Acute Rejection in the Late Post-transplantation Period

Nonadherence of some degree to the appropriate immunosuppressive regimen plays a role in most late acute rejections, and should always be considered when they occur. Because many patients do not admit to missing doses of medications (doctors to underprescribing!), it is difficult to know how often noncompliance causes acute rejection and graft failure. Late rejection sometimes arises because of inadequate dosing of medications or because of the tendency of providers to wean medications in the late post-transplant period, or because of loss, or inadequate medication insurance coverage (see Chapter 21). Although it is always prudent to limit the exposure to immunosuppression to the minimum amount required to prevent rejection, determining the appropriate amount of immunosuppression for optimal graft outcomes may be challenging. Current methods for immune monitoring are crude, at best, and cannot reliably inform whether a given immunosuppression regimen is adequate. Therefore, although immunosuppression reduction may be considered in some patients in the late post-transplant period, patients who reduce doses of immunosuppression should be monitored carefully for signs of graft dysfunction. Periodic screening for development of donor specific antibodies may be considered for those on reduced immunosuppression and may be a marker for inadequate immunosuppression. The treatment of late acute rejection episodes is discussed in Chapter 6.

Recurrent and *De Novo* Renal Disease

The problem of recurrent glomerular disease after transplantation is largely an unsolved one. The reported incidence of recurrence of the original renal disease in the allograft is variable, as is the resultant risk for graft failure. Much of the variation is based on differences in the duration of follow-up and on differences in the frequency with which patients undergo biopsies of their native kidneys and the transplant. As graft failures from death and rejection decline, the apparent incidence of graft failure from recurrent disease may increase. It is also frequently difficult to establish whether some diseases represent recurrences or *de novo* glomerular disease. For patients who did not have a specific biopsy diagnosis of the cause of their native kidney disease, the diagnosis may become evident in the pathology of their transplant biopsy.

The incidence of recurrent and *de novo* glomerular diseases among a large cohort in the Renal Allograft Disease Registry (RADR) was approximately 3% over a mean follow-up period of 5.4 years. Diagnoses were:

Focal segmental glomerulosclerosis (FSGS) (34%)
Immunoglobulin A (IgA) nephropathy (13%)
Diabetes (11%)
Membranoproliferative glomerulonephritis (MPGN) (11%)
Membranous nephropathy (10%)
Hemolytic uremic syndrome or thrombotic thrombocytopenic purpura (5%)
Other (16%)

There was a significant increase in graft failures among the recurrent and *de novo* disease groups (55%) when compared with the others (25%). In a small cohort of two-haplotype–matched living-related donor transplants followed for a mean of over 8 years, the incidence of recurrent disease was 15%, and was 27% in patients with glomerulonephritis as the diagnosis of the original kidney disease. The higher incidence of disease recurrence in this study may reflect the lack of competing graft loss to rejection in well-matched recipients exposed to relatively long follow-up.

In data from large registries, it may be more difficult to discern the incidence of disease recurrence than to define the outcome of patients after recurrent disease has been diagnosed. In a group of more than 1,500 Australian patients with biopsy-proven glomerulonephritis who were followed for 10 years, the incidence of graft loss as a consequence of any kind of glomerulonephritis was 8%. FSGS is clearly the form of glomerular disease most commonly associated with recurrence and graft loss, and patients who have lost a prior transplant because of recurrent FSGS are at much higher risk. Early recognition of recurrent FSGS is particularly important because it may respond to plasmapheresis. The prevention and management of recurrent FSGS, which is most common in children, is discussed in detail in Chapter 17. Dense deposit disease and C3 glomerulopathy frequently recur and are associated with poor graft survival, although newer therapies, such as eculizumab, may eventually prove to alter their prognosis. Membranous glomeru-lonephritis can present as *de novo* disease but probably recurs in 5% to 10% of patients. The presence of anti-phospholipase A2 receptor antibody prior to transplant is associated with post-transplant recur-rence. Histologic recurrence of IgA nephropathy is common. Allograft failure to IgA nephropathy is higher than once reported and may be as high as 25%. Henoch–Schönlein purpura recurs in a high proportion of patients and leads to graft failure in about 25%. Antiglomerular basement membrane disease recurs in 10% to 25% of patients but rarely causes graft failure.

Role of Nonadherence in Late Allograft Failure

The frequency of nonadherence with immunosuppressive medications is difficult to measure, but it is probably more frequent than reported. As a group, transplant recipients may be especially reluctant to admit to nonadherence if they believe that doing so might jeopardize their chances of ever receiving another transplant. Some patients may admit to nonadherence and seek financial assistance in obtaining their medica-tions (see Chapter 21). Nonadherence may also manifest as a failure to keep scheduled appointments or as inconsistent immunosuppressant drug levels. Patients who fail to have their serum creatinine measure-ments performed regularly are more likely to have late graft failure.

Patients may become nonadherent with medications for a number of reasons. They may harbor the false belief that taking medication regularly is unnecessary. This belief may be reinforced by several years of an uneventful post-transplantation course. Many patients believe that the effects of immunosuppression continue indefinitely, even when doses of medications are missed. Such patients are more likely to be nonadherent than are patients who have a better understanding of the duration of the action of immunosuppressive medications. Some patients may become nonadherent because they fear the adverse effects of medication more than they fear graft rejection. This is particularly true of adolescents, who abhor the social stigma of the body habitus changes caused by corticosteroids and, to a lesser extent, cyclosporine.

Patients may simply forget to take doses of medication. In a survey of 100 members of the Transplant Recipient International Organiza-tion (TRIO), less than 30% were taking fewer than 5 medications, and 35% reported taking 10 to 20 different medications daily. Most of the medications require multiple daily doses (In general, studies show that the number of times a day that patients must take medications is a stronger predictor of nonadherence than is the total number of medications). Of those surveyed, 25% admitted missing doses of medi-cations, and 55% of these gave forgetfulness as the reason. It is likely that the members of the TRIO represent a highly motivated popula-tion of transplant recipients. Only 35% of the participants were kidney transplant recipients, and recipients nonrenal organs may suffer lethal consequences if their grafts fail.

Nonadherence increases the risk for late graft loss three- to fivefold and may be the most common cause of late graft loss. Nonadherence can lead to graft failure through several different mechanisms. Patients who receive inadequate immunosuppression because of nonadherence may develop acute or chronic rejection that leads to graft failure, with the development of DSA being a potent etiologic factor. Nonadherence with clinic visits and laboratory follow-up can also contribute to late graft failure. Acute rejection in the late post-transplantation period rarely presents with signs and symptoms until it is far advanced. Thus, to be successfully treated, acute rejection must be detected early, which can only be done by detecting increases in serum creatinine levels soon after they occur. It follows that patients who do not see physicians and who do not have frequent measurements of serum creatinine levels are less likely to have rejection detected at an early stage, when it is treatable. It also follows that it is the responsibility of transplant physicians and transplantation team members to constantly reinforce to patients the importance of adherence and to make every effort to facilitate adherent behavior by minimizing the complexity of the medication protocol and other aspects of long-term post-transplantation follow-up.

MANAGEMENT OF THE ABANDONED GRAFT

In the event that premature death does not intervene, at some point most allografts will eventually fail. Once failure is deemed inevitable, a decision process should be mapped out with the patient so as to minimize unnecessary complications and prepare for ESKD options. This decision process is similar to that faced at the time when CKD was first diagnosed. Patients, and family members, may be reluctant to accept the inevitability of loss of their transplant and should be counseled sympathetically. Reversible causes of graft dysfunction should be identified, hypertension and mineral metabolism controlled, and dialysis access prepared when relevant. Studies have suggested that these basic steps are often neglected or delayed in transplant patients, possibly out of a sense of "denial" by patients or their caregivers. Ideally, a repeat transplant will be available, most likely from a living donor, in which case preparation should be made to attempt preemptive retransplantation (see Chapter 8), and low-intensity immunosuppression maintained. Blood transfusion should be avoided if at all possible to prevent sensitization.

Immunosuppression of the failing allograft is discussed in Chapter 6. Once dialysis has commenced, the decision process regarding the management of immunosuppression depends on a number of factors: a core principle being, the less the better.

1. If the graft has been removed, all immunosuppression should be stopped, though low-dose prednisone may be required for several weeks to avoid adrenal suppression.
2. If the graft has been in place for a prolonged period and is small and echogenic, immunosuppression can typically be stopped in a stepwise manner over several weeks.
3. If the graft has been lost more rapidly or suddenly, and is still of normal size, a slower reduction of immunosuppression may be wise.
4. For patients who continue to pass significant amounts of urine, it may be wise to maintain low levels of immunosuppression (low-dose CNI or MMF) since the quality of life of dialysis patients who still have residual GFR is improved.

5. Dialysis providers should never forget that an abandoned allograft is present in their patients. Grafts that have been abandoned may still manifest their presence, sometimes years after their function has been lost, in a process that can be deemed "rejection of the rejected graft." Clinically this may present with constitutional symptoms, an enlarged and tender graft, hematuria, and elevated inflammatory markers. These symptoms may respond to a transient intensification of immunosuppression. Allograft nephrectomy may be required (see Chapter 9).

6. Allograft nephrectomy, or the need for allograft nephrectomy, often leads to an exaggeration of sensitization with the inherent difficulty in achieving repeat transplantation. It should be avoided if possible.

7. If a re-transplant is imminent, it is be reasonable to maintain low-intesity immunosuppression so as to avoid developing HLA sensitization.

Selected Readings

Blosser C. A call to action: the need for improves transplant screening guidelines. Am J Transplant 2017;17:9–10.

Bramham K, Nelson-Piercy C, Gao H, et al. Pregnancy in renal transplant recipients: a UK national cohort study. Clin J Am Soc Nephrol 2013;8:290–298.

Cosio F, Cattran D. Recent advances in our understanding of recurrent primary glomerulonephritis after kidney transplantation. Kidney Int 2017;91:304–314.

Cruzado JM, Moreno P, Torregrosa JV, et al. A randomized study comparing parathyroidectomy with cinacalcet for treating hypercalcemia in kidney allograft recipients with hyperparathyroidism. J Am Soc Nephrol 2016;27:2487–2494.

Engels EA, Pfeiffer RM, Fraumeni JF Jr, et al. Spectrum of cancer risk among US solid organ transplant recipients. JAMA 2011;306:1891–1901.

Gill J, Wright A, Delmonico F, et al. Towards improving the transfer of care of kidney transplant recipients. Am J Transplant 2017;17:54–59.

Gonzales MM, Bentall A, Kremers WK, et al. Predicting individual renal allograft outcomes using risk models with 1-year surveillance biopsy and alloantibody data. J Am Soc Nephrol 2016;27:3165–3174.

Group SR, Wright JT Jr, Williamson JD, et al. A randomized trial of intensive versus standard blood-pressure control. N Engl J Med 2015;373:2103–2116.

Guidicelli G, Guerville F, Lepreux S, et al. Non-complement-binding de novo donor-specific anti-HLA antibodies and kidney allograft survival. J Am Soc Nephrol 2016;27:615.

Gupta G, Fattah H, Ayalon R, et al. Pre-transplant phospholipase A2 receptor autoantibody concentration is associated with clinically significant recurrence of membranous nephropathy post-kidney transplantation. Clin Transplant 2016;30:461.

Hosseini-Moghaddam SM, Alhomayeed B, Soliman N, et al. Primary Epstein–Barr virus infection, seroconversion, and posttransplant lymphoproliferative disorder in seronegative renal allograft recipients: a prospective cohort study. Transpl Infect Dis 2016;18:423–430.

Huang E, Poommipanit N, Sampaio MS, et al. Intermediate-term outcomes associated with kidney transplantation in recipients 80 years and older: an analysis of the OPTN/UNOS database. Transplantation 2010;90:974–979.

Iyer SP, Nikkel LE, Nishiyama KK, et al. Kidney transplantation with early corticosteroid withdrawal: paradoxical effects at the central and peripheral skeleton. J Am Soc Nephrol 2014;25:1331.

Lamb KE, Lodhi S, Meier-Kriesche HU. Long-term renal allograft survival in the United States: a critical reappraisal. Am J Transplant 2011;11:450.

Lefaucheur C, Viglietti D, Bentlejewski C, et al. IgG donor-specific anti-human HLA antibody subclasses and kidney allograft antibody-mediated injury. J Am Soc Nephrol 2016;27:293–304.

Mathur A, Chang Y, Steidley D, et al. Patterns of care and outcomes in cardiovascular disease after kidney transplantation in the United States. Transplant Dir 2017;3:e126.

Morken NH, Diaz-Garcia C, Reisaeter AV, et al. Obstetric and neonatal outcome of pregnancies fathered by males on immunosuppression after solid organ transplantation. Am J Transplant 2015;15:1666–1673.

Murakami N, Riella LV, Funakoshi T. Risk of metabolic complications in kidney transplantation after conversion to mTOR inhibitor: a systematic review and meta-analysis. Am J Transplant 2014;14:2317–2327.

Naylor KL, Garg AX, Hodsman AB, et al. Long-term changes in bone mineral density in kidney transplant recipients. Transplantation 2014;98:1279–1285.

Nickerson P, Rush D. Beginning at the beginning to prevent the end. J Am Soc Nephrol 2015;26:1477.

Pedrollo EF, Corrêa C, Nicoletto BB, et al. Effects of metabolic syndrome on kidney transplantation outcomes: a systematic review and meta-analysis. Transpl Int 2016;29:1059–1066.

Pham P, Everly M, Faravardeh A, et al. Management of patients with a failed kidney transplant. World J Nephrol 2015;4:148–159.

Quinlan SC, Pfeiffer RM, Morton LM, et al. Risk factors for early-onset and late-onset posttransplant lymphoproliferative disorder in kidney recipients in the United States. Am J Hematol 2011;86:206–209.

Rose C, Schaeffner E, Frei U, et al. A lifetime of allograft function with kidneys from older donors. J Am Soc Nephrol 2015;26:2483.

Sellares J, de Freitas DG, Mengel M, et al. Understanding the causes of kidney transplant failure: the dominant role of antibody-mediated rejection and nonadherence. Am J Transplant 2012;12:388.

Snanoudj R, Royal V, Elie C, et al. Specificity of histological markers of long-term CNI nephrotoxicity in kidney-transplant recipients under low-dose cyclosporine therapy. Am J Transplant 2011;11:2635.

Tait BD, Susal C, Gebel HM, et al. Consensus guidelines on the testing and clinical management issues associated with HLA and non-HLA antibodies in transplantation. Transplantation 2013;95:19.

Trappe R, Oertel S, Leblond V, et al. Sequential treatment with rituximab followed by CHOP chemotherapy in adult B-cell posttransplant lymphoproliferative disorder (PTLD): the prospective international multicentre phase 2 PTLD-1 trial. Lancet Oncol 2012;13:196.

Versele EB, Van Laecke S, Dhondt AW, et al. Bisphosphonates for preventing bone disease in kidney transplant recipients: a meta-analysis of randomized controlled trials. Transpl Int 2016;29:153.

Wiebe C, Gibson IW, Blydt-Hansen TD, et al. Rates and determinants of progression to graft failure in kidney allograft recipients with de novo donor-specific antibody. Am J Transplant 2015;15:2921.

Wyld ML, Clayton PA, Jesudason S, et al. Pregnancy outcomes for kidney transplant recipients. Am J Transplant 2013;13:3173.

Yanik EL, Clarke CA, Snyder JJ, et al. Variation in cancer incidence among patients with esrd during kidney function and nonfunction intervals. J Am Soc Nephrol 2016;27:1495.

12

Infections in Kidney Transplantation

Joanna M. Schaenman and
Bernard M. Kubak

Infection remains a significant cause of morbidity and mortality in renal transplant recipients. Compared to other solid-organ transplant candidates, the elective nature of kidney transplantation facilitates the opportunity to enhance clinical, nutritional, and prevention strategies (e.g., vaccination; identification of occult infectious processes; preemptive screening; assessing pretransplant immune function) to decrease infectious complications, and possibly decrease future rejection episodes as well. Infections related to transplant surgical complications, redo-transplantation, reexploration(s), donor-transmitted infections, acquisition of nosocomial pathogens, and reactivation of latent infectious processes can impact graft function and outcome. Graft dysfunction or chronic rejection requiring augmented immunosuppression increases the risk for infection in general, requiring increased surveillance and clinical suspicion. Systemic infections with immunomodulating viruses (e.g., cytomegalovirus and other human herpesviruses, hepatitis C) may also stimulate alterations in immunity and rejection, directly and indirectly. The predominant infectious syndromes encountered in the kidney transplant recipients include genitourinary infections, pneumonia, wound and abdominal fluid collection infections, device-related infections, and disseminated or organ-specific viral diseases.

This chapter highlights the infectious disease issues in kidney transplant recipients, post-transplantation infection prophylaxis, and the recognition and treatment of common and emerging infectious syndromes with appropriate antimicrobial therapy to minimize allograft toxicity.

GENERAL GUIDELINES FOR INFECTION RECOGNITION

Table 12.1 summarizes the risk factors for infection in the pretransplantation and post-transplantation periods. Recognition of the following factors may assist in the identification of the causative pathogen and the initiation of empiric antimicrobial therapy before laboratory confirmation:

1. *Timing of an infectious episode after transplantation*: Most infections occur in the first month after transplantation and are typically related to technical complications of the surgery or invasive medical devices and most commonly involve the genitourinary tract.

   During months 1 to 6, infections associated with postoperative complications or with enhanced immunosuppression can develop, persist, or recur. Augmented immunosuppression is associated with

Risk Factors for Infection in Renal Transplant Recipients

Pretransplantation

- Medical conditions (renal failure, diabetes, malnutrition, disorders of immune function, older patients)
- Immunosuppression for chronic conditions (corticosteroids, cyclophosphamide)
- Unrecognized or inadequately treated infection in the recipient
- Colonization with unusual or resistant organisms (e.g., VRE in stool, MRSA in nares or on skin, drug-resistant Enterobacteriaceae or *Pseudomonas* in genitourinary tract, gastrointestinal tract, and upper respiratory tract; acquisition of yeasts on mucocutaneous and other mucosal surfaces)
- Preoperative antibiotic exposures (e.g., increased infection risk for *Clostridium difficile* and antibiotic-resistant organisms)
- Duration and frequency of hospitalizations

Perioperative

- Complexity of surgery and requirement for reexploration
- Prolonged operative time
- Graft injury or prolonged ischemia, acute graft failure
- Bleeding or multiple blood transfusions
- Graft infection (donor) or unrecognized infection in the donor
- Perioperative bacteremia or sepsis
- Microbial contamination of preservation fluid of graft
- Retained foreign bodies

Post-transplantation

- Acute graft failure or dysfunction, requirements for augmented immunosuppression and prolonged cytolytic therapies
- Early reexploration or retransplantation
- Complicated postoperative management, development or worsening of comorbid medical conditions (hyperglycemia, hepatic disease, respiratory insufficiency, altered sensorium)
- Infection with immunomodulating viruses (CMV, HHV, respiratory viruses)
- Prolonged catheters, genitourinary stents, or mechanical ventilation
- Bladder-drained procedure, enteric-drained procedure (pancreas, kidney–pancreas transplantation), pancreas transplantation after kidney transplantation
- Anastomotic breakdown or leaks, development of fluid collections, devitalized tissues, hematomas
- Leukopenia, thrombocytopenia, acquired hypogammaglobulinemia
- Prolonged antibiotic therapy, acquisition of antibiotic-resistant healthcare pathogens
- Corticosteroids: maintenance dose and pulses
- Hospital exposures: construction, ventilation, and water supply
- Selected occupational, gardening, and recreational activities: composting, exposure to decaying vegetation, hunting
- Lack of appropriate hand hygiene by caregivers
- Use of inhaled marijuana

CMV, cytomegalovirus; HHV, human herpesvirus; MRSA, methicillin-resistant *Staphylococcus aureus*; VRE, vancomycin-resistant *Enterococcus*.

an increased risk for infection with immunomodulating viruses, such as cytomegalovirus (CMV) and other human herpesviruses (HHV), hepatitis B virus (HBV), hepatitis C virus (HCV), and Epstein–Barr virus (EBV), which enhance susceptibility to opportunistic infections by altering the expression of inflammatory mediators and cytokines by a complex interrelated cascade. These viruses can facilitate a permissive environment for opportunistic pathogens, especially fungi; prominent pathogens include *Aspergillus, Pneumocystis, Cryptococcus,* among others, bacteria, and other pathogens including *Listeria monocytogenes, Nocardia,* and *Toxoplasma.* CMV and other human herpesviruses also exert an immunomodulating effect implicated in acute allograft rejection, chronic rejection, and post-transplantation lymphoproliferative disorder (PTLD).

Patients who have reached month 6 after transplantation without treatment for rejection or reoperation can generally be categorized as having successful graft outcome with stable long-term maintenance immunosuppression, and lower infectious risks. Recipients with poor graft function, rejection treatments requiring intensified immunosuppression, or persistently altered genitourinary dysfunction and physiology can lead to CMV, nosocomially-acquired infections, and reactivation of infectious foci. Infections in patients with long-term successful allografts are typically similar to those reported in the community for nontransplant patients; however, with chronic immunosuppression, the risk for opportunistic infections remains.

2. *The net state of immunosuppression* is a semiquantitative assessment that reflects the complex interaction of the following factors:
   1. The dose, duration, and temporal sequence of immunosuppressive therapy, including augmented immunosuppression for episodes of rejection.
   2. The types of immune suppression used for induction, maintenance, desensitization, and/or treatment for rejection. Antilymphocyte antibody preparations such as antithymocyte globulin (ATG) or alemtuzumab lead to severe deficits in cell-mediated immunity, while antibody-directed therapies such as bortezomib or rituximab can impair B cell and humoral immunity. The impact of newer agents such as mTOR inhibitors and the T-cell costimulation inhibitor belatacept is an area of ongoing study.
   3. Quantitative immunodeficiency, including leukopenia, thrombocytopenia, and low immunoglobulin levels.
   4. Breach of skin and tissue barriers by foreign bodies (e.g., urinary and venous catheters, ureteral stents), nonhealing wounds, fluid collections, and devitalized tissues.
   5. Metabolic abnormalities: hyperglycemia, uremia, liver failure, and malnutrition and disorders of absorption.
   6. Infection with immunomodulatory viruses.
3. *The infectious history of the donor,* specifically any infectious syndromes and pathogen that can be directly transmitted with the allograft (see Chapter 4, Part I).
4. *Recipient history of infections and exposures*: mycobacterial infections (tuberculosis and nontuberculous mycobacteria), fungal infections, hepatitis viruses, human immunodeficiency virus (HIV),

varicella-zoster virus (VZV), CMV, or EBV; immune-altering conditions such as surgical or functional asplenia; concurrent chronic pretransplantation medical conditions including rheumatologic disorders, such as systemic lupus erythematosus, that require immunosuppressive therapy, diabetes mellitus, chronic pulmonary diseases (e.g., COPD, bronchiectasis, pulmonary fibrosis), substance or injection drug use, liver dysfunction, malnutrition, and potential risk for exposure to geographically restricted endemic mycoses, toxoplasmosis, tuberculosis, and *Strongyloides* species. In addition, increased patient age and its associated immune senescence is an independent risk factor for increased rates of infection and death after transplantation. The delay between listing for transplantation and actual receipt of a kidney allograft can further complicate the evaluation process. Prospective candidates can acquire new infections during this waiting period and/or modify their infectious risk factors.

5. *The acquisition of community and healthcare-associated pathogens*: *Streptococcus pneumoniae*, Enterobacteriaceae, multidrug-resistant gram-negative organisms, and *Pseudomonas* species, methicillin-resistant *Staphylococcus aureus* (MRSA), and vancomycin-resistant *Enterococcus* (VRE). Pretransplantation dialysis patients and kidney recipients may be colonized by bacteria and yeasts on their skin, sinopulmonary system, and gastrointestinal tract related to frequent contact with healthcare settings and antimicrobial exposure(s). In the setting of graft dysfunction, postoperative surgical complications, or rejection, these colonizing organisms have the potential to cause invasive infection. Identifying these colonizing organisms and, when appropriate, determining antimicrobial susceptibility may help to direct empiric antimicrobial therapy if clinical infection develops.

6. *Factors that delay or confound the diagnosis of infection in the recipient* include an impaired host inflammatory response; the delay in clinical diagnosis because of the lack of classical clinical and radiologic signs associated with infection and inflammation compared with the immunocompetent host; the rapid progression of infections in this context, particularly with altered anatomy, lymphatic drainage, and physiology after transplantation; the failure to recognize high-risk patient characteristics (e.g., diabetes, enhanced and prolonged immunosuppression, multiple antibiotic courses); and delays in laboratory diagnosis and limited rapid diagnostic assays for fungal, mycobacterial, and viral diseases.

PRETRANSPLANT SCREENING: DONOR AND RECIPIENT

Untreated or unrecognized infections in the recipient can become clinically apparent in the post-transplantation period. These can include intravascular device infection, pneumonia, periodontal disease, intra-abdominal, hepatobiliary, or genitourinary tract infection. During pretransplantation screening, the identification of latent or active infections in the recipient can lead to a reappraisal of transplant candidacy or to alterations in standard post-transplantation antimicrobial therapy.

For the living donor, a careful history of potential latent infections should be ascertained, and any active infection should be treated when appropriate. Donation should be deferred until the respective infection is properly assessed and resolved.

It may be difficult to differentiate among an infection acquired from the allograft, from an exogenous source, or from reactivation of latent disease in the recipient. The following infectious agents have been implicated in transmission from the donor allograft: aerobic Gram-positive and Gram-negative bacteria, anaerobic bacteria, *Mycobacteria* species, *Toxoplasma* species, and *Strongyloides* species; HIV, CMV, HBV, HCV, herpes simplex virus (HSV), VZV, EBV, and West Nile virus (WNV), viruses implicated in central nervous system infection; and fungi including *Candida* species, *Histoplasma capsulatum*, *Coccidioides immitis*, *Cryptococcus neoformans*, *Aspergillus* species, and *Scedosporium apiospermum*. Serious complications of donor allograft-transmitted infections include bacteremia, fungemia, disruption of the vascular anastomoses, formation of "mycotic" (microbial) aneurysms, and infective endocarditis. The risk for donor-transmitted infection can be reduced by careful screening and epidemiologic evaluation (see Chapter 4, Part I).

Screening of Potential Deceased Organ Donors for Transmissible Disease

Postoperative infections can arise from inadequate or incomplete donor screening. The donor's medical and social history should include information on exposure risks based on birth or residence in areas with endemic infection, such as tuberculosis and the endemic fungal and parasitic infections. In addition, the cause of death and complications of prolonged intubation and hospitalization can result in donor infection. Public Health Service (PHS) guidelines can identify donors at "increased risk" for transmission of HIV, HBV, and HCV based on behaviors and exposures associated with increased prevalence of infection including injection drug use, history of incarceration, sex for money or drugs, or hemodialysis. Large-volume donor blood transfusion can lead to hemodilution, limiting the accuracy of donor serum testing; calculations should be performed by organ procurement agencies. Donors identified as PHS increased risk are mandated to undergo nucleic acid testing (NAT) for HBV, HCV, HIV, decreasing, although not eliminating, the chances of transmission of disease during the "window period" of infection. The organ procurement organization should provide results of donor microbiology cultures, and NAT or PCR-based testing, serum serologies, and history of infections, including upper and lower urinary tract infection (UTI) and bacteremia that may not be confirmed by the laboratory until after transplantation in some cases. Communication of pending donor infection results is essential between the organ procurement organization and transplant center. Because many deceased donor kidneys may be recovered from patients in intensive care units, occult bacteremia or UTI should be excluded by appropriate cultures. In the case of donor-associated bacteremia, appropriate antimicrobial therapy should be administered to the recipient typically for 14 days, and follow-up blood cultures should be obtained to exclude endovascular infection of the vascular anastomosis. Although rare, this complication has been associated with donor-derived bloodstream infection with *S. aureus, Pseudomonas aeruginosa*, other gram-negative bacilli, and *Candida* and *Aspergillus* species. During the allograft recovery and transplantation, microbial contamination of the preservation media can occur. In such cases, appropriate antimicrobial therapy should be administered to the recipient, typically for 14 days. Syphilis has been transmitted by solid-organ transplantation, but is not a contraindication to organ donation since the recipient can receive treatment appropriate to the presumed stage of donor syphilis infection. Deceased donor kidneys have been transplanted successfully from donors with localized, nongenitourinary infections, including pneumonia and meningitis. However, donors with active fungal infection, especially bloodstream and genitourinary infections, unspecified viral infections, suspicion of encephalitis, or ambiguous causes of infectious death should be avoided. In addition, it is optimal that potential donors from relevant endemic areas be screened for parasitic infections including *Trypanosoma cruzi* and *Strongyloides*. During periods of increased incidence of WNV, this infection should ideally be screened for in both living and deceased donors.

As of this writing, the World Health Organization has designated injection with the mosquito-borne Zika virus to be an international health emergency because of its likely relationship to microcephaly and Guillain–Barré syndrome. Sexual transmission has been reported and though transmission via organ transplantation has not been described, a history of travel to South and Central America with a febrile illness and a rash should raise concern.

Transplant Candidate Screening for Infectious Disease

Evaluation of the transplant candidate for infection risk should include a history of antibiotic allergies and nature of reaction, a dental examination, and assessment for remote or active infection, including a urine culture and chest radiograph (Table 12.2). Patients with polycystic kidney disease who have been treated for infected polycystic kidneys should have repeatedly negative urine cultures. Pretransplantation polycystic nephrectomy is occasionally required (see Chapter 8). Patients requiring current immunosuppression, such as those with rheumatologic disease or vasculitis, or those who are previous transplant recipients, should be subject to special scrutiny as their risk for infection is higher than that for the general chronic kidney disease population. The candidate should be evaluated for potential risk for exposure to *Mycobacterium tuberculosis* or endemic mycoses, including history of prior residence or travel to high-risk areas, purified protein derivative (PPD) skin test, blood interferon-gamma release assay (IGRA), such as the quantiferon gold test, and, if indicated, serologic testing for *C. immitis* or antigen testing for *H. capsulatum*, especially if the chest radiograph demonstrated calcified or noncalcified granuloma. Living donors should have an IGRA test for tuberculosis if they have risk factors based on behavior or previous travel or residence in endemic areas, and urine acid-fast bacillus

TABLE 12.2	Transplant Candidate Screening

Underlying medical conditions (see Chapter 7)

Antibiotic and medication allergies and adverse reactions

Chest radiograph (e.g., any evidence of active infiltrates, old granulomatous lesions, scarring)

Dental assessment

History of sexually transmitted diseases, high-risk behaviors, injection drug usage

Purified protein derivative (PPD) skin test or interferon-gamma release assay (IGRA); history of tuberculosis risk factors and exposures

Urine culture

Routine serologic testing:

    Cytomegalovirus (CMV) IgG antibody

    Epstein–Barr virus (EBV) antibody panel

    Herpes simplex virus (HSV) and varicella-zoster virus (VZV) IgG antibodies

    Hepatitis B virus (HBV) surface antigen (HBsAg), core antibody (HBcAb IgM and IgG), surface antibody (HBsAb)

    Hepatitis C virus (HCV) IgG antibody

    HIV 1 and 2 antibody

    Rapid plasma reagin (RPR) or TP-PA (*Treponema pallidum* particle agglutination) test for syphilis

Special serologic testing (based on epidemiologic risk factor or exposure history):

    Coccidioides IgM and IgG antibody by enzyme immunosorbent assay (EIA)

    Histoplasma immunodiffusion antibody or urine antigen

    Human T-cell lymphotropic virus (HTLV-I/II) antibody

    Strongyloides antibody

    Trypanosoma cruzi antibody

(AFB) stain and mycobacterial cultures should be obtained if there is a history compatible with disseminated tuberculosis. PPD skin test is a second-choice option for those without access to IGRA testing. The higher incidence of indeterminate test results in patients with end-stage renal disease (ESRD) may confound the tuberculosis risk assessment, so it is critical to assess for a history of latent or active tuberculosis or compatible chest radiograph and to administer isoniazid prophylaxis, if indicated. The 2003 American Thoracic Society and Centers for Disease Control and Prevention (CDC)/Infectious Diseases Society of America guideline recommends treatment of latent tuberculosis with isoniazid (5 mg/kg/day, maximum of 300 mg daily for adults) plus pyridoxine (vitamin B_6) for 9 months. Patients who previously completed an adequate treatment course for latent or active tuberculosis typically do not require additional antituberculous therapy after transplantation. However, this diagnosis should be considered if infectious complications occur post-transplant. Preoperative antibody testing, when appropriate, should include CMV, VZV, EBV, HSV-1 and -2, and HIV-1 and -2; anti–hepatitis B virus surface antibody (anti-HBsAb), surface antigen (HBsAg), and core antibody (HBcAb); and HCV antibody (see Chapter 12); and testing for endemic mycoses and parasites when appropriate.

Specific Serologic Testing
Cytomegalovirus
The seroprevalence of CMV ranges from 40% to 97%, depending on the population screened, and increases with age. Most adult dialysis patients have detectable immunoglobulin G (IgG) antibody to CMV. The CMV antibody status of the donor and recipient should be ascertained. A CMV-seronegative recipient (R–) of a CMV-seropositive donor (D+) is at the highest risk for developing subsequent CMV infection and disease. After transplantation, these recipients should receive antiviral prophylaxis, typically for 6 months, and careful clinical and laboratory monitoring for evidence of CMV viremia. Recipients receiving antilymphocytic therapy may require antiviral prophylaxis rather than preemptive monitoring as well. Although CMV-seropositive recipients (D+/R+, D–/R+) have a lower risk for CMV disease, a similar prevention strategy should be employed, based on the individual patient risk factors and net state of immunosuppression. The clinical implications of the CMV infection are discussed in "Viral Infections" and summarized in Table 12.3.

Epstein–Barr Virus
Both EBV-seronegative recipients of grafts from EBV-seropositive donors and EBV-seropositive recipients may be at increased risk for PTLD, particularly if they receive prolonged or repeated courses of antilymphocytic therapy (see Chapter 11). EBV mismatch occurs more commonly in pediatric kidney recipients. In high-risk patients, the quantitative EBV viral load can be assessed by polymerase chain reaction (PCR). The costimulation inhibitor belatacept carries a black-box warning excluding use in EBV D+/R– patients owing to observed increased PTLD risk during Phase 3 studies.

TABLE 12.3 Risk for CMV Infection and Disease without CMV Prophylaxis by Donor and Recipient CMV Serostatus

Donor	Recipient	Terminology	Cytomegalovirus Antibody Status		
			Infection (%)	Disease (%)	Pneumonitis (%)
+	–	Primary infection	70–88	56–80	30
–	+	Reactivation	0–20	0–27	Rare
+	+*	Reactivation or superinfection	70	27–39	3–14
–	–		Zero†	—	—
±	+	With antirejection, ALA plus conventional immunosuppression‡	—	65	—

*The source of infection and disease may be a new virus strain from the donor or latent virus in the recipient.
†Inadequate or incorrect donor–recipient screening, or viral acquisition during recent peritransplantation periods may result in false-negative serologies; in this case, recent serologies are recommended.
‡Results with conventional immunosuppression: cyclosporine or tacrolimus, azathioprine (or mycophenolate mofetil), prednisone, and antilymphocyte antibody (ALA).
(Data from Davis CL. The prevention of cytomegalovirus disease in renal transplantation. Am J Kidney Dis 1990;16:175–188; Hartmann A, Sagedal S, Hjelmesaeth J. The natural course of cytomegalovirus infection and disease in renal transplant recipients. Transplantation 2006;82:S15–S17.)

Other Human Herpesviruses

Other HHVs of significance to organ transplant recipients include HSV-1 and -2, VZV, and HHV-6 and HHV-8. HHV-6 has been implicated as a cofactor for CMV and other infections. HHV-8 may cause transplant-associated Kaposi sarcoma and EBV-negative lymphoproliferative disease. Generally, screening for HHV-6 and -8 is not performed before transplantation.

Hepatitis B and C

The detection of chronic HBV and HCV infection in both transplant donors and recipients has improved with newer laboratory methods to detect viral-specific antibodies, antigens, and nucleic acids. One of the most important pretransplant assessments is for presence of hepatitis B immunity, as measured by detectable HBV surface antibody. Evaluation of HCV infection in donor and recipient has been transformed in past years by the advent of treatment regimens with curative ability. Each center should assess their respective experience in the evaluation and treatment of patients with hepatitis C infections in evaluating candidacy of these patients. Liaisons with specialists in hepatitis should be a component of transplant recipient assessments. The impact of latent or active HBV and HCV infection on transplant candidacy and kidney donation is discussed in Chapter 13. Particular attention should be paid to the impact of the new and dramatically effective treatments for HCV.

Human Immunodeficiency Virus

All potential transplant donors should be tested for HIV-1 and -2 antibody. A history of any increased-risk behaviors must be obtained, because transplant-derived HIV infection has been associated with acute infection in the seronegative "window" period or associated with massive blood transfusion and false-negative donor HIV antibody test results (see Chapter 4). Routine donor HIV antibody testing and performance of HIV NAT testing in PHS increased risk donors (see above) has reduced the risk for infection to an almost negligible degree. For recipients with HIV, outcomes after kidney transplantation approach those of HIV-negative recipients, with ongoing improvements with the advent of newer antiretroviral regimens with decreased risk for drug–drug interaction with the calcineurin inhibitors (CNIs). The HIV Organ Policy Equity (HOPE) Act, signed into law in 2013, has opened the door for HIV-positive to HIV-positive transplantation, currently only under the supervision of an institutional-review board approved clinical trial.

Human T-Lymphotropic Viruses

Human T-lymphotropic virus 1 (HTLV-1) is more common in individuals from the Caribbean and Japan. Blood products, organ transplants, and intimate contact can transmit HTLV-1. Clinical syndromes include HTLV-1–associated myelopathy or tropical spastic paraparesis and adult T-cell leukemia and lymphoma virus. HTLV-1 myelopathy has been reported after transplantation from an infected donor. HTLV-2 is serologically similar to HTLV-1, but disease association is under investigation. Because of low prevalence of infection in the US population, this serology testing is no longer mandatory under United Network for Organ Sharing (UNOS) guidance but may be indicated for donors or recipients from high-endemicity areas.

West Nile Virus
WNV is a vector-borne flavivirus transmitted from the bite of an infected mosquito, and much less commonly through blood and transplanted organs. In late 2002, the CDC confirmed the transmission of WNV to organ recipients from a single donor with serious consequences to the recipients. First-generation serologic and PCR assays are available. The epidemiology of WNV has changed rapidly, so the extent of risk to the donor pool and recipients remains under investigation. During summer and autumn months, it is prudent to avoid organs from donors from an area with active WNV infection who have symptoms of a viral illness, especially encephalitis or meningitis. Screening by PCR and serology testing can help identify donors at risk for transmission of WNV disease.

Coccidioidomycosis and Histoplasmosis
Candidates who have resided in at-risk geographic areas should be tested for *C. immitis* IgM and IgG antibody by enzyme immunoassay (EIA) or *H. capsulatum* antibody by immunodiffusion or serum or urine antigen during transplant evaluation. Because of the substantial risk for reactivation, recipients with a history of prior infection with endemic fungi or who have detectable antibodies should receive prophylactic azole antifungal therapy following renal transplantation typically for an indefinite period after transplantation.

Strongyloides and Trypanosoma cruzi
Donors and candidates from parts of the world where these parasitic diseases are endemic should be screened by serology testing prior to transplantation. Donors or recipients with positive serology testing should receive two doses of ivermectin, separated by a 2-week interval, to eradicate parasites from the gastrointestinal tract. Kidney transplant donors with positive *T. cruzi* testing may be used, but recipient will be at risk for possible disease transmission and should be monitored post-transplantation. Recipients with positive *T. cruzi* serology should also be monitored by PCR testing to detect reactivation after transplantation.

Transplant Candidate and Recipient Immunization
Vaccine-preventable infections are a major source of morbidity following solid-organ transplantation. During the transplant evaluation, the candidate's immunization history should be carefully reviewed and immunizations updated. Current adult and pediatric immunization schedules are available at http://www.cdc.gov/vaccines/recs/schedules/default.htm, and updated recommendations for vaccination of solid-organ transplant recipients were published in 2016 and are summarized in Table 12.4.

Unless there are contraindications, VZV-seronegative transplant candidates should receive two doses of live varicella vaccine, and seropositive candidates 60 years or older should receive a single dose of live zoster vaccine to decrease the risk for varicella disease. Other live attenuated vaccines, such as measles, mumps, and rubella (MMR)

TABLE 124 Recommended Immunizations for Pediatric and Adult Transplant Candidates and Recipients

Vaccine	Inactivated/Live Attenuated (I/LA)	Pediatric/Adult (P/A)	Recommended before Transplantation	Recommended after Transplantation	Frequency of Administration
Haemophilus influenzae B	I	P	Yes	Yes	3 doses
Hepatitis B	I	P/A	Yes	Yes	3 doses
Hepatitis A	I	P/A	Yes	Yes	2 doses
Human papillomavirus	I	P/A	Yes	Yes	3 doses, ages 11–26 yr
Influenza, injected	I	P/A	Yes	Yes	Yearly
Measles, mumps, rubella (MMR)	LA	P	Yes	No	2 doses
Meningococcal (conjugated or polysaccharide vaccine)	I/I	P/A	Yes	Yes	1 dose*
Polio, inactivated	I	P	Yes	Yes	4 doses
S. pneumoniae (conjugated and polysaccharide vaccine)	I/I	P/A	Yes	Yes	See footnote†
Tetanus, diphtheria, acellular pertussis (Td/Tdap)	I	P/A	Yes	Yes	3 doses of Tdap in childhood, 1 dose of Td every 10 yr‡
Varicella	LA	P/A	Yes	No	See footnote§
Zoster	LA	A	Yes	No	See footnote‖

*Indicated for adults with anatomic or functional asplenia or terminal complement component deficiencies, preadolescents, first-year college students living in dormitories, and others determined to be at risk.

†Children older than 5 years should receive 23-valent pneumococcal polysaccharide vaccine (Pneumovax). Children younger than 2 years should receive three doses of conjugated pneumococcal vaccine (Prevnar). Pneumovax should be repeated for patients 65 years of age or older, at least 5 years after the last Pneumovax dose, and 1 year after Prevnar vaccination.

‡Tdap (Adacel) should replace a single dose of Td for adults younger than 65 years who have not previously received a dose of Tdap.

§Children and nonimmune adults should receive two doses of varicella vaccine (Varivax).

‖Adults older than 60 years should receive a single dose of zoster vaccine (Zostavax).

and varicella, should be administered no later than 4 to 6 weeks before transplantation to minimize the possibility of vaccine-derived infection in the post-transplantation period. Ideally, household contacts of transplant recipients should be fully immunized to protect the transplant recipient. Live vaccines should be avoided before transplantation in candidates receiving immunosuppressive therapy and following solid-organ transplantation. Other live attenuated vaccines, including Bacillus Calmette-Guérin, oral polio, and live attenuated influenza vaccine, should also be avoided.

Inactivated vaccines are safe to administer to transplant recipients and include hepatitis A and hepatitis B, intramuscular influenza A and B, 23-valent unconjugated and 13-valent conjugated pneumococcal, *Haemophilus influenzae* B, inactivated polio, diphtheria-acellular pertussis-tetanus (Tdap), and polysaccharide or conjugated meningococcal vaccines. Annual influenza vaccination is recommended for transplant candidates and recipients. The anecdotal risk of rejection with influenza immunization has not been substantiated in randomized trials of solid-organ transplant recipients, whereas influenza infection in these patients is associated with higher morbidity and mortality, graft rejection, and prolonged viral shedding. Immunization with meningococcal and inactivated polio vaccines may be appropriate for special risk situations, including travel or occupational risk. An accelerated schedule for hepatitis B immunization can be used before and following transplantation, especially if the organ is from a donor positive for anti-HBsAb. Following hepatitis B immunization, anti-HBsAb levels should be measured to document seroconversion.

PATHOGENESIS AND DIAGNOSIS OF INFECTION IN KIDNEY ALLOGRAFT RECIPIENTS

Post-transplant infections impact both on patient morbidity and mortality and allograft function. Approximately 80% of infections in kidney transplant recipients are bacterial. Tables 12.5 and 12.6 summarize the syndromes and microbial pathogens commonly encountered in kidney transplant recipients. Infections occurring during the first month are typically associated with donor-derived infections or nosocomial infections including technical complications of the surgery or indwelling medical devices and most commonly include genitourinary tract infection, bacteremia, surgical-site infection, pneumonia, and intra-abdominal infection. Risk of infection is also increased after treatment for rejection.

Infections in kidney transplant recipients can be difficult to diagnose because concomitant immunosuppression and alterations in the immune response attenuate the usual clinical signs and symptoms of infection such as fever and leukocytosis. High clinical suspicion and prompt administration of empiric antimicrobial therapy are essential for effective treatment and prevention of infectious complications. Resistant infections or coinfection with more than one pathogen should be considered in an immunocompromised patient, especially when failing to respond to targeted antimicrobial therapy. Increased patient age is another risk factor for infection.

TABLE 12.5

Commonly Encountered Bacterial Pathogens in Renal Transplant Recipients Listed by Site of Infection

Intra-abdominal	Septicemia	Urinary Tract	Pneumonia	Wound	Dermatologic (Cellulitis)
Enterobacteriaceae Enterococcus sp. Anaerobes (Bacteroides sp.)	Enterobacteriaceae Pseudomonas aeruginosa Staphylococcus aureus (methicillin-sensitive and methicillin-resistant strains)	Enterobacteriaceae P. aeruginosa Enterococcus sp.	Enterobacteriaceae, P. aeruginosa Streptococcus pneumoniae, S. aureus (methicillin-sensitive and methicillin-resistant) Mixed flora from aspiration	Mixed infection Enterobacteriaceae P. aeruginosa	Staphylococcus sp. Streptococcus sp. Enterobacteriaceae
S. aureus	Enterococcus sp. (vancomycin-sensitive and vancomycin-resistant strains)	—	Nocardia sp.	Enterococcus sp.	P. aeruginosa (ecthyma)
Mixed infection	Rare: anaerobes (Bacteroides sp.)	—	Legionella sp.	S. aureus	Atypical Mycobacterium sp. (nodules)
—	Rhodococcus sp.	—	Mycobacterium tuberculosis, atypical Mycobacterium sp., Rhodococcus sp. (rare)	Anaerobes (Bacteroides sp.)	

	Sinopulmonary	Genitourinary Tract	Gastrointestinal System	Central Nervous System	Dermatologic
	Aspergillus, Cryptococcus	*Candida*	CMV, HSV, adenovirus	*Cryptococcus, Aspergillus*	*Candida*, dermatophytes (*Microsporum, Trichophyton Epidermophyton*), *Malassezia*
	Less common: Mucormycosis, *Coccidioides, Histoplasma, Scedosporium* (*Pseudallescheria*)	Less common: *Aspergillus* (rare)	Less common: EBV	Less common: *Coccidioides, Scedosporium*	Less common: *Cryptococcus, Aspergillus, Coccidioides, Histoplasma*, phaeohyphomycosis
	Pneumocystis	CMV, adenovirus, polyomavirus, papillomavirus	*Candida, Aspergillus*, Mucormycosis	CMV, HSV, VZV, West Nile virus, (rare: EBV, JC virus)	HSV, VZV
	CMV, community-acquired respiratory viruses	—	—	—	—
	Less common: EBV, VZV	—	—	—	—

CMV, cytomegalovirus; EBV, Epstein–Barr virus; HSV, herpes simplex virus; VZV, varicella-zoster virus.

TABLE 12.6 Commonly Encountered Nonbacterial Pathogens in Renal Transplant Recipients Listed by Site of Infection

Urinary Tract Infection

Genitourinary infection is the most common complication after kidney transplantation both early and late after transplantation, with reported incidence ranging up to 75%, with variation in reported rates likely resulting from differences in case definitions. In the immediate post-transplant period, the risk for genitourinary infection is directly related to complications of the surgical procedure, such as urine leaks, wound hematomas, and lymphoceles, that can result in bacterial superinfection and abscess formation. Genitourinary tract manipulation during transplantation, urinary catheters, ureteral stents, anatomic abnormalities (e.g., ureterovesicular stenosis, ureteral stricture, vesicoureteric reflux, bladder augmentation), and neurogenic bladder also predispose to post-transplantation UTI, as do increased patient age, female sex, and need for dialysis after transplantation. Early catheter removal decreased the incidence of UTI in renal allograft recipients. Asymptomatic bacteriuria has been reported in close to 60% of kidney transplant recipients in the first month after transplantation, and frequent episodes are associated with development of pyelonephritis and development of acute rejection. However, the bacteriuria may resolve without treatment, and it is not clear whether treatment results in decreased incidence of graft pyelonephritis; however, these patients should be monitored for progression to invasive infection.

A clean-catch midstream urine specimen should be submitted for urinalysis and quantitative bacterial and fungal culture. In renal transplant recipients, lower levels of bacteriuria may be associated with a significant risk for systemic infection. In addition, asymptomatic bacteriuria and infection are associated with development of impaired graft function and/or acute cellular rejection via cytokine activation, immune dysregulation, and direct kidney injury. Infection may be more difficult to eradicate when associated with ureteral stents that can lead to formation of biofilm. If possible, the stent should be removed. Infected perigraft fluid collections or devitalized tissues often require percutaneous or open incision, in addition to directed antimicrobial therapy, to resolve the infection. Infections owing to multidrug-resistant organisms are more likely to recur. Patients with recurrent UTI should undergo anatomic assessment including evaluation for possible ureteral reflux, presence of urinary stones, and for women, gynecologic exam. Use of methenamine and vitamin C for prophylaxis may reduce the frequency of infection recurrence.

Bacteremia and Candidemia

Among renal transplant recipients, the urinary tract is the most common primary site of infection associated with secondary bacteremia. Among patients with bloodstream infections, poor outcome is associated with Gram-negative species, multidrug-resistant organisms, and *Candida* species, especially when the empiric antimicrobial therapy is inappropriate or delayed. Some studies suggest that bacterial sepsis increases the risk for CMV infection because of high levels of tumor necrosis factor-α (TNF-α) or dysregulated immune response to CMV in the context of serious bacterial infections.

For detection of bloodstream infection, two sets of blood cultures should be obtained before initiation of antimicrobial therapy, but immediate treatment should not be delayed to prevent the occurrence of sepsis and shock. Candidemia is associated with high-dose corticosteroids for rejection; vascular, drainage, or urinary catheters; total parenteral nutrition; gastrointestinal inflammation or perforation; and diabetes mellitus. Fungal blood cultures may decrease the time to obtaining a positive blood culture result, but are no more sensitive than routine bacterial blood cultures for detection of *Candida* species. If intravascular catheter-associated bacteremia is suspected, the device should be removed and the catheter tip should be cultured.

Pneumonia

Bacterial pneumonia is the most common life-threatening infection in kidney transplant recipients. The risk for pneumonia is increased among patients who require prolonged intubation, those with structural lung disease, and those with diminished gag reflex, prolonged nasogastric tube use, or impaired diaphragmatic function that increases the risk for aspiration. Hospital environmental exposure to certain species from contaminated water or aerosols, including *Legionella* and *Pseudomonas,* also increase the risk for pneumonia.

Diagnostic specimens for post-transplantation pneumonia may include blood, expectorated sputum, tracheal suction, bronchoalveolar lavage (BAL) fluid, transthoracic fine-needle aspirate, and, occasionally, lung biopsy. Blood cultures may assist in the etiologic diagnosis of pneumonia because 10% to 15% of patients with pneumonia have secondary bacteremia. Fiberoptic bronchoscopy with BAL and transbronchial biopsy is valuable in the diagnosis of severe pneumonia, especially when the episode is associated with an accessible pulmonary lesion. The diagnostic yield of BAL has been reported as 36% for kidney and liver transplant recipients with pulmonary infections. *Legionella* species can be cultured using charcoal media, and *Legionella pneumophila* group 1 antigen can be detected in urine specimens. Respiratory specimens should be obtained for fungal culture and stain using a sensitive method such as calcofluor staining. Fluorescein-labeled monoclonal antibody staining of BAL or sputum specimens increases the sensitivity for detection of *Pneumocystis jiroveci*. *Nocardia* species can be identified presumptively when modified acid-fast staining reveals delicately branching filamentous and beaded gram-positive rods. Acid-fast staining of respiratory specimens, biopsy specimens, nodules, and lymph nodes may reveal mycobacterial forms. Once there is growth detected on culture, specific DNA probes for *M. tuberculosis* and *Mycobacterium avium* complex can confirm the diagnosis of infections associated with these species. PCR-based testing for influenza and other community-acquired respiratory viruses from nasopharyngeal swab or BAL fluid can identify pathogens in viral pneumonitis, and from BAL fluid or biopsy for CMV qualitative PCR testing.

Chest computed tomography (CT) is valuable in the diagnosis of infectious pneumonia and can be used to guide percutaneous or thoracoscopic biopsy of suspicious lesions. As many as 10% of immunocompromised patients with pneumonia will have normal chest X-ray, with abnormalities apparent only on CT. Concurrent immunosuppression and attenuated inflammatory response can modify the radiographic appearance and progression of pneumonia in transplant recipients. Noninfectious etiologies of pulmonary infiltrates are frequent in transplant recipients and include atelectasis, aspiration (early), contusion, hemorrhage, infarction or emboli, malignancy, capillary leak, and pulmonary edema.

Intra-abdominal Infections

Preexisting medical conditions unrelated to ESRD, such as diverticulosis or biliary disease, can become apparent in the post-transplantation period. Immunosuppression, including corticosteroids, increases the risk for diverticulitis and colonic perforation and gastric perforation by diminishing mucosal immune surveillance, mucosal integrity, and fibroblastic activity. Thrombocytopenia is also implicated in this pathophysiology. Hypoperfusion of the gastrointestinal mucosa, from hypotension or use of vasopressor agents, also increases the risk for mucosal translocation, perforation, and secondary sepsis. History of infections related to peritoneal disease may also increase the risk of post-transplant complications.

Surgical Site and Other Infections

The incidence of surgical site infection following kidney transplantation ranges from 2% to 25%. These infections typically occur within 3 weeks after transplantation and are usually related to technical complications and recipient factors, such as obesity and diabetes. The infection can involve the perinephric space or cause mycotic aneurysms at the site of the vascular anastomosis. Rarely, allograft nephrectomy is required. In pancreas–kidney transplant recipients, pancreatic abscess with Gram-negative organisms or fungi may require surgical drainage or graft removal.

Diagnosis of infection associated with surgical wounds, skin nodules, or necrotic ulcers should include aspiration of any drainable material, a deep swab specimen from the site, and a biopsy specimen, when appropriate. Gram stain, aerobic and anaerobic bacterial culture, and fungal and acid-fast stains and cultures should be performed. Percutaneous or open drainage may be necessary in case of infected perigraft collections, hematomas, or urinomas.

Culture of fluid collections should be performed in patients with unexplained fever or other signs and symptoms of infection in the early postoperative period. In most circumstances, percutaneous or open drainage of infected fluid collections or hematomas is necessary for resolving the infection. Ultrasound or CT guidance can assist in localization and drainage catheter placement. Failure to remove an infected device or drain the infected fluid collections may lead to prolonged antimicrobial therapy and an increased risk for resistance, treatment failure, drug toxicity, and graft dysfunction. Patients with diarrhea, colitis, or abdominal symptoms who have received antibiotic therapy should have stool specimens collected for *Clostridium difficile* PCR or toxin A and B detection. Other causes of diarrhea after transplantation include bacterial infection owing to *Campylobacter* or *Salmonella*, viral infection owing to CMV, norovirus, or rotavirus, and parasitic infections. Mycophenolate-induced mucosal changes may occur concurrently, complicating the diagnosis.

Approach to the Kidney Transplant Recipient with Fever

The differential diagnosis of fever in the kidney transplant recipient is broad and includes infection, graft rejection, drug allergy, and noninfectious systemic inflammatory response (e.g., pancreatitis, pulmonary embolism, or transfusion reaction). Although fever may accompany acute rejection, most patients with rejection are afebrile. Temperature elevations may occur during treatment of rejection with polyclonal antibodies as a result of cytokine release (see Chapter 6). A detailed history and physical exam should be undertaken to try to establish any possible localizing symptoms or findings. For the patient with fever and sepsis, diagnostic testing and empiric antibiotic therapy should be initiated promptly.

MICROBIAL ETIOLOGY, TREATMENT PRINCIPLES, AND SPECIFIC THERAPY

Bacterial Infections

The bacterial pathogens in the early post-transplantation period are similar to those causing healthcare-associated infections in the nontransplant surgical population (Tables 12.5 and 12.6). In the early post-transplantation period, Enterobacteriaceae, *Staphylococcus*, and *Pseudomonas* species are the most commonly isolated healthcare pathogens and increasingly are multidrug resistant. Aerobic Gram-negative bacilli constitute nearly half of all pathogens detected by blood culture, and infection is associated with a 2-week mortality rate of over 10%. Secondary bacteremia most commonly arises from the urinary tract, lung, abdomen, or surgical wound. Urinary tract infections among renal allograft recipients should be considered complicated UTIs and treated for a sufficient length of time to prevent systemic spread of infection. Although uncommon, infective endocarditis in the early post-transplantation period has been associated with *S. aureus,* coagulase-negative *Staphylococci, Escherichia coli, Acinetobacter* species, *Enterococcus* species including VRE, *Pseudomonas* species, and *Candida* species. Most of these episodes are associated with intravascular devices or surgical-site infection.

Aerobic Gram-negative bacilli, including Enterobacteriaceae, such as *E. coli* and *Klebsiella* spp., and *P. aeruginosa*, are the most common organisms causing pneumonia and UTIs in kidney transplant recipients. Additional pathogens include *S. aureus* and enterococci (pneumonia and UTI), *S. pneumonia* (pneumonia), and *Candida* species (UTI). Increasingly, *Klebsiella pneumoniae* and *E. coli* strains with resistance to extended-spectrum cephalosporins are associated with nosocomial UTIs. Patients with history of methicillin-resistant *S. aureus* (MRSA) colonization are more likely to experience invasive infection owing to this pathogen. While *S. aureus* is always significant when isolated from blood, coagulase-negative *Staphylococcus* when positive from a single blood culture may possibly represent skin contamination; however, true bacteremia from this organism may be seen in immune-compromised patients and/or those with indwelling catheters. Vancomycin has long been the treatment of choice for methicillin-resistant Staphylococci; newer agents with activity against drug-resistant gram-positive organism include daptomycin, linezolid, tedizolid, telavancin, and oritavancin.

The most common bacterial organisms causing surgical-site infection include *Staphylococcus* and *Streptococcus,* aerobic gram-negative bacteria, especially *E. coli, Enterobacter* species, *Pseudomonas* species, and enterococci.

Vancomycin-Resistant Enterococcus

Rates of VRE colonization among solid-organ transplant recipients range between 11% and 63%, and infection has been reported to occur in up to 16% of patients. Most VRE infections occur within the first month after transplantation and include bacteremia, intra-abdominal and biliary tract, urinary tract, and surgical wounds. Risk factors for VRE infection include VRE colonization, prolonged hospitalization, and intensive care unit stays; broad-spectrum antibiotics; renal insufficiency and hemodialysis; prolonged operative time; and reoperation. It is uncertain whether VRE infection is an independent risk factor for death or simply a marker for debilitated, immunocompromised patient. Multiple positive blood cultures indicate significant bacteremia and prompt directed therapy.

VRE colonization can be seen in open wounds, urine, and stool and should be interpreted accordingly. VRE colonization may persist for months to years in kidney transplant patients. Recommendations to decrease the risk for VRE colonization and infection include limiting the use of vancomycin and broad-spectrum antibiotics, especially those with anaerobic activity; surveillance cultures to detect VRE stool colonization; and meticulous hand hygiene.

Management of VRE should include removal of infected medical devices, drainage of fluid collections, and relieving urinary or biliary obstruction. Linezolid, tedizolid, quinupristin-dalfopristin (for *Enterococcus faecium* only), daptomycin, and tigecycline are active against VRE strains that are not susceptible to ampicillin and also can be used for treatment of susceptible enterococcal infections in a patient with a penicillin and vancomycin allergy. Linezolid can result in cytopenias, especially with concurrent marrow-suppressing immunosuppressive regimens, and requires close monitoring. Adverse metabolic effects can also be observed.

Multidrug-Resistant Gram-Negative Infections

Extended-spectrum beta-lactamase (ESBL) producing bacteria include *Klebsiella pneumoniae* and *E. coli.* These ESBL enzymes confer resistance to most beta-lactam antibiotics via a variety of mechanisms. Laboratory detection is based on demonstrated resistance to beta-lactam drugs such as ceftriaxone or cefepime, and the inability of beta-lactamase inhibitors to block this resistance. Treatment with pipercillin-tazobactam is not recommended because of reported treatment failures; the treatment of choice is a carbapenem such as meropenem, imipenem, or ertapenem. For UTI without pyelonephritis or bacteremia, oral fosfomycin may be an option; however, resistance to this drug can develop with prolonged exposure. A new class of resistant organisms is the carbapenemase-producing Enterobacteriaceae (CRE), which are growing in prevalence in Europe, Asia, and the Middle East, as well as North America. These infections are associated with prior colonization and use of invasive devices, and have demonstrated high mortality rates. Combination therapy with at least two effective antibiotics based on susceptibility testing results is the cornerstone of effective treatment. *Acinetobacter* and *Pseudomonas* remain the other species of gram-negative bacteria, which can also cause difficult-to-treat MDR infections.

Clostridium difficile Infection

Diarrhea occurs in about 13% of kidney transplant recipients, most commonly within 2 weeks after transplantation and is associated with an infectious agent in approximately 40% and medications in 35%. Of infectious etiologies, *C. difficile* is the most common agent. *C. difficile*–associated syndromes include asymptomatic carriage, diarrhea, pseudomembranous colitis, intestinal perforation, and toxic megacolon. The latter two complications are more common in infection associated with the hyper-toxin–producing epidemic strain of *C. difficile*. Most *C. difficile* infections are acquired nosocomially through either the hands of healthcare workers or from spore-contaminated environmental surfaces. Risk factors include administration of broad-spectrum antianaerobic antimicrobial therapy; prolonged hospitalization; female gender; treatment for rejection; and intra-abdominal graft placement. *C. difficile* infection may result in fluid and electrolyte abnormalities and can lead to malabsorption of medications, including immunosuppressive agents. Oral metronidazole (500 mg 3 times daily) is the preferred first-line treatment for mild-to-moderate *C. difficile* infection. Oral vancomycin (125 to 250 mg 4 times daily) should be used for severe disease (e.g., occurring in the intensive care unit, in persons older than 60 years of age, or associated with hypoalbuminemia or white blood cell count $>15,000/mm^3$) or if metronidazole fails. Fidaxomicin is a relatively new oral agent with *C. difficile* activity which may be less likely to permit recurrence of infection. In patients with severe gastrointestinal dysmotility or ileus, oral agents may not reach the colonic mucosa and intravenous metronidazole should be administered along with oral vancomycin. Fecal microbiota transplantation is a new therapy, which may have utility in preventing recurrent disease.

Listeriosis

In renal transplant recipients, infection with *L. monocytogenes* most commonly presents as meningoencephalitis or septicemia but also may cause febrile gastroenteritis. Infection typically occurs 6 or more months after transplantation. Intravenous ampicillin (2 g every 4 hours for 2 weeks) should be used to treat bacteremia. Meningitis should be treated with high-dose ampicillin. Repeat lumbar puncture should be performed to document cure. Many sporadic cases of listeriosis are associated with ingestion of processed meats. Patients should be instructed to eat only properly cooked meats and pasteurized dairy products.

Nocardiosis

The frequency of *Nocardia* infections varies between 0.7% and 3% in solid-organ transplant recipients. Although the prophylactic use of trimethoprim-sulfamethoxazole (TMP-SMX) has decreased the incidence of *Nocardia* infection, *Nocardia* species should be considered in the differential diagnosis of infection occurring in the setting of early rejection, enhanced immunosuppression, neutropenia, and uremia. There are at least 12 species within the genus of *Nocardia*, with *N. asteroids* complex, *N. brasiliensis*, *N. otitidiscaviarum*, and *N. transvalensis* most commonly associated with infection among transplant recipients. *Nocardia* infection most commonly presents 1 to 6 months after transplantation with acute or subacute pneumonia, but hematogenous spread to the brain, skin and subcutaneous tissues, bone, and eye has been reported. After pulmonary disease is established, dissemination to the brain is common, and cerebral CT or magnetic resonance imaging (MRI) of the brain should be performed. High-dose TMP-SMX (15 mg/kg of trimethoprim in two to four divided doses, depending on the severity of illness) is the treatment of choice for most *Nocardia* species infections. However, resistance has been reported, and antimicrobial susceptibility testing is recommended. Other agents, including imipenem, amikacin, second- and third-generation cephalosporins, minocycline, and quinolones, may be used with TMP-SMX or in combination in place of TMP-SMX when treating serious *Nocardia* infection. Amikacin should be used with caution in the renal transplant patient because of the risk for nephrotoxicity. Surgical debridement and drainage may be required to manage brain abscesses or empyema. Because of the substantial risk for relapse in the setting of ongoing immunosuppression, treatment should be for at least 12 months and radiographic monitoring of the sites of infection should be performed at regular intervals. Following treatment, secondary prophylaxis with TMP-SMX should be considered.

Legionellosis

Legionella species infections have been reported in kidney transplant recipients. Risk factors include repeated corticosteroid boluses, prolonged mechanical ventilation, and exposure to *Legionella*-contaminated hospital water supplies. *L. micdadei* and *L. pneumophila* commonly cause pneumonia, but extrapulmonary involvement, including culture-negative endocarditis and renal, hepatic, and central nervous system infection, have been reported. Signs and symptoms of *L. pneumophila* infection include a nonproductive cough, a temperature-pulse dissociation, elevated hepatic enzymes, diarrhea, hyponatremia, myalgias, and altered mental status. Radiographic findings include alveolar or interstitial infiltrates, cavities, pleural effusions, or lobar consolidation. Diagnosis can be confirmed by culture on special media or direct-fluorescent antibody testing of sputum, tissue, or bronchoalveolar fluid. In addition, a urinary antigen test should be performed; this test has a reported 70% sensitivity and 100% specificity for *L. pneumophila* serogroup 1. Delayed treatment is associated with increased mortality, and empiric treatment should be administered in suspected cases. Macrolides, quinolones, tetracyclines, and TMP-SMX have *in vitro* activity against *Legionella* species. Duration of treatment ranges from 14 to 21 days, depending on severity of illness.

Rhodococcus

Rhodococcus equi is an aerobic gram-positive coccobacillus that can cause infection in animals and in immunocompromised hosts, including renal transplant recipients. *Rhodococcus* most commonly causes pulmonary infection months to years after transplantation. Presentations include nodular or cavitary necrotizing pneumonia and empyema that may be confused with pulmonary tuberculosis. Aspiration of pulmonary nodules may reveal granulomatous inflammation with foamy macrophages with intracellular coccobacilli. Other clinical syndromes include sepsis, osteomyelitis, skin nodules, pericarditis, and lymphadenitis. Effective agents include quinolones, vancomycin, carbapenems, doxycycline, erythromycin, and TMP-SMX; β-lactams may be ineffective. Recurrences can occur, and surgical drainage may be required.

Mycobacterial Infection

Tuberculosis (TB) and nontuberculous mycobacteria (NTM) are potential causes of serious infection in renal allograft recipients that may present as early as the first post-transplantation month. The incidence of active tuberculosis is estimated to be 1% to 4% following renal transplantation and is higher in those who resided in or traveled to a country with a high prevalence of TB infection. Radiographic presentations of pulmonary infection with *M. tuberculosis* and NTM include multilobar disease, focal infiltrates and nodules, empyema, pleuritis, or a combination of findings.

In the transplant population, atypical presentations of *M. tuberculosis* and NTM disease may delay diagnosis and contribute to morbidity. These may include dermatologic presentations, diseases of bone and joints, soft tissues, visceral (e.g., ureter, bladder, and gynecologic), ocular, and central nervous system. Special vigilance for reactivation tuberculosis is warranted, especially among transplant recipients with a prior history of mycobacterial infection, with old granulomatous disease on chest radiograph, or from countries with high TB prevalence. Up to 40% of renal transplant recipients with reactivation tuberculosis will present with disseminated infection, with involvement of the skin, skeleton (bone and joint), or central nervous system. Finding granuloma in biopsy specimens from extrapulmonary sites should suggest disseminated disease. Because of the increase in multidrug-resistant (MDR) strains, appropriate therapy should include four agents: isoniazid (INH), rifampin (RIF) or rifabutin (RBT), pyrazinamide (PZA), and ethambutol (EMB) for 2 months or until susceptibility test results are available followed by up to 10 months of INH and RIF. Rifampin is a strong inducer of the cytochrome P450 CYP3A enzyme leading to near-undetectable levels of CNIs even with dose adjustment. Therefore, rifabutin is typically the preferred rifamycin compound in the setting of solid-organ transplantation; however, its use will still require dose adjustment of tacrolimus or cyclosporine with close monitoring of drug levels. Adverse effects associated with antituberculous agents include hepatitis (INH > PZA > RIF/RBT), peripheral neuritis and optic neuropathy (INH, EMB), gastrointestinal intolerance (INH, RIF, RBT, EMB, PZA), and neutropenia (RIF/RFB > ETH).

Infection with NTM, including *M. kansasii, M. fortuitum, M. chelonei, M. xenopi, M. marinum, M. haemophilum,* and *M. abscessus,* has been reported in renal transplant recipients. These pathogens can be cultured from sputum, lung tissue, skin, bone, and other disseminated sites. Many of the NTM are intrinsically resistant to standard antituberculous agents, and susceptibility testing should be performed against standard tuberculous agents, quinolones, macrolides, cephalosporins, and linezolid. Treatment typically includes combinations of agents for prolonged durations (e.g., longer than 12 months). Patients with osteomyelitis and extensive soft tissue disease may require surgical intervention. *M. fortuitum* may cause bloodstream infection associated with intravascular devices and prompt device removal is critical.

Mixed Infections

Concurrent bacterial, fungal, and viral infections most often occur in the setting of repeated episodes of rejection and resultant enhanced; postoperative healthcare-associated infections (e.g., pneumonia or intra-abdominal abscess); or immunomodulation from CMV or other virus infection, particularly respiratory viruses and hepatitis C.

ANTIMICROBIAL THERAPY

Antimicrobial therapy is given for the following indications:

- *Prophylaxis:* Antimicrobial agents are used to prevent a commonly encountered infection in the immediate postoperative period (e.g., surgical prophylaxis).
- *Empiric therapy:* Antimicrobials are administered without identification of the infecting pathogen.
- *Specific therapy:* Antimicrobials are administered to treat an infection with a diagnosed pathogen.

Surgical Prophylaxis

Preoperative antimicrobial prophylaxis reduces the frequency of surgical-site infection. The agent should have activity against skin pathogens (e.g., Staphylococci, Streptococci) and urinary tract pathogens (*E. coli, Klebsiella,* and *Proteus* species). Cefazolin (1 to 2 g based on body weight) generally is preferred and should be administered within 1 hour of the surgical incision. The choice of antimicrobial agent for renal transplant prophylaxis should also be based on institution-specific antimicrobial susceptibility patterns and a careful review and history of drug allergies. Vancomycin is an alternative agent for patients with penicillin allergy or history of MRSA colonization or infection. Surgical prophylaxis should be given as a single dose or discontinued after no more than 24 hours to minimize the risk for toxicity and superinfection, and limit cost.

Empiric and Directed Antibacterial Therapy

For patients with suspected bacterial infection, the choice of empiric therapy should be guided by the following considerations: potential sites of infection; prior culture and susceptibility results; recent antimicrobial exposure; time since transplantation; the severity of renal and hepatic dysfunction; and the net state of immunosuppression. Initial empiric therapy should include one or more broad-spectrum antibacterial agents. Commonly used agents for empiric therapy include third-generation cephalosporins, β-lactam and β-lactamase inhibitor combinations, carbapenems, fluoroquinolones, or vancomycin, if line-associated infection is suspected. When *P. aeruginosa* is suspected or documented, combination therapy with an antipseudomonal penicillin (i.e., piperacillin), carbapenem, ceftazidime, or cefepime, plus an aminoglycoside or antipseudomonal fluoroquinolone (i.e., ciprofloxacin, levofloxacin) is recommended for initial therapy pending sensitivity testing results and potentially to limit the emergence of resistance. Aminoglycosides, although generally active against Gram-negative bacteria, should be used with caution in renal allograft recipients because of the increased risk for nephrotoxicity. When the culture and sensitivity results are available, therapy should be modified to treat the infection with a narrow-spectrum agent to limit the risk for superinfection with multidrug-resistant organisms, toxicity, and cost. Especially in the setting of severe disease, sensitivity testing for the newer anti-infectives such as ceftazidime/avibactam and others should be performed. Potential interactions between antimicrobials and immunosuppressive agents are discussed in Chapter 6.

FUNGAL INFECTIONS

Despite ongoing refinements in immunosuppressive therapy, graft preservation, and surgical techniques, fungal infections remain a significant cause of morbidity and mortality in renal transplant recipients (Table 12.7). Although the incidence of fungal infections in renal transplant recipients is less than that reported for other solid-organ transplant recipients, the mortality from fungal infections remains high and is related to the pathogenicity of the organisms, site of infection, impaired host inflammatory response, limited diagnostic tools, potential for rapid clinical progression, failure to recognize a high-risk patient, and comorbidities, such as renal failure and diabetes mellitus.

Colonization with yeasts and molds occurs frequently in transplant candidates with ESRD and after transplantation because of exposure to broad-spectrum antibacterial agents, domiciliary and hospital exposures, immunosuppressive therapy, especially corticosteroids, and the presence of urinary catheters and endotracheal tubes. Isolation of *Candida* species from cultures of stool, respiratory, and urine samples occurs commonly in kidney transplant recipients receiving corticosteroids and broad-spectrum antimicrobials and does not necessarily imply infection. However, repeatedly positive fungal cultures from a single or from multiple sites may herald invasive candidiasis in the appropriate clinical setting.

Candida species, *Aspergillus* species, *P. jiroveci*, and *Cryptococcus* species are the most common fungal pathogens reported in renal transplant recipients. Endemic fungi including *Histoplasma*, *Coccidioides*, and *Blastomyces* may also cause invasive disease in transplant patients living in endemic areas. Mucormycosis is a rare but potentially lethal fungal infection caused by *Rhizopus*, *Lichtheimia* (formerly *Absidia*),

TABLE 127

Incidence and Distribution of Invasive Fungal Infections (IFIs) among Kidney Transplant Recipients

Organ Transplant	Incidence of IFI (%)	Proportion of IFI (%)				Mortality (%)			
		Aspergillus	Candida	Cryptococcus	Other Fungi	Aspergillus	Candida	Cryptococcus	Other Fungi
Renal	0–20	0–26	76–95	0–39	0–39	20–100	23–71	0–60	55
Pancreas and pancreas–kidney	6–38	0–3	97–100	—	—	100	20–27	—	—

Data derived from several series using varying definitions of fungal infection between 1980 and 1999.

and *Mucor* species, among others, and remains difficult to treat despite the availability of new antifungal therapies. Hyaline molds other than *Aspergillus* may also cause disease, such as *Scedosporium, Fusarium,* and *Penicillium.* Dematiaceous molds or phaeohyphomycoses can cause both systemic and locally invasive infection, when on the extremities often at areas of past or recent trauma. Fungi colonizing the upper respiratory tract and sinuses may rapidly become invasive.

Donor-transmitted fungal infection is uncommon among kidney transplant recipients, but cases of *Candida, Aspergillus, Histoplasma, Coccidioides, Cryptococcus,* and *Scedosporium* species have been reported, usually associated with unrecognized infection within the donor allograft or in the blood compartment. All donors should be evaluated for evidence of active or occult fungal infection, particularly in the blood and urine.

Candida infections occur most commonly during the first month following transplantation and are usually associated with transplant surgical technical complications, early rejection, diabetes mellitus, simultaneous kidney–pancreas transplantation, and enhanced immunosuppression. *Candida* infection is most commonly associated with an endogenous source of colonization. *C. albicans* is the most common species, followed by *C. glabrata, C. tropicalis,* and *C. parapsilosis.* Speciation is clinically useful because non-*albicans Candida* species vary in *in vitro* susceptibility to amphotericin B, azoles, and echinocandins. Sites of *Candida* infection include mucocutaneous candidiasis and esophagitis; wound infections; cystitis, pyelonephritis, and ureteral obstruction by candida elements or "fungal ball"; intra-abdominal infections, including infected perigraft fluid collections or peritonitis; and intravascular device–associated fungemia. Renal parenchymal infection most often results from candidemia and hematogenous spread, although ascending infection from the bladder can occur. Candiduria is typically asymptomatic, but may be associated with cystitis or upper tract infection. Patients with genitourinary tract stents and recurrent funguria often require removal of foreign body to eradicate the infection.

The risk for fungal infection after simultaneous pancreas–kidney (SPK, see Chapter 16) and pancreas-after-kidney (PAK) transplantations is much greater than after kidney transplantation alone and is similar to that found in liver transplant recipients. More than 45% of these infections are caused by *Candida* species. Risk factors include older donor or recipient age, bladder versus enteric drainage (SPK recipients), retransplantation versus primary transplantation (PAK recipients), and vascular graft thrombosis. Bladder drainage of pancreatic secretions and longer duration of urinary catheterization favor urinary tract colonization with *Candida* species and early postoperative fungal UTIs. Fungal infection of the pancreatic allograft is associated with a high risk for graft loss and mortality rates as high as 20%.

The period of 1 to 6 months after kidney transplantation is marked by opportunistic, relapsed, and residual fungal infection. Opportunistic fungal infections, such as *Cryptococcus,* endemic mycoses, aspergillosis, and mucormycosis, most commonly occur 6 or more months after transplantation. Conditions that intensify the net state of immunosuppression may shift the timeline for fungal infection forward. *Cryptococcus* often presents as meningitis but may cause space-occupying brain lesions; pulmonary, dermatologic, skeletal, organ-specific disease; aspergillosis—pneumonia and other tissue-invasive forms, including genitourinary, central nervous system, rhinocerebral, gastrointestinal, skin, wound, and musculoskeletal disease, and includes both *C. neoformans* and *C. gattii*, which no longer appears to be limited to only tropical and subtropical regions. The endemic fungus *Coccidioides* may cause pneumonia, meningitis, musculoskeletal, and skin involvement, while *Histoplasma* can cause pneumonia, fibrosing mediastinitis, skin, and disseminated disease. *Penicillium marneffei* and *Scedopsorium* cause pneumonia and disseminated disease, similar to *Aspergillus* species. Mucormycosis often manifests as pulmonary, rhinocerebral, and cutaneous disease.

Patients at risk for aspergillosis include those receiving repeated courses of enhanced immunosuppression for rejection and those with chronic graft dysfunction, diabetes, comorbid medical illnesses, or CMV infection. Diagnosis of *Aspergillus* infection depends on a high clinical suspicion, isolation of *Aspergillus* species from a sterile body site or repeated isolation from the respiratory tract, and typical radiographic findings. Radiologic appearances of pulmonary aspergillosis in kidney transplant recipients include nodules, diffuse or wedge-shaped opacities, empyema, or cavitary forms. Serial measurement of *Aspergillus* galactomannan in the serum may aid in the early diagnosis of invasive aspergillosis in the high-risk setting.

Prophylaxis

During induction or periods of enhanced immunosuppression, oral, nonabsorbable, or topical antifungal agents, such as clotrimazole or nystatin, typically are administered to prevent mucocutaneous *Candida* infection. Although prophylaxis with a systemic antifungal agent is not recommended after uncomplicated renal transplantation, it may be indicated in those with persistent candiduria. In such cases, an azole or echinocandin can be administered for a duration proportional to the risk for fungal infection. Renal transplant recipients with a history of prior treatment of an endemic mycosis or radiographic evidence of old, "healed" granulomatous disease associated with coccidioidomycosis or histoplasmosis may benefit from long-term (lifelong) prophylaxis with an appropriate azole.

Treatment

Historically, invasive candidiasis, cryptococcosis, coccidioidomycosis, histoplasmosis, and aspergillosis were treated with amphotericin B (AmB) deoxycholate. Because of inherent toxicities and intolerance, newer agents have increasingly been used in renal transplant recipients. The lipid formulations of amphotericin B are all associated with lower risks for nephrotoxicity, metabolic derangements, and infusion-associated side effects than is AmB. Higher therapeutic dosages can be administered, and broad-spectrum antifungal activity is generally maintained. However, delayed toxicity may be observed even with the lipid-conjugated formulations of AmB.

Voriconazole appears to be superior to conventional AmB for the treatment of invasive aspergillosis and also has *in vitro* activity against a wider range of organisms. Available in both intravenous and oral formulations, the drug is generally well tolerated, but some patients experience visual hallucinations, photosensitivity, and increased incidence of skin cancer. Oral posaconazole has excellent activity *in vitro* against *Candida*, *Aspergillus,* and *Mucor* species, and is now available in an intravenous form. Isavuconazole is a newer agent with similar spectrum to posaconazole, but experience in solid-organ transplant recipients is limited to date. Although itraconazole has good *in vitro* activity against *Aspergillus* species, its use is generally reserved for treatment of less-severe aspergillosis or maintenance therapy following initial response to lipid amphotericin or voriconazole and for treatment of endemic mycoses. Fluconazole is the first-line agent for the treatment or prevention of reactivation coccidioidomycosis in renal transplant recipients. The long-term use of fluconazole may be associated with the development of fungal resistance or tolerance, as well as with the risk for fungal superinfection with *C. glabrata, C. krusei,* or *C. tropicalis.* Fluconazole and 5-flucytosine can be used for cryptococcal disease; 5-flucytosine may be problematic to use owing to its side-effect profile including cytopenias and renal insufficiency. All of the azoles impair CNI metabolism and increase CNI blood levels (see Chapter 5), and their use may require a reduction in cyclosporine or tacrolimus dose of 30% to 50%.

The echinocandins, including caspofungin, anidulafungin, and micafungin, inhibit synthesis of fungal cell wall protein β_{1-3} glucan and are fungicidal for *Candida* species, including fluconazole-resistant species. Available only as intravenous formulations, the echinocandins are effective, well tolerated, and have few drug–drug interactions. As a result, they increasingly are being used to treat serious infections associated with non-*albicans Candida* species in transplant recipients. Coadministration of caspofungin with tacrolimus results in modest (about 20%) reduction in tacrolimus levels and an increased incidence of abnormal liver function tests with cyclosporine.

The development of any serious fungal infection in a transplant recipient mandates a critical evaluation of the immunosuppressive regimen. The corticosteroid dose should be minimized, the blood levels of cyclosporine and tacrolimus should be kept in the low therapeutic range, and other immunosuppressive agents often can be discontinued temporarily. Clinical treatment failure for life-threatening fungal infection despite appropriate antifungal therapy may warrant discontinuation of immunosuppression at the cost of graft loss.

Pneumocystosis

P. jiroveci (formerly *carinii*) pneumonia (PJP) most often occurs 2 to 6 months after transplantation in patients not receiving prophylaxis. It typically presents with fever, nonproductive cough, arterial–alveolar mismatching, and diffuse interstitial infiltration or focal air space consolidation on chest radiograph. Unusual presentations are possible in renal transplant recipients, including pulmonary mass lesions. BAL with transbronchial biopsy and staining is a highly sensitive method of identifying pulmonary disease. First-line treatment is with TMP-SMX 15 to 20 mg/kg for 21 days. Treatment of severe disease should include adjunctive steroids as for HIV-infected persons with PJP (60 mg/day initially, then taper). Second-line agents include intravenous pentamidine (4 mg/kg/day), dapsone-trimethoprim (100 mg dapsone daily with trimethoprim 100 mg twice daily), or clindamycin plus primaquine (600 mg 4 times daily clindamycin with 30 mg base daily primaquine). Adverse effects of trimethoprim include nephrotoxicity, pancreatitis, and bone marrow suppression. Dapsone is associated with hemolytic anemia in patients with glucose-6-phosphate dehydrogenase deficiency. Mild-to-moderate PJP can be treated with atovaquone (750 mg orally twice daily for 21 days) in patients allergic to TMP-SMX. Prophylactic agents, in order of efficacy, include TMP-SMX (single-strength tablet 3 times weekly), monthly aerosolized pentamidine, daily dapsone, and daily atovaquone. Prophylaxis against disease should be reinstituted following augmentation of immunosuppression, such as steroid bolus or ATG administration for acute rejection. Patients reporting sulfa allergies should be questioned regarding the nature of their reaction; desensitization may be possible with mild reactions. For those with severe allergies, dapsone should also be avoided, and PJP prophylaxis provided using atovaquone.

VIRAL INFECTIONS

Viral infections are a major problem in allograft recipients, most commonly in the first months after transplantation. Clinical disease can occur later, especially after intensification of immunosuppression or physiologic insults that increase the net state of immunosuppression. EBV-related lymphoproliferative disorder is discussed in Chapter 11.

Cytomegalovirus

CMV infection occurs primarily after the first month of transplantation with an estimated incidence of 30% to 78% if antiviral prophylaxis is not administered, depending on the serologic status of the donor and recipient (Table 12.3). CMV can be transmitted by the allograft, through blood products, or by sexual contact and establishes lifelong latency after primary infection. Among all organ transplants, renal transplant recipients have the lowest risk for CMV disease in the absence of antiviral prophylaxis, whereas pancreas and kidney–pancreas transplant recipients are at substantially higher risk. In general, the dose, duration, agents, and intensity of immunosuppression determine the risk for CMV among transplant recipients. Specific risk factors include CMV donor-positive–recipient-negative mismatch and the use of lymphocyte-depleting preparations for induction or rejection therapy (see Chapter 6). Other risk factors include comorbidities, patient age, and leukopenia.

Active CMV infections may be symptomatic or asymptomatic and are characterized by viral replication with expression of a CD4+ and CD8+ T-cell response to CMV. Primary CMV infection represents infection in the previously uninfected seronegative host, whereas secondary CMV infection represents infection in a previously infected seropositive host caused by either reactivation of latent endogenous virus, or superinfection with new virus strain. CMV disease refers to symptomatic acute CMV infection and includes CMV syndrome (fever, fatigue, leukopenia or thrombocytopenia, and detectable CMV viremia) and end-organ CMV disease (e.g., pneumonitis, hepatitis, or gastrointestinal involvement such as colitis or enteritis, or involvement of the allograft itself).

In addition to the direct effects of CMV disease, CMV replication is associated with indirect effects of immune modulation and dysregulation, and can culminate in opportunistic infection and allograft injury or rejection. Host mediators implicated in reactivation of CMV include TNF-mediated activation of NF-κB, catecholamines, and proinflammatory prostaglandins, leading to intermediate–early gene expression. CMV infection induces antiendothelial cell antibodies that contribute to both acute and chronic graft dysfunction, and the proinflammatory effect of viral replication can induce cellular migration and proliferation, upregulation of adhesion molecules, and proinflammatory cytokines such as IFN-γ and TNF-α. CMV disease most commonly presents as a viremic syndrome, manifest by fever, malaise, and leukopenia or thrombocytopenia. Pneumonitis is the most serious manifestation of CMV disease and is characterized by dyspnea, hypoxemia, interstitial infiltrates, and the detection of CMV by PCR on BAL or by histopathology on transbronchial biopsy. CMV upper and lower gastrointestinal disease includes esophagitis, cholecystitis, duodenitis, hepatitis, and colitis. Diagnostic endoscopy can reveal solitary or multiple mucosal ulcerations with hemorrhage. Tissue specimens should be stained for CMV using immunofluorescent anti-CMV antibody and examined for inclusion bodies. CMV retinitis is uncommon in transplant recipients and can be diagnosed by direct funduscopy. Central nervous system CMV disease can include meningitis, encephalitis, or transverse myelitis and can be diagnosed by PCR testing of CSF. Neurologic disease caused by other neurotropic opportunistic pathogens, and drug toxicities, should be simultaneously investigated. Multiorgan involvement can be observed in disseminated CMV disease.

Diagnosis

Historically, tissue-invasive CMV disease was diagnosed by histopathology, but this approach can be associated with diagnostic delays or inadequate specimen collection. Detection of serum CMV IgM or IgG antibody by EIA is useful for pretransplantation screening and for documenting seroconversion but is of no utility in the diagnosis of CMV disease. Culture-based methods include conventional tissue culture and shell vial centrifugation and can be performed on blood, urine, cerebrospinal fluid (CSF), respiratory secretions, or other tissue specimens. Staining shell vial culture with monoclonal antibody against early CMV viral antigens at 48 hours can decrease the time to diagnosis, but this method has been largely replaced by PCR-based methods. Previously, detection of CMV pp65 antigen in peripheral blood lymphocytes by a semiquantitative fluorescent assay was utilized as more rapid than traditional culture methods, but is less sensitive than quantitative PCR and supplanted by DNA-based techniques.

Quantitative detection of CMV DNA from blood or CSF using PCR is most commonly used to diagnose CMV disease associated with viremia and to monitor response to antiviral therapy. Because of variability in CMV viral load testing when measured in copies/mL, an international standard for CMV was developed and approved by the World Health Organization, with results reported in international units (IU) per milliliter. PCR-based methods are also used to detect mutations associated with drug resistance. Qualitative CMV DNA detection by PCR is extremely sensitive and can be applied to nonblood samples such as tissue or BAL fluid.

Treatment

Effective antiviral agents for CMV prophylaxis and treatment have substantially decreased the morbidity and mortality associated with CMV disease. Oral valganciclovir (900 mg twice daily) has been demonstrated to have comparable safety and efficacy to intravenous ganciclovir for clearing CMV viremia and resolving clinical disease in solid-organ transplant patients with mild-to-moderate CMV disease. Patients with high CMV viral loads (e.g., $>5 \times 10^5$ IU/mL) or severe tissue-invasive disease, and those who fail to achieve a reduction in viral load after 7 or more days of oral valganciclovir treatment should be treated with intravenous ganciclovir (5 mg/kg every 12 hours). Patients with CMV disease should receive at least weekly monitoring of blood viral load, and antiviral therapy should be continued until there is suppression of viremia, typically 14 to 21 days. After successful suppression of viral replication, an additional course of suppressive therapy, valganciclovir 900 mg once daily, may be continued for an additional 1 to 3 months, or longer if indicated. Dose adjustments are indicated for renal insufficiency. Oral ganciclovir (1,000 mg 3 times daily) is an alternate suppressive therapy, but is limited by poor absorption limiting serum levels. Adverse effects of ganciclovir include reversible, dose-related granulocytopenia and thrombocytopenia, fever, rash, nausea, myalgias, abnormalities in liver enzyme determinations, and, rarely, pancreatitis. Drug interactions include an increased seizure risk when used in combination with imipenem, and additive marrow suppression with azathioprine, mycophenolate, and TMP-SMX.

Anecdotal experience in treating refractory CMV disease suggests that the addition of CMV hyperimmune globulin (CMVIG) or pooled intravenous immune globulin (IVIG) to ganciclovir may improve the clinical response; however, randomized-controlled data are lacking. Foscarnet is indicated for treatment of UL97-mutant ganciclovir-resistant CMV disease; however, caution is indicated because of nephrotoxicity. Supervision by an infectious disease practitioner and transplant pharmacist is suggested; concurrent fluid and mannitol administration can decrease side effects while maintaining anti-CMV efficacy. Cidofovir is a third-line agent for CMV disease treatment for ganciclovir-resistant CMV strains, and should also be used with caution because of nephrotoxicity, especially with concurrent use of CNIs. New anti-CMV compounds in Phase III trials include letermovir and brincidofovir, which may offer avenues for effective treatment without bone marrow suppression.

Prevention

Regimens to limit the risk for CMV disease and to improve patient and allograft survival vary from center to center and are based on the CMV serostatus of the donor and recipient and an assessment of the net state of immunosuppression. In practice, two strategies are used for CMV prevention: universal prophylaxis and preemptive therapy. Universal prophylaxis involves administering antiviral therapy to all at-risk patients immediately after transplantation for a defined duration dependent on the perceived duration of risk and net state of immunosuppression. Preemptive or targeted therapy involves monitoring patients at regular intervals for early evidence of CMV replication by CMV quantitative PCR monitoring. Patients with laboratory evidence of early CMV replication are treated with antiviral therapy to prevent progression to symptomatic disease. The approach of universal prophylaxis may be more useful for patients at high risk for CMV disease, such as the CMV donor-positive (D+) recipient-negative (R−) patient or those receiving ATG for induction of immune suppression, whereas preemptive therapy may be more useful for patients at low or intermediate risk for CMV disease. Patients receiving kidney/pancreas transplants should receive prophylaxis rather than preemptive therapy. Antiviral agents currently used for universal prophylaxis include intravenous or oral ganciclovir, oral valganciclovir, and high-dose valacyclovir. Valganciclovir, the L-valine ester of ganciclovir, is the preferred agent, and is administered at a dose of 900 mg/day by mouth for CMV prophylaxis and produces similar area-under-the-curve values to intravenous ganciclovir (5 mg/kg/day) and much higher values than oral ganciclovir (3 g/day). Length of prophylaxis should be a minimum of 3 months for R+ transplant recipients, and 6 months for D+/R− recipients, in whom this longer course of prophylaxis resulted in decreased rates of early and late CMV disease as compared with 3 months of valganciclovir prophylaxis. Antiviral prophylaxis should be started as early as possible after transplantation.

CMV-positive transplant patients who are treated with antilymphocytic agents, or who require multiple treatments for rejection, have a high incidence of symptomatic CMV disease. Although controlled trials are lacking, intravenous ganciclovir (5 mg/kg/day) or valganciclovir (900 mg once daily) administered during antilymphocyte antibody treatment or intensified immunosuppression courses followed by a period of oral valganciclovir may reduce this risk. Ganciclovir, valganciclovir, and valacyclovir require dosage adjustment for decreased creatinine clearance. In patients with neutropenia, dose adjustment is not recommended in the setting of normal renal function; granulocyte-colony stimulating factor (GCSF) can be used to permit tolerance of prophylaxis or treatment regimens. Antiviral prophylaxis against CMV is not required for D−/R− transplant recipients as long as they receive CMV-negative blood or leuko-depleted blood products. These patients should receive acyclovir or valacyclovir for HSV and VZV prophylaxis for the first 3 to 6 months after transplantation.

Herpes Simplex Virus and Varicella-Zoster Virus

HSV infection typically develops within the first 6 weeks after transplantation in patients not receiving antiviral prophylaxis and most commonly involves mucosal surfaces. Infection occasionally can disseminate to visceral organs and cause esophagitis, hepatitis, and pneumonitis. Most infections are caused by reactivation of endogenous latent virus, although primary infection transmitted from the allografts has been described. Both acyclovir and ganciclovir are active against herpesviruses *in vitro,* and both are useful in the treatment or prophylaxis of HSV. Alternative agents include valacyclovir and famciclovir. Acyclovir can be given intravenously or orally for mucocutaneous infections. For treatment of HSV encephalitis, a higher dosage is given by slow infusion to prevent crystallization within the renal tubules.

Herpes zoster ("shingles") develops in about 10% of adult renal transplant recipients and may involve two or three adjoining dermatomes. Infection is usually caused by reactivation of latent disease. Unless there are contraindications, VZV-seronegative transplant candidates should receive two doses of live varicella vaccine, and seropositive candidates 60 years or older should receive a single dose of live zoster vaccine prior to transplantation to decrease the risk for varicella disease following kidney transplantation.

Acyclovir, famciclovir, and valacyclovir can be used for the treatment of herpes zoster and primary varicella infection. Primary varicella and rarely disseminated zoster can cause pneumonia, encephalitis, disseminated intravascular coagulation, and graft dysfunction. Intravenous acyclovir (10 mg/kg every 8 hours as a slow infusion) should be given for the treatment of primary varicella and disseminated zoster. Oral acyclovir, valacyclovir, or famciclovir may be appropriate for treatment of mild dermatomal zoster. Following exposure to a person with primary varicella or zoster, transplant recipients who are susceptible or nonimmune to VZV should be given VZV immune globulin as soon as possible for maximal effectiveness but no later than 96 hours after exposure.

Other Human Herpesviruses

HHV-6, -7, and -8 may reactivate following renal transplantation. Although more than 90% of adults are seropositive for HHV-6 and 7, only 0% to 5% are seropositive for HHV-8. Neither serology nor PCR of peripheral blood lymphocytes can reliably distinguish active from latent infection with these viruses, and routine monitoring or treatment of asymptomatic individuals is not recommended. HHV-6 reactivates in 31% to 55% of all solid-organ transplant recipients, most commonly occurring during episodes of acute rejection, associated with CNI toxicity, and during the first 4 weeks after transplantation. Reactivation of HHV-6 is associated with CMV disease and can cause hepatitis, pneumonitis, and encephalitis. Symptomatic HHV-6 infection should be treated with ganciclovir and reduction of immunosuppression. HHV-8 seroconversion occurs in up to 12% of seronegative kidney transplants, usually within 3 months of transplantation, and can be primary or transmitted from the donor kidney. HHV-8 infection is associated with Kaposi sarcoma, which occurs with a median of 30 months after transplantation. Diagnosis is supported by pathology and by the presence of HHV-8 DNA sequences in involved tissue. Treatment consists of radiation and chemotherapy. The clinical significance of primary or reactivation HHV-7 infection is poorly characterized.

Adenovirus

Adenovirus can cause hemorrhagic cystitis, fever, renal dysfunction, and, rarely, dissemination with pneumonia, hepatitis, and
death. After transplantation, secondary infection may result from
primary infection from an exogenous source or from transmission
from the renal allograft. Disseminated disease is more common
after primary infection. Definite diagnosis is by kidney biopsy
that typically reveals interstitial nephritis, tubular necrosis, and
ground-glass–like intranuclear viral inclusion bodies in tubular
cells. Reduction of immunosuppression and supportive care are
important components of therapy. Cidofovir is the antiviral agent
of choice, but should be used with caution given its association with
significant nephrotoxicity and neutropenia; however, its use should
be considered in cases of severe, progressive, or disseminated disease.
Typical regimens are either 1 mg/kg 3 times weekly or 5 mg/kg/wk
for 2 weeks followed by 5 mg/kg every other week, with concurrent
administration of probenecid and intravenous hydration to try to
meliorate nephrotoxicity.

BK Virus

Polyomaviruses associated with human disease include BK virus
and JC virus. BK virus causes latent infection of the kidney uroepi-
thelium with reactivation during immune suppression; it may cause
tubulointerstitial nephritis and ureteral stenosis or stricture. Up to
90% of adults are seropositive worldwide. Rates of detection in urine
or blood in renal transplant recipients range between 20% and 60%.
Risk factors for infection and disease include donor seropositivity,
degree of immune suppression, use of tacrolimus and mycophenolate
mofetil, and allograft rejection. BK viuria or viremia precedes development of BK virus association nephropathy (BKN), an important
cause of loss of allograft function with a presentation at a median
of 9 months after transplantation. Definitive diagnosis requires a
renal biopsy with immunohistochemistry staining for presence of
polyoma virus. Monitoring for BK virus in the plasma by DNA PCR is
more specific for diagnosis of BK nephropathy than is detection with
urine specimens. However, the detection of BK virus DNA in urine
specimens may provide the first evidence of polyomavirus infection
in the patient. As an effective BK virus-specific immune response is
essential for disease control, management of BK virus replication and
BKN involves reduction of immunosuppression with close monitoring
for rejection. Recommended protocols include either 50% reduction
or cessation of mycophenolate mofetil, followed by dose reduction
of CNI if this change is not effective. The approach of protocolized
screening or urine or blood plus reduction of immune suppression
has been shown to effectively decrease incidence of BKN after kidney
transplantation. Although a variety of medical therapies including
fluoroquinolones, leflunomide, and cidofovir have been proposed
for prevention or treatment of BK viremia and BKN, none has demonstrated clear benefit. There is limited data to suggest the possible
benefit of IVIG in treatment of BKN.

Influenza Types A and B, Parainfluenza Virus, and Respiratory Syncytial Virus

Community-aquired respiratory viruses may cause significant morbidity and mortality in renal transplant recipients. These seasonal viruses can be transmitted by virus-laden respiratory droplets and aerosols by direct person-to-person contact or by contact with contaminated environmental surfaces. Renal transplant recipients may be the "sentinel" cases for a community influenza outbreak. Community respiratory virus disease usually presents with upper respiratory tract symptoms and fever, myalgias, arthralgias, anorexia, and mucosal inflammation. Illness ranges from mild upper respiratory illness, to bronchiolitis, viral pneumonia with respiratory failure, and superinfection with fungal or bacterial pathogens, such as *S. aureus, Streptococcus* species, and Gram-negative bacilli. Simultaneous CMV reactivation may occur as a result of immunomodulation. Rapid detection of virus-infected upper respiratory cells (e.g., nasopharyngeal swabs or washing, respiratory secretions) using a respiratory virus PCR panel for detection can facilitate the diagnosis, appropriate isolation, and treatment of patients with viral respiratory infections.

All renal transplant recipients should receive annual immunization with inactivated influenza vaccine. The vaccine is safe and confers high seroprotection (range; 79% to 93%) similar to normal, healthy volunteers. Live, intranasal influenza vaccine should not be administered to renal transplant recipients or their household contacts. Vaccination can be safely performed as early as 3 to 6 months after transplantation; although it is less likely to be effective this early after transplantation, this approach may be appropriate in the setting of the start of the respiratory virus season. The neuraminidase inhibitors oseltamivir and zanamivir are active against most influenza A and B and are effective if started within 36 to 48 hours after onset of symptoms. They result in a modest decrease in the duration of illness and significantly decrease the risk for secondary bacterial complications. Because of the high prevalence of resistant influenza A virus, amantadine and rimantadine should no longer be used for treatment or prophylaxis of influenza. During severe community or institutional outbreaks of influenza, susceptible persons should be vaccinated and antiviral prophylaxis administered for 2 weeks until antibodies develop.

RSV pneumonitis may respond to oral or aerosolized ribavirin delivered in a controlled contained administration system given over 24 hours. Parainfluenza virus (types 1 to 4) is a paramyxovirus; it can occur during fall and winter months, or sporadically. Disease spectrum in renal transplant recipients can mimic influenza and can include mild upper respiratory disease, pneumonia, and death. Diagnosis of community-acquired respiratory virus is primarily via PCR-based respiratory virus panel testing. Treatment options are limited for parainfluenza infection, although there is some anecdotal data supporting ribavirin use and new agents for treatment are in development. Human metapneumovirus is another community-acquired respiratory virus with similar ability to cause sometimes severe pneumonitis in transplant recipients. In addition to supportive care, patients with respiratory virus infection may benefit from IVIG administration, especially in the setting of hypogammaglobulinemia.

Parvovirus

In transplant recipients, parvovirus B19 infection is a cause of refractory severe anemia, pancytopenia, thrombotic microangiopathy, fibrosing cholestatic hepatitis, encephalitis, and graft dysfunction. Parvovirus occurs in up to 23% of renal transplant recipients with severe anemia, and 80% of infections occur within the first 3 months of transplantation. Donor transmission has been reported. Of note, the classical skin rash is often not seen in immunocompromised hosts. Examination of bone marrow reveals typical giant proerythroblasts, and the diagnosis should be confirmed by detection of B19 virus DNA in serum by PCR assay. Some patients may have concurrent CMV disease. Treatment consists of high-dose IVIG (0.5 mg/kg/day for 5 to 10 days) and reduction of immunosuppression, for recurrent or persistent disease.

West Nile Virus

The clinical manifestation of WNV in the immunocompetent host typically consists of 3 to 6 days of malaise, anorexia, arthralgia, vomiting, nausea, rash, and lymphadenopathy. In elderly or immunocompromised individuals, more severe neurologic manifestations can occur, including encephalitis or meningitis, mental status changes, seizures, optic neuritis, muscle weakness, flaccid paralysis, and movement disorders. Symptoms that begin in the first 2 weeks after transplantation suggest transmission through the allograft, whereas symptoms that begin later suggest community acquisition. Diagnosis is confirmed by detection of WNV IgM antibody or WNV PCR in the serum or CSF. Treatment includes reduction of immunosuppression and supportive care. IVIG anecdotally has been associated with improvement in some severely ill transplant patients. Interferon-α-2b and ribavirin have activity *in vitro* against WNV. All transplant recipients from at-risk areas should limit the risk for mosquito exposure by using insect repellents and insecticide-impregnated long-sleeved clothing while outdoors during summer months. Sometimes fatal cases of donor-derived infection have been reported.

Human Papillomavirus

Human papillomavirus causes cutaneous and anogenital warts and is associated with cervical intraepithelial neoplasia, squamous cell carcinoma, and anogenital carcinoma. Premalignant skin and cervical lesions are more common and progress more rapidly to cancer among organ transplant recipients. Cutaneous warts, keratotic skin lesions, and anogenital warts should be monitored and referred for early dermatologic or colorectal evaluation, biopsy, and treatment. Treatments include topical keratolytic and caustic agents, topical and oral retinoids, imiquimod, podophyllin, 5-fluorouracil, bleomycin, physical ablation, and investigational immunotherapies.

PARASITES

Toxoplasmosis

Toxoplasma gondii is a parasitic zoonosis that may cause disease in patients with deficiencies in T-cell–mediated immunity, such as renal transplant recipients. About 10% to 40% of US residents are positive for past exposure to this infection, with higher rates approaching

90% in those from endemic areas including sub-Saharan Africa and Latin America. The disease can manifest as fever, lymphadenopathy, leukopenia, encephalitis, chorioretinitis, pneumonia, endocarditis, and hepatitis. It progresses to sepsis and death, if treatment is not initiated. Seronegative recipients are at risk for disease if they receive an organ from a seropositive donor. Protection against disease is obtained when using trimethoprim-sulfadoxine or dapsone as *Pneumocystis* prophylaxis. Diagnosis is made using PCR-based strategies, by demonstration of the parasite in tissue samples, or by classical radiologic findings for central nervous system disease. First-line treatment consists of pyrimethamine, folinic acid (leucovorin), and sulfadiazine. Multiple alternative treatment regimens exist.

Chagas Disease

T. cruzi is a parasite endemic to Central America and can cause disease after transplantation by reactivation or donor-derived infection, even from noncardiac organs including kidney transplant. There is typically no indication for treatment of patients with chronic infection; however, patients with history of exposure as measured by positive antibody testing or recipients of *T. cruzi* positive organs can be screened by PCR testing after transplantation. Fever, cutaneous involvement, and myocarditis are common manifestations of infection or reactivation of disease. Treatment of acute disease is with benznidazole or nifurtimox.

Strongyloides

Strongyloides stercoralis is an intestinal nematode, which is endemic to tropical and subtropical areas worldwide, as well as temperate areas including Eastern Europe and the southeastern United States. As described above, patients born or spending time in endemic areas should be screened for and treated if appropriate, prior to transplantation. Post-transplant infection can result from reactivation or donor-derived infection. The most feared clinical manifestation is hyperinfection syndrome with disseminated disease, when immunosuppression permits accelerated larvae production with migration and an elevated parasite burden causing pulmonary manifestations and bacterial sepsis when gram-negative rods are spread by the parasite during migration, reaching a mortality rate of 70%. Eosinophilia may or may not be seen during immune suppression. Diagnosis is via serologic testing, stool O&P, and identification of larva from respiratory secretions, CSF, urine, blood, or other tissue specimens. Ivermectin is the drug of choice, either daily dosing in cases of hyperinfection, or two doses separated by 2 weeks in the situation of asymptomatic or mild disease.

Selected Readings

Angarone M, Ison MG. Diarrhea in solid organ transplant recipients. Curr Opin Infect Dis 2015;28:308–316.

Ariza-Heredia EJ, Beam EN, Lesnick TG, et al. Impact of urinary tract infection on allograft function after kidney transplantation. Clin Transplant 2014;28:683–690.

Elfadawy N, Flechner SM, Liu X, et al. The impact of surveillance and rapid reduction in immunosuppression to control BK virus-related graft injury in kidney transplantation. Transplant Int 2013;26:822–832.

Fischer SA, Lu K; the AST Infectious Diseases Community of Practice. Screening of donor and recipient in solid organ transplantation. Am J Transplant 2013;6:9–21.

Fishman JA. Infections in organ-transplant recipients. N Engl J Med 2007;357: 2601–2614.

Green M. Introduction: infections in solid organ transplantation. Am J Transplant 2013;(13, suppl 4):3–8.

Hartmann A, Sagedal S, Hjelmesaeth J. The natural course of cytomegalovirus infection and disease in renal transplant recipients. Transplantation 2006;82:S15–S17.

Hirsch HH, Randhawa P; the AST Infectious Diseases Community of Practice. BK Polyomavirus in solid organ transplantation. Am J Transplant 2013;(13, suppl 4): 179–188.

Humar A, Lebranchu Y, Vincenti F, et al. The efficacy and safety of 200 days valganciclovir cytomegalovirus prophylaxis in high-risk kidney transplant recipients. Am J Transplant 2010;10:1228–1237.

Huprikar S, Shoham S; the AST Infectious Diseases Community of Practice. Emerging fungal infections in solid organ transplantation. Am J Transplant 2013;(13, suppl 4): 262–271.

Kumar R, Blumberg EA, Danziger-Isakov L, et al. Influenza vaccination in the organ transplant recipient: review and summary recommendations. Am J Transplant 2011;11:2020–2030.

Limkemann AJ, Wolfe L, Sharma A, et al. Outcomes of kidney transplants and risk of infection transmission form increased infectious risk donors. Clin Transplant 2016;30:886–893.

Locke JE, Mehta S, Reed RD, et al. A national study of outcomes among HIV-infected kidney transplant recipients. J Am Soc Nephrol 2015;26:2222–2229.

Muñoz L, Santin M. Prevention and management of tuberculosis in transplant recipients: from guidelines to clinical practice. Transplantation 2016;100:1840–1852.

Origüen J, Lopez-Medrano F, Fernando-Ruiz M, et al. Should asymptomatic bacteriuria be systematically treated in kidney transplant recipients? Results from a randomized controlled trial. Am J Transplant 2016;16:2943–2953.

Pagalilauan GL, Limaye AP. Infections in transplant patients. Med Clin North Am 2013;97(4):581–600.

Razonable RR, Humar A; The AST Infectious Diseases Community of Practice. Cytomegalovirus in solid organ transplantation. Am J Transplant 2013;(13, suppl 4): 93–106.

Schwartz BS, Mawhorter SD; the AST Infectious Diseases Community of Practice. Parasitic infections in solid organ transplantation. Am J Transplant 2013;(13, suppl 4): 280–303.

Seem DL, Lee I, Umscheid CA, et al. Excerpt from PHS guideline for reducing HIV, HBV and HCV transmission through organ transplantation. Am J Transplant 2013;13:1953–1962.

13 Kidney Transplantation and Liver Disease

Suphamai Bunnapradist, Paul Martin, and
Fabrizio Fabrizi

Liver dysfunction is common in patients undergoing kidney transplantation. Renal transplant candidates are at increased risk for a number of hepatic diseases, most notably chronic hepatitis C (HCV), which remains more common in end-stage kidney disease (ESKD) patients than the general population. A series of measures including vaccination have diminished the risk of hepatitis B transmission in dialysis units although outbreaks of HBV infection continue to occur, typically reflecting failure to adhere to precautions to limit its spread. However, because of their frequent comorbidities such as diabetes, patients with advanced chronic kidney disease (CKD) are also at risk of other etiologies of liver disease such as nonalcoholic fatty liver disease (NAFLD). Ineffective erythropoiesis owing to CKD may result in hepatic iron deposition. Other considerations in this population include drug-induced liver injury common in patients with CKD who are often prescribed multiple medications.

Routine assessment of the renal transplant candidate includes standard liver biochemical tests in addition to serologic testing for HBV and HCV infection. Liver enzyme levels are typically spuriously low in dialysis patients, so the presence of liver disease may not be apparent. The differential diagnosis of hepatic dysfunction in the adult renal transplant candidate includes chronic viral hepatitis as well as the full spectrum of adult liver diseases. These include NAFLD related to diabetes mellitus and hyperlipidemia; drug-induced hepatotoxicity; passive hepatic dysfunction owing to congestive heart failure; and chronic viral hepatitis. Appropriate evaluation of the renal transplant candidate with chronic viral hepatitis includes assessment of viral replication, liver histology, and consideration of antiviral therapy. Availability of effective and well-tolerated oral regimens for HCV will facilitate the treatment of HCV in this population as had happened for HBV previously.

Before approving renal transplant candidacy, the workup needs to establish the etiology of any concomitant hepatic dysfunction and its severity. Alcohol consumption should be quantified as well as excluding the consumption of potentially hepatotoxic herbal products. As discussed below, liver biopsy may be appropriate after ultrasound to exclude unrecognized biliary tract disease.

RENAL TRANSPLANT RECIPIENTS WITH VIRAL HEPATITIS: HEPATITIS B

Diagnostic Tests and Their Interpretation
Table 13.1 describes the key diagnostic tests for hepatitis B virus and their interpretation. Serum hepatitis B surface antigen (HBsAg) is the first detectable serum marker in acute HBV infection. After an

TABLE 13.1	Tests for Hepatitis B Virus
Tests	**Interpretation**
HBsAg (Hepatitis B surface antigen)	HBV infection
IgM Anti-HBc (Antibody to hepatitis B core antigen)	Acute or recent HBV infection
IgG Anti-HBc (Antibody to hepatitis B core antigen)	Chronic or remote HBV infection
HBsAb (Antibody to hepatitis B surface antigen)	Immunity to HBV (vaccine-induced or a result of prior infection)
HBe (Hepatitis B e antigen)	Active replication
HBV DNA (HBV viremia)	Active replication

incubation period of up to 140 days, the patient may develop symptoms such as malaise and anorexia, or even become frankly icteric. By this time, other serum markers of HBV infection appear, including antibody to the hepatitis B core antigen (anti-HBc). Hepatitis B core antigen (HBcAg) is present exclusively in nuclei of infected hepatocytes, but the corresponding antibody circulates in blood. During acute HBV infection, anti-HBc antibody is predominantly immunoglobulin M (IgM). Over the subsequent 6 months, IgM levels decline, whereas IgG anti-HBc levels persist. Although anti-HBc is not a neutralizing antibody, it is the most durable marker of prior HBV infection. With successful resolution of acute HBV, protective antibody against HBsAg (anti-HBs) appears, signifying immunity against HBV. Anti-HBs antibody tends to decline and even disappear over time, leaving an "isolated" core antibody (IgG anti-HBc) as the only marker of prior HBV infection. If HBsAg persists for more than 3 months, serum HBV DNA and hepatitis B e antigen (HBeAg) levels should be obtained to assess the level of active viral replication.

Natural History
Important prognostic factors determining likelihood of developing chronic infection is age of HBV acquisition and host immunity. Approximately 5% of infected immunocompetent adults fail to recover from acute HBV infection and develop chronic HBV. In the latter individuals, HBsAg persists in serum, and anti-HBs fail to appear. Chronicity is also more likely in individuals with impaired immune response such as the elderly and patients with ESKD. Symptomatic acute HBV with jaundice is more likely to lead to successful clearance of HBV infection than subclinical acute HBV. This apparent paradox is explained by the prominent role host immunity plays in the expression of the clinical course of HBV. The immune response during icteric acute HBV infection results in liver injury with a more vigorous response producing symptoms, but also a greater likelihood of spontaneous recovery compared with symptomatically milder acute HBV. Two phases of chronic HBV infection follow. In the early months and years of chronic HBV infection, the "replicative" phase occurs, which is often accompanied by necro-inflammatory changes in the liver with elevated serum aminotransferase levels. The "replicative

phase" is characterized by active viral replication: HBeAg and high titers of HBV DNA are present in serum. The second phase of chronic HBV infection is the "nonreplicative" phase, which is often heralded by a transient increase in aminotransferase levels. The nonreplicative phase follows HBeAg clearance. With HBeAg loss, antibodies to HBeAg appear in serum, HBV DNA levels decrease, and, generally, liver disease activity subsides both biochemically and histologically. After HBeAg clearance, infectivity is much reduced, but low levels of HBV DNA may persist for variable periods of time. Although these patients usually have persistently normal alanine transaminase (ALT) and aspartate transaminase (AST) levels and absent or lower serum HBV DNA ($<2,000$ IU/mL), they still are at risk for developing progressive liver disease triggered by immunosuppression after renal transplantation. The HBV genome shows significant heterogeneity and various mutant forms of HBV have been identified in which amino acid substitutions at crucial sites in the viral genome occur. An important subset of patients clears HBeAg and develops the corresponding anti-HBe antibody, but they continue to have active replication with strongly positive serum HBV DNA with elevated transaminases. This HBeAg-negative form of chronic HBV is characterized clinically by a less likely sustained response to antiviral therapy than is found in chronically infected patients who remain HBeAg positive. The HBeAg-negative form of chronic HBV, a later stage of chronic HBV infection, is becoming more prevalent as vaccination programs reduce the incidence of acute HBV infection.

HBV infection is a major cause of morbidity, with as many as 350 million people infected worldwide, resulting in an estimated 1 million deaths per year. Despite the availability of a vaccine since the early 1980s, HBV remains a major cause of chronic hepatitis, cirrhosis, and hepatocellular carcinoma. Large-scale immigration to Western Europe and North America from areas of higher prevalence of chronic HBV such as Asia and sub-Saharan Africa has resulted in reservoirs of HBV infection in areas with large immigrant populations. Several HBV genotypes have been identified. Specific HBV genotype may be associated with more severe liver disease; for instance, genotype C, common in Asians, confers a high risk for the development of cirrhosis and hepatocellular carcinoma and genotype A are more likely to respond to interferon to induced HBeAg seroconversion. However, HBV genotyping has not yet been recommended as part of routine clinical practice to guide management.

Prevention of HBV acquisition in dialysis centers has been an important aspect of its management in patients with ESKD. The incidence and prevalence of HBV infection in dialysis patients in developed countries have fallen since the mid-1970s as a result of strict attention to relatively simple precautions. Outbreaks of HBV infection in dialysis units are now usually a result of nonadherence to these precautions, which include serologic surveillance, isolation of HBV-infected patients, use of dedicated dialysis machines, and rigorous disinfection. HBsAg rates remain higher in patients on dialysis in less developed countries where HBV remains prevalent in the population as a whole. Despite the availability of HBV vaccination since the early 1980s, many patients on chronic dialysis have not been vaccinated. Although response to vaccination with development of protective levels of anti-HBs is not universal in this population, at least 60% of chronic dialysis patients do respond adequately. Hepatitis B vaccine should be recommended in all candidates with no previous exposure, and anti-HBV titer should be checked to confirm immunity. Subcutaneous administration or higher or repeated doses should be considered in patients with inadequate response. Periodic antibody testing should be considered because of a higher rate of loss of anti-HBs in uremic patients.

HBV Disease Progression after Renal Transplantation
The prevalence of HBV infection among renal transplant candidates has decreased because of the success of efforts to limit spread of HBV infection in the dialysis population and widespread use of hepatitis B vaccine. Because of concern about post-transplantation progression of liver disease, HBV infection had been regarded as a relative contraindication to renal transplantation before introduction of effective oral therapy. Recognized risk factors for progression of HBV-related liver disease include: longer duration of infection; high serum levels of HBV DNA; genotype C; coinfection with hepatitis C or D; HIV coinfection; and therapeutic immunosuppression. Immunosuppression may increase HBV replication by various mechanisms, including diminished activity of cytotoxic T lymphocytes. In addition, the HBV genome contains a glucocorticoid-responsive element that augments HBV replication. Azathioprine and the calcineurin inhibitors (CNIs) may also enhance HBV replication.

The adverse effect of immunosuppressive therapy on HBV infection has been recognized in several clinical settings. Severe, even fatal, HBV reactivation is noted in patients who receive systemic chemotherapy. Reactivation of HBV has been observed in renal transplant recipients with markers of resolved HBV infection with reappearance of HBsAg in serum despite its absence before transplantation.

The adverse effect of HBsAg seropositivity on patient survival in renal transplant recipients had been well established before effective and well-tolerated oral antiviral agents were licensed. With effective long-term suppression of HBV infection with oral therapy, excellent patient and graft survivals are now possible.

Evaluation of Kidney Transplant Candidates with HBV
Figure 13.1 illustrates an approach to the kidney transplant candidate with a diagnosis of HBV. Liver biopsy is recommended in the evaluation of renal transplant candidates with HBsAg because it is often difficult, on noninvasive testing, to gauge the severity of liver disease. As noted earlier, aminotransferase levels may be spuriously normal despite necroinflammatory changes on liver biopsy in the presence of CKD. Desmopressin acetate (DDAVP) should be administered by intravenous infusion at the time of percutaneous biopsy to counteract uremic platelet dysfunction. If there is clinical concern about the presence of cirrhosis, a transjugular liver biopsy with measurement of portal pressures can provide additional prognostic information. If the hepatic venous pressure gradient is <10 mm Hg, complications of portal hypertension such as variceal hemorrhage are unlikely to develop in compensated cirrhosis.

The decision concerning transplant candidacy in HBsAg-positive patients should be based on both liver histology and evaluation of HBV

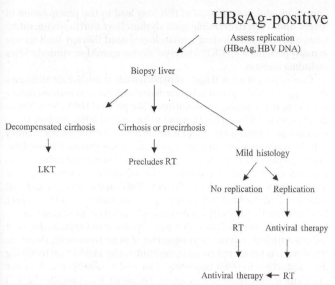

FIGURE 13.1 Approach to the workup of the kidney transplant candidate with viral hepatitis B. HBV, hepatitis B virus; LKT, combined liver-and-kidney transplant; RT, renal transplant.

replication by serum markers (i.e., HBeAg and HBV DNA). The absence of serum marker of replication, that is, HBV DNA or HBeAg positivity, before transplantation, however, does not preclude reactivation of HBV infection after transplantation. In patients with well-compensated cirrhosis without varices on endoscopy or other evidence of hepatic, isolated renal transplant is reasonable. However, if major complications of cirrhosis have supervened, combined liver–kidney transplant is recommended (see below). In patients with intact renal function, antiviral therapy with suppression of HBV replication can lead to regression of even advanced fibrosis. In transplant candidates with active HBV replication, pretransplant antiviral therapy should be initiated to prevent disease progression by suppressing HBV replication. Importantly, even in the absence of cirrhosis, there is an increased risk of hepatocellular carcinoma in patients with chronic HBV infection, so twice-yearly ultrasound is indicated for screening before and after renal transplant. Although liver biopsy has been the gold standard for evaluating disease severity in chronic viral hepatitis, unless equivocal evidence of cirrhosis is present, therapeutic decisions, especially in chronic HCV infection, are increasingly being based on transient elastography ("Fibroscan") which provides noninvasive assessment of severity of fibrosis.

Antiviral Therapy
The options for antiviral therapy for HBV have expanded with several licensed oral agents in addition to interferon (IFN). Although IFN and pegIFN are efficacious in the treatment of chronic HBV, their use is contraindicated in renal transplant recipients because the

immunomodulatory actions of IFN may lead to the precipitation of severe and often irreversible graft dysfunction. Furthermore, interferon side effects including hematologic-based therapy limit its use in many patients with CKD who typically have multiple comorbidities including anemia.

Currently licensed oral agents are nucleoside or nucleotide analogues that suppress HBV replication by interfering with the reverse transcriptase activity of HBV, causing termination of the proviral DNA chain. These drugs suppress HBV replication and reduce necro-inflammatory activity. They are well tolerated and have no adverse immunomodulatory activity so they can be also used post- as well as prerenal transplant. Prolonged use of lamivudine, the first licensed oral agent to treat HBV, is associated with the development of antiviral drug resistance, and it has been replaced by newer oral agents. Entecavir is effective and well tolerated and does not induce antiviral resistance unless the patient has had prior therapy with lamivudine or related drugs. Dosage reduction is required in renal insufficiency. Tenofovir, in contrast, does not induce antiviral resistance irrespective of prior treatment. However, tenofovir has been implicated in nephrotoxicity in addition requiring dose reduction in renal impairment as well as osteopenia. A newer pro-drug formulation of this agent, tenofovir alafenamide ("TAF") reduces these side effects.

RENAL TRANSPLANT RECIPIENTS WITH VIRAL HEPATITIS: HEPATITIS C

Interpretation of Diagnostic Tests

Table 13.2 describes diagnostic tests for HCV and their interpretation. Serologic testing is the initial screening tool for HCV infection. Third-generation enzyme-linked immunosorbent assays (ELISAs), now widely used, have excellent specificity and sensitivity, including in patients with CKD. Confirmation of HCV requires detection of HCV viremia (HCV RNA) in serum by reverse-transcriptase polymerase chain reaction (PCR). A PCR test should be performed if there is unexplained transaminitis

TABLE 13.2	Tests for Hepatitis C Virus	
Tests	**Uses**	**Comments**
Anti-HCV ELISA 3.0	Initial diagnosis	Excellent sensitivity
HCV PCR qualitative TMA	Confirmation of HCV infection	Helpful in dialysis of seronegative patients
HCV PCR quantitative	Assessment of viral load	Less sensitive than qualitative tests; more reproducible than qualitative tests; useful for monitoring response to IFN
HCV genotyping	Treatment decision	Role in predicting responsiveness to IFN

ELISA, enzyme-linked immunosorbent assay; IFN, interferon; PCR, polymerase chain reaction.

or if a clinical concern about HCV infection remains despite negative serologies. Development of anti-HCV may be delayed for several weeks in acute HCV although serum HCV RNA is already detectable.

Natural History

Chronic HCV infection remains prevalent in the hemodialysis population due in part to nosocomial spread in hemodialysis units. HCV infection and its potential complications are a frequent cause of concern in potential renal transplant recipients. Because the natural history of HCV extends over decades rather than years, adverse consequences of chronic HCV infection in patients followed for a short period of time may not be apparent. CKD patients have higher morbidity and mortality rates than do the general population because of their comorbidities such as diabetes and systemic hypertension. As a result, the long-term consequences of HCV infection had been difficult to assess in this population. Evaluation of HCV infection in renal transplant candidates is further complicated by the observation that aminotransferase levels in the dialysis population are usually lower than the nonuremic population. Dialysis patients who are HCV viremic have aminotransferase levels greater than those who are not HCV viremic, although typically, the values are still within the "normal "range. A series of meta-analyses have conclusively established that HCV infection in the hemodialysis population results in excessive morbidity and mortality related to liver disease. Several major HCV genotypes and subtypes have been identified; they differ little in clinical expression but vary somewhat in their responsiveness to viral agents.

Disease Progression after Renal Transplantation

The frequency of HCV infection among renal transplant recipients is influenced by various factors, including prior blood transfusion, history of previous transplantation, type and duration of pretransplant renal replacement therapy, history of IV drug use and geographic origin. Most anti-HCV–seropositive renal transplant recipients have persistent HCV viremia. HCV RNA titers increase markedly as a result of post-transplant as a result of immunosuppression. Post-transplant HCV-related liver disease is often progressive. Factors implicated in more rapid progression include alcohol abuse, HBV and HIV coinfection. Liver disease was more aggressive in recipients who acquired acute HCV at the time of transplantation, before screening for HCV was available, because they experienced liver injury at a time of maximum immunosuppression. It is unclear whether choice of initial CNI affects the progression. Although cyclosporine at high concentrations has an inhibitory effect on HCV replication, the benefit of cyclosporine over tacrolimus in the clinical setting is unclear. Azathioprine and antilymphocyte agents to treat rejection have been implicated in more severe liver disease in HCV-infected recipients. Administration of high-dose steroids and antilymphocyte antibodies may be used after a critical evaluation of potential risk and benefit, especially the risk for accelerating the course of liver disease. With availability of effective oral agents to treat HCV disease, progression of liver disease post renal transplant is now less of a concern.

Detailed studies have documented an adverse effect of HCV infection on patient survival after kidney transplantation alone and after combined kidney–pancreas transplantation. However, the outcome of HCV-infected kidney transplant recipients is better than for matched patients who remain on dialysis. Recipients of a first deceased donor transplant have an initially greater perioperative risk for death than those who remain on dialysis therapy but unequivocal long-term benefits.

Glomerulonephritis and mixed cryoglobulinemia related to HCV have been reported after transplantation and can lead to graft loss. HCV infection is implicated in the development of new-onset diabetes after transplantation (NODAT), itself a risk factor for recipient death and graft loss (see Chapter 11). In HCV-positive renal transplant recipients, an overall incidence of NODAT of 40% has been reported. The figure may be even higher if tacrolimus is used for immunosuppression and if other risk factors are present. Successful treatment of HCV is anticipated to reduce the risk of NODAT.

Evaluation of Renal Transplant Recipient with HCV

Figure 13.2 illustrates an approach to the evaluation of renal transplant candidates with HCV. Liver biopsy has been an integral part of the evaluation of liver disease in kidney transplant candidates with HCV because of concern that reliance on clinical and biochemical findings may underestimate its severity. As noted earlier for HBV, transient elastography is likely to play an increasing role in evaluation of liver disease in renal transplant candidates. Patients with minimal to mild chronic fibrosis (stages I and II) can proceed safely to renal transplant without concern for hepatic decompensation. Pretransplant treatment of hepatitis C will abort progression of liver disease and protect the graft against HCV-related glomerulonephritis. However, eradication

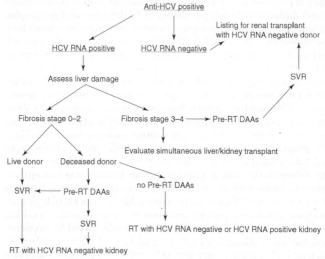

FIGURE 13.2 Approach to the workup of the kidney transplant candidate with viral hepatitis C. HCV, hepatitis C virus; LKT, combined liver-and-kidney transplant; RT, renal transplant.

of HCV infection before renal transplant precludes the recipient from receiving a graft from a deceased HCV-seropositive donor: the benefit being a considerably shorter time on the waiting list. For this reason, HCV-positive kidney transplant candidates who do not have a living donor are generally recommended to delay antiviral therapy until they have received a deceased donor kidney, likely from a HCV-positive donor.

Potential HCV-positive recipients who are suspected to be cirrhotic require transjugular pressure measurements and liver biopsy as outlined for HBV. If portal hypertension is absent or mild with a hepatic venous pressure gradient <10 mm Hg despite the presence of extensive fibrosis or cirrhosis, renal transplant alone is appropriate with treatment of HCV. For decompensated cirrhotic patients, combined liver–kidney transplantation is a consideration (see "Kidney and Liver Transplantation").

Status of Antiviral Therapy for HCV

Progress in the treatment of HCV has been dramatic. The major goals of treatment are to induce a sustained virologic response (SVR) and reverse fibrosis. SVR is defined as absence of HCV viremia 12 or more weeks following completion of antiviral therapy. Interferon-based therapy has become obsolete with the development of a variety of direct antiviral regimens with excellent tolerability. Unlike HBV therapy, which is administered long-term and is suppressive rather than curative in most patients, HCV treatment is curative with finite treatment regimens of 8 to 24 weeks. The appropriate duration of therapy is determined by viral genotype, load, severity of liver disease, and whether the patient has failed prior attempts at therapy. The current approach to treatment of HCV involves a combination of oral agents active against different parts of the HCV replicative cycle. The first-generation direct-acting antiviral agents (DAAs), telaprevir and boceprevir, have now been superseded by more effective and better-tolerated second-generation oral agents. The HCV genome encodes for several proteins, structural and nonstructural. HCV NS5B is a polymerase which is highly conserved and a key target for antiviral agents. Sofosbuvir inhibits this enzyme and has been a crucial component in several regimens which also incorporate agents active against other parts of the HCV replicative cycle. A concern with sofosbuvir has been accumulation of it and its metabolites in patients with severe impairment of renal function. In addition, drug–drug interactions with amiodorone have resulted in reports of bradycardia. Other regimens which do not include sofosbuvir contain NS5A inhibitors as well as NS3/4A inhibitors. However, an increasing number of clinical studies have confirmed the efficacy and tolerability of newer agents in the CKD population. Further details can be obtained at www.hcvguidelines.org where regular updates are available as well as recommendations about dose adjustment of CNIs in the event that HCV treatment is deferred until after renal transplant. With currently licensed drugs, the majority of HCV-infected renal transplant candidates and recipients can be cured. Remaining challenges include spontaneous and treatment-induced viral mutations, overall lower response rates for HCV genotype 3 infection, drug-to-drug interactions, and the requirement for ribavirin with some of these newer regimens.

CAUSES OF LIVER DISEASE IN RENAL TRANSPLANT RECIPIENTS

Viral infections, such as herpes simplex virus (HSV) and cytomegalovirus (CMV), and drug hepatotoxicity should be considered in the differential diagnosis of post-transplantation hepatic dysfunction. Patients should be questioned about ingestion of alcohol and hepatotoxic drugs. Specific inquiry should be made about use of herbal and health food store products. Serum aminotransferase levels should be rechecked after the patient has abstained from potential toxic substances. A low-grade, transient elevation of serum aminotransferases is commonly seen in the first few months post-transplant and is likely owing to drug-induced hepatotoxicity. If hepatic dysfunction persists or is more marked, a thorough workup, including liver biopsy, is indicated. Fatty liver is now an emerging cause of liver failure especially in patient with diabetes and metabolic syndrome.

An important consideration in a transplant recipient with unexplained hepatic dysfunction is viral hepatitis acquired from the donor graft. This should be excluded by appropriate serologies and molecular testing. In patients who received a kidney from Public Health Service (PHS) increased risk donors (see Chapters 5 and 12), interval testing according to PHS increased risk donor guideline should be followed. Intermittent hepatic dysfunction may result from biliary colic, and pain might not be prominent in older or sicker patients. Ultrasound is the initial investigation.

THE DECEASED KIDNEY DONOR WITH POSITIVE HEPATITIS SEROLOGIES

Donor HBsAg positivity has historically precluded kidney donation in the United States and elsewhere. However, the availability of effective hepatitis B therapy suggests that outcomes may be acceptable with appropriate recipient selection. The use of organs from HBsAg-negative, anti-HBc antibody–positive deceased donors also has the potential to transmit HBV infection because of amplification of minute quantities of residual HBV DNA by immunosuppression. The rate of transmission is significantly higher in hepatic recipients than in other solid-organ recipients. In contrast, use of a renal graft from an IgG anti-HBc antibody–positive donor is associated with a very low risk for infection transmission, and these kidneys can be safely considered for donation, especially for recipients who have been successfully immunized with HBV vaccine. If an anti-HBc ("core")–positive organ is used in an HBV-naïve recipient, considerations include the use of oral antiviral prophylaxis at least for 1 year post-transplant. If the potential donor is IgM anti-HBc–positive, recent acute HBV is likely even in the absence of HBsAg with possibly a greater risk for HBV transmission.

Transmission of HCV by renal transplantation has been unequivocally demonstrated with occasionally severe acute, even fatal, hepatitis. There are wide variations in the rate of transmission of HCV from anti-HCV–positive donors, which may reflect several factors, including donor HCV viral load and the technique used for preservation of donor grafts. The rate of transmission of HCV from HCV-infected donors appears to be much higher if flush preservation instead of pulsatile perfusion is used. The role of HCV genotyping of donor and recipient is less well established.

Transplantation of kidneys from anti-HCV–positive donors into anti-HCV–positive recipients appears safe. However, among anti-HCV–positive recipients, those who received anti-HCV–positive kidneys may have a somewhat worse survival rate than did recipients of anti-HCV–negative kidneys. This observation, however, may reflect other factors including recipient selection. HCV infection is more common in deceased donors than in the general population. For an HCV-positive renal transplant candidate, the waiting time for an organ may be considerably shortened by the acceptance of a kidney from an HCV-positive donor. Because survival following renal transplantation is enhanced compared with survival on chronic dialysis, HCV-positive transplant candidate should be encouraged to accept an HCV-positive graft rather than wait for an organ from an HCV-negative donor. The benefits and risks of accepting an HCV-positive graft must be carefully discussed with HCV-positive transplant candidates.

COMBINED LIVER-AND-KIDNEY TRANSPLANTATION

Kidney dysfunction is extremely common in patients with advanced liver disease. Its true frequency and severity are hard to measure because of the unreliability of creatinine-based estimates of GFR in patients with advanced liver disease. Cystatin C-based estimates may be better; radionuclide estimates of GFR (see Chapter 14) are better still though they are infrequently performed. The Model for End-Stage Liver Disease (MELD) score for organ allocation in liver transplantation is derived from the serum sodium, INR, and bilirubin, and assessment of renal function as expressed by the serum creatinine or need for chronic dialysis. Following the introduction of the MELD score, the number of recipients of simultaneous liver–kidney (SLK) transplants has more than doubled in the United States. Over times, given the shortage of livers for transplantation, mean MELD scores at the time of liver transplant have risen so that a potential liver transplant recipient is increasingly likely to have renal dysfunction.

The allocation of the kidney in patients receiving an SLK is determined by the allocation of the prime organ—the liver (similarly for heart–kidney and pancreas–kidney) so that the kidney allocation takes priority over allocation to those waiting for a kidney transplant alone. As a result, paradoxically, patients waiting for an SLK will likely wait considerably less for their kidney than if they were waiting for a kidney transplant alone. A particular challenge has been establishing the objective criteria for SLK. On clinical grounds, it is difficult to predict which patients with decompensated liver disease and renal dysfunction, even if severe enough to require renal replacement therapy pretransplant, will ultimately become dialysis dependent following liver transplant. Recipient survival is diminished in liver transplant recipients who required long-term dialysis post-transplant, while the allocation of kidneys to liver transplant recipients whose own kidneys are destined to recover is clearly wasteful, particularly given the great shortage of kidneys for those in need of a kidney transplant alone.

An additional concern is that renal grafts allocated to SLK recipients often are obtained for donors with a lower kidney donor profile index ([KDPI], see Chapter 5) and thus greater graft expected longevity. Furthermore, since multi-organ donor allocation takes precedence over kidney-alone allocation, access of highly sensitized renal candidates with high panel reactive antibody levels to renal grafts is limited despite the fact that they have high priority in kidney-alone allocation. Experience has shown considerable inconsistency across the United States regarding the policy for SLK.

A number of efforts have been made to develop criteria for performing SLK.

Readers are referred to Nadim et al. in Selected Readings and to Table 13.3 and its source document. Each of these documents attempts

TABLE 13.3 Proposed Indications for Combined Kidney-and-Liver Transplantation

If the Candidate's Transplant Nephrologist Confirms a Diagnosis of:	Then the Transplant Program Must Document in the Candidate's Medical Record:
CKD with a measured or calculated GFR less than or equal to 60 mL/min for greater than 90 consecutive days*	*At least one* of the following: • That the candidate has begun regularly administered dialysis as an ESKD patient in a hospital-based, independent non–hospital-based, or home setting. • That the candidate's most recent measured or calculated creatinine clearance (CrCl) or GFR is less than or equal to 35 mL/min at the time of registration on the kidney waiting list.
Sustained acute kidney injury	*At least one* of the following: 1. That the candidate has been on dialysis for at least 6 consecutive weeks. 2. That the candidate has a measured or calculated CrCl or GFR less than or equal to 25 mL/min for at least 6 consecutive weeks and this is documented in the candidate's medical record every 7 days beginning with the date of the first test with this value. 3. That the candidate has any combination of #1 and #2 above for 6 consecutive weeks.
Metabolic disease	An additional diagnosis of *at least one* of the following: 1. Hyperoxaluria 2. Atypical HUS from mutations in factor H and possibly factor I 3. Familial nonneuropathic systemic amyloid 4. Methylmalonic aciduria

*CKD may occur simultaneously with CLD in patients as a consequence of various forms of glomerulonephritis (related to IgA, HBV, and HCV), diabetes, CNI toxicity from a prior liver transplant, and prolonged acute kidney injury.
(Reprinted with permission from Organ Procurement Transplantation Network (OPTN), Richmond, VA, 2017.)

to address the relative unpredictability of kidney function recovery after peri-liver transplant hepato-renal syndrome and acute kidney injury.

The "Safety Net" for Kidney Allocation Post Liver Transplant

Given the difficulty of predicting which candidates for liver transplant are destined to develop ESKD, a proposal has been made to give patients whose kidneys are not functioning (or eGFR <20 mL/min) between 2 and 12 months post liver transplant, a degree of increased priority in obtaining a deceased donor kidney transplant. The so-called "safety net" or "rescue option" is designed to provide transplant teams the security in knowing that if kidney function does not recover, their patient will not have to wait many years to obtain a kidney, and hence to relieve the pressure to perform SLK when a liver transplant alone may suffice.

Living donor kidney transplantation is also an option if an appropriate living donor is available.

Futility

Pretransplant mortality may approach 50% in some centers where the waiting times for liver transplantation are prolonged and the MELD scores at the time of transplant are very high (>40). These unfortunate patients are likely to have had prolonged ICU stays, to be intubated, deeply encephalopathic, septic, and requiring vasoconstrictor support of blood pressure. In the surviving patients who undergo SLK, mortality rates are high and prolonged delayed kidney graft function may be irreversible in up to 20%. For this reason, and to avoid prolonged suffering and unnecessary wastage of organs, the difficult decision that the transplant is futile may need to be made and comfort measure employed (see Lunsford et al. in Selected Readings). Patients who have been waitlisted for an SLK, but whose condition deteriorates while waiting, should be reassessed at regular intervals to ensure that the SLK has not become futile.

A more favorable scenario, where SLK or kidney transplant alone is contraindicated, may occur in patients who are potential kidney transplant candidates, but have chronic liver disease of a degree that is deemed to contraindicate kidney transplant alone, yet is not of a severity that would indicate candidacy for a liver transplant. Many of these patients' liver function will inevitably deteriorate and their MELD scores rise to a transplantable level. In the interim, they are better served by remaining on dialysis, even though they may feel frustrated and "trapped" by liver function "too bad" for a kidney, but "too good" for a liver. Effective antiviral therapies will hopefully make this scenario less frequent.

Immunologic Protection

Liver transplantation appears to provide a form of immunologic "protection" to concomitantly transplanted organs. This allograft-enhancing effect of the liver on other transplanted organs from the same donor can be demonstrated even for patients with a positive pretransplant crossmatch. Several immunologic mechanisms for this phenomenon have been proposed, including the development of anti-idiotypic antibodies to major histocompatibility complex (MHC) class I and class II antibodies, the absorption of lymphocytotoxic antibodies onto reticuloendothelial cells of the liver allograft, and a soluble MHC class I molecule, which is principally made in the liver, that may inhibit cytotoxic T-lymphocyte activity. Another important mechanism may be the development of hematopoietic chimerism occurring after liver transplantation, resulting in tolerance.

There are practical implications to the protective effect of the concomitant liver transplantation. It may not be necessary to routinely crossmatch unsensitized patients before LKT, though US programs are now required to do so. If the crossmatch is positive in a sensitized patient, the LKT may not necessarily be contraindicated, and some programs progress with transplantation with the addition of a perioperative infusion of intravenous immune globulin (see Chapter 6). The intensity of immunosuppression after liver transplantation alone is generally less than that after other organ transplants, and before the era of effective antiviral therapy, fear of recurrent disease was greater than the fear of rejection.

Polycystic Kidney and Liver Disease

Liver cysts (PLD) are extremely common in polycystic kidney disease (PKD), occurring in over 50% of PKD patients over the age of 50 years. The cysts are typically asymptomatic and clinically insignificant. Occasional however, massive, painful cystic enlargement of the liver can occur with abdominal distension, early satiety, and even malnutrition. Liver function, however, is typically unimpaired. Symptomatic relief can sometimes be obtained by cyst drainage or deroofing. For some of these patients, the best option is hepatectomy and SLK. Because the MELD score of PLD/PKD patients is low, priority for allocation of a liver is likely to be low. In these circumstances, application can be made for a "MELD-exception" by which allocation points are added over time until an SLK is allocated. A similar policy is in effect for a patient with liver cancer. Though surgically challenging, because of the massive size of the liver and kidneys, the surgical prognosis of PKL/PKD patients is good because of maintained liver function and effective coagulation. The decision to remove the native kidneys is usually made at the time of transplantation, depending on their size and relative proportions.

KIDNEY AFTER LIVER TRANSPLANTATION

CKD develops in close to 20% of OLT recipients at 5-year follow-up and is associated with an increased risk of death after transplantation. The etiology of renal failure is typically multifactorial and includes progression of preexisting renal disease, perioperative renal damage, CNI toxicity, nephrotoxic effects of other drugs, hypertension, HCV with associated glomerulonephritis, and diabetes. Renal transplantation may be a consideration in otherwise robust liver transplant recipients who develop ESKD to avoid the higher complication of immunosuppression in this population. Those with hepatitis C–associated glomerulonephritis should be treated with the goal of eradication of the virus and to prevent recurrence.

Selected Readings

Bhamidimarri KR, Czul F, Peyton A, et al. Safety, efficacy and tolerability of half-dose sofosbuvir plus simeprevir in treatment of hepatitis C in patients with end stage renal disease. J Hepatol 2015;63:763–765.

Bunnapradist M, Danovitch GM. Marginal quality kidneys for simultaneous liver-kidney transplantation: to pass or double down? Liver Transpl 2017;23:7–8.

Del Bello D, Ross MJ, Huprikar S. Hepatitis C virus infection and kidney transplantation: newer options and a brighter future ahead? Kidney Int 2015;88:223–225.

Fabrizi F, Martin P, Messa P. New treatment for hepatitis C in chronic kidney disease. Kidney Int 2016;89:988–994.

Formica RN, Aeder M, Boyle G, et al. Simultaneous liver-kidney allocation policy: a proposal to optimize appropriate utilization of scarce resources. Am J Transplant 2016;16:758–766.

Levitsky J, O'Leary JG, Asrani S, et al. Protecting the kidney in liver transplant recipients: practice-based recommendations from the American Society of Transplantation Liver and Intestine Community of Practice. Am J Transplant 2016;16(9):2532–2544.

Lok AS, McMahon BJ, Brown RS Jr, et al. Antiviral therapy for chronic hepatitis B viral infection in adults: a systematic review and meta-analysis. Hepatology 2016;63:284–306.

Lunsford K, Bodzin D, Markovic D, et al. Avoiding futility in simultaneous liver-kidney transplantation: analysis of 331 consecutive patients listed for dual organ replacement [published online ahead of print May 6, 2016]. AnnSurg. 2016.

Morales JM, Fabrizi F. Hepatitis C and its impact on renal transplantation. Nat Rev Nephrol 2015;11:172–182.

Nadim M, Sung R, Davis C, et al. Simultaneous liver-kidney transplantation summit: current state and future directions. Am J Transplant 2012;12:2901–2908.

Pham P, Lunsford K, Bunnapradist M, et al. Simultaneous liver-kidney transplantation or liver transplantation alone for patients in need of liver transplantation with renal dysfunction. Curr Opin Organ Transplant 2016;21:194–200.

Roth D, Nelson DR, Bruchfeld A, et al. Grazoprevir plus elbasvir in treatment-naive and treatment experienced patients with hepatitis C virus genotype 1 infection and stage 4-5 chronic kidney disease (the C-SURFER study): a combination phase 3 study. Lancet 2015;386:1537–1545.

Ruebner R, Goldberg D, Abt PL, et al. Risk of end-stage renal disease among liver transplant recipients with pretransplant renal dysfunction. Am J Transplant 2012;12:2958–2965.

Tapper EB, Castera L, Afdhal NH. FibroScan (vibration-controlled transient elastography): where does it stand in the United States practice. Clin Gastroenterol Hepatol 2015;13:27–36.

Wong F, Leung W, Al Beshir M, et al. Outcomes of patients with cirrhosis and hepatorenal syndrome type 1 treated with liver transplantation. Liver Transpl 2015;21:300–307.

Yilmaz VT, Aliosmanoglu I, Erbis H, et al. Effects of hepatitis B surface antigen (HBsAg) positivity of donors in HBsAg(+) renal transplant recipients: comparison of outcomes with HBsAg(+) and HBsAg(-) donors. Transpl Infect Dis 2016;18:55–62.

Diagnostic Imaging in Kidney Transplantation, and Biopsy Technique

Steve S. Raman and Nagesh Ragavendra

The most commonly utilized imaging modalities for renal transplant evaluation are ultrasound (US), nuclear medicine renal scintigraphy, computed tomography (CT), and magnetic resonance imaging (MRI). US provides mostly gross and vascular anatomic information and scintigraphy provides mostly physiologic information, whereas CT and MRI provide an unparalleled degree of anatomic information with increasing levels of physiologic information with the use of intravenous contrast.

IMAGING EVALUATION OF THE LIVING KIDNEY DONOR

The clinical evaluation of the living kidney donor is discussed in Chapter 7. Imaging provides detailed vascular anatomic information regarding the number and branching pattern of the renal arteries and veins, and is used to determine technical feasibility and surgical planning (Fig. 14.1). CT angiography (CTA) has replaced catheter angiography

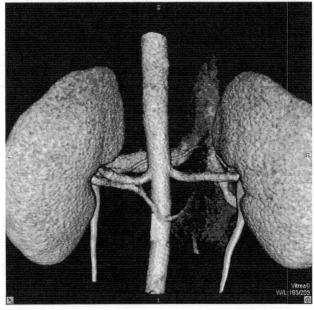

FIGURE 14.1 Computed tomographic angiogram of renal arteries with volume-rendered reformation. Posterior vantage with aorta on **left**, demonstrating two left renal arteries.

as the gold standard for this indication. In CTA, intravenous iodinated nonionic contrast is injected rapidly (4 to 5 cc/sec), after which multi-detector helical imaging is initiated at peak contrast concentration in the aorta using an intermittent sampling technique known as bolus tracking (approximately 20 to 30 seconds after injection) with thin beam collimation (0.5 to 3 mm) for high spatial resolution volumetric data acquisition that can processed for a variety of displays, including multiplanar projections and three-dimensional volume surface rendering and maximal and minimal intensity display.

MR angiography (MRA) is best performed on 1.5 to 3.0T scanners with high-performance gradient coils and multichannel-phased array coils. It is traditionally performed with intravenous gadolinium chelates at 0.1 to 0.2 mmol/kg and is used to delineate renal vascular anatomy without radiation, with almost no risk of nephrotoxicity with one-tenth the contrast dose as multiple detector CT (MDCT). MRA is generally comparable to CTA for detection of major arteries and veins but may be slightly inferior for detection of smaller accessory vessels. Other relative disadvantages of MRA include somewhat lower spatial resolution, lack of reliable imaging of calcification and air, greater operator, protocol, and scanner dependence, and greater sensitivity to artifacts including motion.

The use of intravenous gadolinium chelates are relatively contraindicated in patients with impaired renal function (eGFR < 30 mL/min) and in dialysis patients to avoid nephrogenic sclerosing fibrosis (NSF), a fibrosing disorder of the skin, muscles, visceral surfaces, and organs leading to contractures, muscle weakness, and organ dysfunction. Fortunately, as a result of the precautions introduced after recognition of the relationship between gadolinium and NSF, no new cases of this disorder have been reported for several years. The iron therapy agent ferumoxytol is an alternative imaging agent to gadolinium that may be administered safely to patients with impaired renal function. Non-contrast MRA can also be performed using phase contrast or time of flight techniques. However, phase contrast imaging is time consuming, and time of flight imaging may truncate peripheral arteries, especially when tortuous in course.

Imaging the living donor evaluates renal size, presence of congenital renal anomalies, incidental lesions, calcifications, stones, evidencel of scarring from infection, number and branching patterns of the renal arteries and veins, and the renal collecting system. Also evaluated are the other organs for incidental disorders. Generally, the kidney with a single long left renal artery and vein with major branch vessels near the renal hilum is preferred for harvest. In the event of anatomic abnormalities, the donor is left with the more normal kidney.

IMAGING EVALUATION IN THE EARLY POST-TRANSPLANT PERIOD
Allograft Size
In the early post-transplant period, an increase in renal allograft size occurs both in normal allografts and in a variety of acute processes. The normal renal allograft can increase in volume by up to 30% in the first 2 post-transplant months, usually stabilizing by 6 months. Allograft size in itself is not a reliable indicator of allograft dysfunction.

Collecting System Dilation

Collecting system dilation is graded subjectively as minimal, mild, moderate, or severe and is caused by both obstructive and nonobstructive etiologies. In the immediate postoperative period, self-limited edema at the ureteroneocystostomy site can cause mild obstruction, and mild collecting system dilatation may persist despite. Extrinsic processes such as compression by a peritransplant fluid seroma, hematoma, urinoma or lymphocele are also common (Fig. 14.2). Less common sources of obstruction include intrinsic causes such as a blood clot, calculus, fungus ball, or an intraluminal sloughed papilla. Nonobstructive causes include a distended bladder, transplant ureteral stricture from vascular insufficiency or rejection, BK virus infection, and a prior obstructive cause that has resolved. The absence of collecting system dilation does not exclude the possibility of obstruction.

Obstruction may be seen as progressive collecting system dilatation on serial US, or delayed excretion on renal CT, MR, or scintigraphy that does not respond to administration of diuretics such as intravenous furosemide, with an excretion half-time of more than 20 minutes (normal is less than 15 minutes).

Peritransplant Fluid Collections

Peritransplant fluid collections consist of blood, urine, lymph, or pus and manifest as nonspecific fluid collections on cross-sectional imaging and generally as photopenic regions on renal scintigraphy although urine leaks will collect radiotracer progressively. Although hematomas tend to dense on CT with variable T1 signal on MR, the consistency of the fluid collection cannot reliably be determined on imaging and generally requires imaging-guided fluid aspiration for laboratory analysis. A specimen gram stain, culture, and creatinine should always be sent

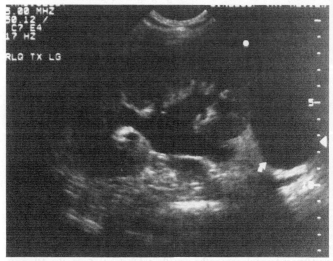

FIGURE 14.2 Sonogram demonstrating hydronephrosis secondary to peritransplant fluid collection.

to exclude infection and urine leak, respectively. Some abscesses may have gas from anaerobic organisms. Complications include allograft collecting system obstruction and iliac vein compression resulting in lower extremity edema.

Hematomas

Hematomas are the most common peritransplant fluid collections in the immediate postoperative period, related to the surgery itself, allograft pseudoaneurysm rupture, or as a complication of biopsy performed to evaluate for transplant rejection. Hematomas may be subcapsular or extra-renal in location and are usually self-limited and resolve spontaneously. Occasionally, a hematoma may be large enough to cause allograft collecting system obstruction.

The imaging appearance of a hematoma depends on the age of blood products, appearing echogenic on US and hyperdense on CT in the acute phase and progressively decreasing in echogenicity on US and density on CT as hemolysis occurs. The signal characteristics of blood products on MR are more complicated, depending on the evolving concentrations of hemoglobin, deoxyhemoglobin, and methemoglobin. They may evolve from T1 hyperintense to T1 hypointense.

Urinomas

Urinomas result from urine extravasation from the allograft pelvis, ureter, or ureteroneocystostomy due to incomplete bladder closure, ureterovesicular anastomotic leak, collecting system ischemia, collecting system rupture from pressure related to severe obstruction, or as a complication of biopsy. Cystography can be performed to determine whether the bladder is the source of leak. The resulting urine leak may be extraperitoneal, intraperitoneal, or both, with urine ascites as a complication of intraperitoneal leak.

Urinomas appear as simple hypoechoic fluid collections usually adjacent to the allograft lower pole on US, as peritransplant fluid collections isodense to that of collecting system fluid on CT, and as peritransplant fluid collections isointense to that of urine seen within the bladder on MR imaging. If urine leakage is active, a contrast-enhanced CT or MR may be acquired in the delayed phase to confirm presence of urine within the peritransplant fluid collection. Similarly, renal scintigraphy may demonstrate an increasingly active accumulation of radiotracer in the urine within the peritransplant fluid collection (Fig. 14.3). Otherwise, ultrasound-guided fluid aspiration may be obtained for creatinine analysis (see Chapter 10).

Lymphoceles

Lymphoceles are the most common peritransplant fluid collection. They result from renal or extraperitoneal lymphatic disruption during allograft harvesting or during transplantation (see Chapter 9) and usually accumulate several weeks to months after surgery. The incidence of lymphocele formation is reported to be higher when rapamycin is used for post-transplantation immunosuppression (see Chapter 6). Small lymphoceles are common and usually asymptomatic, whereas larger ones can cause allograft collecting system obstruction.

Lymphoceles usually appear as septated hypoechoic fluid collections with low-level internal echoes inferior and medial to the allograft on US

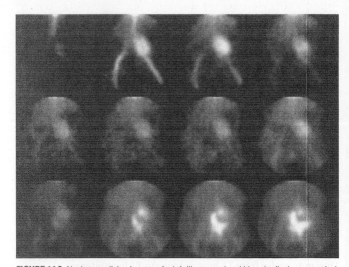

FIGURE 14.3 Nuclear medicine images of a left iliac transplant kidney (radiopharmaceutical: ^{99m}Tc diethylenetriaminepentaacetic acid [DTPA]). The **top left** image shows activity in the abdominal aorta and the beginning of the transplant. The next two images show prompt visualization of the kidney, reflecting normal tracer concentration. In the **bottom row**, enlarging irregular activity is seen between the kidney and urinary bladder, indicative of urinary extravasation.

(Fig. 14.4), as hypodense fluid collections on CT, and as T1 hypointense, T2 hyperintense fluid collections on MRI.

Abscesses

Abscesses usually result from infection of preexisting peritransplant fluid collections and generally occur 4 to 5 weeks after transplantation. Abscesses appear as complicated fluid collections, usually cystic with a thick wall surrounding a central cystic area, which may the containing

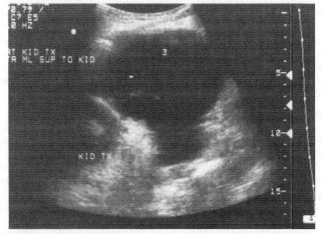

FIGURE 14.4 Sonogram demonstrating lymphocele (*3*) with septations (*arrowhead*).

low-level internal echoes with posterior acoustic enhancement and increased peripheral hyperemia on US. Occasionally, gas is present within abscesses from gas-forming anaerobic bacteria and appears as echogenic foci with indistinct shadowing or ring-down artifact. Similarly, abscesses usually appear as heterogeneous fluid collections that may contain gas on CT (Fig. 14.5). Both US and CT enable rapid diagnosis and provide imaging guidance for aspiration and drainage. Of note, the absence of imaging features characteristic of an abscess does not exclude the presence of infection.

Although image guided aspiration, catheter drainage and lavage is the most efficient method to detect and treat abscesses; in rare cases, variety of radiotracers may be used to detect occult infection, including labeled white blood cells, lymphocytes, antileukocyte antibodies, and Gallium. These tracers are injected intravenously and localize to areas of occult infection or inflammation, especially if collections are deep and intravenous iodine and gadolinium enhanced scans are contraindicated. The dose administered and half-life of the attached radionuclide determine the timing of optimal imaging after injection, which ranges from 2 to 24 hours for ^{99m}Technetium, 1 to 2 days for

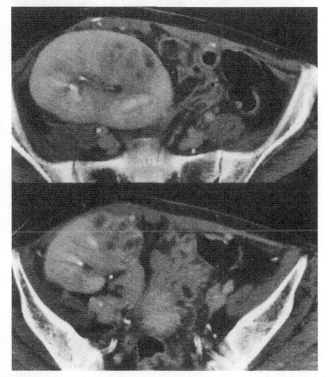

FIGURE 14.5 Abscess in a renal allograft. There is a heterogeneous mass on contrast-enhanced computed tomography. Many small compartments preclude percutaneous drainage. Renal function was surprisingly well preserved. Abscess resolved after intensive antibiotic therapy.

[111]Indium, and 1 to 3 days for [67]Gallium. Of note, scintigraphy results must be interpreted with caution in the presence of rejection, since rejecting transplants may also take up these radiotracers.

Acute Rejection

Acute renal transplant rejection requires a biopsy for definitive diagnosis but has a number of variable imaging appearances, including allograft enlargement, increased or decreased cortical echogenicity, loss of corticomedullary differentiation, prominent hypoechoic medullary pyramids, decreased renal sinus echogenicity, scattered areas of heterogeneously increased echogenicity (presumably hemorrhagic foci) (Fig. 14.6), and/or thickened urothelium on US. Presence of these US findings must be correlated with clinical and laboratory endpoints including elevations in serum creatinine and urinary volume.

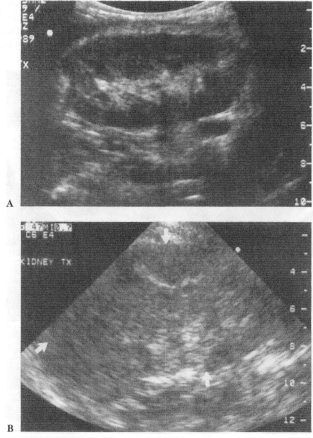

FIGURE 14.6 A: Sonogram of normal transplant kidney. **B:** Sonogram of transplant undergoing rejection reveals graft enlargement, decreased echogenicity of renal sinus (compare to echogenic sinus in **A**), and obscured corticomedullary delineations. Margins of graft are marked by *arrows*.

Chronic Rejection

In chronic rejection, renal function deteriorates gradually. The allograft is usually decreased in size with increased cortical echogenicity, cortical thinning, and elevated RI on US. Angiography may demonstrate decreased number of renal arteries with narrow caliber and irregular lumen, associated with decreased, heterogeneous renal perfusion. Renal scintigraphy shows decreased perfusion, decreased cortical uptake with shift of the renogram peak to the right, and decreased excretion.

Duplex Ultrasound

Duplex US (or more accurately, triplex US if gray scale, color, and pulsed sonographic imaging are employed simultaneously) combines two-dimensional gray scale images with flow information in the form of color, pulsed, or power Doppler. These techniques utilize the same sound waves as real-time imaging but measure the frequency and energy of the Doppler shift from the echoes interacting with flowing blood, allowing determination of flow presence, velocity, and direction (power Doppler does not assess the latter two).

Color Doppler US provides an estimate of the mean velocity and direction of flow within a vessel by color coding the information and displaying the color superimposed on gray scale images. Pulsed Doppler allows a sampling volume to be positioned in a vessel visualized on the gray scale image and provides a spectrum or graph of frequencies translated as an average velocity of blood flow within the Doppler sampling gate plotted as a function of time. A read-out of absolute velocities and calculation of resistive index (RI) and pulsatility index (PI) are obtained using a spectrum from pulsed Doppler. Of note, because the Doppler equation calculated by the machine software uses the angle between the beam axis and the vessel to calculate velocity and the angle of insonation is estimated by the sonographer, and should be less than 60 degrees. Larger angles may yield spurious velocities.

Power Doppler (also known as amplitude or energy map) measures the power of the Doppler signal and displays a greater range of signal strengths, thus allowing improved sensitivity to flow and visualization of smaller vessels. Power Doppler is displayed as a single color map of flow superimposed on gray scale images but does not provide velocity or directional information.

Resistive Index

Vascular resistance (impedance) is measured as the percent reduction of the end-diastolic flow compared with the systolic flow. The RI is calculated as peak systolic velocity (PSV) minus end-diastolic velocity (EDV) divided by PSV, and the PI is calculated as the PSV minus EDV divided by the mean velocity. These two parameters are often elevated in rejection (Fig. 14.7); however, elevated RIs and PIs can be seen in any cause of renal dysfunction and are nonspecific. For example, an elevated RI (greater than 0.9) has been reported not only in rejection but also in severe acute tubular necrosis (ATN), renal vein obstruction, subcapsular hematoma ("Page" kidney), other causes of obstruction, calcineurin-inhibitor toxicity, and pyelonephritis. The RI is also correlated with established cardiovascular risk factors.

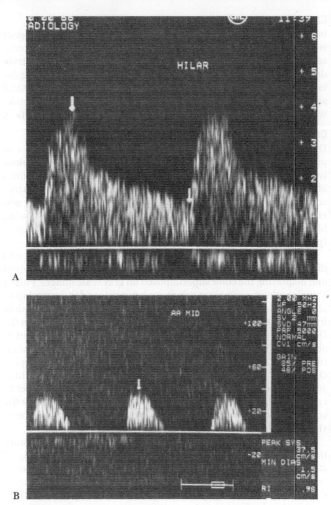

FIGURE 14.7 A: Normal pulsed-gate Doppler spectrum from kidney transplant with considerable flow throughout diastole and normal resistive index ($RI = 0.65$). **B:** Doppler spectrum of graft undergoing acute rejection with no diastolic flow ($RI = 1$). This is a nonspecific indicator of graft dysfunction.

Despite being nonspecific as an indicator of rejection, the renal transplant RI is a valuable predictor of long-term allograft performance; a RI of 0.8 or greater at 3 months after transplantation has been reported to be associated with poor subsequent allograft function.

NUCLEAR MEDICINE IMAGING OF GRAFT FUNCTION AND DYSFUNCTION

Dynamic renal scintigraphy is performed most commonly with ^{99m}Tc-mercaptotriglycine (MAG3), which is cleared from plasma by tubular several ... Different radiopharmaceuticals are summarized in Table 14.1.

Renal scintigraphy assesses the presence of functioning renal parenchyma, the arterial and venous flow, and the drainage of urine from the collecting system. Typical ... image characteristics include ... In ... ... will represent an area of injury (see later).

TABLE 14.1   Radiopharmaceuticals for Use in the Quantification and Evaluation of Renal Transplant Function or Morphology

Radionuclide		Biologic Compound	Percentage	Physiologic or Biochemical Mechanism	Imaging	Application	Comment
^{99m}Tc	DTPA	Diethylenetriaminepentaacetic acid	>90	Glomerular filtration, no resorption	Yes	Flow and function	Plasma binding higher than MAG3
^{99m}Tc	MAG3	Mercaptoacetyltriglycine	>95	Tubular secretion	Yes	Flow and function	Most commonly used
^{99m}Tc	DMSA	Dimercaptosuccinic acid	7–14	Excreted into urine, binds to SH groups in cortical tubule cells	Yes	Parenchyma	Pyelonephritis, infarct, scar
^{67}Ga	Ga	Gallium citrate	—	Localizes in sites of inflammation, and certain neoplasms	Yes	Inflammation	Nonspecific
^{111}In or ^{99m}Tc	WBC	White blood cells	—	Localizes in inflammatory tissue	Yes	Infection	—
^{111}In		Lymphocytes	—	Localizes in inflammatory tissue	Yes	Rejection	Difficult to extract and label

ERPF, effective renal plasma flow; Ga, gallium; GFR, glomerular filtration rate; I, iodine; In, indium; Tc, technetium; WBC, white blood cell count.

secretion. Other available radiopharmaceuticals are summarized in Table 14.1.

Renal scintigraphy assesses three phases of renal function: the angiographic phase for vascular flow and renal perfusion, the parenchymal phase for renal cortical tracer uptake, and the excretory phase for tracer clearance and ureteral system integrity. A time-activity curve is generated, depicting the activity in the transplant kidney as a function of time. Planar images of a normally functioning renal transplant are shown in Figure 14.8A, with corresponding curves in Figure 14.8B.

Acute rejection is seen as decreased perfusion, decreased tracer uptake within the transplant, and decreased tracer clearance with high background activity (Fig. 14.9). A potential confounder is calcineurin inhibitor nephrotoxicity, which can have a similar appearance on renal scintigraphy.

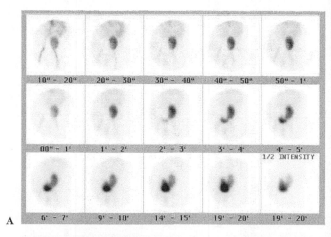

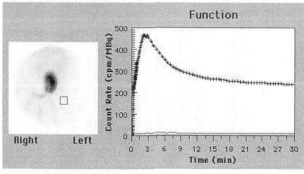

FIGURE 14.8 A: Dynamic images of a normal functioning transplant. The *top row* shows flow-perfusion images, each of 10 seconds' duration. The *middle* and *bottom rows* are 1-minute images taken during the subsequent 20 minutes. **B:** Regions of interest are drawn around the kidney and background (*box*) and curves generated of the activity within that region as function of time.

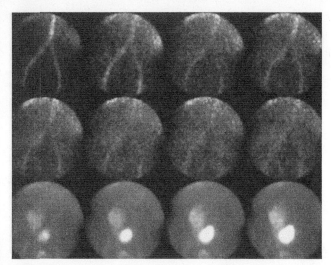

FIGURE 14.9 Nuclear medicine images of a transplanted kidney in rejection (radiopharmaceutical: ^{99m}Tc mercaptotriglycine [MAG3]). Note the poor perfusion to the transplant, that is, delayed renal visualization in the initial images of the *top two rows* (5 seconds per image). The *bottom row* shows poor function (4 minutes per image). Overall, reduced function is represented by high surrounding background tissue activity, poor parenchymal washout of accumulated tracer, and reduced collecting system or urinary bladder activity.

ATN is seen as normal perfusion, normal tracer uptake within the transplant, and lack of tracer clearance into the collecting system and bladder, with consequent high background activity (Fig. 14.10). The time-activity curve shows tracer uptake that reaches a plateau after 3 to 6 minutes, without decrease in tracer uptake due to lack of excretion. These findings are consistent with the pathophysiology of ATN, in which renal blood flow is preserved relative to glomerular filtration.

VASCULAR COMPLICATIONS

Renal Arterial Thrombosis

Renal arterial thrombosis (RAT) is overall uncommon, but frequently leads to graft loss. It usually occurring in the early postoperative period due to faulty surgical anastomosis, thrombogenic state, severe acute rejection, or progression of preexisting stenosis to thrombosis.

US shows absent arterial and venous blood flow within the allograft, and renal scintigraphy shows lack of perfusion, lack of cortical tracer uptake, and lack of tracer excretion with high background activity (Fig. 14.11). Of note, hyperacute rejection, acute cortical necrosis, and renal vein thrombosis may have similar scintigraphic findings. RAT is seen as nonvisualization or abrupt truncation of the transplant renal artery, or as global lack of perfusion of the renal allograft on CTA and MRA.

Acute renal infarction is seen as segmental lack of flow on US (Fig. 14.12), as wedge-shaped photopenic defects on renal scintigraphy, and as wedge-shaped areas of nonenhancement on contrast-enhanced CT and MR.

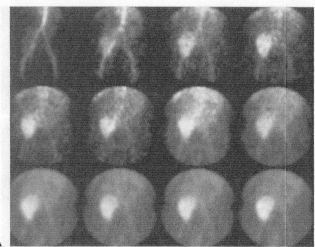

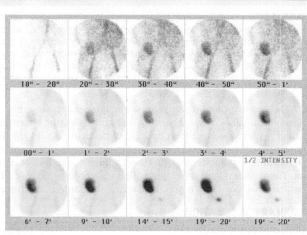

FIGURE 14.10 A: Nuclear medicine images of acute tubular necrosis. Note the well-preserved perfusion in the transplant, that is, prompt renal visualization in the initial six images. Concentration of tracer by the transplant is maintained, but there is no excretion and no collecting system or urinary bladder activity. Radiopharmaceutical: ^{99m}Tc diethylenetriaminepentaacetic acid (DTPA). **B:** Study performed with ^{99m}Tc mercaptotriglycine (MAG3) as radiopharmaceutical. *Top row* is the flow-perfusion phase (10 seconds per image). *Middle and bottom rows* show 1-minute images with normal renal concentration. There is visualization of tracer in the bladder in the last two frames, indicative of minimal function. Note the superior quality of ^{99m}Tc MAG3 over ^{99m}Tc DTPA in panel A.

Renal Vein Thrombosis

Renal vein thrombosis is an uncommon complication that usually occurs in the first week after transplantation and is seen as high-impedance renal arterial waveforms with a spiked systolic component, reversed and prolonged diastolic flow, and lack of venous flow on US (Fig. 14.13).

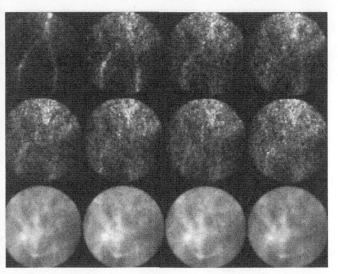

FIGURE 14.11 Nuclear medicine images of a transplanted kidney with renal artery thrombosis. Note the absence of renal perfusion, that is, nonvisualization of the transplant in the *top two rows*. In addition, there is no activity in the collecting system and bladder. Background tissue activity remains high, indicative of absent excretion. Radiopharmaceutical: ^{99m}Tc diethylenetriaminepentaacetic acid (DTPA).

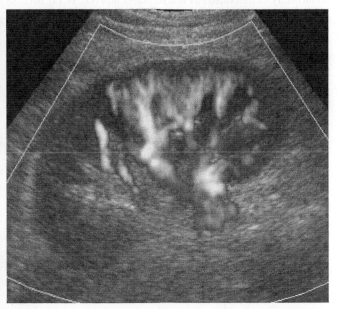

FIGURE 14.12 Color Doppler image reveals flow to most of the kidney, with absence of flow to area in upper pole, compatible with hypoperfusion and possible ischemia.

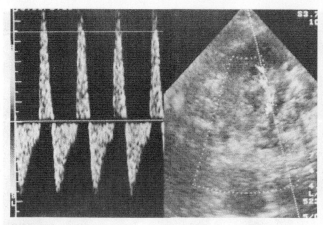

FIGURE 14.13 Duplex sonogram of transplant renal vein thrombosis demonstrates reversed flow in diastole and a spike-like systolic peak. No venous flow was detectable in the kidney, renal hilum, or location of the renal vein.

Reversal of diastolic flow alone is a nonspecific finding that is reflective of increased arterial impedance within the allograft and may also be seen in severe obstruction, acute rejection, and ATN.

Renal Artery Stenosis

Renal artery stenosis (RAS) is seen on US as a segmental region of flow abnormality with elevated PSV and turbulent flow (Fig. 14.14). Because the normal range of PSV values in a transplant renal artery is variable, an elevated ratio (greater than 3) of PSV in the renal artery compared

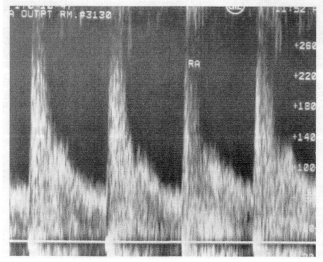

FIGURE 14.14 Renal artery stenosis. Doppler spectrum demonstrates focal elevated peak systolic velocity (faster than 260 cm/sec), with mild spectral broadening at the anastomosis.

to that in the external iliac artery is more reliable than the various proposed threshold values of PSV ranging from 100 to 300 cm/sec.

Importantly, estimation of PSV is dependent on the angle of insonation (should be less than 60 degrees) used by the sonographer, and the correct angle can be difficult to obtain when the renal artery is tortuous, resulting in spuriously elevated PSVs. Therefore, elevated PSVs without associated turbulence in a region where the accuracy of angle correction is equivocal should be interpreted with skepticism. Due to this potential pitfall, angiography may be considered to confirm the presence of RAS (see Chapters 10 and 11).

CTA or MRA can also be used to confirm RAS. Their advantages over Doppler US are the ability to provide a broad overview of all the inflow, outflow, and branch vasculature and to image other areas of potential arterial stenosis, such as in the iliac artery proximal to the anastomosis. Both CTA and MRA more reproducibly determine the diameter, circumference, and length of stenosis and enable multiplanar reconstructions in multiple projections to better detect eccentric stenoses. MRA has additional advantages over both CTA and catheter angiography since both gadolinium and ferumoxytol intravenous contrast are nonnephrotoxic compared to iodinated contrast and lacks ionizing radiation.

Arteriovenous Fistulas

Arteriovenous fistulas may arise after transplant biopsy. They are usually self-limited and resolve spontaneously but can cause persistent hematuria or hypertension. They are seen as an area of artifactual color assignment in the renal parenchyma on color Doppler US (Fig. 14.15). This finding is thought to be caused by high-velocity flow in the fistula, which causes localized turbulence and vessel wall vibrations that are

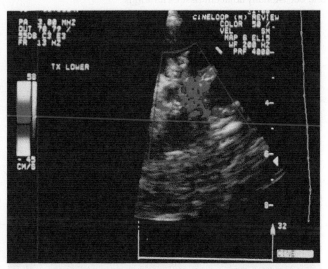

FIGURE 14.15 Postbiopsy arteriovenous fistula. Color Doppler image shows an area of random color assignment. Pulsed-gate Doppler analysis revealed high-velocity, low-resistance arterial flow and arterialization of the venous waveform.

transmitted to the perivascular parenchyma. The vibrating interfaces in the perivascular tissues produce phase shifts in the reflected sound waves and result in random color assignment in this region, the Doppler equivalent of a bruit. Confirmation of an arteriovenous fistula is achieved by performing pulsed Doppler waveform analysis and demonstrating high-velocity, low-resistance flow in the supplying artery and arterialization (highly pulsatile flow) of the waveform in the draining vein. A focal intra-renal arterial stenosis can also produce high-velocity flow and tissue vibration, mimicking an arterio-venouf fistula (AVF); however, the associate venous waveform changes are not seen.

Although Doppler US is the initial imaging examination of choice to assess for AVF, angiography may also be considered, especially to determine the extent of the fistula and for treatment planning, as super selective occlusion of segmental or interlobar arterial branches is possible using a variety of occlusive devices, including steel coils and detachable balloons. CTA and MRA can also be used to diagnosis AVF but are potentially limited by spatial resolution.

Pseudoaneurysms

Intra-renal transplant pseudoaneurysms are usually a complication of central needle biopsy, whereas the less common extra-renal transplant pseudoaneurysms are usually a consequence of a faulty surgical anastomosis or adjacent infection. Extra-renal pseudoaneurysms are at much higher risk for spontaneous rupture and are therefore treated as a relative surgical emergency. Pseudoaneurysms may be associated with AVFs. Both intra- and extra-renal pseudoaneurysms appear as spherical fluid collections that may or may not contain thrombus on US. Color Doppler reveals a swirling internal flow pattern (Fig. 14.16) and occasionally adjacent tissue vibrations.

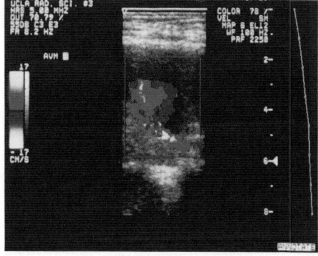

FIGURE 14.16 Pseudoaneurysm. Gray scale image demonstrated a cystic lesion, and color Doppler image shows swirling internal flow.

INVESTIGATIONAL NONCONTRAST MR TECHNIQUES

There are several promising new MR techniques for which further investigation is necessary before their implementation into routine clinical use.

Noncontrast MR can provide microstructural and physiologic information relying on techniques such as blood oxygenation level-dependent (BOLD) imaging, diffusion weighted imaging (DWI), and diffusion tensor imaging (DTI). In BOLD imaging and DWI, endogenous substances such as deoxyhemoglobin and water molecules are used as intrinsic "contrast" agents, respectively.

BOLD imaging capitalizes on the direct relationship between oxygen consumption and deoxyhemoglobin concentration to create a signal map from the susceptibility produced by deoxyhemoglobin, such that areas of increased oxygen consumption show high signal. In DWI, restricted water molecules generate high signal. In renal allograft dysfunction, the oxygen consumption decreases while the deoxyhemoglobin concentration decreases, with consequent loss of signal. Similarly, ischemic areas result in restricted diffusion of water molecules with consequent gain of signal. Using these MRI techniques bypasses concerns regarding renal or systemic toxicity related to intravenous contrast agents. Of note, BOLD imaging has been shown to be influenced by hydration status and may be compromised by susceptibility artifact from adjacent bowel.

DTI provides microstructural information inferred from diffusion and its anisotropy, or direction of diffusion. Normally functioning kidneys have an organized, radial orientation of tubules, collecting ducts, and blood vessels in the medulla, and DTI tractography reveals these tightly packed tracts. Conversely, in impaired allografts, DTI shows a reduced number and density of these tracts, reflecting microstructural alterations in allograft dysfunction.

Ferumoxytol-enhanced MRA provides long-acting, nonnephrotoxic, nongadolinium imaging of the entire arterial and venous system, enabling a reliable assessment of blood flow and vascular structural abnormalities.

Core Needle Biopsy of the Transplanted Kidney

INDICATIONS

Percutaneous renal transplant allograft needle biopsy is most frequently performed to help determine the etiology of graft dysfunction when clinical evaluation and noninvasive diagnostic tests are nonspecific, and commonly is performed to distinguish ATN from acute rejection and nephritis. In addition, renal transplant biopsy may be performed at predetermined intervals after transplantation (protocol biopsies) as part of routine surveillance for subclinical rejection (see Chapter 10) or as part of clinical trials evaluating immunosuppressive drugs. Additional indications for biopsy are discussed in Chapters 10 and 11.

TECHNIQUE

Preparations for transplant biopsy are similar to those for native renal biopsy. There is much less risk of bleeding: the transplant kidney is more superficial than the native kidney and does not move with respiration.

Prior to any biopsy, all anticoagulants including antiplatelet agents should be stopped according to their half-lives, and basic serum laboratory values for hemoglobin, hematocrit, platelets, prothrombin time, partial thromboplastin time, and INR should be checked. For patients taking low-dose aspirin, a 3- to 5-day abstinence is usually required; though in urgent circumstances biopsies are sometimes performed without discontinuation. For patients receiving clopidogrel (Plavix), a 5-day period of abstinence is generally required.

Severe anemia, thrombocytopenia (platelets < 50,000), and/or coagulopathy should be corrected prior to biopsy. A blood urea nitrogen of greater than 50 mg/dL has been associated with bleeding complications and should be corrected if possible. Blood pressure should be controlled at a level of less than 160 mm Hg systolic and/90 mm Hg diastolic. Informed consent is required, with specific discussion regarding the potential risks of biopsy-induced hemorrhage and graft injury (see "Complications" section).

Because of its superficial location, the renal graft can be potentially localized by palpation. However, ultrasound guidance is preferred because it provides direct visualization of the renal graft and the targeted biopsy site in the cortex. This reduces the frequency of inadequate specimen collection as well as of complications.

In addition, ultrasound can detect perinephric fluid collections and graft hydronephrosis. Any perinephric fluid collection should be aspirated prior to biopsy due to the potential inability to tamponade the biopsy site adequately in the presence of a perinephric fluid collection. Significant hydronephrosis should also be decompressed prior to biopsy because the hydronephrosis itself may be the cause of the graft dysfunction. In addition, a postbiopsy blood clot may exacerbate the degree of obstruction.

In general, the cortex of the upper or lower pole of the renal graft is targeted for biopsy since the microscopic and electro microscopic evaluation are centered around the glomerulus. The skin overlying the targeted biopsy site is anesthetized with 1% lidocaine, and a dermatotomy is made to facilitate passage of a 17-gauge introducer into the renal cortex and an automatic spring-loaded 18-gauge core needle biopsy device is inserted coaxially to retrieve cortical tissue. Two tissue samples are usually adequate. An on-site cytologist may examine the specimens immediately after acquisition to confirm the adequacy of sample acquisition based on the number of glomeruli.

After biopsy-device withdrawal, procoagulants such as blood patch or gelfoam pledgets may be injected via the cannula and manual compression may all be applied to achieve hemostasis. A follow-up US is performed approximately 5 minutes after hemostasis to detect any bleeding. Postbiopsy orders should include bed rest for 3 to 6 hours with observation of vital signs every 15 minutes for at least 2 hours and then hourly for several hours. Given stable vital signs and absent macroscopic hematuria, outpatients may return home on the same day of biopsy.

COMPLICATIONS

Major complications after needle biopsy include perinephric hematoma or hematuria. Extensive perinephric hematomas may rarely result in renal compression necessitating angiographic embolization, surgical exploration, and/or graft nephrectomy. Perinephric hematomas may also cause ureteral obstruction requiring decompression by means including percutaneous nephrostomy. Macroscopic hematuria occurs approximately 3% of renal biopsies. While transient macroscopic hematuria is common and is of little clinical significance, patients may occasionally require blood transfusion, placement of a bladder catheter for clot drainage, and even hospitalization. Arteriovenous fistulas may result from renal biopsy. They may be detected as an incidental finding on color and spectral Doppler sonography and are usually observed rather than treated with angiographic embolization.

Complications that require hospitalization, transfusion, operative, or interventional radiologic procedures have been described to occur after approximately 2% of transplant biopsies (see Morgan et al. in Selected Readings). They are more common after "for cause" biopsies compared to protocol biopsies.

Selected Readings

Broome D, Girguis M, Baron P, et al. Gadodiamide-associated nephrogenic systemic fibrosis: why radiologists should be concerned. Am J Roentgenol 2007;188: 586–592.

Bruno S, Ferrari S, Remuzzi G. Doppler ultrasonography in post-transplant renal artery stenosis: a reliable tool for assessing effectiveness of revascularization? Transplantation 2003;76:147–153.

Fan WJ, Ren T, Li Q, et al. Assessment of renal allograft function early after transplantation with isotropic resolution diffusion tensor imaging. Eur Radiol 2016;26: 567–575.

Ismaeel MM, Abdel-Hamid A. Role of high resolution contrast-enhanced magnetic resonance angiography (HR CeMRA) in management of arterial complications of the renal transplant. Eur J Radiol 2011;79:122–127.

Liam Y, Kock MC, Ijzermans JN, et al. Living renal donors: optimizing the imaging strategy—decision- and cost-effectiveness analysis. Radiology 2003;226:53–62.

Martin L, Boris R. Interventional therapy of vascular complications following renal transplantation. Clin Transpl 2006;20:55–59.

Morgan T, Chandran S, Burger I, et al. Complications of ultrasound-guided renal transplant biopsies. Am J Transplant 2016;16:1298–1305.

Park SY, Kim CK, Park BK, et al. Assessment of early renal allograft dysfunction with blood oxygenation level-dependent MRI and diffusion-weighted imaging. Eur J Radiol 2014;83:2114–2121.

Radermacher J, Mengel M, Ellis S, et al. The renal artery resistive index and renal allograft survival. N Engl J Med 2003;349:115–124.

Tublin ME, Bude RO, Platt JF. The resistive index in renal Doppler sonography: where do we stand? Am J Roentgenol 2003;180:885–892.

Xiao W, Xu J, Wang Q, et al. Functional evaluation of transplanted kidneys in normal function and acute rejection using BOLD MR imaging. Eur J Radiol 2012;81: 838–845.

The gold standard for assessing structural abnormalities in the kidney transplant is routine histopathology of a biopsy or transplant nephrectomy. Immunofluorescence or immunohistochemistry and electron microscopy also provide important information for identifying changes of antibody-mediated rejection and glomerular lesions.

CORE-NEEDLE BIOPSY

Indications and Technique

Kidney transplant biopsies are most frequently performed at times of graft dysfunction when the etiology cannot be accurately elucidated by clinical or noninvasive means. Protocol biopsies are performed at predetermined intervals after transplantation at some centers in an attempt to recognize so-called subclinical rejection (see Chapter 10); they may also be required as part of clinical trials for the evaluation of new immunosuppressive drugs. More precise clinical indications for biopsy are reviewed in Chapters 10 and 11. Transplant programs may vary in their reliance on biopsies and the clinical setting in which biopsies are performed.

Since transplant biopsies are now routinely performed with ultrasound guidance and/or location, the technical aspects of the transplant biopsy procedure itself are described in Chapter 14.

Specimen Handling

Detailed methods for handling tissue specimens are beyond the scope of this chapter. All specimens should be divided so renal cortex is collected for each of the three traditional methods of evaluating renal parenchyma: light microscopy, immunofluorescence, and electron microscopy. In selected instances, rapid processing or frozen section of the tissue collected for light microscopy can be performed when an immediate assessment of allograft morphology is necessary for initiating or modifying therapy.

TRANSPLANT REJECTION

Traditionally, three major forms of rejection are recognized: hyperacute, acute, and chronic. Each has reasonably distinctive changes, although acute and chronic rejection may be present simultaneously resulting in a mixture of histopathologic features, and must be considered in the context of its pathogenesis: antibody or cell-mediated injury. Table 15.1 lists the pathologic findings in the major lesions responsible for functional impairment of the graft.

T A B L E 15.1   Histopathologic Findings in the Major Causes of Allograft Dysfunction

Type	Interstitium	Tubules	Glomeruli	Arteries
Acute cell-mediated rejection	Edema, lymphocytes ± monocytes, plasma cells	Lymphocytes, epithelial cell injury, sometimes reactive atypia	No specific lesions	Swollen endothelium, intimal lymphocytes
Acute antibody-mediated rejection	Edema; monocytes and neutrophils in PTC; often PTC C4d	Often epithelial cell injury	Monocytes, neutrophils, endothelial swelling, ± thrombi	May be endothelial swelling, intimal monocytes, fibrinoid necrosis, arteriolar thrombi
Acute tubular injury	Edema, ± small numbers of lymphocytes	Epithelial cell flattening, loss of brush borders, individual cell necrosis, regenerative atypia	Normal	Normal
Acute calcineurin inhibitor toxicity	Edema	Isometric vacuoles, ± individual cell necrosis	May be capillary thrombi	Normal ± arteriolar thrombi
Chronic rejection	Fibrosis ± lymphocytes, monocytes; PTC basement membrane multilayering	Atrophy, dropout	Transplant glomerulopathy (GBM double contours)	Intimal fibrosis, often with monocytes, lymphocytes, foam cells in sclerotic intima
Chronic calcineurin inhibitor toxicity	"Striped" fibrosis	Atrophy	Ischemic collapse, focal and segmental or global glomerulosclerosis	Peripheral nodular hyaline arteriolopathy

GBM, glomerular basement membrane; PTC, peritubular capillary.

Hyperacute Rejection

Hyperacute rejection is produced by preformed cytotoxic antibodies against the graft. Nowadays this is a rare occurrence with all transplant centers routinely performing pretransplantation crossmatches to detect such antibodies (see Chapter 3). It is typically manifest shortly after vascular anastomosis is established. Early changes are prominent margination of leukocytes, mainly neutrophils, within the glomerular and peritubular capillaries. This is followed by widespread vascular thrombosis, predominantly affecting glomeruli, arterioles, and interlobular arteries, often with neutrophils incorporated in the thrombi. The kidney becomes cyanotic, slightly edematous, and flaccid, and urine production suddenly ceases or does not begin at all. If the kidney is not removed immediately, extensive tubular necrosis ensues, followed after 24 hours by numerous cortical and medullary infarcts. Immunofluorescence may disclose capillary and arterial wall immunoglobulin G (IgG) or IgM, C3, and fibrin, with fibrin also in the thrombi. Peritubular capillary C4d (see *Antibody-Mediated* Rejection below) deposition occurs after 24 to 72 hours if the kidney remains viable during this time.

Hyperacute rejection needs to be differentiated from other circumstances in which extensive vascular thrombi occur. The differential diagnosis includes physical perfusion-related injury to vascular endothelium and injury caused by cold-reacting IgM antibodies against blood cells. Both of these conditions rarely may manifest in the immediate posttransplantation period and may produce entrapment of leukocytes in thrombi. It is only in hyperacute rejection, however, that neutrophils are typically and regularly incorporated in the thrombi. Recurrent hemolytic uremic syndrome and acute thrombotic microangiopathy associated with calcineurin inhibitor (CNI) administration (discussed later under "Calcineurin Inhibitor Nephrotoxicity") are characterized by thrombi, but these usually lack incorporated leukocytes and generally occur later after transplantation.

Acute Rejection

There are two immunopathologic forms of *acute rejection*: cell-mediated rejection (CMR; also referred to as T-cell–mediated rejection or cellular rejection), and antibody-mediated rejection (ABMR, or AMR). While these forms of acute rejection involve different pathogenic mechanisms, they are not mutually exclusive and not infrequently occur simultaneously (mixed rejection); there is also evidence that acute CMR is a risk factor for the development of *de novo* antibodies against the graft and subsequent AMR.

Acute Cell-Mediated Rejection

Acute CMR is mediated primarily by T lymphocytes. The characteristic lesions of acute CMR may involve tubules and interstitium, arteries, or both. The diagnosis of acute CMR is established by light microscopy, although at times, routine immunofluorescence and electron microscopic evaluation may be helpful for the differential diagnosis. In the tubulointerstitial form of acute CMR, the cortical interstitium is diffusely or focally edematous and infiltrated by numerous leukocytes, most of

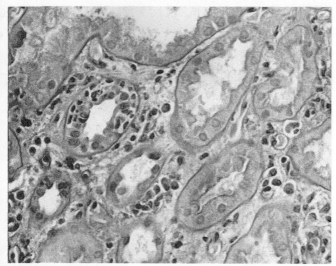

FIGURE 15.1 Acute cell-mediated rejection, tubulo-interstitial type (Banff 2007 type 1B). There are interstitial lymphocytes and some plasma cells with accompanying interstitial edema, and focally severe tubulitis with multiple lymphocytes in the most severely involved tubular cross-section (periodic acid–Schiff ×400).

which are mature and activated T lymphocytes (CD4, CD8), with variable numbers of monocytes and plasma cells (Fig. 15.1). Eosinophils and neutrophils may be present but are not typically found in large numbers; the presence of intratubular neutrophils should raise the possibility of an acute bacterial infection (pyelonephritis) and eosinophil-rich infiltrates primarily near the cortico-medullary junction and in the outer medulla suggest the possibility of a drug-induced interstitial nephritis. Peritubular capillaries contain lymphocytes that may be seen migrating into the interstitium; it is important to recognize that leukocytes within these capillaries are not specific for AMR (see below). A characteristic lesion, called *tubulitis,* occurs, whereby lymphocytes infiltrate the tubules, often with associated reactive or degenerative changes of tubular epithelial cells. Tubulitis is best demonstrated with periodic acid–Schiff (PAS) and silver methenamine stains that highlight tubular basement membranes, and allow the pathologist to definitively identify lymphocytes that are within the tubule. In severe cases, tubular basement membranes may be disrupted. For tubulitis to have diagnostic significance, the inflammation should be documented in nonatrophic tubules. The significance of tubulitis solely in atrophic tubules remains unclear.

In the vascular form of acute CMR, lymphocytes and monocytes are found beneath the endothelium of arteries, but only in rare cases do the inflammatory cells extend into the muscularis (Fig. 15.2). Endothelial cells are swollen and may be detached from the vascular wall, but arterial wall necrosis usually is not a feature of CMR, and should instead suggest AMR or mixed rejection. These arterial lesions are

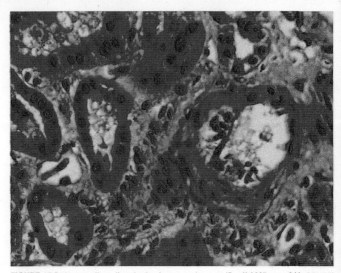

FIGURE 15.2 Acute cell-mediated rejection, vascular type (Banff 2007 type 2A). A small artery contains mononuclear leukocytes directly beneath the endothelium. Also note the interstitial inflammation and edema (hematoxylin and eosin ×400).

referred to as *intimal arteritis* or *endarteritis* and often, but not always, occur in concert with tubulointerstitial acute CMR. Note that only vascular lesions involving arteries are diagnostic of CMR, although some pathologists also consider similar lesions in arterioles as indicative of, or at least suspicious for, CMR; lesions involving veins are nondiagnostic. In biopsies demonstrating CMR, immunofluorescence may disclose fibrin in the interstitium. C4d staining is negative within peritubular capillaries. When acute cell-mediated rejection is treated successfully, the interstitial inflammatory infiltrate diminishes rapidly, whereas edema, tubular inflammation, and tubular cell damage may persist for a longer interval.

Most biopsies showing acute CMR are performed for an indication of acute or persistent graft dysfunction; however, lesions of acute CMR may be seen in protocol biopsies of normally functioning grafts (subclinical acute CMR). Although early studies suggested that such subclinical lesions, if not treated, were associated with graft scarring and loss of function, this is less certain in the current era of immunosuppressive therapy.

It has become standard to grade CMR according to the *Banff working classification* (so-named after the first workshop on the topic in Banff, Canada in 1991). The classification has undergone several revisions since its initial development (thus the term "working classification"); the most recent update of the classification of CMR (Banff '07) is shown in Table 15.2. The Banff classification defines three types, or grades, of acute CMR: type 1, which is purely tubulointerstitial; type 2, in which there is intimal arteritis, with or without concurrent tubulointerstitial lesions, and type 3, with transmural arteritis and/or necrosis of

TABLE 15.2	Banff 2007 Diagnostic Criteria for Acute Cell-Mediated Rejection

No acute rejection. Absence of tubulitis or intimal arteritis, with or without interstitial inflammation.

Borderline (suspicious) changes. Mononuclear cell infiltrate involving 10% or more of the nonscarred cortical interstitium, but not meeting the threshold for diagnosis of type 1 acute rejection due to:
- Insufficient tubulitis (<5 lymphocytes in most severely involved tubular cross-section)
- Insufficient inflammation (<25% of nonscarred cortex inflamed)

Type 1 Acute Rejection
Interstitial inflammation in ≥25% of nonscarred cortical tissue with:
1A. Moderate tubulitis (5–10 lymphocytes in most severely involved tubular cross-section or group of 10 tubular epithelial cells, excluding atrophic tubules)
1B. Severe tubulitis (>10 lymphocytes in most severely involved tubular cross-section or group of 10 tubular epithelial cells, excluding atrophic tubules)

Type 2 Acute Rejection
Intimal arteritis, with or without interstitial inflammation and/or tubulitis, with:
2A. Less than 25% luminal occlusion in the most severely involved artery (mild to moderate intimal arteritis)
2B. ≥25% luminal occlusion in the most severely involved artery (severe intimal arteritis)

Type 3 Acute Rejection
Transmural arterial inflammation and/or arterial fibrinoid change and necrosis of medial smooth muscle cells with accompanying lymphocytic inflammation

(Adapted from Solez K, Colvin RB, Racusen LC, et al. Banff 07 classification of renal allograft pathology: updates and future directions. Am J Transplant 2008;8:753–760.)

medial smooth muscle cells. Within the categories of type 1 and type 2 acute CMR, lesions are divided into mild-to-moderate (1A, 2A) and severe (1B, 2B) forms. A number of studies have found these different types or grades of acute CMR to be highly predictive of response to immunosuppressive therapy and graft survival, with an order (best to worst) of 1A > 1B, 2A > 2B > 3. Biopsies showing interstitial inflammation and tubulitis but without sufficiently severe inflammation (i.e., involving ≥10% but <25% of the cortex) and/or tubulitis (with ≥1 but <5 lymphocytes in the most severely involved tubular cross-section) are classified as *borderline* for CMR. The borderline category remains problematic for clinicians as some of these lesions, if untreated, behave clinically as CMR although the majority do not, and there are no specific morphologic features that differentiate between these. Perhaps molecular approaches will be useful in identifying which borderline lesions need to be treated as CMR (see Chapter 3). Another apparent shortcoming of the Banff classification is that it specifies that only interstitial inflammation in nonscarred areas of the cortex should be graded, although some recent studies indicate that inflammation in areas of interstitial fibrosis is a much stronger predictor of poor graft outcomes than interstitial fibrosis alone. This will likely be addressed in future iterations of the classification.

Acute Antibody-Mediated Rejection

Acute AMR is caused by circulating antibodies directed against the graft—*donor-specific antibodies (DSA)* (see Chapter 3). Most often, the DSA are directed against HLA antigens expressed on endothelial cells within the graft, although much less commonly antibodies against non-HLA antigens are involved. Unlike the case with hyperacute rejection where the antibodies are present at the time of transplantation, in acute AMR the DSA develop under two potential scenarios: a memory response where there is a "rebound" humoral immune response against an antigen present on the graft to which the recipient had been previously exposed (e.g., through a blood transfusion, pregnancy, or previous transplant), and a *de novo* humoral response against the graft. The rebound response, sometimes referred to as type 1 AMR, is often seen in highly sensitized recipients who undergo pretransplant desensitization to remove antibodies against the donor kidney prior to transplantation, and most often occurs early post-transplantation. By contrast, AMR caused by *de novo* DSA, termed type 2 AMR, most often occurs after the first year post-transplantation, sometimes much later, and not infrequently in the context of patient nonadherence with immunosuppressive medications. As with acute CMR, acute AMR may be seen in the context of graft dysfunction or on protocol biopsies of normally functioning grafts (subclinical AMR); it is well documented that subclinical AMR, if untreated, can lead to development of chronic rejection and chronic graft dysfunction.

The hallmark of acute AMR, whether of type 1 or type 2, is *microvascular inflammation and injury*, involving the glomerular and peritubular capillaries. Histologically, this is primarily manifest as two lesions: *glomerulitis and peritubular capillaritis*. Glomerulitis involves margination of leukocytes—primarily monocytes/macrophages and neutrophils—within the glomerular capillaries with associated swelling of glomerular endothelial cells, partially or completely occluding capillary lumina (Fig. 15.3). This process is most often focal and segmental, although in severe cases most or all glomeruli may be extensively involved. Peritubular capillaritis involves margination of leukocytes—primarily monocytes/macrophages and neutrophils—within cortical peritubular capillaries (Fig. 15.4); as with glomerulitis, the process can be focal or diffuse. Less frequently seen morphologic lesions in acute AMR are thrombotic microangiopathy (TMA), most typically with fibrin thrombi within the glomerular capillaries and/or arterioles, and fibrinoid necrosis of the walls of arterioles and small arteries. Recent studies have also shown that intimal arteritis may be a manifestation of acute AMR as well as of acute CMR, although cases of AMR where intimal arteritis is the sole histologic lesion are rare. Finally, there is a small number of cases of AMR where the major histologic lesion present is acute tubular injury; in such instances, it is crucial that other potential causes of tubular injury are excluded before this injury is attributed to an effect of antibodies directed against the graft. It should be recognized that several of the morphologic lesions of acute AMR—glomerulitis, peritubular capillaritis, TMA, and arterial/arteriolar fibrinoid necrosis—are also seen in hyperacute rejection (see above). This is not surprising since hyperacute rejection is also caused by antibodies directed against the graft.

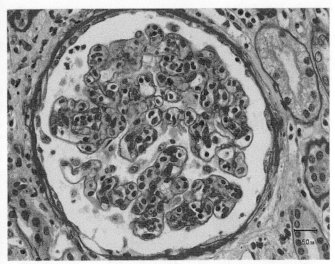

FIGURE 15.3 Severe transplant glomerulitis. Glomerular capillary lumens are filled with leukocytes, including monocytes and lymphocytes, occluding many of the capillary lumina. There is also swelling of glomerular endothelial cells (periodic acid–Schiff ×400).

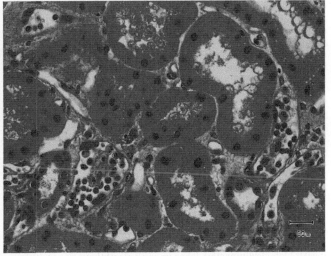

FIGURE 15.4 Peritubular capillaritis. The peritubular capillaries are filled with multiple leukocytes, including monocytes, lymphocytes, and a small number of neutrophils. Note the relative lack of inflammation in the adjacent interstitium and tubules; this biopsy showed antibody-mediated rejection without concurrent cell-mediated rejection (hematoxylin and eosin ×400).

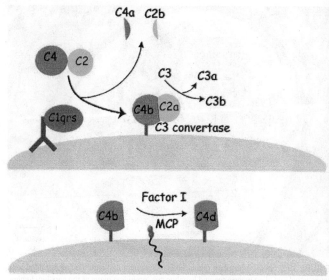

FIGURE 15.5 Complement activation and formation of C4d. Binding of complement-fixing antibodies to a cell surface recruits C1qrs complexes. C1qrs cleaves and activates C4 and C2. C4b formed in this way may form covalent bonds with the cell surface and associate with C2a to form C4b2a, the classical complement pathway C3 convertase. C4b2a catalyzes cleavage of C3 and C5, amplifying complement activation **(top)**. C3 convertases are controlled by various mechanisms. One mechanism involves cleavage of C4b by factor I plus membrane cofactor protein (MCP) or C4-binding proteins as cofactors to yield C4d, which is catalytically inactive. Although C4d is catalytically inert, it can interact with C4d receptors on B cells and follicular dendritic cells. These interactions may help to regulate humoral immune responses **(bottom)**. (From Platt JL. C4d and the fate of organ allografts. J Am Soc Nephrol 2002;13:2417–2419, with permission.)

Importantly, none of the above histologic lesions are specific for acute AMR, and these may be seen in the context of other causes of endothelial injury including, but not limited to, acute CNI nephrotoxicity and recurrent TMA (e.g., atypical hemolytic-uremic syndrome). Thus, it is crucial that DSA be demonstrated in the patient's serum at the approximate time of biopsy for a definitive diagnosis of AMR to be made. In addition, the majority of biopsies with acute AMR will demonstrate *C4d deposition* within peritubular capillaries. C4d is a split product of C4 involved in the classical complement cascade. Its formation is illustrated in Figure 15.5 and the accompanying legend. Although C4d itself is biologically inactive, it becomes covalently bound to peritubular capillary endothelium or basement membrane collagen, serving as a marker for recent complement activation. C4d may be demonstrated in biopsy specimens by indirect immunofluorescence performed on frozen sections of fresh tissue or immunohistochemistry performed on sections of formalin-fixed, paraffin-embedded tissue. The immunofluorescence method using frozen sections is the more sensitive of the two, with a positive result indicated by linear staining within peritubular

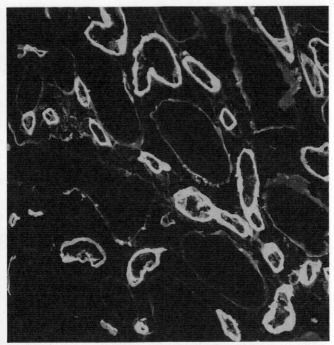

FIGURE 15.6 C4d staining in peritubular capillaries. Indirect immunofluorescence using a mouse monoclonal antibody against C4d followed by fluorescein-conjugated anti-mouse IgG shows strong linear staining in the walls of peritubular capillaries. Tubular basement membranes are recognized by weak, nonspecific staining (×400).

capillaries of the cortex and/or medulla (Fig. 15.6). With this method, glomerular staining is not specific and is seen in most biopsies, most often in the mesangium. The treatment and prognosis for acute AMR are different from those for CMR (see Chapters 6 and 10).

As with acute CMR, there are also Banff criteria for diagnosis of acute AMR, the most recent of which were developed in 2013 (Table 15.3). The diagnosis of acute AMR requires three components: *histologic evidence* (glomerulitis, peritubular capillaritis, intimal or transmural/necrotizing arteritis, or acute tubular injury without other apparent cause); *evidence of recent antibody interaction with graft endothelium* (C4d staining in at least 10% of peritubular capillaries by immunofluorescence or any peritubular capillary C4d staining by immunohistochemistry, or at least moderate microvascular inflammation [glomerulitis and/or peritubular capillaritis]); *and serologic evidence* in the form of DSA. Unlike the case with acute CMR, the Banff classification does not specify types or grades of ABMR that correlate with severity, although lesions of glomerulitis and peritubular capillaritis are graded as mild, moderate, or severe based on the fraction of glomeruli involved and the number of leukocytes within the most severely involved peritubular capillary cross-section, respectively. For diagnosis

TABLE 15.3	Banff 2013 Classification of Antibody-Mediated Rejection (ABMR) in Renal Allografts

Acute/Active ABMR; All Three Features Must be Present for Diagnosis

1. Histologic evidence of acute tissue injury, including one or more of the following:
   - Microvascular inflammation (glomerulitis and/or peritubular capillaritis)
   - Intimal or transmural arteritis
   - Acute thrombotic microangiopathy, in the absence of any other cause
   - Acute tubular injury, in the absence of any other apparent cause
2. Evidence of current/recent antibody interaction with vascular endothelium, *including at least one of the following*:
   - Linear C4d staining in peritubular capillaries (in at least 10% of capillaries by immunofluorescence on frozen sections, or in any capillaries by immunohistochemistry on paraffin sections)
   - At least moderate microvascular inflammation (mild glomerulitis AND peritubular capillaritis, at least moderate glomerulitis OR peritubular capillaritis; at least mild glomerulitis must be present when there is acute cell-mediated rejection)
   - Molecular markers, such as increased expression of endothelial-associated transcripts
3. Serologic evidence of donor-specific antibodies (HLA or other antigens)

Chronic, Active ABMR; All Three Features Must be Present for Diagnosis

1. Morphologic evidence of chronic tissue injury, including one or more of the following:
   - Transplant glomerulopathy by light microscopy and/or EM, if no evidence of chronic thrombotic microangiopathy
   - Severe peritubular capillary basement membrane multilayering (requires EM)
   - Arterial intimal fibrosis of new onset, excluding other causes
2. Evidence of current/recent antibody interaction with vascular endothelium, *including at least one of the following*:
   - Linear C4d staining in peritubular capillaries (as with acute/active ABMR, above)
   - At least moderate microvascular inflammation (as with acute/active ABMR, above)
   - Molecular markers, such as increased expression of endothelial-associated transcripts
3. Serologic evidence of donor-specific antibodies (HLA or other antigens)

C4d Staining without Evidence of Rejection; All Three Features Must be Present for Diagnosis

1. Linear C4d staining in peritubular capillaries (as with acute/active ABMR, above)
2. No glomerulitis, peritubular capillaritis, transplant glomerulopathy, thrombotic microangiopathy, peritubular capillary basement membrane multilayering, or acute tubular injury (in the absence of another apparent cause for this)
3. No acute cell-mediated rejection (Banff 2007 type 1A or greater) or borderline changes

(Adapted from Haas M, Sis B, Racusen LC, et al. Banff 2013 meeting report: inclusion of C4d-negative antibody-mediated rejection and antibody-associated arterial lesions. Am J Transplant 2014;14:272–283.)

of peritubular capillaritis, there must be leukocytes in at least 10% of cortical peritubular capillaries and at least three cells in one or more such capillaries. While mild glomerulitis *or* peritubular capillaritis is sufficient for diagnosis of acute AMR in the presence of C4d and DSA, in the absence of C4d there must be mild glomerulitis *and* peritubular capillaritis or at least moderate glomerulitis or peritubular capillaritis if only one of these is present.

The Banff classification for AMR (Table 15.3) also recognizes instances in which C4d staining is present in the absence of histologic lesions of AMR (or CMR). These are most often seen with *ABO-incompatible transplants* and antibodies against blood group antigens. Biopsies of ABO-incompatible grafts are often C4d-positive and, when there are no accompanying histologic findings of rejection, the C4d staining is clearly not associated with any short- or long-term deleterious effect on graft outcome. However, when this finding is associated with DSA against HLA antigens, its significance remains unclear and, in fact, there is some recent, albeit preliminary, evidence that in such cases C4d staining without histologic lesions of rejection may represent a *forme fruste* of acute AMR.

Differential Diagnosis of Acute Cell-Mediated Rejection

Other forms of acute interstitial nephritis may have many of the same structural lesions as acute CMR, including infectious interstitial nephritis (viral, bacterial) and drug-induced acute interstitial nephritis. Certain viral and bacterial interstitial nephritides may be characterized by a mononuclear, rather than polymorphonuclear, infiltrate, thereby simulating rejection. Because of the negligible role of neutrophils in acute CMR, their presence should be taken to signify acute infection, most often bacterial (particularly with intratubular neutrophils), or acute AMR (with neutrophils within glomerular and/or peritubular capillaries), especially when recent infarction is excluded. Multiple interstitial plasma cells and the presence of nuclear atypia within tubular epithelial cells may be seen in acute CMR, but may also signify a viral infection, particularly polyoma (BK) virus infection as discussed later in this chapter (and Chapter 12). This is true even in the absence of diagnostic viral inclusions. A high index of suspicion for BK virus infection is always advisable, especially with biopsies performed during the period from 1 to 2 months to 1 to 2 years post-transplantation, as treatment for acute rejection can cause a worsening of the viral infection. Likewise, post-transplant lymphoproliferative disorders (PTLDs) can mimic acute CMR, particularly polymorphous PTLDs that lack the severe cytologic atypia of frank lymphomas. As with BK virus infections, a high index of suspicion for PTLDs is advisable; immunohistochemical staining for T (CD3) and B (CD20) lymphocytes is a reasonable approach as most PTLDs are B-cell lesions, whereas acute CMR is primarily a T-cell–mediated process. As noted earlier, drug-induced interstitial nephritis often involves the region of the cortico-medullary junction and outer medulla, and may have a prominent component of eosinophils and sometimes granulomas. However, extreme caution should be made in diagnosing drug-induced interstitial nephritis with inflammatory lesions meeting Banff criteria for acute CMR, type 1A or greater. Some biopsy specimens with CNI toxicity may have focal interstitial lymphocytic perivenous infiltrates, but these are not associated with significant tubulitis or interstitial edema. Intimal arteritis, if present, is always helpful in resolving the differential diagnosis of an inflammatory infiltrate in a renal allograft biopsy, although it should be cautioned that rejection and nonrejection infiltrates may occur concurrently.

Differential Diagnosis of Acute Antibody-Mediated Rejection

As noted above, microvascular inflammation and injury are not specific for acute AMR. Thus, staining for C4d should be performed on *all* renal allograft biopsies and routine testing for DSA is also strongly advisable, especially in sensitized patients and whenever AMR is in the differential diagnosis. The necrotizing arteritis that may be seen in acute AMR may be indistinguishable from a systemic necrotizing arteritis, but recurrence of vasculitic lesions in the transplant is rare and other findings (e.g., glomerular necrotizing lesions and crescents in ANCA vasculitis) are often helpful in resolving this differential.

Chronic Changes in the Allograft

Although the term *chronic allograft nephropathy* (CAN) had been popular in the past, it is nonspecific, lacks precision, is not well understood, and certainly does not indicate causality; consequently it has fallen out of favor. Morphologically, chronic abnormalities include, but are not limited to, interstitial fibrosis and tubular atrophy (IF/TA). These are features of many of the chronic processes which may affect the allograft and include chronic rejection, chronic CNI toxicity, hypertension and nephrosclerosis, chronic obstruction, bacterial and viral infections, recurrent diseases, and others. In many instances, it is possible to distinguish one process from the others by microscopic examination of kidney tissue (biopsy or nephrectomy); when distinguishing features are not present, use of the nonspecific but descriptive term *IF/TA* is appropriate. As noted above, CAN is no longer part of the vocabulary of transplant pathology. It is unfortunate that many studies dealing with therapy and prognostic indicators in the recent past have used it without reference to specific biopsy features to allow precise classification of the lesions, thereby obscuring potentially important data. In this section, the important entities responsible for chronic damage are described separately. Table 15.1 summarizes some of these.

Chronic Rejection

Although the Banff classification mentions chronic CMR, this lesion remains poorly defined. The morphologic lesions that are commonly recognized as being associated with chronic rejection are primarily lesions of chronic AMR: *transplant glomerulopathy, peritubular capillary basement membrane multilayering, and transplant arteriopathy.*

Transplant glomerulopathy (TG) is the most recognizable lesion of chronic AMR, although only about 75% of such lesions can be definitely linked to coexisting or previous DSA. Multiple studies have demonstrated a strong association of TG with DSA, particularly antibodies against class II HLA. In addition, TG has been shown to be strongly

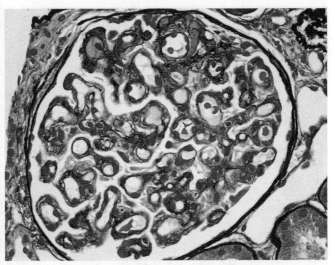

FIGURE 15.7 Transplant glomerulopathy. Numerous glomerular basement membrane double contours are evident on the silver stain. There is very segmental glomerulitis at about 9 o'clock (periodic acid–methenamine silver ×400).

associated with poor graft outcomes, particularly when combined with positive C4d staining. TG is manifest histologically as double contours of the glomerular capillary basement membrane (GBM), best demonstrated on PAS and silver stains (Fig. 15.7). By light microscopy, TG is only rarely seen in biopsies performed during the first 6 months post-transplantation, even in patients with prior documented episodes of acute ABMR, and is uncommon before 1 year post-transplantation. However, early lesions of TG, manifest by the triad of glomerular endothelial cell swelling, subendothelial electron-lucent widening, and early GBM duplication, may be seen by electron microscopy (EM), even during the first few weeks post-transplantation (Fig. 15.8). There is strong evidence that in patients not treated for AMR, these early ultrastructural lesions will progress to overt TG. Accordingly, these early ultrastructural lesions have been incorporated into the most recent version of the Banff classification for AMR (Table 15.3), and the Banff group recommends performing EM, where feasible, on all renal allograft biopsies from sensitized recipients and on all biopsies performed ≥6 months post-transplantation.

Peritubular capillary basement membrane multilayering (PTCBML) (Fig. 15.9) can be viewed as the peritubular capillary equivalent of TG. In both cases, one can envision antibody-mediated endothelial injury leading to separation of the endothelial cells from the underlying basement membrane, with these cells then laying down new basement membrane matrix. However, unlike TG, PTCBML can only be diagnosed by electron microscopy. In addition, the correlation between PTCBML and DSA or evidence of prior acute ABMR is not as strong as with TG, and the findings of studies examining this correlation are

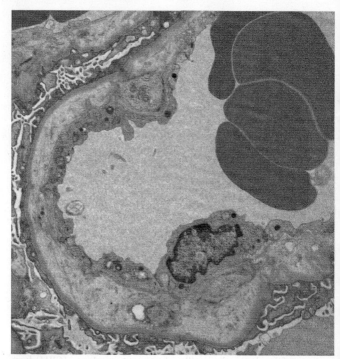

FIGURE 15.8 Early transplant glomerulopathy: electron microscopy. This glomerular capillary shows endothelial cell swelling with loss of fenestrations, prominent subendothelial electron-lucent widening, and early duplication of the glomerular basement membrane, evident just beneath the endothelium. Note the absence of electron-dense, immune complex deposits (uranyl acetate and lead citrate stain, original magnification ×10,000).

more variable. While it is reasonably established that PTCBML with seven to eight circumferential basement membrane layers in the most severely involved capillary and with five or more layers in at least two other capillaries is highly correlated with DSA and prior acute ABMR, the significance of lesser degrees of PTCBML is much less clear.

Transplant arteriopathy is characterized by arterial intimal thickening, usually with inflammatory cells (monocytes/macrophages, lymphocytes, and sometimes foam cells) within the thickened intima. This latter feature, as well as the frequently circumferential nature of transplant arteriopathy, are somewhat helpful in distinguishing this lesion from arteriosclerosis (either donor disease or developing owing to post-transplant hypertension), although these are by no means specific and recent studies have shown that arterial intimal fibrosis without such features may, in some cases, be related to DSA. Some cases of transplant arteriopathy may reflect chronic CMR rather than or in addition to chronic AMR, and it is not unusual to see an artery with both endarteritis and intimal fibrosis with leukocytes in the sclerotic intima. One useful means to help determine if a lesion of arterial intimal

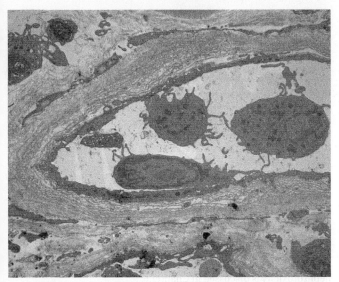

FIGURE 15.9 Peritubular capillary basement membrane multilayering. Electron microscopy shows multiple circumferential layers of the peritubular capillary basement membrane. The lumen contains several cells with an ultrastructural appearance consistent with monocytes/macrophages (uranyl acetate and lead citrate stain, original magnification ×10,000).

fibrosis, with or without leukocytes within the intima, represents chronic rejection as opposed to arteriosclerosis is by comparison with previous biopsies of the same allograft, if these are available.

The Banff classification for AMR (Table 15.3) defines two forms of chronic AMR: chronic, active AMR and chronic AMR. Both require the presence of one or more of the above lesions, and DSA. The main difference between these is that chronic, active AMR shows evidence of recent antibody interaction with the endothelium, in the form of peritubular capillary C4d staining or moderate microvascular inflammation (glomerulitis and/or peritubular capillaritis), whereas chronic AMR does not. In addition, diagnosis of chronic, active AMR requires demonstration of DSA at the approximate time of the biopsy, while any documented DSA post-transplantation is sufficient for diagnosis of purely chronic AMR.

Glomerular and vascular lesions of chronic rejection are typically accompanied by changes in the tubulointerstitial compartment, namely interstitial fibrosis and tubular atrophy (IF/TA), with or without accompanying interstitial mononuclear cell inflammation.

Differential Diagnosis

As noted above, TG is not specific for chronic AMR, and evidence indicates that this may be seen in several other contexts including hepatitis C infection (possibly with associated anti-cardiolipin antibodies), chronic TMA, whether *de novo* (e.g., owing to CNI nephrotoxicity) or recurrent, and possibly even chronic CMR. Thus, the clinical, pathologic, and serologic context in which TG is observed is crucial for a proper diagnosis. Of course, double contours of the GBM may also be seen in the context of recurrent or *de novo* glomerulonephritis (GN); such lesions are typically either immune complex-mediated or complement-mediated (C3 glomerulopathy). While "pure" TG is easily distinguished histologically from active GN owing to the glomerular hypercellularity associated with the latter, it should be cautioned that early lesions of recurrent or *de novo* GN may show relatively little glomerular hypercellularity, and that the combination of TG and glomerulitis may mimic active GN histologically. It is thus important to perform routine immunofluorescence and EM to resolve this differential diagnosis.

OTHER PATHOLOGIC TRANSPLANT LESIONS

Calcineurin-Inhibitor Nephrotoxicity

Cyclosporine and tacrolimus produce similar renal structural and functional effects, and the pathologist cannot differentiate between the nephrotoxic effects of these two drugs. Interestingly, sirolimus may induce similar morphologic features. The pathogenesis of CNI nephrotoxicity is discussed in Chapter 6.

Acute Toxicity

There are few specific pathologic findings of acute CNI nephrotoxicity, with the transplant dysfunction likely secondary to alterations in renal blood flow. Histologic findings are of tubular abnormalities including relative luminal dilation, epithelial cell flattening, and necrosis of individual proximal tubular cells. The most specific finding is of clear, small isometric vacuoles in proximal tubular cell cytoplasm, often involving many cells of only few tubular profiles (Fig. 15.10) and most often the straight portion of the proximal tubule (S3 segment, best represented in deeper portions of the cortex). If carefully sought, these can be identified in some patients and are more common with higher drug levels. However, many biopsies from patients with toxicity do not show such vacuoles, and they may be seen in other settings such as following IVIG infusion or contrast dye administration. The interstitium has modest or no edema and there is minimal inflammation with the exception of small perivenous lymphoid aggregates which lack associated tubulitis. Focal tubular calcifications or giant mitochondria also may be present, but are not of diagnostic help.

Vascular Effects

Several vascular lesions are ascribed to the CNIs. *Arteriolopathy* consists of a variety of abnormalities that occur separately or together. There initially are vacuolization and necrosis of individual myocytes with lost smooth muscle cells subsequently replaced with large plasma protein precipitates. These arteriolar insudates (hyalinization/hyalinosis) are characteristically nodular occurring on the outer (peripheral) aspect of afferent arteriolar walls (Fig. 15.11). These arteriolar insudates may occur early after transplantation if there has been severe vascular injury as detailed below, although typically are found after months of drug administration. In contrast, in hypertension, the insudative lesions usually

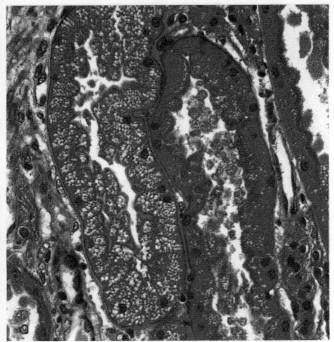

FIGURE 15.10 Proximal tubule with cytoplasmic small isometric vacuoles in all epithelial cells in a patient with acute calcineurin-inhibitor nephrotoxicity. Note that the cells of the adjacent proximal tubule do not contain the vacuoles (masson trichrome ×400).

are subendothelial or within the muscularis. Cessation or reduction of the cyclosporine dose has resulted in amelioration or resolution of the arteriolopathy in some patients, although sampling variability and poor intraobserver reproducibility limit these observations.

Thrombotic Microangiopathy
TMA is an idiosyncratic, uncommon, but well-recognized complication of CNI administration and also has been associated with mTOR inhibitors; its clinical diagnosis and manifestations are discussed in Chapters 5 and 9. Typically, bland thrombi are present within lumens of arterioles and/or glomerular capillaries, are focal in distribution, and seldom are associated with tissue necrosis. More severe lesions result in arterial and arteriolar features of TMA including muscular hypertrophy and mucoid intimal thickening, endothelial cell swelling and fibrin in the walls and/or lumens, rarely with cortical necrosis (Fig. 15.12). Glomeruli may have ischemic capillary wall wrinkling and collapse or capillary double contours with or without a lobular appearance, mimicking TG or, infrequently, certain forms of glomerulonephritis.

Chronic Toxicity
The changes of chronic CNI nephrotoxicity are similar to chronic renal ischemia. In their purest form, they consist of focal (*striped*)

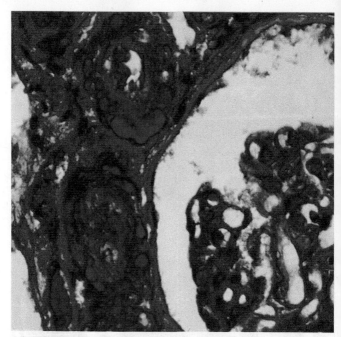

FIGURE 15.11 Calcineurin-inhibitor–associated arteriolopathy. The arteriole has plasma protein insudates (hyalinization/hyalinosis) in a nodular pattern along the outer aspect of the hypertrophied muscularis (masson trichrome ×400).

interstitial fibrosis/tubular atrophy without inflammation (Fig. 15.13). The interstitium may show a generalized increase of collagen types III and IV with lesser increases in type I. The diagnosis is supported by finding concurrent nodular peripheral afferent arteriolar hyalinosis and enlarged juxtaglomerular apparatus. Glomerular ischemic collapse, segmental glomerulosclerosis or complete glomerulosclerosis also may be present. While there are no definitive histologic features of chronic CNI toxicity, the combination of the above changes in the presence of normal arteries is highly suggestive of this lesion.

Differential Diagnosis
In acute CNI toxicity, proximal tubular cell isometric vacuolization is the only feature with any specificity. However, similar vacuoles may be observed in patients treated with IVIG if prepared in sorbitol or dextrans (such preparations should be avoided), in kidneys exposed to volume expanders such as mannitol, following intravenous contrast for imaging studies or in patients with nephrotic syndrome and tubular reabsorption of lipid.

Nodular arteriolar hyalinization is not a specific lesion and is particularly common in diabetic patients, which is a key differential diagnosis. Histologic features of CNI-induced TMA are similar to those seen in TMA owing to other causes including *de novo* or recurrent thrombotic

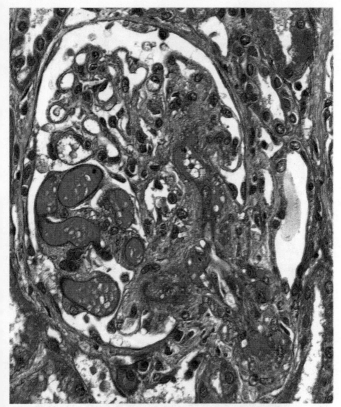

FIGURE 15.12 Calcineurin-inhibitor–induced thrombotic microangiopathy. The arteriole has thickening of the muscular wall and fibrin in the lumen with thrombosis of glomerular capillaries segmentally. Note the outer nodular hyalinization on the right side of the arteriole (masson trichrome ×400).

thrombocytopenic purpura (TTP) and atypical hemolytic uremic syndrome, antiphospholipid syndrome, and TMA in the setting of AMR. TMA in the setting of AMR usually has associated microvascular injury with capillaritis and there is often (but not always) C4d deposition in peritubular capillaries; patients with these findings should be assessed for DSA. Antiphospholipid syndrome with anticardiolipin antibodies has been associated with hepatitis C virus infection in transplant recipients. In some settings, a full hematologic assessment may be required to determine the underlying cause of the TMA.

In subacute to chronic renal injury, the differentiation between nonspecific interstitial fibrosis/tubular atrophy, nephrosclerosis, and chronic CNI nephrotoxicity may be difficult, and transplant kidneys with and without CNI exposure demonstrate similar renal lesions. Arterial fibrosis with or without inflammation, indicating chronic rejection and nephrosclerosis, respectively, may coexist with CNI toxicity, further

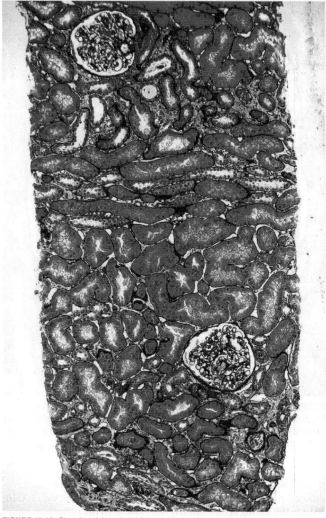

FIGURE 15.13 Chronic calcineurin-inhibitor nephrotoxicity characterized by focal "striped" tubular atrophy and interstitial fibrosis without inflammation (periodic acid–methenamine silver ×200).

complicating the diagnosis. There is much overlap of chronic allograft changes owing to these insults, and it has been suggested that chronic renal transplant failure is unlikely to be a result of CNI toxicity alone.

Acute Tubular Necrosis

Acute tubular necrosis (or more correctly, acute tubular injury) in transplants is similar histologically to the lesion found in native kidneys with tubular luminal dilatation, epithelial cell flattening, loss of proximal

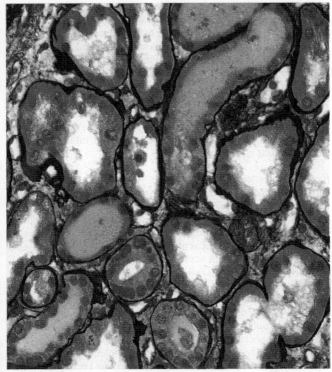

FIGURE 15.14 Acute tubular injury. The tubule in the center is incompletely lined by epithelial cells, with a sloughed degenerated cell and cytoplasmic debris in the lumen. A tubular cell mitotic figure is present at the bottom left. There is mild interstitial edema without inflammation (periodic acid–methenamine silver ×325).

cell brush borders, and in some cases overt necrosis of epithelial cells as well as sloughing of pyknotic and nonpyknotic epithelium into tubular lumens (Fig. 15.14). It is most often encountered in a biopsy performed within the first month or so after transplantation in the clinical setting of delayed graft function (see Chapter 10); however, all insults resulting in tubular necrosis in the native kidney can injure the transplant kidney in the same manner. In addition to the usual changes of tubular injury noted above, interstitial edema and focal interstitial lymphocytic infiltrates may be present but without tubular inflammation. When regeneration ensues, there are mitotic figures in tubular epithelial cells.

Infections

The transplanted kidney may be involved with a variety of infections, but only a small number are regularly identified on renal biopsy. These include acute infectious interstitial nephritis (pyelonephritis) owing to bacterial, and less often fungal, infections in which neutrophils infiltrate the interstitium and tubules, with tubular cell necrosis and neutrophils admixed with cellular debris in tubular lumina (*tubular microabscess*). Viral infections typically evoke a mononuclear tubulointerstitial nephritis which may be morphologically similar to cell-mediated acute rejection, but frequently has a prominent plasma cell component. Polyomavirus infection is the most common infectious organism identified in renal transplant biopsies, and is described below. Viruses observed far less frequently in renal biopsies include cytomegalovirus (CMV), which requires identification of intranuclear or cytoplasmic inclusions and confirmation by immunohistochemical staining. Even less common is adenovirus infection, characterized by focal but severe necrosis of the tubulointerstitium including sloughed necrotic tubular cells with viral cytopathic changes.

Human Polyomavirus Infection

Human BK polyomavirus is the most common infectious agent identified in renal transplant biopsies (see Chapter 12). The infection presents clinically as an elevated creatinine level with biopsy findings of tubulointerstitial nephritis; identification of the virus is critical as an erroneous diagnosis of acute rejection may result in increased immunosuppression with worsening of the viral infection. Polyomavirus preferentially infects collecting duct epithelium with medullary involvement often predominating relative to the renal cortex. The tubulointerstitium may contain a minimal inflammatory infiltrate or display patchy or diffuse brisk inflammation including prominent plasma cells and lymphocytic tubulitis, depending on the viral load in the kidney. There is minimal-to-extensive tubular atrophy/interstitial fibrosis relative to the chronicity of the viral infection. Tubular cells contain large basophilic intranuclear inclusions occasionally with central clearing, and undergo necrosis and sloughing into the tubular lumina (Fig. 15.15). Polyomavirus may induce tubular basement membrane immune complex deposits and, in the absence of a known cause such as lupus, this finding warrants a careful search for the virus. Immunohistochemical staining with polyomavirus monoclonal antibody confirms the diagnosis, and in our view should be performed on all biopsies showing the combination of nuclear atypia in tubular epithelium and interstitial inflammation. This recommendation is made because not all biopsies with polyomavirus infection will show diagnostic inclusions, and in consideration of the potential clinical consequence of misdiagnosing such an infection as acute rejection. Acute CMR and polyomavirus infection may occur concurrently and this presents a diagnostic challenge. In the absence of intimal arteritis, this dual diagnosis may be suggested by the presence of interstitial inflammation and tubulitis in cortical areas remote from infected tubular epithelium, using both histologic findings and immunohistochemistry to define the latter. Polyomavirus infection may occur in the ureter where it induces ureteric stenosis (see Chapter 9).

Several classification schemes for polyomavirus nephropathy have been suggested to provide clinical correlative and prognostic information. The most recent was developed by a Banff working group incorporating the degree of intrarenal viral load and extent of parenchymal scarring. Grade 1 indicates early disease with no significant inflammation, minor

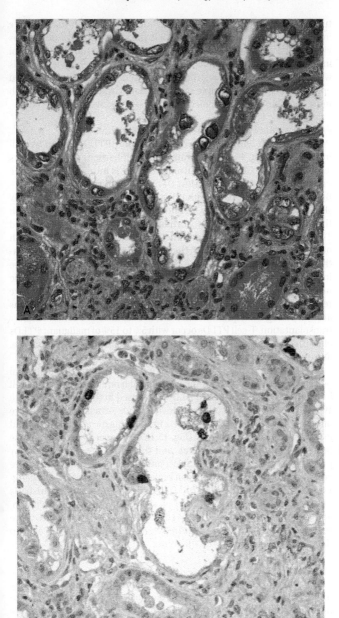

FIGURE 15.15 Polyoma virus infection. **A:** Tubular cells are enlarged with intranuclear viral inclusions characterized by a ground-glass appearance and focal nuclear clearing. There is an adjacent interstitial lymphocytic inflammatory infiltrate (hematoxylin and eosin ×325). **B:** Immunoperoxidase stain for SV40 (polyomavirus) showing positive brown staining in infected tubular epithelial cell nuclei (×325).

tubular injury, and few intranuclear inclusions which may require immunostaining to identify. Grade 2 is florid disease with numerous viral inclusions, tubular cell necrosis and sloughing, tubulointerstitial inflammation, and less than 50% fibrosis. In grade 3, there is sclerosis with more than 50% interstitial fibrosis and fewer residual infected epithelial cells with variable inflammation. Grade 3 correlates with more renal functional impairment at biopsy and worse outcome.

Post-transplant Lymphoproliferative Disorder

Post-transplant lymphoproliferative disorder (PTLD) has an overall incidence of 1% to 2% in renal transplant recipients; its clinical aspects are discussed in Chapter 11. Intragraft PTLD is more common in the first 2 years post-transplant. Most PTLDs are associated with Epstein–Barr virus (EBV) infection, with EBV transformed lymphocytes usually showing B-cell markers. EBV secondarily infects B lymphocytes, which then undergo malignant transformation. The coincident diminished T-cell surveillance owing to immunosuppression allows the outgrowth of the transformed cells, which then develop into the lymphoproliferative disorder. In some cases, the transformed cells themselves may be immunosuppressive through release of viral IL-10. Risk factors include primary EBV infection and the intensity of the immunosuppressive regimen. Up to 30% of PTLDs may be EBV-negative, and these lesions are increasing in frequency with a later onset at 50 to 60 months after transplantation. T-cell PTLDs occur with 5% to 15% of malignant PTLDs classified as T/NK-cell lymphoma and typically are EBV-negative, although infrequent EBV-driven T-cell lesions do occur.

   PTLD encompasses a spectrum of lymphocyte features from atypical polyclonal proliferations to frankly malignant lymphomas or plasma cell lesions. The classification of PTLD was revised in the year 2008 by the World Health Organization (Table 15.4). The abnormal lymphocytes are often large, with cleaved, noncleaved, immunoblastic and plasmacytoid features with mitotic activity (Fig. 15.16). These cells occur in dense infiltrates or nodular aggregates, and there may be irregular patchy parenchymal necrosis without interstitial edema. Some cases have concurrent acute CMR which can make the diagnosis more challenging, particularly in the earlier PTLD lesions. Immunohistochemistry is necessary to determine lymphoid subsets and light-chain restriction, and *in situ* hybridization for EBV (EBER) should be performed. Gene rearrangement studies are required in a limited number of cases to determine clonality and classification.

De novo Glomerulopathies

There are glomerular lesions that occur post-transplant, which may or may not impact graft survival. As for native renal biopsies, immunofluorescence and electron microscopy are necessary for accurate diagnosis, and it is suggested that tissue is collected for these modalities in all transplant biopsies. *Focal and segmental glomerulosclerosis* (FSGS) including perihilar, NOS and collapsing variants, likely is the most common *de novo* glomerular disease, typically occurring more than 1 year after transplantation. The histology is similar to that seen in the native kidney relative to the variant present. It is likely a

TABLE 15.4	Classification of Post-transplant Lymphoproliferative Disorders (PTLD)

Early lesions
    Infectious mononucleosis-like PTLD
    Plasmacytic hyperplasia
Polymorphic PTLD
Monomorphic PTLD (classified by lymphoma they resemble)
    B-cell neoplasms*
        Diffuse large B-cell lymphoma
        Burkitt lymphoma
        Plasma cell myeloma
        Plasmacytoma-like lesion
        Other
    T-cell neoplasms
        Peripheral T-cell lymphoma, NOS
        Hepatosplenic T-cell lymphoma
        Other
Classical Hodgkin lymphoma-type PTLD

*Indolent small B-cell lymphomas are not considered PTLDs.
(Adapted from Swerdlow SH, Campo E, Harris NL, et al. Post-transplant lymphoproliferative disorders. In: Swerdlow SH, Campo E, Harris NL, et al, eds. *WHO Classification of Tumours of Haematopoietic and Lymphoid Tissue.* Sterling, VA: Stylus Publishing, 2008.)

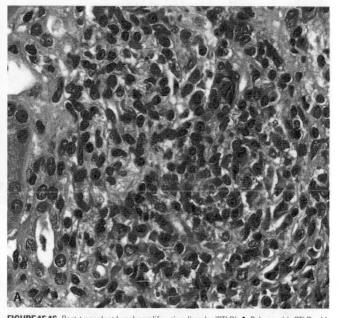

FIGURE 15.16 Post-transplant lymphoproliferative disorder (PTLD). **A:** Polymorphic PTLD with atypical B lymphocytes that had no light-chain restriction on immunohistochemical staining. **B:** Monomorphic PTLD, diffuse large B-cell lymphoma type. The lymphocytes are atypical with enlarged nuclei and prominent nucleoli. **C:** Monomorphic PTLD, plasma cell myeloma type. The plasma cells show restricted staining for kappa light chain (hematoxylin and eosin ×450).

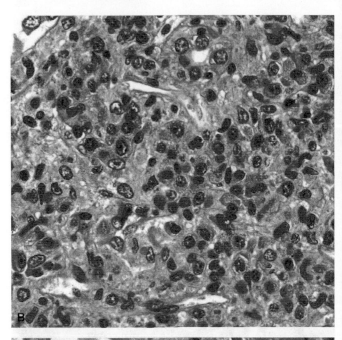

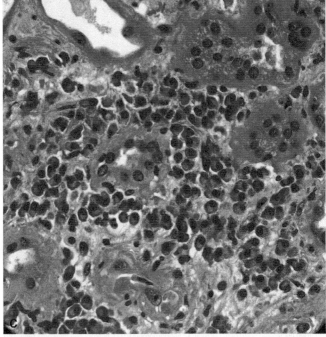

FIGURE 15.16 (*continued*)

secondary process owing to reduced renal mass, hypertension, medications, infections, etc. and imparts a negative impact on renal survival. *De novo membranous nephropathy* is found in approximately 2% of adult renal transplants. Phospholipase A2 receptor (PLA2R) staining is almost always negative, supporting the reported associations with a variety of infectious, alloimmune, and other forms of injury rather than the *de novo* occurrence of "primary" membranous nephropathy. The morphology is the same as in the native kidney, and it is suggested that PLA2R staining or serologic testing be performed to exclude recurrent disease. As patients with low-grade proteinuria are being biopsied more frequently to assess for early AMR, the membranous nephropathy may be in a very early stage. Post-transplant diabetes may result in *de novo* diabetic glomerulosclerosis, which tends to develop more rapidly compared with diabetic nephropathy in the native kidney. Although rare, antiglomerular basement membrane antibody nephritis can arise in a normal kidney transplanted into a patient with Alport syndrome (see Chapter 8) with subsequent graft failure. Other forms of *de novo* glomerulonephritis are uncommon.

Recurrent Disease
Glomerular Lesions

A variety of glomerulonephritides may recur after transplantation, but only a small number tend to be clinically significant with regard to graft function and survival (see Chapter 11). Overall, 6% to 20% of renal allograft recipients develop *de novo* or recurrent glomerular lesions. However, it is difficult to determine the incidence of recurrent glomerular disease accurately, as up to 85% of native kidneys are not biopsied and the original disease is not known. FSGS has a 30% to 50% recurrence rate. When FSGS recurs early (hours to weeks after transplantation), it is associated with extensive podocyte foot process effacement and reduced allograft survival. Older allografts also are at risk for recurrent FSGS with less explosive proteinuria and more variable foot process effacement. The risk of recurrence is unrelated to the initial variant of FSGS (tip lesion, perihilar, collapsing, etc.), although the recurrent FSGS often, but not always, is the same variant as that observed in the native kidney. Other recurrent glomerulonephritides associated with graft loss include forms of membranoproliferative glomerulonephritis (MPGN), most often those related to infections (e.g., hepatitis C) and complement abnormalities (C3 glomerulonephritis and dense deposit disease). The data for MPGN are muddied, as there is a recent histologic reclassification of this disease based on pathogenesis rather than morphology. Still, the data that are available suggest that there is a high rate of recurrence of immune complex MPGN with a significant impact on graft survival. C3 glomerulopathy and dense deposit disease, lesions of complement dysregulation, are reported to recur in 67% and up to 100% of patients, respectively, with approximately two-thirds of these patients losing their kidneys to the recurrent disease. IgA nephropathy commonly recurs as glomerular immune deposits, much less frequently induces symptomatic disease, and rarely leads to graft loss. Recurrent membranous nephropathy typically occurs within 1 year after engraftment. It can recur within weeks in patients with circulating antibodies against PLA2R at the time of transplantation, and frequently is in an early morphologic stage (Churg and Ehrenreich stage I). Identification of PLA2R in subepithelial deposits in the native kidney biopsy and in the transplant biopsy, or anti-PLA2R antibodies in patient serum at the time of biopsy, will help determine if the disease is recurrent. Up to 50% of patients transplanted for end-stage lupus nephritis will develop nonspecific clinically insignificant immune complex glomerulonephritis or mesangial lupus nephritis in the renal transplant; however, proliferative lupus nephritis seldom recurs and there is no impact on graft survival. Other glomerulonephritides such as anti-glomerular basement membrane antibody nephritis and ANCA-vasculitis with crescentic glomerulonephritis rarely recur.

Other Lesions

Systemic diseases that are still active in a transplant recipient may damage the renal allograft in the same manner as the native kidney. Amyloidosis, Bence Jones cast nephropathy (myeloma kidney), light-chain deposition disease, and oxalosis can recur, often with significant graft dysfunction. Atypical hemolytic uremic syndrome, associated with alternative complement pathway dysregulation, may recur in up to 90% of patients depending on the underlying abnormality. The features of recurrent thrombotic microangiopathy are identical to those of *de novo* disease, requiring historical and clinical correlation to determine the underlying pathogenesis. Recurrent diabetic nephropathy occurs more quickly than diabetic injury to the native kidney, with typical features including glomerular basement membrane thickening, diffuse and nodular glomerulosclerosis, and hyalinization of both afferent and efferent arterioles. There may be associated proteinuria, but diabetic nephropathy alone is infrequently responsible for graft loss (see Chapter 16).

NEW TECHNIQUES IN EVALUATING TRANSPLANT DYSFUNCTION

The evaluation of acute and chronic renal allograft dysfunction is an area ripe for the application of new technologies, including genetic profiling with microarrays or RNA sequences, metabolomics, and proteomics. Several studies have examined sets of differentially expressed gene transcripts from biopsy samples or peripheral blood cells to identify those that can define types of rejection or provide precision treatments for transplant recipients. Microarray studies on biopsy tissue have proven useful in helping to verify that AMR can occur in the absence of C4d deposition, resulting in an update of the Banff classification for AMR (Table 15.3). More recent molecular studies have validated this classification's threshold for microvascular inflammation in the diagnosis of C4d-negative AMR. Other microarray studies on biopsy tissue have defined specific transcript sets associated with acute CMR, acute AMR, and the presence of DSA. The former of these has promise toward potentially eliminating the troublesome borderline category in the Banff classification for CMR (Table 15.2). There is also evidence that combining the molecular and standard histopathologic approaches to renal transplant biopsy diagnosis gives more accurate results than either approach alone, although this needs to be validated by studies at additional centers and subjected to cost–benefit analysis. Others have applied a systems biology approach to transplant patients, integrating genomic and proteomic data to identify candidate biomarkers for the diagnosis and monitoring of transplant rejection. Molecular assessment also has been applied to implantation biopsies to determine the risk of early graft dysfunction. These studies show promise, but data are complex and sometimes conflicting; there is much more work needed to create clinically useful algorithms for patient selection and management.

KIDNEY DONOR HISTOPATHOLOGY

The gap between the supply and demand for kidneys from deceased donors has led to the increasing use of organs from "marginal" and "extended criteria" donors (terms that have now been replaced in the United States by the Kidney Donor Profile Index—KDPI: see Chapters 4 and 5). Histopathology of these kidneys often is requested as a guide to the potential viability of a particular organ. The most common clinical situations in which donor pathology is requested are for older donors, donors with a history of hypertension or vascular disease, or donors with prerecovery evidence of renal dysfunction. Baseline histology may be required in clinical trials evaluating new immunosuppressive drugs. The time constraints imposed by the need for rapid decision making prevent routine histopathologic processing of biopsy material. Frozen-section techniques may impair diagnostic precision, and rapid-processing techniques are preferred. A superficial wedge biopsy specimen often is provided; however, the subcapsular parenchyma frequently has chronic changes and is not representative of the whole organ. Additionally, arteries may be absent from superficial biopsy specimens, precluding adequate evaluation for arteriosclerosis. Therefore, such specimens should be interpreted with caution.

A number of histologic scoring systems have been suggested for determining the suitability of a kidney for transplantation. Parameters variably included in histologic scores are percentage of globally sclerosed glomeruli, the extent of interstitial fibrosis with or without tubular atrophy, and the severity of sclerotic vascular disease. More than 20% global glomerulosclerosis is often used to determine if kidneys are discarded and such kidneys have a decreased 1-year survival rate. However, despite a correlation of predicted outcomes with renal parenchymal scarring, standard guidelines for determining graft suitability from histologic findings have not been established and vary across centers. Composite scores including histologic and clinical features are likely to be better predictors both of delayed graft function and of long-term outcomes. There is also evidence that, when histologic scoring of preimplantation biopsies is done by experienced renal pathologists rather than general surgical pathologists, correlation of pathology with subsequent graft function is improved and discard rates of marginal kidneys are reduced.

Selected Readings

Azancot MA, Moreno F, Salcedo M, et al. The reproducibility and predictive value on outcome of renal biopsies from expanded criteria donors. Kidney Int 2014;85:1161–1168.

Baid-Agrawal S, Farris AB III, Pascual M, et al. Overlapping pathways to transplant glomerulopathy: chronic humoral rejection, hepatitis C infection, and thrombotic microangiopathy. Kidney Int 2011;80:879–885.

Djamali A, Kaugman DB, Ellis TM, et al. Diagnosis and management of antibody-mediated rejection: current status and novel approaches. Am J Transplant 2014;14:255–271.

Dorr C, Wu B, Guan W, et al. Differentially expressed gene transcripts using RNA sequencing from the blood of immunosuppressed kidney allograft recipients. PLoS One 2015;10:e0125045. doi:10.1371/journal.pone.0125045.

Gaston RS, Cecka JM, Kasiske BL, et al. Evidence for antibody-mediated injury as a major determinant of late kidney allograft failure. Transplantation 2010;90:68–74.

Gunther OP, Shin H, Ng RT, et al. Novel multivariate methods for integration of genomics and proteomics data: applications in a kidney transplant rejection study. OMICS 2014;18:682–695.

Haas M. Chronic allograft nephropathy or interstitial fibrosis and tubular atrophy: what is in a name? Curr Opin Nephrol Hypertens 2014;23:245–250.

Haas M, Sis B, Racusen LC, et al. Banff 2013 meeting report: inclusion of C4d-negative antibody-mediated rejection and antibody-associated arterial lesions. Am J Transplant 2014;14:272–283.

Kreepala C, Famulski KS, Chang J, et al. Comparing molecular assessment of implantation biopsies with histologic and demographic risk assessment. Am J Transplant 2013;13:415–426.

Lefaucheur C, Loupy A, Vernerey D, et al. Antibody-mediated vascular rejection of kidney allografts: a population-based study. Lancet 2013;381:313–319.

Naesens M, Kuypers, D, Sarwal M. Calcineurin inhibitor nephrotoxicity. Clin J Am Soc Nephrol 2009;4:481–508.

Ponticelli C, Moroni G, Glassock RJ. *De novo* glomerular diseases after renal transplantation. Clin J Am Soc Nephrol 2014;9:1479–1487.

Sar A, Worawichawong S, Benediktsson H, et al. Interobserver agreement for polyomavirus nephropathy grading in renal allografts using the working proposal from the 10th Banff conference on allograft pathology. Human Pathol 2011;42:2018–2024.

Sellares J, Reeve J, Loupy A, et al. Molecular diagnosis of antibody-mediated rejection in human kidney transplants. Am J Transplant 2013;13:971–983.

Sis B, Jhangri G, Bunnag S, et al. Endothelial gene expression in kidney transplants with alloantibody indicates antibody-mediated damage despite lack of C4d staining. Am J Transplant 2009;9:2312–2323.

Snanoudj R, Royal V, Elie C, et al. Specificity of histological markers of long-term CNI nephrotoxicity in kidney-transplant recipients under low dose cyclosporine therapy. Am J Transplant 2011;11:2635–2646.

Solez K, Colvin RB, Racusen LC, et al. Banff '05 meeting report: differential diagnosis of chronic allograft injury and elimination of chronic allografts nephropathy. Am J Transplant 2007;7:518–526.

Solez K, Colvin RB, Racusen LC, et al. Banff 07 classification of renal allograft pathology: updates and future directions. Am J Transplant 2008;8:753–760.

Sprangers B, Kuypers DR. Recurrence of glomerulonephritis after renal transplantation. Transplant Rev 2013;27:126–134.

Wiebe C, Gibson IW, Blydt-Hansen TD, et al. Evaluation and clinical pathologic correlations of *de novo* donor-specific HLA antibody post kidney transplantation. Am J Transplant 2012;12:1157–1167.

Wohlfahrtova M, Viklicky O. New strategies for evaluating the quality of kidney grafts from older donors. Transplant Rev 2015;29:212–218.

16

Options for the Diabetic Kidney Transplant Candidate

Gerald S. Lipshutz

Pancreas transplantation is the ultimate intensification of insulin therapy because it normalizes glucose levels far better than any other strategy available for the treatment of type 1 diabetes mellitus. There are three major types of whole-organ pancreas transplantation: simultaneous pancreas and kidney transplant (SPK), pancreas transplantation after kidney transplantation (PAK), and pancreas transplant alone (PTA). SPK is the most commonly performed of the three. The potential benefits of SPK in a patient with type 1 diabetes and chronic or end-stage kidney disease (CKD, ESKD) are improved quality of life, prevention of recurrent diabetic nephropathy, freedom from exogenous insulin with euglycemia, normalization of glycosylated hemoglobin, lack of frequent whole-blood glucose monitoring, lack of dietary restrictions, and stabilization or improvement in secondary complications. These benefits of SPK are the basis of its acceptance as an appropriate therapy for patients with type 1 diabetes mellitus and renal failure. The trade-off for the patient is the operative risk and the need for chronic immunosuppression.

The challenges of pancreas transplant are reflected in prolonged initial admissions and high rates of rehospitalization (more than 50% of patients within the first month). Pancreas transplantation is associated with a higher incidence of rejection compared with kidney transplant alone, reflecting the relatively high immunogenicity of the pancreatic allograft.

In this chapter, the medical and technical issues concerning pancreas transplantation are presented. The indications for, technical differences between, and management of the different methods of pancreas transplantation are discussed together with a consideration of the therapeutic decision-making faced by patients and their physicians and surgeons. Unless otherwise stated, "diabetes" will refer to type 1 diabetes mellitus, though in the United States insulin-dependent type 2 diabetes patients (defined as C-peptide > 2 ng/mL) with kidney failure may qualify for an SPK if their body mass index (BMI) is less than 30 kg/m^2. Only approximately 6% of patients wait-listed for an SPK fall into this category. Figure 16.1 illustrates the whole-organ transplantation options available for diabetic patients with advanced renal disease.

HISTORY OF PANCREAS TRANSPLANTATION

The first human pancreas transplant was performed in 1966 by William Kelly and Richard Lillehei at the University of Minnesota. The major

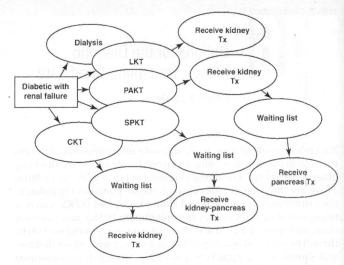

FIGURE 16.1 Options for diabetics with renal failure. A diabetic patient with renal failure can choose one of five treatment strategies: dialysis, living kidney transplantation (LKT), pancreas after living kidney transplantation (PAKT), simultaneous pancreas and kidney transplantation (SPKT), or deceased donor kidney transplantation (CKT). (From Knoll GA, Nichol G. Dialysis, kidney transplantation, or pancreas transplantation for patients with diabetes mellitus and renal failure: a decision analysis of treatment options. J Am Soc Nephrol 2003;14:500–515, with permission.)

surgical challenge that needed to be overcome was a method of pancreatic exocrine drainage. A duct-ligated segmental pancreatic allograft and a deceased donor kidney were transplanted into a 28-year-old diabetic woman with ESKD. Post-transplantation immunosuppression was azathioprine and prednisone. A pancreatic fistula complicated the patient's postoperative course and both the kidney and pancreas were removed about 2 months later. Subsequently, the patient died from a pulmonary embolus. The second patient, a 32-year-old, was transplanted 2 weeks after the first recipient. The patient suffered from rejection and was treated with steroid boluses and graft irradiation. The patient died from sepsis 4 months post-transplant.

Although these initial results were poor, they were encouraging in that these early transplantation experiences did demonstrate that glucose control without exogenous insulin was possible. The procedure established that endogenous secretion of insulin with normal feedback mechanisms could occur with a whole-organ vascularized pancreas transplant. As will be discussed below, in the ensuing decades most of the technical details associated with pancreas transplantation were solved and the various forms of whole-organ pancreas transplantation became increasingly popular, though the procedure was always challenging from both surgical and medical perspectives. Some of that popularity has waned in the last decade, producing what has been termed "an alarming crisis of confidence" in pancreas transplantation (see Stratta et al in Selected Readings).

SOME TRENDS IN DIABETES, DIABETIC KIDNEY DISEASE, AND PANCREAS TRANSPLANTATION

Diabetes mellitus is an enormous health problem worldwide, affecting as many as 135 million people. In the United States, it affects about 6% of the population (18 million individuals), with at least half being unaware that they have the disease. It accounts for more than 160,000 deaths each year in the United States, and massive expenditure. After decades of relentless rise, the total number of new cases of all forms of diabetes in the United States has finally started to decline. The rate of new cases fell by about a fifth from 1.7 million in 2008 to 1.4 million in 2014, likely related to improved eating habits and increased physical activity. The prevalence of type 1 diabetes in the United States is estimated to be 1,000,000 people, with 30,000 new cases diagnosed each year.

At the turn of the 19th century, a patient diagnosed with type 1 diabetes had an average life expectancy of 2 years. However, with the isolation and development of insulin as a treatment for diabetes, the disease has been changed from one that is rapidly fatal to a chronic disease with the potential for multiple secondary complications within 10 to 20 years after disease diagnosis. These include blindness, cardiovascular disease (CVD), dyslipidemia, cerebrovascular disease, amputation, and life-span reduction.

The different forms of diabetes mellitus are the leading causes of ESKD, accounting for about one-half of the newly wait-listed candidates each year. About 40% to 45% of the ESKD population have diabetes, and most have type 2 diabetes. The incidence of ESKD as a consequence of type 2 diabetes is increasing in countries with a Western diet and lifestyle, though in the United States, the rate of new ESKD cases caused by diabetes has remained quite stable since 2000, reaching 152 per million population in 2010. Because of the prevalence of diabetes in the population, the number of diabetic patients with new ESKD has surpassed the number of patients with ESKD from all other primary diagnoses and has most commonly lead to kidney transplantation in adult Whites, Asians, and Native Americans. In addition to ESKD, major complications in these patients include retinopathy, which is the second leading cause of blindness in all persons, and peripheral vascular disease. Ten percent of diabetic patients require a major amputation in their lifetime. Life expectancy is about one-third lower in diabetic patients compared with nondiabetic patients, and CVD is the leading cause of death. Some encouragement may come from the fact that in the period 2008 to 2014 the rate of new cases of diabetes fell by 20% in the United States, perhaps reflecting effort at improving diet and addressing juvenile obesity.

For some patients with diabetes, the treatment of choice is a whole vascularized pancreas transplantation. As of the end of 2010, more than 35,000 pancreas transplantations had been performed worldwide, and through 2010, more than 24,000 pancreas transplantations were performed in the United States. Since 2000, the 1-year patient survival rates for SPK, PAK, and PTA have been 95% to 97%, and the 1-year pancreas graft survival rates have been 85%, 78%, and 77%, respectively.

The number of pancreas transplants performed each year in the United States has decreased substantially.

The different types of pancreas transplantation are now allocated from a single waiting list, though SPK transplants take priority over kidney transplants alone (see Chapter 5). In 2016, approximately 800 SPKs were performed, approximately 80% of the number performed a decade earlier. In 2016, 215 PAKs and PTAs were performed, a nearly 70% drop over the previous decade. Despite the smaller number of transplants, the number of active SPK wait-listed patients has declined to approximately 1800 as of early 2017. The pancreas donor risk index, a measure of the quality of the donated organ, steadily decreased over the decade prior to 2016, as the frequency of most risk donor factors declined and the quality of the organs increased. Head trauma is the most common cause of death for pancreas donors; transplantation of pancreata following death by circulatory criteria (DCD, see Chapter 4, Part I) is now rarely performed.

There are several potential reasons for declining trend in the numbers of pancreas transplants. Better treatment of diabetes with newer insulin preparation and more widespread use of insulin pumps have reduced demand. Given that pancreas transplantation is most frequently an elective "quality of life" procedure, the tolerance for complications by both patients and transplant teams is understandably low. Regulatory agencies in the United States set high standards for outcomes that not all programs can achieve, likely making some "gun-shy." Pancreas transplantation requires rigorous training of both surgical and medical professionals, and there is concern that as the number of transplants fall, this training will become less available. The surgical aspects of pancreas transplantation are particularly demanding, there being three consecutive procedures, ideally performed by the same surgical team: pancreas recovery from the donor, back-table preparation of the organ, and implantation into the recipient described under "Surgical Technique" below.

SURGICAL OPTIONS FOR THE TYPE 1 DIABETIC PATIENTS

SPK transplantation is the major pancreas transplant option for type 1 diabetic patients with advanced renal disease or ESKD (see Fig. 16.2). Its major advantage is that there is only one surgical intervention and one source of foreign human leukocyte antigen (HLA) to which the patient is exposed. Chronic immunosuppressive therapy is similar to that of a kidney transplant alone. As in PAK transplantation, however, many patients have already suffered substantial secondary diabetic complications, and the extent to which these complications will reverse or stabilize is uncertain. Regardless, SPK transplantation is established as a therapeutic and effective procedure, and not only is it life-prolonging for the appropriately selected diabetic patient, it is also life-enhancing, with a significant overall improvement in quality of life over kidney transplantation alone. Among pancreas recipients, those with an SPK transplant have the best pancreas graft survival rates: approximately 85% at 1 year and 50% at 10 years.

PAK transplantation is an option for the diabetic patient who is already the recipient of a well-functioning kidney allograft. A second major intra-abdominal surgery is required together with intensification

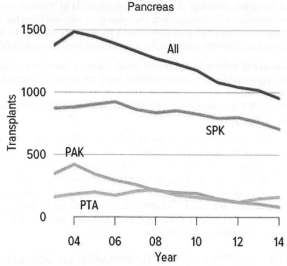

FIGURE 16.2 All pancreas transplant recipients, including adult and pediatric, retransplant, and multiorgan recipients. (From Kandaswamy R, Skeans MA, Gustafson SK, et al. Pancreas. Am J. Transplant 2016;(16, suppl 2):47–68, with permission.)

of the immunosuppressive regime in place of the kidney transplant. This can negatively affect postoperative renal function and exaggerate the inherent risk of infectious complications. PAK transplantation is typically considered in patients with a living kidney donor, in which case the kidney is placed in the left iliac fossa in anticipation of pancreas transplantation in the future. The graft survival rate for PAK recipients at 1 year is approximately 80%, with a 10-year survival rate of 30%.

PAK recipients have already suffered significant secondary diabetic complications. Other than making these recipients insulin independent, it is uncertain whether a well-functioning pancreatic allograft will have any additional benefit in the long term. Overall, the results of PAK transplantation are worse than those of SPK transplantation, likely related to difficulties in diagnosing pancreatic allograft rejection because the kidney (owing to differing HLA) is now longer available as surrogate to assess for rejection by biopsy. It is the second most common pancreas transplant operation. In 1999, Medicare approved reimbursement for pancreas transplantation for patients with ESKD (i.e., those receiving an SPK and PAK but not PTA), thus making the procedure available for a much larger population of patients.

Transplantation of the pancreas alone (PA) in the preuremic recipient is the least commonly performed whole-organ pancreas transplants. It is a therapeutic option for diabetic patients with minimal to no renal dysfunction, who have brittle diabetic control despite the administration of insulin. Many also have hypoglycemic unawareness. In addition to the risks of the surgical procedure itself, the main risks to these patients are the long-term effects of chronic immunosuppression, not only on native renal function but also in the development of atherosclerosis and increased risk for malignancy. One-year graft survival rates for PTA recipients are approximately 80%, with a 10-year rate of close to 30%. The American Diabetes Association (ADA) criteria for PTA are as follows:

1. Consistent failure of intensive insulin-based therapy to establish reasonable glycemic control and to prevent secondary complications
2. Incapacitating clinical and emotional problems with exogenous insulin therapy

There is controversy regarding the survival benefit with PTA because of its associated morbidity and mortality, the need for immunosuppression, and questions about whether secondary complications are prevented. Most centers only consider the procedure in diabetic patients with severe hypoglycemic unawareness or significant secondary complications of diabetes without renal dysfunction. The option of islet transplantation for these patients is discussed later in the chapter.

EVALUATION OF THE PANCREAS TRANSPLANTATION CANDIDATE

Traditionally, pancreas transplantation has been reserved as a therapeutic option for patients with type 1 diabetes mellitus and ESKD. Type 2 diabetes mellitus is thought to result from a combination of resistance to action of insulin and an inadequate compensatory insulin secretory response. Reluctance to consider pancreas transplantation in type 2 diabetic patients stems from concern that existing insulin resistance may limit the benefits of the pancreas allograft. There is a wide variation in the degree of insulin resistance among patients with diabetes that is assumed to be type 2 that has not been well characterized. Some of these patients have detectable C-peptide, are not obese, and can be managed with oral agents and require insulin only later in life. As noted above, a small percentage of the SPK waiting list consists of nonobese type 2 diabetic patients who have a clinical phenotype suggestive of minimal insulin resistance and worsening glucose control. In these selected patients, glucose homeostasis can be achieved that is not different than transplanted type 1 diabetics.

Recipient selection and pretransplant evaluation are essential to avoid significant transplant-related complications. Wait-list candidates should be seen and examined routinely while awaiting organ transplantation. Specific studies should be repeated if the patient remains on the wait-list for a prolonged period of time.

Coronary Artery Disease

Serious vascular complications limit the success of transplantation in diabetic patients. These patients often have multiple cardiovascular risk factors, in addition to the long history of diabetes mellitus. These often include tobacco use, hypertension, hyperlipidemia, family history, and renal failure. Type 1 diabetic patients are at particularly high risk for premature coronary atherosclerotic disease, with as many as 35% dying of coronary artery disease by age 55 years. Coronary artery disease prevalence increases significantly with age and has been found in most diabetic patients older than 45 years. The risk for death in these patients is increased 8- to 15-fold if they also have nephropathy. Not surprisingly, nearly half of diabetic transplant recipients who die within 3 years after transplantation die of a vascular complication, and in pancreas transplant recipients, CVD is the single greatest cause of death.

Diabetic patients with coronary artery disease may not suffer typical anginal symptoms, and thus the possibility of covert coronary artery disease must be considered in every diabetic patient being evaluated for organ transplantation. All patients should undergo some form of evaluation preoperatively. Nuclear perfusion imaging is the most commonly performed screening study, but because of the poor predictive value of noninvasive imaging in diabetic transplant candidates, the precise protocol used is controversial and center specific (see Chapter 8, Part I). In general, young patients who have had diabetes mellitus for less than 25 years, have not smoked tobacco, and lack other cardiovascular risk factors may be evaluated by stress imaging alone. A treadmill nuclear stress test used with thallium or sestamibi scintigraphy or echocardiography is an appropriate initial study. Many diabetic patients with ESKD, however, have poor exercise tolerance and are unable to obtain a rate of 85% of their predicated maximal heart rate. These patients should undergo an adenosine nuclear stress test or a dobutamine stress echocardiogram designed to replicate the effect of exercise stressing on cardiac function.

Positive or equivocal results of noninvasive studies are generally followed by coronary angiography. Patients with coronary lesions amenable to bypass grafting or angioplasty and stent placement should be treated before transplantation. If patients require a postprocedure course of clopidogrel bisulfate, it is preferable that this be completed before undergoing transplantation. The dilemma facing patients who are not yet on dialysis yet require potentially nephrotoxic radiocontrast material for angiography is discussed in Chapter 8. Patients on the waiting list are often recommended to undergo routine annual reassessment with noninvasive stress imaging until transplanted, although the benefit of this commonly used strategy had not been documented. Patients with significant coronary artery disease that is not amenable to interventional cardiology or surgical therapy should not be considered candidates for pancreas transplantation.

The cardiac risk status of diabetic patients should not be forgotten after a successful pancreas or kidney transplant. Risk-factor modification should continue throughout the pretransplant and post-transplant periods. This should include use of statins for elevated low-density lipoprotein cholesterol and total cholesterol with appropriate dose modification for patients receiving calcineurin inhibitors (CNI) (see Chapter 6). Experience in transplant recipients with the new low-density lipoprotein (LDL)–lowering drugs that target the enzyme PCSK9 has not yet been reported. When possible, patients should be started on low-dose β blockade if they do not have hypoglycemic unawareness of other contraindications. β_1-selective blockers are preferable to avoid undesirable side effects. Antihypertensive drugs that do not aggravate insulin sensitivity or lipid metabolism should be selected for treatment of arterial hypertension. β_1 blockers without intrinsic sympathomimetic action are preferable for patients with both diabetes and hypertension and with associated ischemic heart disease, whereas β_1 blockers with intrinsic sympathomimetic action, exerting a vasodilative action, are useful for diabetic hypertensive patients without ischemic heart disease because they do not aggravate insulin sensitivity and lipid metabolism. In addition, daily aspirin and omega-3 and omega-6 fatty acids should be recommended to promote vascular health.

Cerebrovascular and Peripheral Vascular Disease

The increased susceptibility of diabetic transplant recipients for cerebrovascular and peripheral vascular disease mandates particular attention to these issues in the pretransplant evaluation. Approximately 4% of kidney-alone and SPK recipients experience a stroke or transient ischemic attack in the 4 years following surgery, and nearly one-third of these are fatal. Any history of cerebrovascular events or intermittent claudication or findings of carotid or femoral bruits or poor peripheral pulses should be further assessed during patient evaluation. Further consultation with a vascular surgeon may be necessary.

Infections

Patients should be free of significant infections, such as peritonitis, osteomyelitis, or unhealed foot or lower extremity ulcerations at the time of transplantation. Close examination of the patient's feet and lower extremities should be performed at each visit and on admission for organ transplantation. If a patient is admitted to undergo transplantation and a lower extremity ulcer is found, that patient should be discharged and should notify the transplantation center when it is completely healed. Significant dental decay and periodontal disease should also be treated before transplantation. Patients should be informed that if they develop infectious complications while awaiting transplantation, their candidacy will be placed "on hold" until all infectious issues have been resolved.

Preemptive Transplantation

The advantages of predialysis, "preemptive," transplantation for kidney transplant candidates also apply to candidates for SPK. Early transplantation can obviate the need for both temporary and permanent dialysis access and disfigurement of the extremities associated with these procedures, can prevent episodes of congestive heart failure and fluid overload, and can correct hypertension, which may contribute to more rapid vision loss in this group of patients. Some data suggest that early transplantation may slow retinopathy and correct neuropathy. The development of diabetic complications on dialysis may impair the rehabilitation potential after transplantation.

Predialysis diabetic transplant candidates who require coronary angiography risk worsening of renal function and potential dialysis initiation induced by exposure to iodinated contrast agents. This risk of contrast-induced nephropathy has to be carefully weighed against the risks associated with undiagnosed coronary artery disease. Working closely with a cardiologist can be helpful in that the dose of intravenous contrast administered during coronary angiography can be minimized to reduce the risk for precipitating renal failure.

Insulin Requirements

By the time many diabetic patients develop advanced nephropathy or the need for dialysis, their insulin requirements often diminish. Patients receiving peritoneal dialysis may have higher insulin needs owing to the use of dextrose-containing dialysates. Pancreas transplant candidates should have a C-peptide level drawn to confirm they are insulinopenic; however, their history will likely confirm their diagnosis. In type 1 diabetic patients, a C-peptide value should be undetectable, or less than 0.5 ng/mL.

It may be more difficult to achieve adequate postoperative insulin levels in recipients who have a high daily insulin requirement. Obese type 1 diabetic patients may have also developed insulin resistance, and an estimate of the pretransplant insulin requirement may be helpful in assessing the need for exogenous insulin after transplantation. Some glucose intolerance can be seen in the early postoperative period owing to large doses of corticosteroids, carbohydrate intolerance, infusion of medications prepared in 5% dextrose, improved appetite, and the use of a CNI that may lead to periods of elevated blood glucose and increased insulin requirements. Type 1 diabetic patients should expect to be free of exogenously administered insulin after a successful transplantation. Freedom from the use of insulin and strict dietary disciple are the most concrete benefits of successful pancreas transplantation.

DONOR SELECTION

Appropriate pancreas donor selection is key to avoiding complications relating primarily to vascular thrombosis and duodenal enteric leaks. The organ donor for pancreas transplantation is typically in the age range of 10 to 45 years with a traumatic mechanism as the cause of brain death. Donors whose death is defined by cardiac criteria (see Chapter 4) are not suitable for whole-organ pancreas donation. The donor should have had no previous pancreatic surgery or history of pancreatic trauma, or a diagnosis of diabetes mellitus. A HgbA$_{1c}$ level before procurement may help assess for glucose intolerance. Hyperglycemia is a common occurrence during the management of brain-dead patients and does not represent a contraindication to pancreas donation.

An increased incidence of allograft thrombosis and graft loss has been described when the donors are aged greater than 45 years or have died from cerebrovascular accidents. Pancreata originating from older donors have had higher rates of intra-abdominal infections, anastomotic or duodenal leaks, relaparotomy, and decreased graft survival. As a result, caution should be urged in accepting and using pancreata from organ donors older than 45 years. Weight and body mass are also important considerations. Although no strict criteria exist regarding donor weight, some centers consider a donor lower weight limit of 45 kg. This is primarily because of concern of the size of the pancreatic arterial vasculature for construction of the iliac Y-graft and risk for arterial graft thrombosis. Some centers, however, routinely use pancreata from small or even pediatric donors with good outcomes. Donors with a BMI higher than 30 are avoided by many centers because of an increased incidence of fatty infiltration and subsequent increased risk for ischemia-reperfusion injury, infection, pancreatitis, and allograft thrombosis.

PANCREAS TRANSPLANTATION: SURGICAL TECHNIQUE

The surgical procedure can be divided into three stages: (1) organ procurement, (2) back-table pancreas preparation, and (3) pancreas transplantation.

Organ Procurement

Successful and uncomplicated pancreas transplantation requires meticulous allograft procurement and attention to detail in preparing the pancreas on the back table. There is no substitute for a skilled surgeon examining the pancreas during procurement and making an assessment of the suitability of the organ.

After opening the lesser sac, the gastrocolic ligament is divided, and the pancreas is closely examined and palpated. The aorta and venal cava are exposed, followed by division of the right gastroepiploic and pyloric vessels. Some centers perform a bowel decontamination procedure. A nasogastric tube may be advanced into the second portion of the duodenum, and 200 mL of saline and povidone-iodine with amphotericin B is instilled. The short gastric arteries are ligated, the transverse colon is completely mobilized, and the stomach is then divided proximal to the pylorus. The fourth portion of the duodenum is similarly divided, however, just before removal of the pancreas. With careful retraction of the spleen by a no-hands technique, the splenonephric and splenophrenic attachments are carefully divided. The liver is mobilized, and the aorta, vena cava, and inferior mesenteric vein are isolated. The gallbladder is emptied, and the bile duct is divided. The supraceliac aorta is isolated, and heparin is given intravenously. Cannulas are placed into the aorta and inferior mesenteric vein. In coordination with the cardiothoracic team, the aorta is cross-clamped, and preservation solution is instilled along with surface cooling with ice slush. The thoracic organs are then procured, followed by removal of the liver after division of the gastroduodenal artery, portal vein, and splenic artery. The pancreas with spleen attached is then removed (Fig. 16.3). The allograft is kept ice cold in sterile preservation solution until ready to be prepared on the back table.

Back-Table Pancreas Preparation

The back-table preparation of the pancreatic allograft requires careful surgical technique. It can be divided into four steps. First, the distal and proximal duodenum must be shortened to proper length. This is performed while probing the common bile duct at the ampulla to ensure that it is not compromised during duodenal shortening. The ends of the duodenum are generally stapled and then oversewn. The bile duct is ligated. A culture of the excised duodenum should be sent to the laboratory for Gram stain, fungal stain, and bacterial and fungal cultures. Second, arterial reconstruction is required. An arterial Y-graft is used with the donor common iliac–external iliac–internal iliac artery bifurcation. The internal iliac artery is anastomosed to the splenic artery, and the external iliac artery is anastomosed to the superior mesenteric artery. The inferior mesenteric vein is ligated. The portal vein

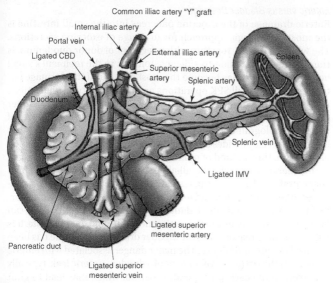

FIGURE 16.3 Anatomy of procured pancreatic allograft before backbench preparation. CBD, common bile duct; IMV, inferior mesenteric vein. (From Lipshutz GS, Wilkinson AH. Pancreas–kidney and pancreas transplantation for the treatment of diabetes mellitus. Endocrinol Metab Clin North Am 2007;36:1015–1038, with permission.)

should be separated from the surrounding tissue. An extension graft is rarely required and should be avoided. Third, extraneous tissue at the periphery of the gland is removed. The hilum of the spleen is carefully dissected, and the splenic artery and vein are transected and tied by suture ligature. The stapled mesenteric vasculature is oversewn. Fourth, the gland should be tested for vascular integrity. Using a syringe with a tapered connector attached, ice-cold preservation solution should be carefully instilled into the common iliac artery and the gland carefully examined from all aspects for evidence of preservation solution extrusion. These should be identified and ligated.

Surgical Implantation Techniques

The main surgical controversies regarding pancreatic transplantation techniques have involved the method of exocrine drainage and vascular drainage. To provide the mass of islets needed to produce insulin and treat diabetes, it is necessary to transplant both the exocrine and endocrine pancreas. During the initial development of pancreas transplantation, procedures including duct ligation and creation of a duodenal button to drain exocrine secretions were tested but were fraught with complications, and these methods in general have been abandoned. Many studies and much interest have been focused on the handling of the exocrine pancreatic secretions. The most commonly used techniques today are enteric drainage and bladder drainage. This situation may change if pancreatic islet transplantation becomes a readily available clinical reality.

Enteric versus Bladder Drainage

Enteric drainage of the exocrine pancreas into the small intestine is the most physiologic approach for drainage of exocrine secretions. The whole pancreas, together with a segment of donor duodenum, is transplanted with a side-to-side anastomosis to the recipient's small bowel (Fig. 16.4). It has become the most popular of the drainage options, with almost all SPK operations and most PAK transplantations and PA performed by this method. Some centers still prefer bladder drainage in PAK transplantation and PA because of the higher rates of pancreatic allograft rejection in these two groups and the option that bladder drainage provides monitor serial urine amylase in the evaluation of rejection: this method of monitoring is lost with enteric drainage.

Bladder drainage of highly alkaline pancreatic secretions with high concentration of amylase can result in fluid and electrolyte abnormalities (volume contraction and metabolic acidosis) and urologic abnormalities (cystitis, urethritis, balanitis, and reflux pancreatitis) that can have a major impact on postoperative morbidity and quality of life. It is largely for these reasons that the bladder drainage technique has been replaced by enteric drainage. The major danger associated with enteric drainage is the risk for development of a duodenoenteric leak, typically occurring in the early postoperative period, which may lead to graft

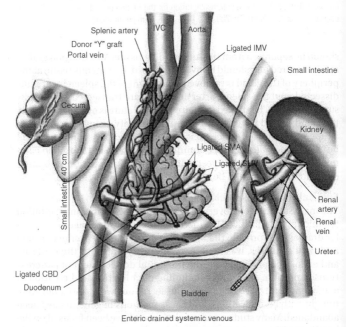

Enteric drained systemic venous

FIGURE 16.4 Systemic venous and enteric-drained pancreatic allograft with kidney on the left. (From Lipshutz GS, Wilkinson AH. Pancreas–kidney and pancreas transplantation for the treatment of diabetes mellitus. Endocrinol Metab Clin North Am 2007;36:1015–1038, with permission.)

loss and intra-abdominal sepsis. The danger of a duodenal leak may be somewhat less when the anastomosis is to the bladder, and the leak can sometimes be managed conservatively by bladder catheterization.

Few centers now choose bladder drainage as their primary method of exocrine drainage. When they do, pancreatic allografts are typically transplanted with a side-to-side pancreatic duodenocystostomy (Fig. 16.4). A disadvantage of senteric drainage of exocrine secretions is the inability to monitor urinary amylase as a means of detecting pancreatic allograft rejection. With current immunosuppressive protocols, however, this disadvantage is a minor one.

Systemic versus Portal Drainage

Most pancreatic allografts are transplanted heterotopically like kidneys in the pelvis using the iliac vasculature (Figs. 16.4 and 16.5). Advantages of this approach include lower rates of allograft thrombosis, easier access to percutaneous biopsy, and the ability to use either the bladder or intestine for drainage of exocrine secretions. With systemic venous drainage, basal and stimulated peripheral serum insulin levels are 2 to 3 times higher than normal because insulin does not undergo first-pass hepatic effect. Patients may be susceptible to peripheral hyperinsulinemia with portal hypoinsulinemia and postprandial hypoglycemia, and some report that the high ambient insulin levels, insulin resistance,

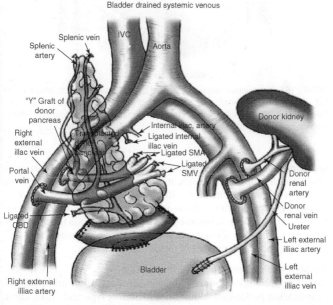

FIGURE 16.5 Systemic venous and bladder-drained pancreatic allograft with kidney on the left. (From Lipshutz GS, Wilkinson AH. Pancreas–kidney and pancreas transplantation for the treatment of diabetes mellitus. Endocrinol Metab Clin North Am 2007;36:1015–1038, with permission.)

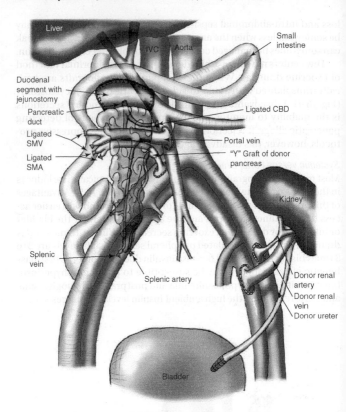

Enteric drained portal venous

FIGURE 16.6 Portal venous and enteric-drained pancreatic allograft with kidney on the left. SMA, superior mesenteric artery; SMV, superior mesenteric vein. (From Lipshutz GS, Wilkinson AH. Pancreas–kidney and pancreas transplantation for the treatment of diabetes mellitus. Endocrinol Metab Clin North Am 2007;36:1015–1038, with permission.)

and abnormal lipoprotein metabolism may accelerate the progression of atherosclerotic CVD in recipients. Portal venous drainage (Fig. 16.6) results in normal insulin levels with improvements in lipoprotein metabolism compared with systemic venous drainage. However, there are higher rates of allograft thrombosis, and percutaneous biopsy, when necessary, is more challenging. In addition, enteric drainage is required owing to cephalic placement of the donor duodenum.

Preoperative and Intraoperative Preparation

After the patient is admitted and a thorough history and physical examination performed, blood draw including type and cross, chest radiography, and an electrocardiogram should be performed. Some centers perform a bowel prep or series of enemas to clear the colon of formed stool. Leukocyte-reduced packed red blood cells should be prepared for the patient. Some centers administer a preoperative dose of aspirin (if the patient is not already receiving it) and an oral antifungal agent. Intraoperative immunosuppression should be ordered and prepared.

While awaiting the transplantation, half the normal dose of insulin should be administered, and serum glucose levels should not exceed 250 mg/dL because of concern for the development of acidemia intraoperatively, leading to intraoperative management difficulties. Preoperatively, blood glucose levels should be monitored every 4 hours and a sliding scale used for dosing regular insulin. Long-acting forms of insulin are avoided, allowing the surgeon to assess pancreatic allograft function in the operating room. Patients should undergo dialysis if there is significant evidence of volume overload or hyperkalemia.

Intraoperatively, patients generally have a nasogastric tube placed, and both arterial access and central venous access are obtained. Some centers have abandoned the routine use of nasogastric tubes. Poor gastrointestinal function may compromise absorption of immunosuppressive therapies, and many centers use intravenous induction agents, lessening the need for early gastrointestinal function to absorb oral immunosuppressants (see "Immunosuppression" below). Slow resumption of bowel function may follow transplantation, and, occasionally, prolonged nasogastric suctioning may be required in cases of a persistent ileus. A broad-spectrum antibiotic is administered (e.g., piperacillin/tazobactam) before skin incision.

Postoperative Complications

Unlike solitary kidney transplantation, in which the allograft is typically placed in a retroperitoneal location, pancreatic allograft placement is intra-abdominal. Because of the length of the operative intervention and the manipulation of the small intestine and anastomosis (whether bladder or enteric drained), an ileus should be expected in the immediate postoperative period. Although studies have shown no significant difference in major postoperative complications in diabetic versus nondiabetic patients, especially with regard to wound complications, postoperative ileus, nausea, and vomiting are common after pancreas transplantation. Because of the use of high-dose corticosteroids with induction agents at some centers, the need for frequent blood sugar monitoring is essential. Some centers use an insulin infusion in the immediate postoperative period. Others do not because following the serum or whole-blood glucose is important in assessing complications that may occur in the early postoperative period, particularly the possibility of allograft thrombosis.

Anastomotic Leak

Duodenal segment leaks in the bladder-drained pancreas recipient most often occur in the first 3 months after transplantation and usually present with the acute onset of abdominal pain and elevation of serum amylase. Diagnosis can be made by performing a cystogram or by nuclear medicine imaging. Treatment is nonoperative in as many as two-thirds of patients, usually requiring prolonged Foley urethral drainage. Resistant cases may require exploration and closure of leakage site or enteric conversion.

The development of an anastomotic leak is the most serious complication of an enteric-drained whole pancreas transplant. Leaks from enteric-drained pancreas transplants are suggested by the sudden onset of severe abdominal pain, rising serum amylase and creatinine levels, and fever. Early duodenal segment leaks tend to result from technical complications or as a result of ischemia. Late duodenal leaks tend to be due to rejection, infection, or ischemia of the duodenal staple line. Leaks do not result in alteration of endocrine function. However, patients present with elevated white blood cell counts, graft tenderness, and fever and generally lead to a pancreaticocutaneous fistula or peripancreatic abscess. These are particularly serious because of the spillage of succus entericus within the abdomen. Computed tomography and percutaneous drainage usually demonstrate a mixed infection of bacteria and often fungus. Broad-spectrum antibiotics are essential, and surgical exploration should be performed without delay. At laparotomy, a decision regarding the extent of the infection, its potential for clearance, and need for removal of the pancreatic allograft must be made. Treatment of the infection, if inadequate, will lead to organ failure, sepsis, and often death of the recipient. Some have converted the allograft to a Roux-en-Y limb when there has been evidence of an anastomotic leak; however, this has not always been successful in salvaging the allograft.

Graft Pancreatitis
Pancreatitis of the allograft is a common postoperative complication and can occur in a variety of settings. It is usually self-limited and resolves early in the patient's postoperative course. Pancreatitis typically occurs as a result of cold ischemic storage and reperfusion injury or from handling during organ recovery. It usually induces a mild hyperamylasemia without significant clinical consequence, is self-limited, and resolves with conservative therapy. In more severe cases, significant ischemia-reperfusion injury can be the cause and can lead to allograft thrombosis, likely because of the effect on the vasculature. Doppler ultrasound studies are essential in evaluating graft dysfunction, and an examination of the arterial waveforms will often demonstrate high-resistive indices with sharp arterial peaks and poor runoff ("water-hammer" pulsations) (Fig. 16.7). Such poor runoff should raise concern of impending allograft thrombosis. In addition to heparinization, octreotide may be effective.

For bladder-drained pancreas transplants, reflux pancreatitis of urine has been described. It is most common in patients with distended neurogenic bladders. It is managed by encouraging more frequent urination, catheter drainage, or self-catheterization to avoid high urinary residuals. α_1-adrenergic receptor blocking agents such as terazosin may be useful in some. Patients with persistent reflux pancreatitis should undergo enteric conversion.

Thrombosis
Graft thrombosis is well recognized and the most common early cause of loss of a pancreatic allograft. It is a devastating complication that can occur in as many as 10% to 20% of pancreatic transplant recipients. It is more common in pancreas as compared to kidney transplantation,

A

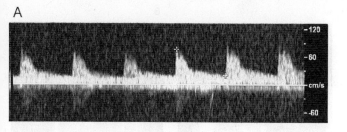

B

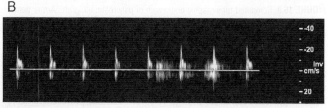

FIGURE 16.7 **A:** Normal arterial waveform with low-resistive index and good runoff in the splenic artery of a pancreatic allograft. **B:** "Water-hammer" pulses are demonstrated in this Doppler waveform indicating a high-resistive index and poor runoff. Note the relative absence of diastolic flow.

in part because the pancreas is a relatively low–blood-flow organ. Most graft thromboses occur in the first week after transplantation. Both donor and recipient factors increase the risk for thrombosis. Recipient factors are the ones that decrease blood flow to the allograft and include pancreatitis, hypotension, acute rejection, and reperfusion injury. Donor factors include older age (>45 years), longer cold ischemia times, and donor death due to a cerebrovascular event.

Thrombosis of a pancreatic allograft may occur in either the arterial or the venous system. Arterial thrombosis may occur in the splenic artery or superior mesenteric artery; it sometimes occurs in both. Arterial thrombosis of the superior mesenteric artery leads to nonviability of the duodenal segment. On exploration, the pancreas appears soft and pale. In general, early on the patient feels no abdominal pain, and there is typically an acute rise in serum glucose with a fall in serum amylase. Even in the face of a patent splenic artery, surgical removal is generally the most appropriate measure because loss of the superior mesenteric arterial blood supply will leave the duodenal segment compromised. In some cases, the most distal end of the superior mesenteric artery or splenic artery may thrombose because these vessels become end arteries and have no outflow at the distal end. Although thrombosis at these locations initially may result in a transient hyperamylasemia, if imaging demonstrates good perfusion of the allograft, these distal thromboses will likely be of no long-term consequence (Fig. 16.8). However, long-term antiplatelet agents would be recommended.

Venous thrombosis usually presents with graft swelling, resulting in symptoms of abdominal pain. Serologically, patients demonstrate

A

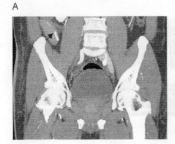

B

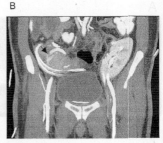

FIGURE 16.8 Computed tomographic angiogram of pancreatic allograft. *Arrow* demonstrates thrombosis of distal splenic artery **(A)** and distal SMA superior mesenteric artery of the allograft **(B)**. Note that the gland is well perfused because of collateral blood flow.

a rise in glucose and amylase. On abdominal exploration, the graft often appears enlarged, dark blue, and engorged. Doppler ultrasound examination is routinely used to examine vascular flow. In the case of venous thrombosis, there is high resistance in the pancreatic arteries with no flow in the pancreatic veins. Pancreatectomy is required.

Prevention and postoperative vigilance are the main measures for addressing the risk for allograft thrombosis. Anticoagulation and antiplatelet drugs are the main measure to prevent graft thrombosis; however, with this, the risk for postoperative bleeding increases. Doppler ultrasound imaging (alternatively computed tomography [CT] angiography or magnetic resonance angiography) should be employed for any indication of early graft dysfunction.

Gastrointestinal Bleeding
Early gastrointestinal bleeding may occur in either the bladder-drained or enteric-drained pancreas transplant recipient. This is typically due to bleeding from the suture line of the duodenal–ileal anastomosis or the duodenal–bladder anastomosis. Causes include ischemia-reperfusion injury of the duodenal mucosa or a bleeding vessel at the suture line of the anastomosis. When heparin or antiplatelet agents are used to decrease the risk for allograft thrombosis postoperatively, bleeding can be evident by a fall in either the hematocrit or the development of melanotic stool. In addition, in uremic patients who have a delay in kidney allograft function, platelet dysfunction may become evident, and bleeding can occur. In both cases, bleeding tends to stop with cessation of anticoagulation, or transfusion of packed red blood cells and platelets in the case of uremia and delayed kidney function. Bleeding in enteric-drained patients usually resolves with such therapy. However, in bladder-drained patients, bladder irrigation may be necessary, and cystoscopy may be required to remove larger clots. Occasionally, open cystotomy may be necessary with fulguration or ligation of a bleeding vessel.

Abscess and Infection
Intra-abdominal infections are much more common after pancreas transplantation than after kidney transplantation and represent a significant cause of mortality if not adequately treated. Peripancreatic

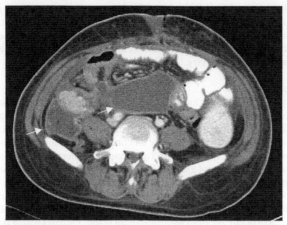

FIGURE 16.9 Computed tomography demonstrates peripancreatic fluid collections.

fluid collections can become infected, and conservative therapy with percutaneous drains and intravenous antibiotics is often adequate (Fig. 16.9). However, persistence or lack of resolution will require consideration of operative exploration and drainage. Pancreatectomy must be considered in these situations. A dangerous and often late complication in patients with peripancreatic abscesses is the development of a mycotic aneurysm and serious and life-threatening bleeding.

Neurogenic Bladder and Urinary Tract Infections

Neurogenic bladder is a frequent complicating factor after transplantation. Urinary tract infections are also more common in diabetic recipients because of the higher incidence of a neurogenic bladder. Chronic intermittent self-catheterization may be necessary in some patients to completely evacuate the bladder. This can be challenging in some owing to vision loss. Prophylaxis with daily trimethoprim-sulfamethoxazole or ciprofloxacin is recommended.

Orthostatic Hypotension

Orthostatic hypotension with supine hypertension is a common result of autonomic neuropathy and may be transiently exacerbated after successful transplantation, particularly if the patient was in a fluid-positive state before transplantation. This condition can be challenging to treat on an outpatient basis. Initial treatment is to recommend increased salt intake in the diet; salty soups and bullion are recommended. If ineffective, patients should be prescribed sodium bicarbonate, up to 1,300 mg taken orally 4 times daily, and fludrocortisone acetate (Florinef), 0.1 to 0.2 mg daily, should be added. Most patients respond to this form of therapy, and over time (typically many months later), fludrocortisone can be weaned and discontinued, and sodium bicarbonate doses can be decreased. If this is ineffective, midodrine (an α-adrenoreceptor agonist), up to 10 mg taken orally 3 times a day, can be added. In some, this may be poorly tolerated because supine hypertension often occurs, resulting in severe headaches. Clonidine can improve orthostatic hypotension, probably by a peripheral venoconstriction effect. Orthostatic hypotension typically resolves as the hematocrit rises; this process can be expedited with erythropoietin injections or packed red blood transfusions, if necessary.

Allograft Rejection

Persistently elevated glucose is a poor sign and a late finding in allograft rejection. It usually implies that the rejection has been ongoing for some time. The diagnosis of pancreas allograft rejection can be difficult to make and can only be confirmed with a percutaneous biopsy. Pancreatic allograft rejection is generally heralded by a rise in the serum amylase, not glucose. In effect, the exocrine pancreas and a rise in serum enzymes are used as a surrogate to diagnose rejection. The islets, in the initial phases of rejection, are spared, and serum glucose remains normal. Only later, when inflammation and destruction of the islets have occurred, does hyperglycemia result. Patients will at times report an acute rise in home monitoring of whole-blood glucose after long periods of not checking their glucose. However, it is likely that allograft rejection began a significant amount of time earlier and that only at that time, when the glucose was checked, was hyperglycemia detected. At this stage, rejection is usually irreversible. Rejection must be recognized early, before the development of hyperglycemia, to prevent complete destruction of islets.

In SPK transplantation, the kidney allograft often shows clinical signs of rejection first before the pancreatic allograft. This is heralded by an acute rise in the serum creatinine such that a kidney biopsy is prompted. Although it is possible to have pancreatic rejection without kidney allograft rejection when recipients have received organs simultaneously and from the same donor, it is uncommon, probably occurring in less than 5% of cases. Thus, when possible, a kidney biopsy should be employed first to determine the cause of graft dysfunction to prevent unnecessary immunosuppression in these patients. A percutaneous kidney biopsy is generally considered a safer procedure for patients because of the intra-abdominal location of the pancreatic allograft and the greater risk for postprocedure hemorrhage. If this is not diagnostic or does not show rejection in the face of elevated pancreatic exocrine enzymes, a pancreatic allograft biopsy should be performed. This is generally performed under ultrasound or computed tomographic guidance. If possible, any antiplatelet agents should be discontinued before biopsy.

The diagnosis of rejection in PAK and PTA transplantation is much more challenging. A rise in serum amylase or lipase could indicate rejection or another nonspecific process. Urine collection for amylase and examination for urinary eosinophils are useful in bladder-drained pancreata. This requires that urinary amylase was followed at routine outpatient visits. However, in these cases, diagnosis also requires a percutaneous biopsy or a transcystoscopic biopsy of the head of the pancreas. Such difficulty in diagnosis in these groups may in part explain their overall worse graft survival compared with SPK recipients and why some centers continue to use bladder drainage in both PAK and PTA patients.

Treatment of pancreatic allograft rejection generally requires antibody therapy (typically, antithymocyte globulin, see Chapter 6), which should, ideally, not be given unless rejection is biopsy proved. A high-dose steroid pulse (5 mg/kg), while often causing an initial decline in serum amylase and lipase, may be followed by rebound rejection because this therapy alone is not effective or long lasting.

IMMUNOSUPPRESSION

Immunosuppressive therapy for whole-organ pancreas transplantation with SPK is not markedly different than that for kidney transplantation alone (see Chapter 6). One-year rates of rejection have steadily decreased and are currently in the 10% to 20% range depending on the type of transplantation and immunosuppressive regimen. Nearly all recipients receive some form of antibody induction, with most receiving maintenance therapy with a tacrolimus–mycophenolate mofetil–low-dose steroid combination. Of the CNIs, tacrolimus is more frequently used than cyclosporine despite the fact that tacrolimus is the more islet-toxic of the two drugs. The preference for tacrolimus is likely because of the undocumented impression that it is more effective and "stronger."

Because of the frequency of acute rejection episodes in SPK transplantation, there is a tendency by most centers to be more aggressive with chronic immunosuppression protocols employed typically as triple immunosuppression postoperatively. Although the combination of tacrolimus, mycophenolate mofetil, and low-dose prednisone is the most common post-transplantation regimen, some centers have developed protocols with steroid withdrawal or are steroid free. Some centers have employed sirolimus in their maintenance regimen. Limited data with a tacrolimus–sirolimus combination have shown excellent short-term outcomes, but attempts to date, except in a few selected cases, of CNI avoidance or minimization have been less successful, overall. In general, maintenance of higher levels of CNI in pancreas transplant recipients is recommended compared with kidney-alone patients.

PAK and PTA recipients are at higher risk for allograft rejection than SPK recipients. This is likely in part explained by not having an HLA-matched kidney present that can be evaluated to help determine the status of the pancreatic allograft. Typical regimens in these patients are based on triple immunosuppression. Some studies with steroid withdrawal and the use of sirolimus in these patients have suggested inferior results.

OUTCOME OF PANCREAS TRANSPLANTATION

There are significant complexities in comparing survival probabilities between diabetic ESKD patients who undergo different renal replacement therapies. Caution is advised in comparing transplant and dialysis groups because they are not strictly comparable; those with the least severe manifestations of diabetes are more likely selected for transplantation of the pancreas, whereas those with morbid manifestations and severe secondary complications are often declined. This is reflected in multiple studies regarding the benefit or detriment of pancreas and renal transplantation versus renal transplantation alone in this patient population. Although both primary and repeat kidney transplantations have been shown to provide greater survival benefit in diabetic patients compared with nondiabetic patients, there have been conflicting reports regarding whether SPK provides additional survival benefit over renal transplantation alone.

Data from the US Scientific Renal Transplant Registry (SRTR) supplemented with data from the US Renal Data System (USRDS) indicate that SPK recipients can be expected to live 15 years longer than type 1 diabetics who were not transplanted and remain on the wait-list. In addition, recipients of an SPK can expect to live 10 years longer than if they were a type 1 diabetic recipient of a deceased donor kidney alone. Overall, the projected extra lifetime gained for all SPK recipients is 23 years; those in the cohort of 18 to 29 years of age are projected to gain as many as 49 years, whereas those of 40 to 49 years of age are expected to gain 19 years. The overall adjusted mortality rates for SPK, living kidney recipients, and deceased donor recipients were 40, 41, and 59 deaths, respectively, per 1,000 patient-years. The results of this analysis suggest that there is a survival advantage with pancreas transplantation for all demographic subgroups except those 50 years or older at the time of transplantation.

With this increased survival, however, there is the additional risk for excess early morbidity and mortality, primarily related to the procedure itself and the risk of complications. SPK recipients were estimated to have a 2-fold increased risk for death after transplantation. In addition, their overall risk for mortality was higher. When compared with wait-list type 1 diabetic patients receiving dialysis, it takes about 100 days for SPK recipients to reach the same relative mortality risk (mortality risk immediately after transplantation is >1.3). This is nearly twice as long as recipients of deceased donor kidneys only (43 days) and 7 times as long as those receiving a living donor kidney (15 days). However, despite this early elevated mortality risk with SPK transplants, with the selection criteria in use today and the current post-transplantation management, diabetic recipients can expect improved longevity with transplantation.

Registry data on the survival of pancreas transplants are less reliable than data on kidney survival. Kidney failure can be clearly defined as a return to dialysis, whereas pancreas failure does not have such a clear endpoint. Intuitively, pancreas failure could be defined as the return of the need to use insulin, since it is the need to use insulin that is the most potent indication for the procedure. In many reports, pancreas failure is self-reported and could represent a variety of "soft" endpoints. In the United States, a definition of pancreas allograft failure has been approved based on a set of criteria including a recipient's average insulin use per kilogram per day: the definition has not yet been implemented, but when it is, a more consistent and accurate of pancreas allograft survival should be available.

In SPK, kidney and pancreas failure often occurs in parallel because of similar pathogenic processes in both organs. If the kidney fails first and the patient returns to dialysis still insulin free, immunosuppression needs to be maintained to keep the pancreas functioning. In these circumstances, pancreatic function often deteriorates; the best way to maintain its function is to transplant another kidney at the earliest.

EFFECT OF PANCREAS TRANSPLANTATION ON DIABETIC COMPLICATIONS

The goal of kidney and pancreas transplantation in diabetic recipients is to restore renal function, normalize carbohydrate metabolism, and establish a state of normoglycemia while improving quality of life for the recipient. Successful transplantation is not only life-enhancing but also lifesaving. It frees patients from exogenous insulin and dietary restrictions and the emotional burden that these carry. In successful pancreas transplantation, quality-of-life improvements include a greater satisfaction with life, a feeling of control and independence, and improved perceptions of both physical and mental health. Although the value of making patients insulin independent is clear, the effectiveness of arresting or reversing secondary complications of chronic diabetes mellitus.

Nephropathy

Studies have demonstrated that renal allografts transplanted into diabetic recipients may demonstrate signs of diabetic nephropathy as early as 2 years after transplantation. The thickness of the glomerular basement membrane has been compared between diabetic recipients of an SPK and diabetic recipients of only a kidney transplant and found to be within the normal range in SPK recipients, whereas it was increased in most diabetic kidney-alone recipients. Although these investigations have limitations, these studies suggest that when patients have prolonged normoglycemia, the recurrence of diabetic glomerulopathy is prevented.

Other studies in PTA patients demonstrate no amelioration of established diabetic nephropathy lesions 5 years after pancreas transplantation; but after 10 years there was reversal of diabetic glomerulopathy in patients with functioning pancreatic allografts. Glomerular and tubular basement membrane width, which was unchanged after 5 years, decreased after 10 years, falling into the normal range for some. Kimmelstiel–Wilson nodular lesions disappeared, and glomerular capillaries previously compressed by mesangial expansion were noted to have reopened in some patients. To put this information in context, it is important to note that failure of a kidney-alone transplant in diabetics is typically *not* solely due to diabetic nephropathy, but due to the same pathogenic mechanism that impacts transplanted kidneys of nondiabetic patients.

In comparing the renal outcome of recipients of SPK and of isolated deceased donor kidney transplants, it must be recalled that the kidney quality of SPK donors tends to be better than that of kidney donors alone. It is this improved quality that is largely responsible for the improved renal outcome of SPK recipients. Patients often request a pancreas transplant in order to "protect" their kidney transplant. Although this is an intuitively logical request, it is important to remind patients that it remains the quality of the kidney, rather than the presence of a functioning pancreas, that is most likely to determine outcome.

Cardiovascular Disease

CVD is the most common cause of mortality in diabetics so that the impact of pancreas transplantation on CVD is an important outcome measure. Hyperlipidemia and other risk factors should be aggressively treated in diabetic transplant recipients, particularly in the presence of coronary artery disease. Improvement in glucose levels reduces risk for microvascular complications. However, there are few prospective studies with a large number of patients examining the relationship between the re-establishment of normoglycemia in long-term diabetic patients and a reduction in cardiovascular mortality.

In general, studies suggest a cardioprotective effect of normo-glycemia established after successful pancreas transplantation. A greater decrease in left ventricular mass and normalization of diastolic dysfunction has been shown in SPK recipients compared with those who underwent kidney transplantation alone. Progression of coronary artery disease, using mean segment diameter loss on coronary angiography, was slower in those with a functioning graft after SPK than in those with pancreatic graft failure. Carotid artery disease also appears to progress slower with SPK than with kidney transplant alone. Vascular disease events and mortality are likely to be less after pancreas transplantation.

Retinopathy

Many studies have examined the impact of pancreas transplantation on existing diabetic retinopathy: most have shown little impact. Recipients with severely impaired vision may note some improvement, although some patients with preexisting severe disease may progress to blindness. Longer duration studies in patients with less-advanced retinopathy and in those who have macular edema have suggested that there may be some improvement after successful pancreas transplantation. In some with preproliferative retinopathy, stability or regression after transplantation was detected, and macular edema improved. However, the improvement in macular edema and subsequent mild visual improvement may in fact be related to a return of normal fluid balance provided by the kidney allograft.

Neuropathy

Focal neuropathies and polyneuropathies are common complications of diabetes mellitus. They affect both the autonomic and somatic nervous systems. Polyneuropathy is disabling, is the most common neurologic complication of diabetes, and is a contributor to foot ulceration. As with other secondary complications of diabetes, extended observation periods may be necessary to recover from the pathologic abnormalities that developed over the previous 20 or more years since the onset of diabetes mellitus in these patients.

Prospective studies of patients with polyneuropathy demonstrate a general trend toward improvement in the motor and sensory nerve conduction studies at 1 year and in autonomic function at 5 years. Patients who had a PTA, SPK, or PAK transplant showed improvement throughout a 10-year follow-up period, demonstrating that the effect was not solely related to correction of uremia. Diabetic autonomic nervous system dysfunction is associated with excess mortality. Some data suggest that patients with moderate neuropathy, but not those with severe neuropathy, who retained a functioning pancreas transplant had longer survival than those whose pancreatic function was lost. Of those who died during the period of observation, the results of cardiovascular autonomic testing were correlated with mortality.

Quality of Life

Multiple studies have reported a better quality of life in successful SPK recipients than in diabetic patients who are recipients of a kidney alone. Patients indicate satisfaction with diet flexibility and health management after pancreas transplantation. They are relieved of the strict dietary restrictions and the emotional burden of frequent blood sugar monitoring and insulin therapy. A significantly higher proportion of recipients of a pancreas transplant are working compared with patients on the waiting list. However, social and diabetes-related worries may persist, partly because a large number of recipients have advanced diabetic end-organ damage such as retinopathy and neuropathy by the time they receive the pancreas transplant.

Despite these anticipated benefits, it is critical that patients have a realistic and educated understanding of the relative risks and benefits of the range of transplant and nontransplant options available to them. Patients and family members may tend to overestimate the benefits and underestimate the risks of the procedures they are facing. It is difficult to quantitate the sense of liberation felt by lifetime diabetic patients who no longer must self-inject insulin and monitor every morsel they eat. Permitting patients that hope, while educating them as to what is involved in achieving it, is at the core of successful pancreas transplantation.

CHOICE OF PROCEDURE

Patients and their physician advocates may be faced with a difficult dilemma when choosing between a kidney transplant alone and an SPK transplant. This dilemma is reflected in the ongoing discussions on this topic in the medical and transplantation literature. SPK transplantation is associated with increased early morbidity but may offer better long-term quality of life and the greater potential for stabilization or improvement of diabetic complications. Most centers recommend kidney transplantation alone when a live donor is available because this option offers the best long-term patient and graft survival: a PAK transplant may follow. Patients choosing between an SPK and a deceased donor kidney transplantation must be thoroughly informed regarding the comparative risks and benefits of the two procedures and, in particular, must have realistic expectations regarding the effect of pancreas transplantation on secondary complications. Patients should also be aware of the fact that, in most regions of the United States, the waiting time for an SPK transplant is less than that for a deceased donor kidney transplant alone, and that a prolonged period of dialysis may expose them to additional risk. Patients seeking an isolated pancreas transplant in the presence of normal or near-normal renal function (PTA or PAK) should be made aware that some data suggest a relative survival disadvantage of this procedure. This survival disadvantage is likely a reflection of the excellent survival of diabetic patients whose renal function is good. The rationale to proceed with an isolated pancreas transplant should be based on the judgment that quality of life will be improved and the survival disadvantage outweighed by avoiding the need for insulin.

TRANSPLANTATION OF PANCREATIC ISLETS

Transplantation of the islets of Langerhans is an appealing alternative to whole-organ pancreas transplantation, primarily because of the lowered risk for surgical complications. Recall that the pancreas is predominantly an exocrine gland and that clusters of endocrine cells, the islets, are scattered throughout the gland. These islets contain the glucose-responsive, insulin-secreting β cells. The autoimmune destruction of these β cells is the cause of type 1 diabetes mellitus. Replacement of the β-cell mass provides the freedom from insulin therapy enjoyed after successful pancreas transplantation, and the exocrine pancreas is unnecessary for insulin independence. Separation of the islets from the exocrine pancreas allows transplantation with minimally invasive techniques. More importantly, islet transplantation does not require vascular and allograft duodenal anastomoses, thus avoiding the major sources of surgical complications.

Until recently, success with islet transplantation has been poor compared with whole-organ pancreas transplantation. The so-called Edmonton protocol generated new optimism for the success of islet transplantation. Using a steroid-free immunosuppression protocol (based on sirolimus, tacrolimus, and daclizumab), insulin independence was achieved in a small group of type 1 diabetic patients, without renal failure, receiving islet transplants alone. The recipients selected for this trial suffered hypoglycemic unawareness or "metabolic instability." The investigators transplanted the islets immediately after isolation, using a radiologically guided, transhepatic portal venous infusion technique. Besides the steroid-free immunosuppression, the success of the Edmonton protocol clearly depended on transplantation of an adequate islet mass, and this often necessitated multiple transplants with islets isolated from two to four donors. Since the original publication of this protocol, several other programs have reported similar experiences, and up to 80% of patients have been reported to remain insulin independent after 2 years. The long-term follow-up from the Edmonton program has been somewhat disappointing. Of the original seven patients followed for up to 12 years, only one remained insulin independent, though the remainder showed evidence of continued islet function. With current protocols based on belatacept (see Chapter 6), it has been claimed that islet transplantation can produce outcomes similar to PA and represents a clinically viable option to achieve long-term insulin independence in selected patients with type 1 diabetes.

Current Status

The knowledge, expertise, and expenses required to isolate a large number of quality human islets for transplantation are substantial. The US Food and Drug Administration (FDA) deems isolated human islets for transplantation a biologic product and requires an approved Investigational New Drug Application and Institutional Review Board approval for investigators conducting clinical islet transplantation research. The FDA also requires that investigators isolating human islets for transplantation use current Good Manufacturing Processes (cGMPs), such as clean room facilities, careful record keeping, and quality controls. Islet transplantation thus remains an experimental technique and is yet to become part of the routine diabetes care. Patients with failed islet transplants may successfully undergo PA transplants.

Islet Isolation

Fundamental steps in the process of islet isolation are procurement of the donor pancreas, transportation to the isolation laboratory, enzymatic digestion of the glandular tissue, separation, and purification of the islets. In most laboratories, it may take one to four donor pancreata to yield enough islets for investigators to consider the mass adequate for a recipient. In the case of a patient who requires three transplants, for example, it may take as many as 12 donor pancreata to provide persistent insulin independence. The preferential allocation of pancreata from the best donors to whole-organ transplantation may explain the multiple organs required to provide adequate islets.

Improved transplant success of islets may result from postisolation culture of the islets for up to 72 hours before transplantation, and this may permit insulin independence with a single donor transplant. The culture period may improve success by providing the time to measure the viability of the islets, time that is not available with immediate transplants. It is not clear whether the culture actually decreases the number of isolations required per recipient. Careful recipient and donor selection may also be factors responsible for allowing single donor success.

Recipient Selection

Like other allografts, islet transplant recipients require immunosuppression to prevent rejection. Therefore, patients are selected for clinical trials based on the risks of immunosuppression compared with ongoing insulin therapy for diabetic control. As with whole-organ pancreas transplantation, more recipients who received islets before the Edmonton protocol received a renal transplant either before or simultaneously with the islet transplant. For these patients, there is a minimal additional risk for immunosuppression for the islet transplant beyond that required for the renal transplant. For this reason, investigators continue to enroll type 1 diabetic patients with renal failure in clinical trials of islet-after-kidney and simultaneous islet-kidney transplantation.

For islet transplantation alone in nonuremic patients, investigators look for severe or even life-threatening problems with blood glucose control to balance the risks of immunosuppression. Hypoglycemic unawareness is a readily documented indication. "Metabolic instability" is a less precise inclusion criterion for clinical trials, but a limited number of fully compliant patients working diligently with an attentive diabetologist clearly manifest this severe problem.

FUTURE DIRECTIONS IN THE SURGICAL TREATMENT OF DIABETES

The declining trend in the use of whole-organ pancreas transplants has been discussed above. For the near future, it is likely that islet transplantation will remain a procedure that is limited in its scope. Enthusiasm for its promotion has been dampened somewhat by the disappointing long-term results. Transplantation tolerance, eliminating the need for long-term immunosuppression, might allow patients to undergo islet transplantation earlier in the course of their disease, providing improved quality of life, and lowering the risk for long-term complications. Encapsulation of the islets within a device that bars the immune response, for example, by preventing recipient immune cells from contacting the islets, is an enticing means to achieve tolerance but has met with limited success to date. From the purely numerical point of view, transplantation of either whole pancreases or islets can never meet the needs of a massive diabetic population. Trials are about to begin on an artificial pancreas consisting of an insulin pump with tubing inserted under the skin, a blood sugar monitor with a wire sensor placed under the skin, and a smartphone loaded with software that determines how much insulin is required based on factors such as food intake, physical activity, stress, metabolism, and sleep. Success with such a technological advance has been long awaited and might well eventually replace the standard surgical options that have been the subject in this chapter.

Selected Readings

Gruessner R, Gruessner A. Pancreas after islet transplantation: a first report of the international pancreas transplant registry. Am J Transplant 2016;2:688–693.

Humar A, Ramcharan T, Kandaswamy R, et al. Technical failures after pancreas transplants: why grafts fail and the risk factors—a multivariate analysis. Transplantation 2004;78:1188–1192.

Kandaswamy R, Skeans M, Gustafson S, et al. OPTN/SRTR 2014 Annual Data Report: pancreas. Am J Transplant 2016;(16, suppl 2):47–68.

Khairoun M, de Koning EJ, van den Berg B, et al. Microvascular damage in type 1 diabetic patients is reversed in the first year after simultaneous pancreas–kidney transplantation. Am J Transplant 2013;13:172.

King E, Kucirca L, McAdams-Dimarco M. Early hospital readmission after simultaneous pancreas–kidney transplantation: patient and center-level factors. Am J Transplant 2016;16:541–549.

Markmann J. Isolated pancreatic islet transplantation: a coming of age. Am J Transplant 2016;16:381–382.

Markmann JF, Bartlett ST, Johnson P, et al. Executive summary of IPITA-TTS opinion leaders report on the future of beta-cell replacement. Transplantation 2016;100:e25–e31.

Nagai S, Powelson J, Taber T, et al. Allograft pancreatectomy: indications and outcomes. Am J Transplant 2015;9:2456–2464.

Neiderhaus S, Leverson G, Lorentzen D, et al. Acute cellular and antibody-mediated rejection of the pancreas allograft: incidence, risk factors and outcome. Am J Transplant 2013;11:2945–2955.

Perkovic V, Agarwal R, Fioretto P, et al. Management of patients with diabetes and CKD: conclusions form a "Kidney Disease Improving Global Outcomes" (KDIGO) controversies conference. Kidney Int 2016;90:1175–1183.

Shapiro AM, Ricordi C, Hering BJ, et al. International trial of the Edmonton protocol for islet transplantation. N Engl J Med 2006;355:1318–1330.

Stratta RJ, Gruessner AC, Odorico JS, et al. Pancreas transplantation: an alarming crisis in confidence. Am J Transplant 2016;16:2556–2562.

Thabit H, Tauschmann M, Allen J, et al. Home use of an artificial beta cell in type 1 diabetes. NEJM 2015;373:2229–2140.

Vendrame F, Hopfner Y, Diamantopoulos S, et al. Risk factors for type 1 diabetes recurrence in immunosuppressed recipients of simultaneous pancreas–kidney transplants. Am J Transplant 2016;16:235–245.

Young B, Gill J, Huang E, et al. Living donor kidney versus simultaneous pancreas-kidney transplant in type 1 diabetes: an analysis of the OPTN/UNOS database. Clin J Am Soc Nephrol 2009;4:845–852.

Kidney Transplantation in Children

Eileen Tsai Chambers, Meghan H. Pearl, and Robert B. Ettenger

Kidney transplantation is universally accepted as the therapy of choice for children with end-stage kidney disease (ESKD). Approximately two-thirds of pediatric patients with ESKD ultimately receive a kidney transplant. Successful transplantation in children and adolescents not only ameliorates uremic symptoms but also allows for significant improvement of delayed skeletal growth, sexual maturation, cognitive performance, and psychosocial functioning. The child with a well-functioning kidney transplant can enjoy a quality of life that cannot be achieved by any form of dialysis therapy.

Current success in pediatric renal transplantation is attributed to improvements in transplantation technology, immunosuppressive therapy, and the provision of age-appropriate clinical care. Transplantation continues to result in better survival than dialysis for pediatric patients of all ages. Five-year survival rates in transplant patients are close to 95%, whereas in dialyzed patients, the survival rates are about 80%. Nevertheless, success in pediatric kidney transplantation remains a challenging undertaking. Children and adolescents are constantly growing, developing, and changing. Each developmental stage produces a series of medical, biologic, and psychological challenges that must be appropriately addressed if truly successful graft outcome and rehabilitation are to be realized.

Much of the statistical data reviewed in this chapter comes from databases that have provided an invaluable resource for the advancement of pediatric transplantation. These databases have enabled the evaluation and extrapolation of data from multiple pediatric renal transplant programs that tend to be small when compared with their adult counterparts. Major databases referred to are the *North American Pediatric Renal Trials and Collaborative Studies* (NAPRTCS), the *Scientific Registry of Transplant Recipients* (SRTR), and the *United States Renal Data System* (USRDS) annual report and data available from the United Network for Organ Sharing (UNOS).

EPIDEMIOLOGY OF END-STAGE RENAL DISEASE IN CHILDREN

Incidence

The incidence and prevalence of treated pediatric ESKD have slowly been declining since 2008. The incident rate of ESKD in children up to 19 years of age peaked in 2003 and decreased to 14 per million U.S. children in 2012. The incidence of ESKD increases with age, with the highest incidence observed in children between 15 and 19 years of age (23 per million). Adolescents represent approximately 50% of treated pediatric ESKD patients.

There is a wide variation by ethnic group in the incidence rates of treated ESKD. The incidence rate for Whites is 16 per 1 million compared to 32 per 1 million in children of other ethnicities. African-American children comprise approximately half (15 per 1 million) of non-White ethnicities. During the past 20 years, incident rates for White pediatric patients have remained constant. For African-American patients and other non-White ethnicities, however, the rates of ESKD have more than doubled. Focal segmental glomerulosclerosis (FSGS) is more prevalent in African-American children (23%), while congenital/urologic abnormalities are more common in Whites and Hispanics (32%). Boys have higher incidence of treated ESKD than girls in all age groups.

Etiology

Congenital, hereditary, and cystic diseases account for about 50% and glomerular diseases for 20% of cases of pediatric ESKD (Table 17.1). Incidence rates for patients with glomerular diseases and patients with congenital, hereditary, and cystic diseases continue on an upward trend.

The most common primary diagnoses remain aplastic, hypoplastic, or dysplastic kidney and obstructive uropathy, each present in about 15% of patients. FSGS is the third most common (12%) and continues to be the most prevalent acquired renal disease. In contrast to adults, ESKD caused by diabetes mellitus or hypertension is rare in children.

Access to Transplantation

Between 1987 and 2017, approximately 12,000 children received over 13,000 transplants in the United States. At the time of transplantation, about half of pediatric recipients of kidney transplants are older than 12 years, 33% are 6 to 12 years of age, 16% are between the ages of 2 and 5 years, and 5% are younger than 1 year of age. About 60% are male, 55% are White, 17% are African American, and 17% are Hispanic.

Pediatric transplantations constitute 4% to 7% of all kidney transplantations in the United States. The number of pediatric kidney transplantations peaked at 899 in 2005 and has remained relatively constant at approximately 750 per year. During the same period, the total number of adult kidney transplantations has remained relatively stable while the number of candidates on the waiting list continues to rise (see Chapter 1, Fig. 1.1).

Efforts to Prioritize Children for Transplantation

Changes have been made to UNOS donor allocation policy over the years in the hope of improving their access to high-quality transplants and hence prevent death and morbidity. Prior to 2005, the majority of pediatric patients received living donor transplants, mainly from parents. In 2005, the allocation of deceased donor transplants was modified to give children priority for deceased donor kidneys from "high-quality" donors younger than 35 years. The number of these kidneys transplanted in children did, indeed, increase. The modification, however, had the unanticipated effect of reducing living donation so that the total number of transplants for children remained essentially stable and fewer deceased donor kidneys were available for adults!

The principle of advantaging children for high-quality deceased donor kidneys has remained in place in the new Kidney Allocation System

TABLE 17.1	Incidence of End-Stage Renal Disease in Pediatric Transplant Patients According to Primary Disease, 2014*	
Primary Renal Disease		**Incidence (%)**
Cystic, hereditary, and congenital disease		**47.1**
Renal hypoplasia, dysplasia		15.8
Congenital obstructive uropathy		15.3
Polycystic disease		3.0
Medullary cystic disease (nephronophthisis)		2.7
Prune belly syndrome		2.5
Congenital nephrotic syndrome		2.6
Drash syndrome		0.5
Alport syndrome, other familial disease		2.2
Cystinosis		2.0
Oxalosis		0.5
Glomerulonephritis (GN)		**20.7**
Focal segmental glomerulosclerosis		11.7
Chronic GN		3.1
Membranoproliferative GN type I		1.7
Idiopathic crescentic GN		1.7
IgA nephropathy		1.2
Membranoproliferative GN type II		0.8
Membranous nephropathy		0.5
Interstitial nephritis, pyelonephritis		**6.8**
Chronic pyelonephritis, Reflux nephropathy		5.1
Pyelonephritis/Interstitial nephritis		1.7
Secondary GN, vasculitis		**6**
Hemolytic uremic syndrome		2.6
Systemic lupus erythematosus		1.5
Henoch–Schönlein purpura		1.0
Wegener granulomatosis		0.6
Other systemic immunologic disease		0.3
Hypertension		**1.3**
Miscellaneous conditions		**0.7**
Neoplasms		0.5
Sickle cell nephropathy		0.1
Diabetes mellitus		0.1
Other		**10.9**
Uncertain etiology		**6.2**

*The study included 11,186 patients younger than 21 years.
Modified from the NAPRTCS 2014 annual report available at www.emmes.com/study/ped.

(KAS) which was implemented in December 2014 (see Chapter 5). In this system, pediatric patients have prioritized access to high-quality kidneys from donors with a kidney donor profile index (KDPI) of less than 35%. However, adult recipients who are highly sensitized with a calculated panel reactive antibody (cPRA) of greater than 99% or adults with multiorgan transplants take priority over pediatric recipients. In the early months after implementation of the KAS, the portion of transplants to pediatric recipients appeared to fall, but then rose toward pre-KAS level. Careful long-term monitoring will determine if children are in fact advantaged, in terms of morbidity and mortality, by these allocation changes.

Timing of Transplantation

Renal transplantation should be considered when renal replacement therapy is indicated. In children, dialysis may be required before transplantation to optimize nutritional and metabolic conditions, to achieve an appropriate size in small children, or to keep a patient stable until a suitable donor is available. Many centers prefer that a recipient weigh at least 10 kg, both to minimize the risk for vascular thrombosis and to accommodate an adult-sized kidney. In infants with ESKD, a target weight of 10 kg may not be achieved until 12 to 24 months of age. At some centers, transplantation has been successful in children who weighed less than 10 kg or who were younger than 6 months.

Preemptive transplantation (i.e., transplantation without prior dialysis) accounts for 25% of all pediatric renal transplantations. The major reason cited by patients and families for the decision to undertake preemptive transplantation is the desire to avoid dialysis. Candidates for preemptive transplantation should have careful psychological assessment before transplantation because there may be a greater tendency for noncompliance in children who have not experienced dialysis. Nevertheless, there appears to be no impairment in graft outcome in pediatric recipients who have undergone preemptive transplantation when compared with those who have undergone dialysis before transplantation, and data suggest improved patient and allograft outcome. The reasons for the improved patient and graft survival are unknown. Because of the waiting time for deceased donors, most preemptive kidney transplants are from living donors.

Patient and Graft Survival

Both patient and graft survival rates have improved steadily since systematic recording began in 1987. Patient survival after transplantation remains superior to that achieved by dialysis for all pediatric age groups. The overall 1- and 5-year patient survival rates are now 99% and 95%, respectively, for all primary transplants, and are comparable for recipients of living and deceased donors. Although patients younger than 2 years of age have lower survival rates, their outcome is steadily improving. Infection accounts for 28% of deaths. Other causes include cardiovascular disease (15%), malignancy (12%), and dialysis-related complications (3%). Nearly half of children who die do so with a functioning graft.

Graft survival rates for pediatric transplants are somewhat better than for adult transplants. The 1- and 5-year graft survival rates are 94% and 83%, respectively, for living donor recipients and 88% and 71%, respectively, for deceased donor recipients. Of the approximately 13,000 pediatric kidney transplantations performed since 1987, approximately 25%% have failed. Chronic rejection accounts for 41% of graft failures, with acute rejection accounting for 10%. Other causes include vascular thrombosis (7%), recurrence of original disease (8%), and patient nonadherence (6%). Chronic rejection remains the most common and ever-increasing cause of allograft failure. Although some causes of graft failure, such as recurrence of the original disease, have remained constant during the past 10 years, loss from acute rejection and graft thrombosis has decreased. Technical issues remain a challenge and are a more common cause of graft loss in children than in adults.

PROGNOSTIC FACTORS INFLUENCING GRAFT SURVIVAL

The following factors are important determinants of the improving graft survival reported in pediatric patients. Long-term renal function is a particularly important consideration in pediatric renal transplantation because of its impact on skeletal growth.

Donor Source

Short- and long-term graft and patient survival rates are better in recipients of living donor transplants in all pediatric age groups. Younger transplant recipients benefit the most from living donor transplantation and enjoy a 10% to 20% better graft survival rate 5 years after transplantation. Shorter cold ischemia time, better human leukocyte antigen (HLA) matches, lower acute rejection rates, and better preoperative preparation help to account for the improved outcome. Marked improvement has been made in deceased donor patient and graft survival related to improved immunosuppression, decreased transfusion requirements, and decreased use of young deceased donors.

Recipient Age

A trend for younger children, especially those younger than 2 years of age, to have lower graft survival rates than older children has been reversed. Some studies even suggest that adult kidneys transplanted into infants, with immediate graft function, may have the longest half-lives of any type of kidney transplant. Pediatric recipients younger than age 11 years who receive living donor transplants now have 5-year graft survival rates of approximately 85%, similar to those of recipients in older age groups. The results for deceased donor recipients are also better in this age group than in adults generally. Recipients 1 to 5 years of age have a 5-year graft survival rate of 75% and recipients 6 to 10 years of age have a 5-year graft survival rate of 73%.

On the other hand, the long-term graft survival rates in adolescents are not as good as those seen in younger children, even though the short-term outcome is similar. The 1- and 5-year graft survival rates for adolescent recipients of living donor kidneys are 94% and 79%, respectively. For deceased donor kidneys, the graft outcomes were 93% and 68%, respectively. Adolescents have the poorest 5-year results of any age group except for recipients 65 years and older. Higher rates of medication noncompliance, loss of medical insurance during transition to adulthood, and a high recurrence rate of FSGS, which is the most common acquired cause of ESKD in this age group, have all been cited as potential causes for the reduced long-term outcome.

Donor Age

For all deceased donor recipients, kidneys from donors 18 to 49 years of age provide optimal graft survival and function. This group is followed next by donors 2 to 17, less than 2, and then greater than 50 years of age.

Grafts from donors younger than 2 years fare more poorly, and grafts from donors older than 50 years fare most poorly. Although transplanted kidneys grow in size with the growth of the recipient, transplantation with deceased donor kidneys from donors younger than 6 years is associated with decreased graft survival. The 5-year graft survival rate for recipients of deceased donor kidneys from donors younger than 2 years of age is approximately 50%, compared with 68% for recipients of grafts from donors 2 to 17. Kidneys from donors 18 to 49 years of age have the best 5-year graft survival of about 73%. Children younger than 5 years receiving a kidney from a donor younger than 2 years have the highest relative risk for graft failure.

Ethnicity
African-American ethnicity is associated with a worse outcome. Five years after transplantation, African-American children have graft outcomes of 61% and 73% for recipients of deceased donor and living-related donor kidneys, respectively. For White and Hispanic recipients, graft survival rates at 5 years are 74% and 70%, respectively, for recipients of deceased donor kidneys, and 84% for living donor grafts. African-American children have not only poorer graft survival but also poorer renal function compared to other ethnic groups.

HLA Matching in Children
In pediatric transplantation, most living donor transplants come from parents. Long-term graft survival is best when the donor is a HLA-identical sibling. When considering transplants from HLA haplotype-identical sibling donors, some studies suggest that there is improved outcome when donor and recipient share "noninherited maternal antigens," as distinct from "noninherited paternal antigens" (see Chapter 3). Additionally, some studies suggest that sharing of HLA-DR and HLA-DQ antigens may decrease the risk of antibody-mediated rejection and may improve long-term allograft survival.

Presensitization
Repeated blood transfusions expose the recipient to a wide range of HLA antigens and may result in sensitization to these antigens, leading to higher rates of rejection and graft failures. The graft failure rate increases by 20% for recipients with more than five blood transfusions before transplantation compared with those who had fewer transfusions. Blood transfusions have become less common since erythropoiesis stimulating agents (ESAs) became an integral part of ESKD therapy. Hemoglobin levels in children on dialysis are lower than levels in their adult counterparts, and there is support for more aggressive management of anemia to forestall transfusions. Sensitization may also result from rejection and failure of a previous transplant, and the risk of graft failure increases by up to 50% for those patients.

Immunologic Factors
Immunologic parameters in younger children are different from those in adults and older children. Such differences include higher numbers of T and B cells, higher $CD4^+$-to-$CD8^+$ T-cell ratio, and increased blastogenic responses. These differences may account for the increased immune responsiveness to HLA antigens and may be partly responsible for the higher

rates of rejection that have been observed in children. With improved understanding and management of immunosuppression in pediatric patients, these higher rates of rejection have been significantly ameliorated.

Technical Factors and Delayed Graft Function

Surgical kidney transplant techniques used in older children are similar to those in adults (see Chapter 9). Placement of the vascular anastomoses depends on the size of the child and the vessels. An extraperitoneal approach is usually accomplished with the venous anastomoses to the common or external iliac vein and the arterial anastomoses to the common or external iliac artery. These vascular anastomoses tend to be more cephalad than for adult transplants.

Small children present difficult operative challenges. The relatively large size of the graft may result in longer anastomosis times, longer ischemia time, and subsequently higher rates of early graft dysfunction. When possible, the transplanted kidney is usually placed in an extraperitoneal location, although with very small children, the placement can be intra-abdominal. The aorta and inferior vena cava are usually used for anastomoses to ensure adequate blood flow, but smaller vessels may be used. Vascular anastomosis may be problematic in a child with a previous hemodialysis access placed in the lower extremities or with a previous kidney transplant. Children should be evaluated thoroughly before transplantation to identify any potential anastomotic difficulties. Unidentified vascular anomalies may lead to prolonged anastomosis times and subsequently higher rates of delayed graft function (DGF) and graft thrombosis.

Occasionally, native kidney nephrectomy is necessary at the time of transplantation. Although this can be done routinely in living donor transplantations in which there is little cold ischemia time, it is preferable to avoid this, when possible, in recipients of deceased donor transplants. Native nephrectomy at the time of transplantation prolongs the surgical procedure and may complicate fluid management and contribute to an increase in DGF.

DGF is discussed in detail in Chapter 10. It occurs in about 5% of living donor and 15% of deceased donor transplants and is associated with a reduced graft survival. In children with DGF, the 5-year graft survival rates are reduced by up to 25%. Risk factors for DGF in children are more than five prior blood transfusions, prior transplantation, prior dialysis, native nephrectomy, African-American ethnicity, donor age greater than 49 years old, and a cold ischemia time of longer than 24 hours.

Antibody Induction

Antibody induction, with either polyclonal or monoclonal antibodies, is used either for prophylaxis against rejection or in a sequential manner to avoid nephrotoxicity resulting from early use of calcineurin inhibitors (CNI) (see Chapter 6). The NAPRTCS database shows a nearly 20% reduction in the proportional hazard of graft loss with the use of antibody induction in living-related transplantation, but surprisingly no significant survival advantage for deceased donor transplantation. Nevertheless, the use of induction agents continues to increase year by year. Depleting antibodies (see Chapter 6) such as rabbit antithymocyte globulin are more commonly used over nondepleting antibodies for induction therapy in pediatric transplants in the United States (Fig. 17.1).

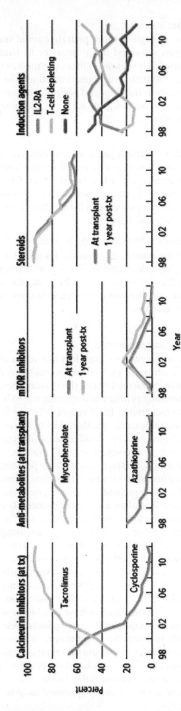

FIGURE 17.1 Immunosuppression use for induction and maintenance therapy in pediatric recipients with kidney transplants, 1998–2012. (Reprinted from Matas AJ, Smith JM, Skeans MA, et al. OPTN/SRTR 2012 Annual Data Report: kidney. Am J Transplant 2014;14 suppl 1:11–44, with permission from John Wiley & Sons, Inc.)

Transplantation Center Volume

Transplant outcome in high-volume pediatric renal transplantation centers has been reported to be superior to that found in lower-volume centers. High-volume centers (defined as the performance of more than 100 pediatric transplantations between 1995 and 2005) reported a lower incidence of graft thrombosis and DGF, improved long-term patient and graft survival, and more frequent use of antibody induction.

Cohort Year

The results of pediatric renal transplantation have been steadily improving such that 1-year and 5-year graft survival results have improved by up to 15% improvement in the last two decades. Graft outcome in transplants from deceased donors performed between 2005 and 2013 is equivalent to the graft survival in living donor transplantation performed between 1996 and 2004.

Recurrent Renal Disease in Pediatric Transplantation

Recurrent disease in the renal graft accounts for graft loss in almost 7% of primary transplantations and 10% of repeat transplantations. This is more than double that reported for adult transplantation. Both glomerular and metabolic diseases can recur, with most recurrences caused by glomerular disease.

Glomerular Diseases

Focal and Segmental Glomerulosclerosis

FSGS is the most common cause of graft loss as a result of recurrent disease. For patients whose original disease was steroid-resistant nephrotic syndrome or confirmed FSGS, the disease recurs in up to 55% of patients undergoing primary transplantation. When the first transplant was lost to recurrence, FSGS recurs in 70% to 85% of those undergoing subsequent transplantation. About 15% to 30% of transplants in patients with the diagnosis of FSGS fail because of recurrence. The mean time to graft failure from recurrence is 17 months.

Recurrence is usually characterized by massive proteinuria, hypoalbuminemia, and nephrotic syndrome with edema or anasarca and hypercholesterolemia. It may present immediately or weeks to months after transplantation. DGF is often a feature of immediate recurrence. Predictors of recurrence include rapid progression to ESKD from the time of initial diagnosis (<3 years), poor response to therapy, younger age at diagnosis, non–African-American ethnicity, and the presence of mesangial proliferation in the native kidney biopsy. A protein permeability factor has been isolated from sera of patients with FSGS, and its concentration found to correlate with recurrence and severity of disease in the transplanted kidney. Candidate molecules associated with recurrent disease in humans include soluble urokinase-like plasminogen activator receptor (suPAR) and a panel of seven antibodies such as anti-CD40. In mice, the co-administration of suPAR and anti-CD40 provoked podocyte injury and proteinuria, suggesting that circulating factors may contribute to a multi-hit process in recurrent FSGS. The search for a defined permeability factor or factors has been a frustrating, and there are no clinically approved assays.

Early post-transplantation recognition of recurrent FSGS is important because plasmapheresis (which may lower the serum levels of presumed protein permeability factors) and high-dose CNI administration may lead to significant reduction in graft loss from recurrence. *In vitro* studies using rat glomeruli show that cyclosporine or tacrolimus, incubated with sera from FSGS patients, will inhibit the proteinuric effect of such sera. Thrice-daily cyclosporine administration may be used in doses that maintain high blood levels (see Chapter 6), and the dose is tapered slowly after achieving remission of the nephrotic syndrome and as cholesterol concentration decreases, or if significant toxicity develops. Some centers have used a high-dose continuous intravenous infusion of cyclosporine with similar improvement, or have used high-dose or thrice-daily administration of tacrolimus. Cyclophosphamide has also been reported to induce remission. Rituximab may prevent recurrence; however, results have been mixed, and its use is more successful in children than in adults. Ofatumumab, a humanized anti-CD20 antibody, has been shown to be useful in a small series of children with nephrotic syndrome refractory to rituximab. Angiotensin-converting enzyme (ACE) inhibitors and angiotensin receptor blockers (ARBs) are used as adjuncts to decrease proteinuria. Plasmapheresis is generally used with a frequency that matches disease severity and is occasionally required on a weekly basis for prolonged periods. Plasmapheresis, in combination with a high-dose calcineurin inhibitor, is reported to be superior to either when given alone. Moreover, LDL plasmapheresis using an absorptive column, which originally was used to treat familial hypercholestremia, has been shown to be effective in a small series of children with FSGS. Abatacept, a co-stimulatory inhibitor that targets B7-1 (CD80) in glomerular, or allogeneic mesenchymal stem cells, has been used in case reports. Although there is currently no consensus on the treatment regimen for FSGS, the protocol outlined in Table 17.2 represents a summation of the UCLA Pediatric Transplant Program

TABLE 17.2	Focal Segmental Glomerulosclerosis Protocol at the Mattel Children's Hospital at UCLA

- Identify the high-risk patient
- Living-related donation if possible (to allow pretreatment and to avoid acute tubular necrosis so that high-dose cyclosporine or tacrolimus can be used)
- All patients on angiotensin-converting enzyme inhibitors or angiotensin receptor blockers as tolerated
- Living donor graft recipients
  - Ten pretransplantation plasma exchanges (1.5 volumes with albumin; fresh-frozen plasma for patients who are coagulopathic)
  - Three post-transplantation plasma exchanges (may need to be extended)
  - Tacrolimus 2 or 3 times daily; aim for trough levels of 12 to 15 ng/mL
- Deceased donor graft recipients
  - Ten post-transplantation plasma exchanges
  - May need to extend the number of plasma exchanges
  - Cyclosporine 3 times daily; aim for trough levels of 200 to 500 ng/mL
- In refractory cases to the above regimen, Rituximab and/or Ofatumumab may be considered

experience. For deceased donor transplantation, recurrence is less in patients on high-dose cyclosporine and post-transplant plasmapheresis. For living-related transplantation, high-dose tacrolimus is effective when combined with more than five plasma exchanges.

Some studies suggest that living-related donor transplant recipients suffer from a higher rate of recurrence. The graft outcome in recipients of living donor grafts with FSGS recurrence is no better than the outcome observed in recipients of deceased donor grafts who have not experienced recurrence. These data have led some pediatric transplantation centers to reduce or discontinue the use of living-related donation for patients with FSGS. However, the controlled settings of living donor transplantation may allow certain benefits in the event that FSGS does recur. The lower incidence of DGF in living donation may permit augmentation of the CNI dose. In addition, the preplanning implicit in living donation permits preoperative and early postoperative plasmapheresis, an approach that may potentially prevent or decrease the severity of recurrent disease.

Alport Syndrome

Alport syndrome, or hereditary glomerulonephritis, is a progressive disease often associated with neurosensory hearing loss and ocular abnormalities such as anterior lenticonus and cataracts. The inheritance pattern can be X-linked, autosomal recessive, and autosomal dominant. The abnormality in almost all patients stems from mutations in the α_3, α_4, or α_5 helices of type IV collagen. In more than 85% of patients, Alport syndrome results from mutations in the *COL4A5* gene on the X chromosome.

Strictly speaking, Alport syndrome itself does not recur; however, antiglomerular basement membrane (anti-GBM) glomerulonephritis occurs in about 3% to 5% of patients after transplantation and can lead to graft loss. The antibodies causing the anti-GBM nephritis are usually directed against the α_5 chain of the noncollagenous portion of type IV collagen in the GBM, but antibodies against the α_3 chain have also been described. The risk appears to be greatest in patients with mutations of *COL4A5* that prevent synthesis of the α_5 chain.

Anti-GBM glomerulonephritis presents as rapidly progressive crescentic glomerulonephritis with linear deposits of immunoglobulin G (IgG) along the basement membrane and commonly leads to graft loss, with rates approaching 90%. It usually occurs within the first post-transplantation year. Asymptomatic cases with linear IgG deposits have also been reported. Treatment consists of plasmapheresis and cyclophosphamide or rituximab, but is of only limited benefit. Retransplantation is associated with a high recurrence rate.

Membranoproliferative Glomerulonephritis

Current classifications of membranoproliferative glomerulonephritis are based upon immunofluorescence staining in renal biopsies described as immunoglobulin mediated, complement mediated, or without immunoglobulin or complement (thrombotic microangiopathy). Cases with immunoglobulin (IgG) and C3 deposition are commonly activated by the classical complement pathway in the setting of Hepatitis B or C infection, autoimmune disease, monoclonal gammopathy, or unknown causes (idiopathic). The risk of post-transplant recurrence for immune-mediated MPGN is significantly reduced when the primary condition is successfully treated or in remission. Clinical manifestations include proteinuria and deterioration of renal function. Cases with C3 deposition are grouped as C3 glomerulopathy and are further subdivided into Dense Deposit Disease (DDD) or C3 glomerulonephritis (C3GN) according to electron microscopy findings. DDD has characteristic osmiophilic intramembranous and mesangial dense deposits while C3GN involves subendothelial and mesangial deposits. C3 glomerulopathy histologically recurs in over 70% of patients with graft loss in up to 50% of patients. The presence of crescents in the native kidney biopsy and persistent proteinuria may predict severe recurrence that often leads to graft loss. There is no proven treatment for recurrence of C3 glomerulopathy in children. Anecdotal case reports describe success with high-dose corticosteroids, mycophenolate mofetil (MMF), or plasma exchange. Eculizumab has been used in a small prospective cohort with partial success; however, long-term studies need to be performed. Cases with thrombotic microangiopathy (TMA) and no complement or immunoglobulin have been associated with hemolytic uremic syndrome, thrombotic thrombocytopenic purpura, antiphospholipid antibody syndrome, malignant hypertension, or radiation nephropathy.

IgA Nephropathy and Henoch-Schönlein Purpura

Recurrence of IgA nephropathy and Henoch–Schönlein purpura (HSP) after renal transplantation occurs with a frequency ranging from 20 to 60%. The immunosuppressive regimen may affect the recurrence rate with anti-thymocyte globulin associated with a decrease in recurrence frequency, whereas steroid withdrawal is associated with an increased risk. Most of the recurrences are asymptomatic, but graft loss may occur, often associated with crescent formation. In children, up to 10% of graft failures have been ascribed to recurrent IgA nephropathy or HSP. There is no effective immunosuppressive therapy for the treatment of recurrent IgA nephropathy. ACE inhibitors and ARBs can be used for reducing proteinuria and preserving renal function.

ESKD in both children and adults is often loosely ascribed to post-streptococcal glomerulonephritis though "post-strep" very rarely causes ESKD. Most of these cases are likely due to unrecognized IgA nephropathy which may become evident with the finding of IgA deposition on immunoflourescent staining of transplanted kidney biopsy specimens.

Hemolytic Uremic Syndrome

Hemolytic uremic syndrome (HUS) accounts for up to 3% of primary renal disease in children leading to ESKD. When considering transplantation in patients whose original cause of ESKD is HUS, care must be directed to the form of HUS the patient has suffered. Current classifications of HUS are evolving into HUS associated with coexisting disease or specific infection versus atypical HUS associated with a mutation in the alternative complement pathway. Coexisting conditions that are associated with HUS include: bone marrow transplantation, solid-organ transplantation, malignancy and/or cancer chemotherapy, autoimmune disorders (SLE, antiphospholipid syndrome, scleroderma, dermatomyositis), medications (calcineurin inhibitors, sirolimus, and anti-VEGF agents), cobalamin C deficiency, and malignant hypertension. Furthermore, specific infections associated with HUS include viral infections such as HIV, parvovirus, influenza A/H1N1, and cytomegalovirus (CMV) and bacterial infections such as Shiga toxin-producing *Escherichia coli* (STEC) and *Streptococcus pneumoniae*. Moreover, a defect in von Willebrand factor cleaving metalloproteinase (ADAMTS13) with either congenital deficiency or antibodies against ADAMTS13 must be ruled out.

Atypical HUS associated with abnormal complement dysregulation has the worst prognosis and in the pre–anti-C5 blockade (Eculizumab) era resulted in 60% disease recurrence and more than 70% graft failure. Patients have genetic defects in factor H, factor I, membrane cofactor protein (MCP), factor B, C3, diacylglycerol kinase ε (DGKE), and thrombomodulin. Pretransplantation genotyping for these mutations is recommended. The risk of post-transplant recurrence is highest for Factor H, Factor B, Factor I and C3 mutations and lowest for MCP, thrombomodulin, and DGKE mutations. The use of CNIs does not appear to trigger HUS recurrence, and their avoidance does not appear to prevent recurrence.

In randomized controlled trials, Eculizumab has successfully been used to treat post-transplant recurrence by decreasing the damage associated with anaphylatoxin C5a and preventing formation of membrane attack complex on cell surfaces. Eculizumab prophylaxis prevents post-transplant recurrence in those patients with the highest risk based on complement mutations. Additionally, prevention of meningococcal infection with vaccination and antibiotic prophylaxis is essential in Eculizumab-treated patients. An acquired factor H deficiency as a result of anti-factor H autoantibodies has been found in some children. Plasma exchange can be used to remove anti-factor H antibodies and immunosuppression with steroids and rituximab used to suppress further antibody production. Combined liver and kidney transplantation is curative for atypical HUS associated with Factor H, C3, and Factor B mutations, which are factors synthesized in the liver, and may be considered under certain circumstances. Living donor transplantation is not advocated for patients with atypical HUS because of the high recurrence rates. In addition, it has been noted that some parental carriers of atypical HUS might not manifest the disease until later in life, and organ donation would put such carriers at excessive risk.

Antiglomerular Basement Membrane Disease
Anti-GBM disease is rare in children. A high level of circulating anti-GBM antibody before transplantation is thought to be associated with higher rate of recurrence. Therefore, a waiting period of 6 to 12 months with an undetectable titer of anti-GBM antibody is recommended before transplantation to prevent recurrence. Reappearance of anti-GBM antibody in the serum may be associated with histologic recurrence. Histologic recurrence has been reported in up to half of cases, with

clinical manifestations of nephritis in only 25% of these cases. Treatment for recurrence includes plasma exchange, cyclophosphamide, and corticosteroids. In refractory cases, Rituximab has been utilized as rescue therapy. Graft loss is rare, and spontaneous resolution may occur.

Congenital Nephrotic Syndrome

Congenital nephrotic syndrome occurs in the first 3 months of life. It can be classified by mutations in the nephrin gene (*NPHS1*), podocin gene (*NPHS2*), or Wilms tumor suppressor gene (*WT1*). Congenital nephrotic syndrome of the Finnish type (CNSF) is an autosomal recessive disease that occurs as a result of a mutation in the *NPHS1* gene. Although it is most commonly seen in Finnish patients, it is also found in other countries. The *NPHS1* gene is located on chromosome 19 and has as its gene product the protein *nephrin*. Nephrin is a transmembrane protein, which is a member of the immunoglobulin family of cell adhesion molecules. It is characteristically located at the slit diaphragms of the glomerular epithelial foot processes. Over 200 mutations of *NPHS1* have been identified in CNSF, but more than 90% of all Finnish patients have one of two mutations—the so-called Fin major and Fin minor mutations.

Infants with CNSF are usually born prematurely and exhibit low birth weight and placentomegaly. CNSF manifests as heavy proteinuria, edema, and ascites, often in the first week of life and always by 3 months of age. Renal histology is nonspecific and shows expansion of glomerular mesangium and dilations in the proximal and distal tubules. Untreated, these children suffer from malnutrition, poor growth, frequent infections, and thromboembolic complications. ESKD occurs invariably by mid-childhood. Corticosteroids do not ameliorate CNSF, but in mild forms, ACE inhibition, together with indomethacin, may be successful. The best therapeutic success has come from the approach of early dialysis, nephrectomy, and transplantation.

De novo nephrotic syndrome has been reported in about 25% of cases. It presents with proteinuria, hypoalbuminemia, and edema that may start immediately or as late as 3 years after transplantation. Patients with post-transplantation nephrotic syndrome have been reported to have the homozygous Fin major genotype. Antibodies against fetal glomerular structures are found in most patients with post-transplantation nephrotic syndrome, and antibodies to nephrin are found in more than 50%. About half of patients with this nephrotic syndrome respond to steroids and cyclophosphamide, Plasma exchange, rituximab and bortezomib, proteasome inhibitor which targets plasma cells, have been useful adjuncts. In the NAPRTCS database, vascular thrombosis and death with a functioning graft (mostly as a consequence of infectious complications) occur in 26% and 29% of cases, respectively, and account for a higher rate of graft failure in this particular group.

Close to 60 mutations in the *NPHS2* gene located on chromosome 1 have been identified and are autosomal recessive. Podocin is a podocyte-adapter protein required for proper targeting of nephrin into the slit diaphragm. Patients who are homozygous for podocin mutations develop early-onset steroid-resistant nephrotic syndrome, usually in infancy or early childhood, and usually progress to ESKD.

Renal histology shows FSGS. Because podocin is a structural component of the glomerular filtration barrier, it was hypothesized that deficient podocin was the cause of renal disease and that recurrence would not occur. However, there are reports of recurrence in recipients from parents who are obligate carriers of *NPHS2* and in patients with heterozygous *NPHS2* mutations. The mechanisms remain unclear. Response to plasma exchange has been favorable.

Although NPHS1 and NPSH2 mutations account for the majority of CNS cases (75%), mutations in *WT1* gene located on chromosome 11p13 account for some cases. *WT1* transcription factor plays a crucial role in the embryonic development of the kidney and genitalia. It is abundantly expressed in podocytes and controls cellular functions, such as nephrin expression. Patients with *WT1* mutations have moderate proteinuria, and renal biopsy reveals diffuse mesangial sclerosis (DMS) of glomeruli. *WT1* mutations can be found in isolated form, or as part of Denys–Drash syndrome. Denys–Drash syndrome is composed of progressive renal disease with nephrotic syndrome and DMS, Wilms tumor, and male pseudohermaphroditism. *WT1* mutations can also be associated with Frasier and WAGR syndromes. Frasier syndrome is composed of nephrotic syndrome with FSGS progressing to ESKD in adolescence or young adulthood, normal female external genitalia, streak (hypoplastic) gonads, XY karyotype, and predisposition to gonadoblastoma. WAGR is composed of Wilms tumor, aniridia, urogenital abnormalities, and retardation. While rare, patients with *WT1* mutations who have received kidney transplants can develop nephrotic syndrome.

Membranous Nephropathy

Membranous nephropathy is uncommon in children, and post-transplantation recurrence is rarely seen. *De novo* membranous nephropathy occurs more frequently and affects up to 10% of transplanted children. It usually presents later than the recurrent disease, which usually becomes apparent within the first two post-transplantation years. The occurrence of *de novo* membranous nephropathy does not appear to affect graft outcome in the absence of rejection.

Systemic Lupus Erythematosus and the Vasculitides

In the pediatric transplant literature, recurrence of systemic lupus erythematosus (SLE) is rarely seen. Recurrence in adults is more common and may not manifest until several years after transplantation. In pediatric nephrology, it is most common to observe lupus nephritis progress to ESKD in adolescence. Because it is standard practice to defer transplantation until SLE has become clinically quiescent, it is likely that the pediatric patient with SLE who receives a kidney transplant may not suffer from recurrence until young adult life.

Antineutrophil cytoplasmic antibody (ANCA)-positive glomerulonephritides can recur in the transplanted kidney. Granulomatosis with polyangitis and pauci-immune glomerulonephritis recur in a small number of patients and can cause graft loss. Treatment with corticosteroids and cyclophosphamide appears to be beneficial, and patients must be monitored carefully for signs of recurrence.

Metabolic Diseases

Primary Hyperoxaluria Type I

Oxalosis results from deficiency of hepatic peroxisomal alanine glyoxylate aminotransferase (AGT). Deficiency of this enzyme leads to deposition of oxalate in all body tissues, including the kidneys, myocardium, and bone. Renal transplantation alone does not correct the enzymatic deficiency, and graft loss is common because of oxalate mobilization from tissue deposits and subsequent deposition in the graft. Therapy with a combined liver-and-kidney transplantation has led to higher rates of success (see Chapter 13). The transplanted liver corrects the enzymatic deficiency and thus prevents further oxalate production. The well-functioning transplanted kidney excretes the mobilized plasma oxalate. Success of this approach is greatly facilitated by immediate graft function with a good diuresis. If possible, combined liver-and-kidney transplantation occurs early in the course of renal disease, preferably before the glomerular filtration rate (GFR) decreases below 15 to 30mL per minute per 1.73 m^2. This serves to optimize outcome and prevent severe complications of the disease that may lead to irreversible morbidity.

Ideally, aggressive hemodialysis before transplantation is employed to decrease oxalate load to safe levels and minimize tissue oxalate deposition. The target plasma oxalate level is less than 50 mg/mL. At transplantation, a large donor kidney is used whenever possible to permit effective excretion of the oxalate burden. Early use of a CNI may be deferred until the serum creatinine falls to the range of 1 to 2 mg/dL. Until this occurs, immunosuppression is accomplished with MMF, corticosteroids, and antibody induction. If early renal transplant dysfunction occurs, daily hemodialysis is continued. When good renal function is established, CNI therapy is begun. In addition, post-transplantation treatment includes pyridoxine, neutral phosphate, citrate, magnesium, and noncalciuric diuretics.

Nephropathic Cystinosis

Transplantation in children with cystinosis corrects the transport defect in the kidney, but not in other organs affected by the disease. Hypothyroidism, visual abnormalities, and central nervous system manifestations are not corrected by transplantation and require ongoing therapy with cysteamine and thyroid hormone. Cystine crystals can be found in the renal graft interstitium within macrophages of host origin. This does not result in recurrence of Fanconi syndrome or graft dysfunction.

Sickle Cell Anemia

The long-term graft survival rate for patients with sickle cell disease is lower, with only about 50% of grafts functioning beyond 3 years after transplantation. The improvement in the hematocrit results in higher numbers of abnormal red blood cells, leading to sickling episodes in the renal graft.

PRETRANSPLANTATION EVALUATION

The evaluation and preparation of a child for transplantation is essentially the same as for an adult (see Chapter 8). There are few absolute contraindications to kidney transplantation in children. Recent or metastatic malignancy and multiorgan failure precludes patients from transplantation. Administration of immunosuppressive medications to immunocompromised children such as those who are HIV positive requires special consideration (see Chapter 12). Patients with severe devastating neurologic dysfunction may not be suitable candidates; however, the wishes of the parents, as well as the potential for long-term rehabilitation, must be considered.

Evaluation of the Potential Living Donor

As a general rule, it is possible to consider an adult donor of almost any size for a child, no matter how young (see Chapter 7). Living donation from siblings is usually restricted to donors older than 18 years, although the courts have given permission for younger children to donate under extraordinary circumstances.

Histocompatibility matching considerations are not different for pediatric recipients of kidneys from living donors than for adult recipients. HLA-identical transplants are optimal and enable the lowest amount of immunosuppression to be used, thereby minimizing steroid and other side effects. The first living donor for a child is usually a one-haplotype–matched parent. Siblings may become donors as they reach the age of consent. When considering transplantation from siblings, data suggest that kidneys from haploidentical donors with noninherited maternal HLA antigens function better in the long term than do those from donors with noninherited paternal HLA antigens (see Chapter 3). Second-degree relatives, zero-haplotype–matched siblings, and nonbiologically-related individuals may also be considered as donors. To enhance matching, especially at HLA class II loci, and potentially prolong allograft survival, recipient–donor pairs can be entered into a paired-exchange program.

Evaluation of the Recipient

The evaluation of the potential pediatric transplant recipient is similar to that performed in adults, but because certain problems occur with more frequency in children, the emphasis may be different. It is important to establish the precise cause of ESKD in children whenever possible. Surgical correction may be required for certain structural abnormalities before transplantation. The precise cause of metabolic or glomerular disease should also be established if possible, because of the possibility of post-transplantation recurrence. Discussions of some common medical, surgical, and psychiatric issues in pediatric transplant candidates follow.

Neuropsychiatric Development

Infants. Infants with ESKD during the first year of life may suffer neurologic abnormalities. These include alterations in mental function, neurocognitive delay, microcephaly, and involuntary motor phenomena, such as myoclonus, cerebellar ataxia, tremors, seizures, and hypotonia. The pathogenesis is unclear, although aluminum toxicity, uremia, prematurity, hypertensive crises, and dialysis-related seizures have been incriminated. Preemptive kidney transplantation or institution of dialysis at the earliest sign of head-circumference growth-rate reduction or developmental delay may ameliorate the problem. Studies describe an improvement in psychomotor delay in some infants with successful transplantation, with a significant percentage of infants regaining normal developmental milestones. Tests of global intelligence show increased rates of improvement after successful transplantation.

Older Children. It is often difficult to assess to what extent uremia contributes to cognitive delay and impairment in older children. Uremia has an adverse, but often reversible, effect on a child's mental functioning, and it may often cause psychological depression. It may be necessary to institute dialysis and improve the uremic symptoms before making a precise assessment of the child's mental function. Initiation of dialysis often clarifies the picture and permits progression to transplantation in situations in which it might otherwise have not seemed feasible. On the other hand, severely delayed children respond poorly to the constraints of ESKD care. A child with a very low IQ cannot comprehend the need for procedures that are often confusing and uncomfortable. In this situation, the family must be involved and supported in the decision to embark on a treatment course that does not include chronic dialysis or transplantation.

Seizures. Up to 10% of young pediatric transplant candidates have a seizure disorder requiring anticonvulsant treatment. Before transplantation, seizures should be controlled, whenever possible, with drugs that do not interfere with CNIs, mammalian target of rapamycin (mTOR) inhibitors, or prednisone metabolism (see Chapter 6). Newer antiepileptic drugs such as levetiracetam (Keppra), gabapentin, pregabalin, and lacosamide are good options because they do not interfere with immunosuppression. Benzodiazepines can be used when circumstances permit. Carbamazepine does reduce CNI and prednisone levels, but its effect is not as strong as that of phenytoin (Dilantin) or barbiturates. Should it prove necessary to use a drug that lowers immunosuppressive drug levels, a moderately augmented dose of prednisone may be given twice daily. The CNI and/or mTOR inhibitor may need dose adjustments to achieve the desired trough levels, which should be monitored closely.

Psychoemotional Status
Psychiatric and emotional disorders are not, by themselves, contraindications to dialysis and transplantation; however, the involvement of healthcare professionals skilled in the care of affected children is mandatory. Primary psychiatric problems may be amenable to pharmacologic therapy and concomitant counseling and should not exclude children from consideration for transplantation. Experience with psychotropic drugs, such as selective serotonin reuptake inhibitors (SSRIs), has been very positive. As with anti-seizure medications, it is important to recognize that certain drugs may interfere with the metabolism of some immunosuppressive medications. This has not been found to be a major issue with SSRIs such as citalopram, escitalopram, and sertraline (discussed in the current chapter).

Nonadherence is a particularly prevalent problem in adolescent transplant recipients. Patterns of medication and dialysis compliance should be established as part of the transplant evaluation. Psychiatric evaluation should be performed in high-risk cases. If nonadherence is identified or anticipated, interventions should be in place before transplantation. These should include both social and psychiatric interventions, where possible. Psychosocial support systems must be identified and nurtured. Frequent medical, psychological, and social work monitoring is crucial if the patient is to be rehabilitated to the point at which the patient is a candidate for transplantation. The best outcomes will be achieved when there is close coordination between the medical and mental health providers. It is particularly important for the transplant and dialysis teams to stay in close communication as they prepare the patient for transplantation.

Cardiovascular Disease
Children and adolescents are unlikely to have overt cardiovascular disease that requires invasive diagnostic workup. Hypertension and chronic fluid overload during dialysis predisposes to left ventricular hypertrophy (LVH), hypertensive cardiomyopathy, and congestive heart failure. LVH may be present in up to 75% of pediatric transplant recipients, and peripheral resistance is often elevated. In children, as in adults, transplantation may be beneficial to cardiac function. Occasionally, the degree of pretransplantation cardiac compromise is so severe that heart transplantation must accompany kidney transplantation.

The importance of hypertension control in children with ESKD cannot be overemphasized. In the pretransplantation evaluation, blood pressure profiles and dialysis management must be carefully scrutinized. In the child who is hypertensive on dialysis, echocardiograms should be performed annually to assess ventricular hypertrophy and valve competence. In patients who require multiple antihypertensive drugs, bilateral nephrectomies may be required before transplantation.

Premature cardiovascular disease is a common feature of adults who have suffered childhood ESKD, and attention to adult cardiovascular disease risk factors in childhood may serve to minimize long-term morbidity and mortality. The coronary vessels of young adult dialysis patients have significant premature calcification (see Chapter 1). This may be the harbinger of atherosclerotic lesions. Control of calcium and phosphorus metabolism in the pretransplantation period is a potential way of ameliorating post-transplantation coronary heart disease. Statins may be indicated, and recommendations for their use in children with CKD have been made by Kidney Disease Improving Global Outcomes (KDIGO).

Infection
Common Bacterial Pathogens. Urinary tract infections and infections related to peritoneal dialysis are the most common sources of bacterial infection in children with ESKD. Aggressive antibiotic therapy and prophylaxis of urinary tract infections in children may effectively suppress infection, although pretransplantation nephrectomy is occasionally required for recalcitrant infections in children with reflux. Peritonitis and related infections with peritoneal dialysis are discussed later (see "Children Receiving Peritoneal Dialysis").

Cytomegalovirus. The incidence of CMV infection increases with age, and young children are unlikely to have developed CMV seropositivity.

CMV IgM and IgG levels should be obtained with the pretransplantation evaluation, and these studies should be considered when planning post-transplantation CMV prophylaxis.

Epstein–Barr Virus. It is important to establish the Epstein–Barr virus (EBV) antibody status of the child. As with CMV, EBV infections and resultant seropositivity increase with age. Primary EBV infection, in the context of potent immunosuppression, may predispose to a particularly aggressive form of post-transplantation lymphoproliferative disorder (PTLD).

Immunization Status. Children should be completely immunized prior to transplantation whenever possible to minimize the risk of preventable infectious diseases. Because children with ESKD have a suboptimal immune response, higher initial doses and antibody titer monitoring with booster doses of vaccines may be required. Live viral vaccines including measles, mumps, rubella, and varicella are contraindicated in the immunosuppressed patient and should be complete prior to transplantation. Vaccination of the immunosuppressed host may fail to induce an adequate immune response, especially with the use of agents, such as MMF, that suppress antibody production. Therefore, nonlive immunizations may be more efficacious when recipients are on low levels of maintenance immunosuppression approximately 6 months to 1 year after transplantation. Injectable influenza vaccine is recommended annually.

Hemostasis

About 7% of graft loss in pediatric patients is caused by graft thrombosis. For this reason, it is particularly important to search for clues of a patient's tendency toward hypercoagulability, such as recurrent hemodialysis access clotting. In pediatric patients, a full workup for thrombotic risk factors includes prothrombin time, partial thromboplastin time, platelet count, protein S level, protein C level, factor V Leiden, antithrombin III level, G20210A prothrombin mutation, homocysteine level, MTHFR T677 mutation, antiphospholipid antibody, anticardiolipin antibody, β_2-glycoprotein 1 level, lipoprotein A level, and factor VIII level. If the thrombophilia workup is positive or pediatric en-bloc kidneys are being utilized, perioperative and long-term anticoagulation can be used to minimize graft thrombosis.

Patients with Glomerulonephritis of Unknown Etiology

Pediatric patients are often referred for pretransplantation evaluation without having had the diagnosis of ESKD established. As noted earlier, recurrence of glomerulonephritis or glomerulopathy is a significant concern in pediatric and adolescent recipients. For this reason, any patient with significant proteinuria or hypertension accompanying ESKD should have a serologic profile that can help classify the diagnosis of ESKD. This includes C3, C4, antinuclear antibody, anti–double-stranded DNA, anti-GBM and ANCA titers.

Urologic Problems

Obstructive uropathy is the cause of ESKD in about 15% of transplanted children. Other causes of ESKD that are commonly associated with abnormalities of the urinary tract, such as reflux nephropathy, neurogenic bladder, prune belly syndrome, and renal dysplasia, account for another 20% of transplanted children. Because of this high frequency, urologic abnormalities should always be considered as a cause of ESKD of uncertain etiology in children and young adults. A history of voiding abnormalities, enuresis, nocturia, or recurrent urinary tract infections may be the only clue to an underlying urologic defect.

The presence of an abnormal lower urinary tract is not a contraindication to transplantation. Urologic problems are best addressed before transplantation. Malformations and voiding abnormalities (e.g., neurogenic bladder, bladder dyssynergia, remnant posterior urethral valves, urethral strictures) should be identified and repaired if possible. Children with urologic disease and renal dysplasia often require multiple operations to optimize urinary tract anatomy and function. Such procedures include ureteric reimplantation to correct vesicoureteric reflux; bladder augmentation or reconstruction; Mitrofanoff procedure (creation of a vesicocutaneous fistula using the appendix to provide for continent and cosmetically acceptable intermittent catheterization); and excision of duplicated systems or ectopic ureteroceles that may cause recurrent infections.

Bladder Augmentation. Urodynamic studies can provide important information about bladder capacity and function and help to define those situations that require bladder augmentation. Bladders that have high intravesical pressures are at risk for producing serious hydronephrosis in a transplanted kidney. Bladder augmentation is often required for patients with posterior urethral valve and some cases with small bladder capacity. Augmentation can be done using dilated ureter tissue, small intestine, or large intestine. Ureteric augmentation provides the best results because the ureteric mucosa is identical to the urinary bladder mucosa. Intestinal or colonic augmentation often requires frequent bladder irrigation and is often complicated by significant mucus secretion that can cause intermittent obstruction of the bladder stoma and lead to frequent urinary tract infections. Augmentation using gastric tissue causes severe dysuria because of the acidity of gastric secretions and has been abandoned in most centers. After bladder augmentation, most children require chronic intermittent catheterization. Forceful hydrodilation as a substitute for bladder augmentation is used at some centers, but most physicians agree that it is very painful and futile, especially in children awaiting deceased donor transplantation.

If a child has a neurogenic bladder, a bladder augmentation, or other voiding abnormality, it is usually possible to teach a parent or the patient clean, intermittent self-catheterization. This can be done in transplant recipients safely and successfully. However, urinary tract infection may occur when catheterization technique is poor. In addition, noncompliance with self-catheterization may lead to partial obstruction and subsequent graft dysfunction.

In some studies, graft outcome in children with urologic problems is inferior to that of children with normal lower urinary tracts. In addition, in recipients with an abnormal bladder, there is an increased incidence of post-transplantation urologic complications and urinary tract infection. Nevertheless, in centers with skilled pediatric urologists, children with ESKD as a consequence of urologic malformations can be successfully transplanted.

Renal Osteodystrophy

Early diagnosis and treatment of nutritional vitamin D deficiency, metabolic acidosis, hyperparathyroidism, osteomalacia, and adynamic bone disease are important in the pretransplantation period. Control of hyperparathyroidism with vitamin D analogues, calcimimetic agents for older children and adolescents or even parathyroidectomy, may be required. Additionally, the endocrine hormone fibroblast growth factor 23 (FGF23) is gaining recognition for its role in bone mineral metabolism and cardiovascular disease. Agents that target FGF23 are under development and may be tested in future clinical trials. Failure to optimize renal osteodystrophy prior to transplantation can lead to hypophosphatemia and limit the growth potential of a successful transplant recipient.

Children Receiving Peritoneal Dialysis

It has been generally accepted that children being treated with peritoneal dialysis have graft and patient survival rates that are similar to those of children receiving hemodialysis, although they may have higher risk for graft thrombosis, as may those children who receive preemptive transplants. The etiology of this observation is not clear. Therefore, a full coagulation workup should be considered before transplantation. Peritoneal dialysis may, in fact, facilitate transplant surgery, especially in very young and small infants. Repeated peritoneal fluid cycling expands the abdomen and creates adequate space for extraperitoneal placement of the relatively large adult kidney. Extraperitoneal placement of the graft is desirable because it may allow for continued peritoneal dialysis after transplantation in the event of DGF, and patients can tolerate oral feeds and medications sooner because of minimal bowel manipulation. However, intraperitoneal graft placement is not an absolute contraindication to post-transplantation peritoneal dialysis, should it become necessary.

A recent episode of peritonitis or exit-site infection in a child awaiting a transplant does not necessarily preclude transplantation. Potential transplant recipients should be appropriately treated for 10 to 14 days and have a negative peritoneal fluid culture off antibiotic treatment before contemplating transplantation. In addition, the preoperative peritoneal cell count should not suggest peritonitis. If a chronic exit-site infection is present at the time of surgery, the catheter should be removed and appropriate parenteral antibiotics administered. An overt tunnel infection should be treated before transplantation. The incidence of post-transplantation peritoneal dialysis-related infections is low. However, peritonitis and exit-site infection should be considered in the differential diagnosis in any child with unexplained fever after transplantation, and early sampling of the peritoneal fluid should be pursued. Such infections typically respond to appropriate antibiotic therapy, although catheter removal may be necessary for recurrent infections. In the absence of infections, the peritoneal catheter may be left in place until good graft function has been established for 2 to 3 weeks.

Nephrotic Syndrome

In children with glomerular diseases, proteinuria usually diminishes as kidney function deteriorates and ESKD ensues. Occasionally, florid nephrotic syndrome may persist, particularly in children with FSGS. Persistence of heavy proteinuria causes a hypercoagulable state and increases the risk for graft thrombosis and thromboembolic complications at the time of surgery. This makes fluid management difficult because of leakage of fluids into the extravascular space, which may lead to DGF and adversely affect graft outcome. Control of heavy proteinuria before transplantation is important and can sometimes be achieved with prostaglandin inhibitors, although renal embolization or bilateral laparoscopic nephrectomy may be required.

In the child with CNSF, unilateral or bilateral nephrectomy is usually performed early in the course of the disease to allow for better skeletal growth while on dialysis and to prevent infectious and thromboembolic complications. Nephrotic syndrome associated with isolated *WT1* mutations or in association with Denys–Drash, Frasier, or WAGR syndromes usually requires early bilateral nephrectomy as part of the prevention and treatment of Wilms tumor.

Pretransplantation Nephrectomy

Nephrectomy should be avoided if possible because leaving the kidneys *in situ* may facilitate fluid management during dialysis, an important consideration for small children in whom fluid balance may be tenuous. Nephrectomy may be indicated for severely hypertensive patients in whom blood pressure control is suboptimal despite optimal fluid removal and use of a multiple antihypertensive agents. Intractable urinary tract infection, in the presence of hydronephrosis or severe reflux, may also require nephrectomy before transplantation. Occasionally, nephrectomy is required to create adequate space for placement of the adult graft in a small infant. This is frequently the case in autosomal recessive polycystic kidney disease, in which the enlarged kidneys occupy the abdominal cavity, and may impair diaphragmatic movement, causing respiratory difficulty.

Portal Hypertension

Portal hypertension may occur in certain forms of ESKD common in children, such as congenital hepatic fibrosis, which may accompany autosomal recessive polycystic kidney disease and nephronophthisis. The manifestations of congenital hepatic fibrosis must be controlled; esophageal varices require sclerotherapy or portosystemic shunting. If neutropenia and thrombocytopenia are present as a result of hypersplenism, surgical shunting, transjugular intrahepatic portosystemic shunt (TIPS), partial splenectomy or splenic embolization may occasionally be required. Occasionally, combined liver–kidney transplantation is indicated for severe complications of portal hypertension in patients with ESKD and congenital hepatic fibrosis.

Prior Malignancy

Wilms tumor is the most common renal malignancy in children and the principal malignancy producing ESKD in children. Post-transplantation recurrence of Wilms tumor has been described in up to 6% of patients. Patients with recurrent Wilms tumor tend to be younger and have a shorter interval from tumor recognition to transplantation. A disease-free period of 1 to 2 years from the time of remission should be observed before transplantation. Premature transplantation has been associated with overwhelming sepsis, which may be related to recent chemotherapy. The presence of a primary nonrenal malignancy is not an absolute contraindication to transplantation, although an appropriate waiting time must be observed between tumor elimination and transplantation (see Chapter 7).

Preemptive Transplantation

Nearly 25% of all pediatric transplantations are now performed without the prior institution of dialysis. The percentage is even higher for recipients of living donors and is much higher than that reported in adults. The incidence of preemptive transplantation is nearly double in White children (31%) compared with African-American (13%) and Hispanic (17%) children. In children and in adults, there is a modest improvement in patient and graft survival for patients who have not received pretransplantation dialysis.

Nutrition

Poor feeding is a prominent feature of uremia in children. Optimal nutritional support is essential. Early gastrostomy or nasogastric tube feeding is often employed to improve caloric intake and promote growth, especially in children started on dialysis therapy at a young age. Because of technical difficulty, increased risk of graft thrombosis, and a resultant possibility of graft loss, a weight of 8 to 10 kg is used as a target weight for transplantation at most centers. This weight may not be reached until 2 years of age, even with the most aggressive nutritional regimens. Transplantation in children weighing less than 5 to 8 kg has been successfully performed at some centers.

PERIOPERATIVE MANAGEMENT OF THE PEDIATRIC RENAL TRANSPLANT RECIPIENT

Preparation for Transplantation

For living donor transplants, some programs commence immunosuppression in the week before the transplant date. A final crossmatch is performed within 1 month of transplantation, and the patient is evaluated clinically to ensure medical stability. Laboratory tests obtained at admission permit detection of metabolic abnormalities that require correction by dialysis. Aggressive fluid removal is discouraged in the immediate preoperative period to reduce the risk for DGF. Preoperative immunosuppression is discussed later.

Intraoperative Management

Methylprednisolone sodium succinate (Solu-Medrol), 10 mg/kg, is given intravenously at the beginning of the operation. Close attention is paid to blood pressure and hydration status in an attempt to reduce the incidence of DGF. Typically, a central venous catheter is inserted to monitor the central venous pressure (CVP) throughout the operation. To achieve adequate renal perfusion, a CVP of 12 to 15 cm H_2O should be achieved before removal of the vascular clamps; a higher CVP may be desirable in the case of a small infant receiving an adult-sized kidney. Dopamine is usually started in the operating room at 2 to 3 µg/kg per minute and increased as required and is continued for 24 to 48 hours postoperatively. It is used to facilitate diuresis and perhaps to effect renal vasodilation. The mean arterial blood pressure is kept above 65 to 70 mm Hg by adequate hydration with a crystalloid solution or 5% albumin and,

TABLE 17.3	Cytomegalovirus (CMV) Prophylaxis Protocol at the Mattel Children's Hospital at UCLA Pediatric Renal Transplant Program	
Donor CMV Status	**Recipient CMV Status**	**Ganciclovir***
Positive	Positive	Yes
Positive	Negative	Yes
Negative	Positive	Yes
Negative	Negative	No

*Ganciclovir is given intravenously initially (2.5 mg/kg daily) until oral intake is tolerated; oral valganciclovir dosing per Table 17.4.

if necessary, the use of dopamine at higher doses. Blood transfusion with packed red blood cells may be required in very small recipients because the hemoglobin may drop as a result of sequestration of about 150 to 250 mL of blood in the transplanted kidney. Mannitol and furosemide may be given before removal of the vascular clamps to facilitate diuresis. Urine volume is replaced immediately with 0.45% or 0.9% normal saline. Occasionally, an intra-arterial vasodilator, such as verapamil, is used to overcome vasospasm that may impair renal perfusion.

Postoperative Management

Because of the small size of young children, fluid management must be fastidious. Urine output should be replaced on a milliliter-for-milliliter basis with 0.45% or 0.9% normal saline continued for 24 to 48 hours. Insensible water losses are replaced with a dextrose-containing crystalloid. Potassium replacement may be required. Dextrose is not added to the replacement solution and is only used as part of the insensible water loss replacement solution. Withholding dextrose in the urine replacement solutions helps to prevent post-transplantation hyperglycemia and osmotic diuresis. The lack of concentrating ability of the newly transplanted kidney accounts for an obligatory high urine output that may be observed in the first few post-transplantation days. As the kidney function improves and the serum creatinine levels fall close to normal values, urinary concentrating ability recovers, and urine output decreases from several liters per day to amounts that begin to match daily fluid intake. At this time, urine output replacement can be stopped, and daily fluid intake is usually set to provide about 150% to 200% of the normal daily maintenance needs, preferably administered orally.

Hypertension is commonly observed. Pain is an important cause of hypertension in the immediate postoperative period, and adequate analgesia may be all that is required to control blood pressure. Hypertension is rarely aggressively corrected in the immediate postoperative period to avoid sudden swings in blood pressure that may impair renal perfusion. Electrolyte disorders encountered early in the postoperative course are discussed elsewhere. Prophylaxis against CMV infection is outlined in Tables 17.3 and 17.4 and in Chapter 12.

PEDIATRIC IMMUNOSUPPRESSIVE PROTOCOLS

Readers are referred to Chapter 6 for a full discussion of transplantation immunosuppressive agents and protocols and to Tables 17.5, 17.6, and 17.7. The construction of the immunosuppressive protocol for pediatric

TABLE 17.4 Valganciclovir (Valcyte) Dosing					
Creatinine Clearance (mL/min/1.73m²), Schwartz Formula	**< 12.5 kg**	**12.5–22.5 kg**	**22.5–35kg**	**35–50 kg**	**≥50 kg**
≥60	14–16 mg/kg PO daily	225 mg PO daily	450 mg PO daily	675 mg PO daily	900 mg PO daily
40–59	7–8 mg/kg PO daily	7–8 mg/kg PO daily	225 mg PO daily	7–8 mg/kg PO daily	450 mg PO daily
25–39	7–8 mg/kg PO every other day	7–8 mg/kg PO every other day	225 mg PO every other day	7–8 mg/kg PO every other day	450 mg PO every other day
10–24	7–8 mg/kg PO twice weekly	7–8 mg/kg PO twice weekly	225 mg twice weekly	7–8 mg/kg PO twice weekly	450 mg PO twice weekly

TABLE 17.5 Steroid Avoidance Immunosuppressive Protocol for Pediatric Kidney Transplantation at the Mattel Children's Hospital at UCLA

Pretransplantation (1 Week in Living Donor Recipients Only)

- MMF: 600 mg/m²/dose twice daily + Famotidine: 1 mg/kg/dose twice daily (maximum, 20 mg twice daily; other H_2 blockers, except cimetidine, or H^+ pump blockers may be used)

Pretransplantation (6 to 24 Hour)

- Rabbit anti-thymocyte globulin 1.5 mg/kg x 4 doses (maximum dose 125 mg) infuse over 6 hr (premedications with Solumedrol 10mg/kg, Benadryl, and Tylenol) MMF: 600 mg/m² PO/IV within 6 hour

Intraoperatively

- Solu-Medrol: 10 mg/kg IV at the beginning of surgery (maximum dose of 1 g)[*]

Immediate Postoperative Period

- MMF: 600 mg/m²/dose IV q 12 hour[†]
- Tacrolimus: 0.15–0.2 mg/kg/d PO divided twice daily to achieve levels of 8–12 ng/mL[‡] + Famotidine or H_2 blocker

Maintenance Therapy

- MMF: 600 mg/m²/dose PO twice daily until tacrolimus levels are adequate; then can switch to 300–450 mg/m²/dose PO twice daily[§]
- Tacrolimus: dose adjusted to achieve the desired trough levels (see Chapter 5, Table 5.8).

[*]Solumedrol taper for rapid withdrawal: 10 mg/kg POD#0, 2 mg/kg POD#1, 1 mg/kg POD#2, 0.5 mg/kg POD#3–5
[†]The drug is given orally when the patient tolerates oral intake.
[‡]Tacrolimus is started once urine output has been established and the serum creatinine level is below 2 mg/dL or less than 50% of its baseline value before transplantation.
[§]The dose can be spread to a 3-times-daily schedule if gastrointestinal symptoms develop early.
H_2, histamine-2; MMF, mycophenolate mofetil.

	Steroid-Based Immunosuppressive Protocol for Pediatric Kidney Transplantation at the Mattel Children's Hospital at UCLA

Pretransplantation (1 Week in Living Donor Recipients Only)
- Prednisone: 0.5 mg/kg daily (minimum = 20 mg/d)
- MMF: 600 mg/m²/dose twice daily[*]
- + Famotidine: 1 mg/kg/dose twice daily (maximum = 20 mg twice daily; other H₂ blockers, except cimetidine, or H⁺ pump blockers may be used)

Pretransplantation (6 to 24 Hour)
- Basiliximab: <35 kg: 10 mg
- ≥35 kg: 20 mg POD 0 and POD 4
- MMF: 600 mg/m² PO/IV within 6 hour

Intraoperatively
- Solu-Medrol: 10 mg/kg IV at the beginning of surgery (maximum dose: 1 g)

Immediate Postoperative Period
- Solu-Medrol: 0.5 mg/kg/d IV (minimum dose = 20 mg/d)[*]
- MMF: 600 mg/m²/dose IV every 12 hour[‡]
- Tacrolimus: 0.15–0.2 mg/kg/d PO divided twice daily to achieve levels of 8–12 ng/mL[†]
- + Famotidine or H₂ blocker

Maintenance Therapy
- Prednisone: dose tapering started 1 week after transplantation and continued to reach a maintenance dose 0.07–0.1 mg/kg/d by 2–3 month
- MMF: 300–450 mg/m²/dose PO twice daily with tacrolimus[‡]
- Tacrolimus: dose adjusted to achieve the desired trough levels (see Chapter 5, Table 5.8)

[*]The drug is given orally when the patient tolerates oral intake.
[†] Tacrolimus is started once urine output has been established and the serum creatinine level is below 2 mg/dL or less than 50% of its baseline value before transplantation.
[‡]The dose can be spread to a 3-times-daily schedule if gastrointestinal symptoms develop early.
H₂, histamine-2; MMF, mycophenolate mofetil.

transplantation is similar to that for adults. Because of the long-term toxicities of corticosteroids, many pediatric renal transplantation centers have moved toward steroid avoidance or withdrawal. It has been estimated that approximately 60% of children receive steroids. Table 17.5 represents one version of a steroid-avoidance protocol that includes rabbit anti-thymocyte globulin, tacrolimus, MMF, and frequent protocol biopsies. Rejection rates with this protocol are low, and growth and renal function are significantly improved. However, there have been few reports of increased incidence of rejection when MMF is held or decreased because of side effects. Unlike steroid-based regimens, it remains unclear whether MMF can be safely held without steroids and therefore another agent such as an mTOR inhibitor or azathioprine should be employed when MMF is not tolerated. Additionally, an increased risk of subclinical BK or CMV viremia has been associated with this regimen. A steroid-free regimen using Alemtuzumab induction followed by maintenance therapy with tacrolimus and MMF has been successful.

| TABLE 17.7 | Guidelines for Drug Dose Tapering in Pediatric Renal Transplant Recipients |

1. Tacrolimus

Minimal or no change is made in the first 4 weeks to allow for faster tapering of prednisone.

Dose reduction should not exceed 10% to 20%.

Tacrolimus and prednisone doses should not be lowered on the same day (risk for precipitating an acute rejection).

Serum creatinine and tacrolimus levels should be checked 2–3 days after each change and before the next change is made.

2. Prednisone

Start tapering the dose 2–3 weeks after transplantation if stable and tacrolimus level is within the desired range.

Initial dose tapering is by 2.5 mg each time, about 10% (may reduce by 5 mg if total dose is >2 mg/kg). Once a 10-mg dose is reached, dose reduction is by 1 mg each time.

Longer periods of time should elapse before further tapering at the lower dose range.

Tacrolimus and prednisone doses should not be lowered on the same day.

Serum creatinine and tacrolimus levels should be checked 2–3 days after each change and before the next change is made.

3. Mycophenolate Mofetil

Dose reduction is only indicated if hematologic or gastrointestinal side effects develop.

Dose reduction is done in 30% to 50% increments.

It can be safely withheld for a few d or up to 3–4 weeks for severe side effects with steroid-based regimens.

A protocol using Basixilimab induction, steroids, CNI, and MMF, and then conversion to an mTOR inhibitor and low-dose CNI at 4 to 6 weeks with complete steroid withdrawal by 6 months has also been effective. Induction therapy with a biologic agent is employed in about 85% of transplant recipients (Figure 17.1). Thymoglobulin can be used to provide adequate initial immunosuppression and allow delayed introduction of the CNI in cases of DGF, or to provide intensified immunosuppression in the highly sensitized transplant recipient. When transplantation is contemplated in a child with prior malignancy, a two-drug regimen, or even monotherapy, may be considered to minimize the effect of recurrent malignancy associated with immunosuppressive drugs. In this situation, the use of antibody induction is generally avoided, and living donation is encouraged to provide the best HLA match.

Corticosteroids

Steroid-avoidance protocols have been successful and safe in children. Retarded skeletal growth is the most important side effect of steroid use. Concerns remain about other familiar side effects, such as hypertension, obesity, diabetes mellitus, hyperlipidemia, osteopenia, and aseptic necrosis. Cosmetic side effects, such as cushingoid facies and acne, may tempt children and adolescents to stop taking their immunosuppressive drugs. Steroids are employed in children in certain circumstances including retransplantation, high panel reactive antibodies (PRAs), recurrent disease, and preexisting use (Table 17.6). However, doses are quickly tapered in children and when possible converted to alternate-day steroids which minimize their toxicity.

Calcineurin Inhibitors

There are some important differences in the use of cyclosporine and tacrolimus between adults and children. Children, particularly those younger than 2 years, may require higher doses than adults when calculated on a milligram per kilogram of body weight basis. The higher dose requirement is believed to be the result of a higher rate of metabolism by the hepatic cytochrome P-450, resulting in faster clearance. Dosing based on surface area, or thrice-daily dosing, appears to provide better therapeutic levels in smaller children and in children in whom metabolism is accelerated (e.g., patients receiving certain anticonvulsant medications). The use of peak-level monitoring of cyclosporine (C2 levels, see Chapter 6) that has been recommended for adults has also been independently validated in children. The recommended drug levels of cyclosporine and tacrolimus for children are similar to those recommended for adults (see Chapter 6). Studies comparing the efficacy of cyclosporine and tacrolimus in children have tended to favor tacrolimus in terms of the incidence of both acute rejection and graft loss. In the NAPRTCS database, there was little difference in acute rejection and graft loss between the two drugs when used in combination with MMF; however, improvement in graft function at 1 and 2 years post-transplantation was observed with tacrolimus. Concern generated from data collected in the late 1980s regarding a much higher incidence of PTLD in children receiving tacrolimus has largely mitigated.

The side-effect profile of the CNIs in children is similar to that seen in adults (see Chapter 6). Hirsutism, gingival hyperplasia, and coarsening facial features may be troublesome in children receiving cyclosporine, particularly Hispanic and African-American children. In the adolescent population, especially girls, these side effects may be devastating, causing severe emotional distress and possibly leading to dangerous noncompliance. Switching to tacrolimus may be helpful, although hair loss may follow. Seizures are observed more commonly in children treated with CNIs than in adults. Neurologic symptoms tend to be more severe with tacrolimus. Children, like adults, are more likely to develop hypercholesterolemia and hypertriglyceridemia with cyclosporine and may be candidates for lipid-lowering agents. Glucose intolerance is less common than in adults and occurs in less than 5% of children; it is more common with tacrolimus. Overt diabetes mellitus may occasionally occur. There has been a steady trend toward using tacrolimus rather than cyclosporine for children (Figure 17.1).

Mycophenolate Mofetil and Sodium Mycophenolate

MMF is used in over 90% of U.S. pediatric renal transplant recipients and has largely replaced azathioprine (Figure 17.1). The capacity of MMF to reduce the incidence of acute rejection episodes relative to azathioprine is similar in children to that described in adults (see Chapter 6).

In children, as in adults, gastrointestinal and hematologic side effects can be troublesome and may respond to dose reduction. Conversion to enteric-coated mycophenolate sodium (Myfortic) gives equivalent dosing as MMF and has been claimed to reduce gastrointestinal side effects. Therapeutic drug monitoring of MMF has been proposed for children but has not achieved widespread use. MMF has been used successfully in children for the treatment of steroid-resistant acute rejection.

mTOR Inhibitors

When used, sirolimus and everolimus are regarded in most centers as second-line agents. The primary difference between the two medications is the shorter half-life of everolimus (see Chapter 6). Reported efficacy and side-effect profiles mimic the adult experience. Several studies have shown beneficial effects of mTOR inhibitors in pediatric renal transplantation including: stabilization of GFR, good graft survival, and a low number of rejections when used in combination with low-dose CNI. However, mTOR inhibition with high-dose CNI must be avoided as an NAPRTCS-sponsored clinical trial revealed an unacceptably high level of PTLD. Side effects of mTOR inhibitors such as hyperlipidemia, impaired wound healing, proteinuria, growth impairment, or reduced testosterone levels are more likely to occur with higher doses.

Biologic Immunosuppressive Agents

The indications for the use of antibody induction are discussed in Chapter 6 and do not differ between adults and children. More than 85% of children are treated with antibody induction, most frequently with depleting agents (Figure 17.1). In pediatric living donor transplantation, there is a 5% advantage in the 5-year graft survival rate when antibody induction is used.

Depleting agents have gained popularity especially in steroid avoidance/withdrawal protocols or in highly sensitized patients. Rabbit antithymocyte globulin (Thymoglobulin) is most commonly used. Thymoglobulin suppresses CD3-, CD4-, and CD8-bearing T cells in pediatric patients and has anti–B-cell effects. Campath 1-H (Alemtuzumab), a humanized, monoclonal antibody directed against CD52 determinants on the surface of human B-, T-cells, natural killer cells, and monocytes, is another depleting agent used in children. The lymphocyte-depleting effects of both thymoglobulin or Campath 1-H may last many months and may predispose to viral infections; thus, close viral monitoring is recommended. Additionally, some studies report an increased risk of late antibody-mediated rejection with Campath 1-H.

The non–lymphocyte-depleting anti-CD25 monoclonal antibody available is basiliximab (Simulect), as daclizumab (Zenapax) is no longer available. Basiliximab is utilized for low-risk patients and for steroid withdrawal. It may be of particular benefit in children because of its effectiveness, ease of administration, and absence of side effects.

ACUTE REJECTION IN PEDIATRIC TRANSPLANTATION

Overall, significant improvements have been achieved in reducing acute rejection episodes in pediatric renal transplantation. They account for approximately 10% of graft failures. With standard immunosuppressive therapy, an acute rejection episode is experienced in about 9% of recipients of living donor transplants and 14% of deceased donor transplant recipients. African-American race, DGF, no antibody induction, and poor HLA matching may predispose to rejection episodes. In children, as in adults, acute rejection is the single most important predictor of chronic rejection. It precedes graft failure from chronic rejection in more than 90% of cases. Chronic allograft failure is the most common cause of graft loss in children.

Diagnosis of acute rejection in the very young transplant recipient is not always straightforward and requires a high index of suspicion. Because most small children are transplanted with adult-sized kidneys, the elevation in serum creatinine may be a late sign of rejection as a result of the large renal reserve compared with the body mass. Significant allograft dysfunction may be present with little or no increase in the serum creatinine level. One of the earliest and most sensitive signs of rejection is the development of hypertension along with low-grade fever. In children, any increase in serum creatinine, especially if accompanied by hypertension, should be considered a result of acute rejection until proven otherwise. Late diagnosis and treatment of rejection are associated with higher incidence of resistant rejections and graft loss.

The differential diagnosis of acute allograft dysfunction in children is similar to that in adults (see Chapter 10). Renal biopsy is the gold standard for diagnosis. The procedure has been shown to be safe in pediatric patients, with a low complication rate. We recommend the administration of DDAVP (0.3 µg/kg given intravenously) 1 hour before the procedure in any child with allograft dysfunction to correct any potential bleeding tendency. Urinalysis and culture, viral surveillance, and ultrasound and radionuclide imaging studies are used to diagnose other causes of graft dysfunction.

Treatment of Acute Rejection

The techniques used to treat acute rejection are similar in children to those used in adults (see Chapter 6). Complete reversal of acute rejection, as judged by a return of the serum creatinine level to baseline, is achieved in about half of children; somewhat less than half achieve partial reversal, and graft loss occurs in the remainder. Complete reversal from acute rejection is even less likely with subsequent rejection episodes or when the rejection is associated with donor specific antibody (DSA).

Corticosteroids

In children, as in adults, high-dose corticosteroid pulses are the first line of treatment of acute rejection, and about 75% of episodes are responsive to treatment. After the diagnosis is made, intravenous methylprednisolone is given in doses that range from 5 to 10 mg/kg per day for 3 to 5 days. After completing therapy, the maintenance corticosteroid is resumed at the prerejection level, or is increased and then tapered to baseline levels over a few weeks. For those on a steroid-avoidance protocol, conversion to low-dose maintenance steroids should be considered. The serum creatinine level may rise slightly during therapy and may not go back to baseline until 3 to 5 days after therapy is completed.

Lymphocyte-Depleting Agents

Thymoglobulin reverse up to 90% of the acute rejection episodes that do not respond to steroids. The standard dose of Thymoglobulin for acute rejection is 1.5 mg/kg/day for 7 to 14 days or can be dosed based on T-cell subsets. Administration through a peripheral vein often leads to vein thrombosis or thrombophlebitis. Therefore, peripherally inserted central catheter line placement is recommended before administration. To avoid allergic reactions, the patient should receive intravenous premedication consisting of methylprednisolone and diphenhydramine hydrochloride (Benadryl) 30 minutes before infusion. Weight-appropriate acetaminophen dosing should be given before and 4 hours after commencement of infusion for fever control. Vital signs should be monitored every 15 minutes during the first hour of infusion and then hourly until infusion is complete.

Side effects of Thymoglobulin in children are similar to those described in adults and include leukopenia and thrombocytopenia, which should be monitored with daily blood counts. The dose should be reduced by 50% for a platelet count of 50,000 to 100,000 cells/mL or a white blood cell count of less than 3000 cells/mL. Administration should be stopped if counts fall lower. Azathioprine, MMF, and sirolimus should be held during the course of treatment because they exacerbate hematologic side effects.

Refractory Rejection

Refractory rejection usually refers to episodes of acute rejection that do not respond to, or reoccur after, treatment with high-dose corticosteroids and lymphocyte-depleting agents. Some cases can be reversed by switching to tacrolimus or adding MMF, if this drug had not been part of the immunosuppressive protocol. Relatively high doses and trough levels are required. Conversion to sirolimus and low-dose CNI is a potential treatment option. If a renal biopsy shows that the refractory rejection has a component of antibody-mediated rejection (as manifested by positive staining for C4d, DSA, and/or histologic changes on kidney biopsy including peritubular capillaritis), therapy with high-dose intravenous immune globulin, Rituximab, and plasma exchange can be successfully used. Additionally, other agents including Bortezomib, Eculizumab, and Tocilizumab, an IL-6 receptor blocker, can be employed for refractory antibody-mediated rejection, although experience is limited in children. Whenever such aggressive immunosuppressive therapy is employed, the risk for opportunistic infections and post-transplantation lymphoma increases. Viral prophylaxis and infection surveillance are critical.

NONADHERENCE IN PEDIATRIC TRANSPLANTATION

Nonadherence is common in pediatric renal transplantation. Across several studies, the incidence of nonadherence among pediatric renal transplant recipients is approximately one-third. Among adolescents greater than 10 years of age, it exceeds 40%. As a result, 23% of late rejection episodes and 32% of allograft losses are associated with nonadherence. Patterns of nonadherence vary from partial adherence to complete nonadherence. Partial adherence ranges from the occasional missed dose to an occasional extra dose. It is most commonly the result of forgetfulness, misunderstanding of a dose change or modification, or the presence of events that lead to the belief that medications are not helping. In children, complete nonadherence is often the result of underlying emotional or psychosocial stress.

Measuring Adherence

Currently, there is no standardized method of detecting adherence. Both indirect and direct methods have been designed. The easiest indirect method is, asking patients directly about their adherence; patients, however, tend to tell physicians what they want to hear. Assessments made by patients of failure to take medications are often accurate, whereas denials of nonadherence are not. Other indirect methods to measure nonadherence include pill counts and assessment of prescription refill rates. The most validated indirect measure of nonadherence is a continuous microelectronic device, which is attached to the cap of the medication bottle, records each opening of the bottle as a presumptive dose and records the time and frequency of taking the medication. Recorded data can then be retrieved and an assessment of adherence made. Direct measures such as directly observed therapy, video directly observed therapy using a cellular device, or detection of an electronic marker added to the drug formulation may be more accurate, but are either impractical or are in early stages of development. A more practical direct measure of nonadherence is drug-level monitoring using the coefficient of variation or standard deviation for medications with stable pharmacokinetics such as CNI and mTOR inhibitors.

Predicting Adherence

Pretransplantation prediction of post-transplantation nonadherence is difficult. Risk factors include a disorganized family structure, insufficient social/emotional support, female sex, adolescence, poor patient/ practitioner communication, high cost of medication, and a history of previous graft loss as a consequence of nonadherence. Personality problems related to low self-esteem, preexisting psychiatric disorder, and poor social adjustment are found with higher frequency in nonadherent patients. Studies indicate that adherence has no correlation with intelligence, memory education, or the number of drugs that a patient takes, although the daily frequency of taking medications may affect adherence greatly. A linear decline in adherence rates has been demonstrated with increasing number of doses per day. Frequent clinic visits may improve adherence. Nonadherence in children must be suspected when there is unexplained diminution in cushingoid features, sudden weight loss, development of *de novo* DSA, or unexplained swings in graft function or trough blood levels of CNI or mTOR inhibitors.

Strategies to Improve Adherence

Education, planning dose regimens, clinic scheduling, communication, and getting patients involved in the medical management are the main strategies. The child should know that the physician is their advocate and is interested in how they take their medications. Providing patients with specific reminders or cues to which the medication can be tied can be of great help. These cues should be simple and preferably part of the patient's daily activities, such as meal times, daily rituals, specific clock times, a certain television program, tooth brushing, shaving, and so forth. For adolescents, the use of technology such as text reminders, cellular phone alarms, social media websites designed for transplantation, or a medication app on their smart phones may be beneficial. Contracting with pediatric patients and rewarding them is another strategy to enhance adherence. Finally, asking the same questions about adherence at each visit and explaining the consequences of nonadherence repeatedly reinforce the compliance message and physician interest.

Psychological Intervention

Behavior modification programs and other means of psychological intervention may be beneficial in some patients. In the pretransplantation period, an ongoing program of counseling should be undertaken in high-risk patients. Clearly defined therapeutic goals should be set while the patient is receiving dialysis, and family problems that are recognized in the pretransplantation period should be addressed before activation on the transplant list or the scheduling of a living donor transplantation. The presence of at least one highly motivated caretaker is a helpful factor in long-term graft success.

Adolescence brings with it rapid behavioral and bodily changes. The adolescent's strong desire to be normal conflicts with the continued reminder of chronic disease that the taking of medication engenders; this tendency is particularly true when medications are taken many times a day and alter the physical appearance. Ambivalence between the desire for parental protection and autonomy, combined with a magical belief in his or her invulnerability, sets the stage for experimentation with nonadherence. Adolescents with psychological or developmental problems may use impulsive nonadherence during self-destructive episodes. The transplantation teams must be aware of these developmental issues so that they can initiate appropriate psychological intervention before the onset of significant nonadherent behavior.

GROWTH

Retarded skeletal growth is a constant feature in children with chronic renal failure and ESKD. The severity of growth retardation is directly related to the age of onset of renal failure; the earlier the onset, the more severe the skeletal growth retardation. Renal osteodystrophy, metabolic acidosis, electrolyte disturbances, anemia, protein and calorie malnutrition, delayed sexual maturation, and accumulation of uremic toxins have all been implicated in the development of growth retardation.

Growth retardation is typically assessed by the *standard deviation score* (SDS) or height deficit score (also known as the *Z score*). These measure the patient's height compared with that of unaffected children of similar age.

Determinants of Post-transplantation Growth

Growth improves after transplantation; however, full catch-up growth is not realized in most patients. The following factors have a major influence on post-transplantation growth.

Age

Children younger than 6 years of age have the lowest standard deviation scores before transplantation, and these children exhibit the best improvement in their SDS after transplantation. Two years after transplantation, infants younger than 1 year of age have an improvement in their SDS by 0.7 standard deviation (SD), compared with an improvement of only 0.5 SD for those between 2 and 5 years of age, and 0.2 SD for those between the ages of 6 and 12 years. Children older than 12 years of age have minimal or no growth after transplantation. Older children occasionally continue to grow into puberty; however, the growth spurt experienced by most growing children at this age may be blunted or lost.

The fact that youngest children benefit the most in statural growth from early transplantation provides a strong argument for expedited transplantation in an attempt to optimize and perhaps normalize stature. In addition, earlier transplantation allows less time for growth failure while receiving dialysis and therefore a lesser requirement for catch-up growth.

Corticosteroid Dose

The precise mechanism by which steroids impair skeletal growth is multifactorial. Steroids may reduce the release of growth hormone, reduce insulin-like growth factor (IGF) activity, directly impair growth cartilage, decrease calcium absorption, or increase renal phosphate wasting. Strategies to improve growth include the use of lower daily doses of steroids, the use of alternate-day dosing, dose tapering to withdrawal, or avoidance. Conversion to alternate-day dosing should be considered in selected, stable patients in whom adherence can be ensured.

Ideally, steroids are withdrawn or avoided. In two randomized controlled trials using tacrolimus-based immunosuppressive regimens, daclizumab induction, and either steroid withdrawal or steroid avoidance, there was a significant improvement in height, especially for young children <5 years of age. More importantly, comparable rate of acute rejection and graft loss at 3 years post-transplantation were achieved between steroid-based and steroid-withdrawal or avoidance groups. Thus, steroid-withdrawal or -avoidance protocols can be successfully employed; however, further long-term studies using alternative forms of induction including Campath 1-H, basiliximab, or thymoglobulin are needed as daclizumab is no longer available.

Growth Hormone

The use of recombinant human growth hormone (rhGH) in pediatric renal transplant recipients significantly improves growth velocity and SDS. Growth velocity almost triples in the first year after starting rhGH therapy, with a slight slowing in the ensuing 2 years of therapy. There is some evidence to suggest that rhGH increases allogeneic immune responsiveness, leading to acute rejection and graft loss in addition to direct adverse effects on graft function. Growth hormone therapy is generally started in prepubertal children at least 1 year after transplantation and continued until catch-up growth is achieved or until puberty ensues. Cyclosporine levels may fall after initiation of rhGH therapy; therefore, CSA levels should be monitored closely and the dose should be increased by 10% to 15% when appropriate.

Allograft Function

A GFR of less than 60 mL per minute per 1.73 m^2 is associated with poor growth and low IGF levels; optimal growth occurs with a GFR greater than 90 mL per minute per 1.73 m^2. Graft function is the most important factor after high corticosteroid dosage in the genesis of post-transplantation growth failure. The immunosuppressive properties of corticosteroids needed to control rejection and preserve kidney function must be balanced against the need to minimize steroids to maximize growth. Thus, an excessive steroid dose leads to impairment of growth and an inadequate dose to impairment of graft function. Administration of high-dose rhGH may induce acceleration of growth even in the presence of chronic graft dysfunction but should be used with caution.

Post-transplantation Sexual Maturation

Restoration of kidney function by transplantation improves pubertal development. This most likely occurs as a result of normalization of gonadotrophin physiology. Elevated gonadotrophin levels and reduced gonadotrophin pulsatility are observed in chronic renal failure, whereas children with successful kidney transplants demonstrate a higher nocturnal rise and increased amplitude of gonadotrophin pulsatility.

Female patients who are pubertal before transplantation typically become amenorrheic during the course of chronic renal failure. Menses with ovulatory cycles usually return within 6 months to 1 year after transplantation, and potentially sexually active adolescents should be given appropriate contraceptive information. Adolescent female transplant recipients have successfully borne children; the only consistently reported neonatal abnormality has been an increased incidence of prematurity and low birth weight. MMF, mycophenolic acid, and mTOR inhibitors should be held in pregnant female transplant recipients owing to their teratogenic effects on the fetus. Corticosteroids, azathioprine, and CNIs can be safely continued. Adolescent males should be made aware that they can successfully father children; however, decrease in spermatogenesis with subsequent infertility has been associated with the use of mTOR inhibitors. No consistent pattern of abnormalities has been reported in their offspring.

Post-transplantation Infections

The reader is referred to Chapter 12 for a full discussion of post-transplantation infections. The spectrum of infections and their presentation may differ somewhat between children and adults, and the following sections focus on these differences. Infection in the immunocompromised child remains the major cause of morbidity and mortality after transplantation and is the most frequent reason for post-transplantation hospitalization.

Bacterial Infections

Pneumonia and urinary tract infections are the most common post-transplantation bacterial infections. Urinary tract infection can progress rapidly to urosepsis and may be confused with episodes of acute rejection. Opportunistic infections with unusual organisms usually do not occur until after the first post-transplantation month.

Viral Infections

The herpesviruses (CMV, herpesvirus, varicella-zoster virus, and EBV) pose a special problem in view of their common occurrence in children. Many young children have not yet been exposed to these viruses, and because they lack protective immunity, their predisposition to serious primary infection is high. The incidence of these infections is higher in children who receive antibody induction therapy and after treatment of acute rejection, and prophylactic therapy is advisable.

Cytomegalovirus. CMV seronegativity is 65% in children compared to 40% in adults, placing them in a high-risk category. The younger the child, the greater the potential for serious infection when a CMV-positive donor kidney is transplanted. CMV infection may have the same effect on the course of pediatric transplantation as on adult transplantation, and various strategies have been proposed to minimize its impact. It has been suggested that seronegative children receive only kidneys from seronegative donors; however, given the frequency of seropositivity in the adult population, this restriction would penalize seronegative children with a prolonged wait for a transplant at a critical growing period. CMV hyperimmune globulin, high-dose standard immune globulin, high-dose oral acyclovir, and oral ganciclovir are all potentially valuable therapeutic options. Ganciclovir is effective therapy for proven CMV infection in children. Valganciclovir has been shown to be effective prophylactic therapy in pediatric transplantation (Table 17.4).

Varicella-Zoster Virus. The most commonly seen manifestation of varicella-zoster virus infection in older pediatric transplant recipients is localized disease along a dermatomal distribution. In younger children, however, primary varicella infection (chickenpox) can result in a rapidly progressive and overwhelming infection with encephalitis, pneumonitis, hepatic failure, pancreatitis, and disseminated intravascular coagulation. It is important to know a child's varicella-zoster antibody status because seronegative children require prophylactic varicella-zoster immune globulin (VARIZIG) within 96 hours of accidental exposure. VARIZIG is effective in favorably modifying the disease in 70% of cases.

A child with a kidney transplant who develops chickenpox should begin receiving parenteral acyclovir without delay; with zoster infection, there is less of a threat for dissemination, although acyclovir should also be used. In both situations, it is wise to discontinue azathioprine, mTOR inhibitor, or MMF until 2 days after the last new crop of vesicles has dried. The dose of other immunosuppressive agents will depend on the clinical situation and response to therapy.

Epstein–Barr Virus. About half of children are seronegative for EBV as compared to 10% of adults. Prospective surveillance studies reveal that 35% to 40% of pediatric renal transplant recipients develop subclinical EBV viremia. EBV viremia usually precedes EBV infections and PTLD in children. Therefore, early identification of EBV viremia with surveillance is recommended.

Polyomavirus. Polyomavirus nephropathy is emerging as an important cause of allograft dysfunction and is discussed in Chapters 10, 11, 12, and 15. Post-transplant BK surveillance with urine or plasma BK is recommended to prevent overt nephropathy. First-line treatment involves immunosuppression reduction and monitoring of graft function and development of DSA is important. Other unproven therapies include leflunamide, ciprofloxacin, IVIG, and cidofovir.

Post-transplantation Antibiotic Prophylaxis

Protocols for post-transplantation antibiotic prophylaxis in children vary from center to center. Most centers use an intravenous cephalosporin for the first 48 hours to reduce infection from graft contamination and the transplant incision. The use of nightly trimethoprim-sulfamethoxazole for the first 3 to 6 months serves as prophylaxis against *Pneumocystis carinii* (PCP) pneumonia and urinary tract infections. Alternative agents for PCP prophylaxis include pentamidine, dapsone, or atovaquone. Prophylactic oral miconazole (nystatin) or fluconazole minimizes oral and gastrointestinal fungal infections. CMV prophylaxis has been discussed. Children who have undergone splenectomy or will receive Eculizumab should be immunized with pneumococcal and meningococcal vaccine. Additionally, these recipients should receive postoperative prophylaxis for both gram-positive and gram-negative organisms, both of which may cause overwhelming sepsis.

Post-transplantation Hypertension and Cardiovascular Disease

Persistent post-transplantation hypertension is a serious problem in children, as it is in adults. Medications including corticosteroids and CNI, especially cyclosporine, have been implicated and many children require multiple medications for blood pressure control. The differential diagnosis is the same as that for adults. It should be emphasized, however, that late-onset hypertension, especially when accompanied by low-grade fever, is commonly the first sign of acute rejection and may be present before any change in the serum creatinine level. Calcium-channel blockers are generally well tolerated in children and are the agents of choice for blood pressure management; however, angiotensin-converting enzyme (ACE) inhibitors may offer long-term reno-protection and should be considered in patients with stable allograft function.

Concern regarding long-term cardiovascular morbidity and mortality has generally been directed toward the older adult post-transplantation population. Young adults who developed chronic renal disease in childhood must also be considered to be at high risk for cardiovascular morbidity. Risk factors should be addressed in children who will hopefully grow to adulthood with their transplants. Serum cholesterol levels are frequently higher than the 189 mg/dL at-risk level for children with transplants. Dietary measures are appropriate to reduce hyperlipidemia and vascular calcification. Recommendations for the use of statin in children have been made by KDIGO.

REHABILITATION OF TRANSPLANTED CHILDREN

Successful reentry into school after transplantation requires coordinated preparation of the child, family or caregivers, classmates, and school personnel. Treatment side effects, social and emotional difficulties, academic difficulties, school resources, and caregiver attitudes all play a role and should be addressed.

Within a year of successful transplantation, the social and emotional functioning of the child and the child's family appears to return to preillness levels. Pretransplantation personality disorders, however, continue to manifest themselves. Within 1 year after transplantation, more than 90% of children attend school, and less than 10% are not involved in any vocational or education programs. Three-year follow-up shows that nearly 90% of children are in appropriate school or job placement. Surveys of 10-year survivors of pediatric kidney transplants report that most patients consider their health to be good; engage in appropriate social, educational, and sexual activities; and experience a good quality of life.

Children carry with them many of the medical consequences of chronic kidney disease into their adult life. Nearly half of adult pediatric transplant recipients are severely short and more than 25% are obese. Rates of hypertension, orthopedic problems, and cataracts are high. Despite these health problems, most of these adult "survivors" report a good quality of life and successful rehabilitation.

Selected Readings

Amaral S, Sayed BA, Kutner N, et al. Preemptive kidney transplantation is associated with survival benefits among pediatric patients with end-stage renal disease. Kidney Int 2016;90:1100–1108.

Barbour S, Gill JS. Advances in the understanding of complement mediated glomerular disease: implications for recurrence in the transplant setting. Am J Transplant 2015;15:312–319.

Bartosh SM, Leverson G, Robillard D, et al. Long-term outcomes in pediatric renal transplant recipients who survive into adulthood. Transplantation 2003;76: 1195–1200.

Cochat P, Rumsby G. Primary Hyperoxaluria. N Engl J Med 2013;369:649–658.

Dharnidharka VR, Fiorina P, Harmon WE. Kidney Transplantation in Children. N Engl J Med 2014;371:549–558.

Holmberg C, Jalanko H. Congenital nephrotic syndrome and recurrence of proteinuria after renal transplantation. Pediatr Nephrol 2014;29:2309–2317.

Hooper SR, Gerson AC, Butler RW, et al. Neurocognitive functioning of children and adolescents with mild-to-moderate chronic kidney disease. Clin J Am Soc Nephrol 2011;6:1824–1830.

Hsiau M, Fernandez HE, Gjerston D, et al. Monitoring nonadherence and acute rejection with variation in blood immunosuppressant levels in pediatric renal transplantation. Transplantation 2011;92:918–922.

Kaidar M, Berant M, Krauze I, et al. Cardiovascular risk factors in children after kidney transplantation—from short-term to long-term follow-up. Pediatr Transplant 2014;18:23–28.

Kranz B, Vester U, Nadalin S, Paul A, et al. Outcome after kidney transplantation in children with thrombotic risk factors. Pediatr Transplant 2006;10:788–793.

Laster ML, Fine RN. Growth following solid organ transplantation in childhood. Pediatr Transplant 2014;18:134–141.

Loirat C, Fakhouri F, Ariceta G, et al. An international consensus approach to the management of atypical hemolytic uremic syndrome in children. Pediatr Nephrol 2016;31(1):15–39.

Neu AM. Immunizations in children with chronic kidney disease. Pediatr Nephrol 2012;27:1257–1263.

Ng YW, Manpreet S, Sarwal MM. Antibody-mediated rejection in pediatric kidney transplantation: pathophysiology, diagnosis, and management. Drugs 2015;75:455–472.

Pape L, Ahlenstiel T. mTOR inhibitors in pediatric kidney transplantation. Pediatr Nephrol 2014;29:1119–1129.

Ponticelli C, Moroni G, Glassock R. De novo glomerular diseases after renal transplantation. Clin J Am Soc Nephrol 2014;9:1479–1487.

Sarwal MM, Ettenger RB, Dharnidharka V, et al. Complete steroid avoidance is effective and safe in children with renal transplants: a multicenter randomized trial with three-year follow-up. Am J Transplant 2012;12:2719–2729.

Savige J, Gregory M, Gross O, et al. Expert guidelines for the management of Alport syndrome and thin basement membrane nephropathy. J Am Soc Nephrol 2013;24:364–375.

Smith JM, Vikas R. Viral surveillance and subclinical viral infection in pediatric kidney transplantation. Pediatr Nephrol 2015;30:741–748.

Suszynski TM, Rizzari MD, Gillingham KJ, et al. Antihypertensive pharmacotherapy and long-term outcomes in pediatric kidney transplantation. Clin Transplant 2013;27:472–480.

Tagliamacco A, Cioni M, Comoli P, et al. DQ molecules are the principal stimulators of de novo donor-specific antibodies in nonsensitized pediatric recipients receiving a first kidney transplant. Transpl Int 2014;27:667–673.

Trachtman R, Sran SS, Trachtman H. Recurrent focal segmental glomerulosclerosis after kidney transplantation. Pediatr Nephrol 2015;30:1793–1802.

Van Arendonk KJ, King EA, Orandi BJ, et al. Loss of pediatric kidney grafts during the "high-risk age window": insights from pediatric liver and simultaneous liver-kidney recipients. Am J Transplant 2015;15:445–452.

Wesseling-Perry K, Bacchetta J. CKD-MBD after kidney transplantation. Pediatr Nephrol 2011;26:2143–2151.

Wesseling-Perry K, Pereira RC, Tsai E, et al. FGF23 and mineral metabolism in the early post-renal transplantation period. Pediatr Nephrol 2013;28:2207–2215.

Zaman RA, Ettenger RB, Cheam H, et al. A Novel Treatment Regimen for BK Viremia. Transplantation 2014;97:1166–1171.

18 Psychiatric Aspects of Kidney Transplantation

Akhil Shenoy and Itai Danovitch

This chapter will describe the psychiatric implications of kidney transplantation. It will cover psychiatric considerations for the donor and recipient evaluation; the psychological perspective on modifiable behaviors such as nonadherence; and management of psychiatric symptoms in patients with end-stage kidney disease (ESKD) and post-transplant.

BACKGROUND

Psychiatric problems are common among persons with chronic diseases, and ESKD is no exception. An inflammatory environment and heightened stress may contribute to mood and anxiety disorders. Simultaneously, a preexisting history of psychological problems is negatively associated with transplant outcomes.

Despite the growing recognition of comorbid psychiatric disorders among patients with ESKD, provision of treatment remains limited. Some degree of depression is common in ESKD patients though less than 20% of them actually receive treatment. Up to 40% of transplant recipients report depressive symptoms. Although in many cases it may be reasonable for the primary medical team to initiate treatment, the complexity of psychiatric issues in transplant recipients often requires subspecialty care. Ideally, the mental health needs of transplant recipients and donors are provided by specialists in transplant psychiatry; however, general psychiatrists with experience taking care of medically ill patients are also well equipped to provide this care.

PSYCHIATRIC ASSESSMENT OF THE TRANSPLANT CANDIDATE

Goals

The pretransplant psychiatric evaluation has two primary goals: The evaluator seeks to optimize outcomes for the patient and assist the transplant team to determine appropriate allocation of a scarce societal resource. The purpose of the evaluation is to assess the psychosocial strengths and vulnerabilities of the transplant candidate, and then to use that assessment to inform a plan of care, as well as to determine current eligibility for transplantation.

A psychosocial evaluation is an essential part of the evaluation of transplant candidates (see also Chapters 8 and 21). Cognitive impairment, mental illness, a history of nonadherence, substance use disorder, and lack of social support are concerns that need to be recognized and addressed, but are not, in themselves, absolute contraindications for kidney transplantation. Many of these risk factors, when detected proactively, can be specifically addressed through therapeutic interventions that improve post-transplant outcomes. It is imperative that the pretransplant evaluation not only identifies risks, but also recommends specific social, psychological, or psychiatric services required to support optimal patient outcomes.

Approach

The evaluating psychiatrist should communicate the evaluation goals at the outset. A constructive introduction from the referring physician or social worker is essential. For many patients, this will be their first meeting with a mental health professional and they may be apprehensive. It is helpful for the patient to understand that a psychiatric evaluation is a standard component of the pretransplant evaluation, that the evaluation will incorporate collateral information from multiple providers and possibly family, and that recommendations will be presented to the transplant team. Collateral information is often secured from the social worker, clinical coordinator, nephrologist, referring physicians, and outside psychiatric providers.

Psychiatric assessment begins with a comprehensive biopsychosocial evaluation. Diagnosing a treatable psychiatric disorder involves assessing a wide range of symptoms across emotional, cognitive, and behavioral domains. However, beyond diagnosis, the evaluating psychiatrist must assess the ability of the patient to adapt to stress, to utilize coping mechanisms, and to adhere to a challenging behavioral and medical management plan. The patient's knowledge and motivation for transplant should be assessed, as well as their expectations of post-transplant care and outcomes. Their history of adherence with medications, dialysis, and other treatment recommendations should be reviewed. Normalizing imperfect adherence may help the patient be open about challenges they have faced, or strategies they have developed to maximize adherence. Asking about missing medications in the past 2 weeks has been shown to be a helpful technique to trigger recollection of specific instances. It is also important to evaluate conditions, such as mental health problems or risky substance use, which can indirectly impact adherence. Barriers to adherence such as cognitive decline, depression, caregiver loss, and stable living arrangements should also be evaluated. Given the prevalence of post-transplant delirium, and the risk of neuropsychiatric sequelae, establishing a baseline assessment of cognitive status and decision-making capacity is also important. Presence of adequate social support has been found to be a consistent prognosticator for post-transplant success. Identifying positive prognostic factors such as coping abilities and resilience enables development of a treatment plan that reinforces a patient's strengths.

Tools

Pretransplant evaluation screening tools can be useful for transplant programs to identify high-risk patients for additional intervention. Two such tools, the Psychosocial Assessment of Candidates for Transplantation (PACT) and the Transplant Evaluation Rating Scale (TERS), were early developments which have been superseded by the Stanford Integrated Psychosocial Assessment for Transplant or SIPAT which has been tested prospectively for the purpose of pretransplant

TABLE 18.1	Components of the SIPAT (Stanford Integrated Psychosocial Assessment for Transplant)

A. Patient's readiness level
   Knowledge of illness
   Knowledge of transplant
   Willingness, desire, and motivation
   Compliance/Adherence
   Lifestyle (diet, exercise, habit)
B. Social support system
   Support system
   Functionality of support
   Living space and environment
C. Psychological stability and psychopathology
   Psychopathology
   Neurocognitive impairment
   Personality
   Truthfulness and deception
   Overall psychological risk
D. Lifestyle and effects of substance abuse
   Alcohol use history and risk of relapse
   Substance use history and risk of relapse
   Nicotine use

evaluation. It covers a wide range of relevant psychosocial concerns to be considered for transplant (Table 18.1). The SIPAT has been shown to have excellent inter-rater reliability and higher scores predict higher rates of psychiatric decompensation and medical hospitalizations. High scores can be used as a trigger for referring for more intensive psychiatric evaluation. Some programs also use a structured questionnaire to assess adherence with dialysis.

LIVING DONATION

The number of patients who are waitlisted for kidney transplant far exceeds the number of cadaveric donors available. Living donors may help meet this demand through traditional direct donation or through networks of paired exchange donation (see Chapter 7). The psychiatric liaison in a kidney transplant program should encourage living donation, but also consider themselves the individual donor's advocate. Mandated advocacy, in the form of the Independent Living Donor Advocate (ILDA), is discussed in Chapters 7 and 21.

The ethical dictum to "do no harm" is the guiding principle in the evaluation of the live donor. In parallel to comprehensive medical screening, psychological vulnerability factors should be identified and addressed accordingly. A psychiatric interview can uncover subtle coercive factors contributing to the donor's decision. The donor may be motivated to correct their feelings of guilt or to repair a troubled relationship. Clarifying the donor's experience with the recipient and their expectations for the future relationship is a critical feature of fully exploring the donor's motivations. Ambivalence prior to donation is associated with postdonation adverse psychosocial consequences. Learning about how the donor arrived at their decision enables an evaluation of their comprehension and rationale, both requirements for informed consent. The motivated donor must be autonomous, informed, voluntary, and have full understanding of the donation process. Along these lines, the psychiatrist should also assesses the donor's knowledge of kidney disease and transplant surgery, their expectations of outcome, and any anticipated economic, social or psychological consequences of the procedure. A Live Donor Assessment Tool (LDAT) has been designed to encompass the various psychosocial concerns for donors (Table 18.2).

Guidelines have also been helpful to direct the psychosocial evaluation of living-unrelated kidney donors where there is heightened concern regarding the nature of their motivation. Programs should be mindful of potential donors who may be exploited or coerced to donate. The psychosocial team can determine if these donors have unrealistic expectations about the donation experience and recipient outcomes. Donors in kidney paired donation (KPD) programs deserve special psychosocial review (see Chapter 7) to help limit "backing out" or reneging from chain. Psychiatrists can comment on the donor's motivation to donate but also assess for severe anxiety and impulsivity which may be barriers to following through as the donor. As their advocate, the psychosocial team should be assessing ambivalence in these potential donors to help them with their decision making. Resolving this ambivalence through motivational interviewing prior to donation has been shown to improve donor outcomes.

As living donation has grown, so has the interest in psychosocial outcomes of donors. Optimism and postdonation physical well-being may better predict higher satisfaction with donation than the recipient outcome. Pain may be associated with lower satisfaction. Nonetheless, multiple studies have reported excellent psychosocial outcomes of traditional "altruistic" donation. The incidence of depression is low,

TABLE 18.2	Components of the LDAT (Live Donor Assessment Tool)

1. Motivation
   Internal and external motivation, types of motives
2. Knowledge
   Knowledge of process and recipient's diagnosis
3. Relationship with the recipient
4. Social support
5. Psychological
   Coercion, anxiety, indecision, impulsivity, ambivalence
6. Expectations
   Optimistic/Realistic (for donor and recipient)
7. Stability in life
   Early life, relationships, employment, financial, stressors, sleep
8. Psychiatric issues
   Symptoms, personality traits, truthfulness
9. Substance abuse
   Alcohol, substances, marijuana, nicotine

arid quality-of-life scores are high. A well-deserved "halo" effect may enhance the sense of well-being that donors enjoy. The converse is observed when donors are paid in what are essentially commercial, rather than medical, transactions.

MANAGING ADHERENCE POST-TRANSPLANTATION WITH A MULTIDISCIPLINARY TEAM

Nonadherence to treatment is the most common preventable cause of organ transplant rejection. Compared with all transplant recipients, kidney transplant patients have the highest nonadherence rates which may account for 25% of graft losses. The pretransplantation psychosocial evaluation is intended to anticipate the challenges to adherence and initiate a plan to address them. A large part of preparing the patient for transplantation is to foster their interest in participation and cooperation with their team. Adherence is defined as following the treatment recommendations (nutritional, pharmacologic, appointments). Fostering and maintaining a strong therapeutic alliance between doctor and patient is integral to adherence. More recently, the term "concordance" has been used to emphasize this agreement.

While nonadherence cannot be predicted reliably prior to transplantation, a history of regular office visits and medication refills is one good indication of future adherence. There are mixed opinions about dialysis adherence being a predictor of medication compliance. Adherence has been shown to wane with time post-transplant and so adherence assessment after the first few years after transplant may be just as important as in the first year. Exploring habits at subsequent visits can help identify nonintentional or environmental barriers to taking medications. A nonjudgmental, collaborative approach may be more fruitful in this endeavor. If intentional nonadherence or other psychological factors are suspected, referral to a psychiatrist or psychologist is appropriate. Emphasis on adherence should be a routine part of each clinic visit.

Patients may reduce their medications on their own owing to actual or feared side effects of immunosuppression. Cosmetic concerns such as hirsutism, hair-loss, or acne may also play a role. Patients may fear malignancy or have other specific beliefs that they cannot feel they can share with staff. The complex post-transplant medication regimes may be a source of unexpressed, and hence unaddressed, financial stress (see Chapter 21). Pessimism, use of avoidant coping strategies, and belief that the medications have a negative effect on general health are also associated with low adherence.

Patients often cite "forgetting" as the main reason for nonadherence. Unintentional nonadherence can be due to forgetfulness or disorganization and environmental interventions may help. Transplant medications can be ordered with calendar packaging and adherence apps on smartphones may be useful, though their value has not been systematically tested. Groups organized to review the specific knowledge of, and behavior related to, immunosuppression has been shown to improve adherence.

A standardized technique to evaluate nonadherence has been recommended. The Medication Level Variability Index (MLVI) may be a powerful predictor of late rejection and an opportunity to direct services for improved adherence. Assessment of both intentional and nonintentional nonadherence will continue to be important as long as immunosuppression medication predicts graft success.

MANAGEMENT OF PSYCHIATRIC DISORDERS IN TRANSPLANT CANDIDATES AND RECIPIENTS

What follows is a symptom-based guide to treatment. With the exception of acute agitation, in most cases, immediately correctable medical contributors need to be addressed before treatment is initiated. Also, given the rapid evolution of pharmacologic agents, new drugs should be checked for interactions against the remainder of each patient's regimen.

Delirium and Agitation

When severe illness overwhelms the brain's capacity to maintain homeostasis, the result is delirium, an acute syndrome characterized by impaired cognition, fluctuating level of consciousness, inattention, and behavioral dysregulation. The psychiatric consultant can assist the primary team in developing a comprehensive differential diagnosis for the underlying cause of delirium (Table 18.3). The behavioral manifestations of delirium may incline some to suspect a psychiatric disorder, but it is critical not to be misled. Psychiatric management of delirium focuses on controlling symptoms. Nonpharmacologic, behavioral management of delirium should be implemented. Antipsychotic medications have been shown to increase risk of all-cause mortality, however, when acute agitation threatens to injure patients or their caregivers, the benefits of an antipsychotic medication may well outweigh the risks.

Postoperative delirium is fairly common in the surgical population. Various medications used in the post-transplant period are associated with neuropsychiatric side effects (Table 18.4). A specific syndrome of posterior reversible encephalopathy syndrome (PRES) has been associated with cyclosporine, tacrolimus, and sirolimus. Characteristic white matter edema in the posterior lobes is seen on cerebral MRI, but frontal lobe involvement can be found in 50% of cases.

Mood

Depression is widespread among patients with ESKD and transplant recipients. Mood disorders can be challenging to diagnose owing to the overlap of neurovegetative symptoms in renal insufficiency and

TABLE 18.3	Common Causes of Delirium in Kidney Transplant Recipients

Acute kidney injury
Drug toxicity
Drug withdrawal
Uremia
Infection
Ischemic stroke
Intracerebral hemorrhage
Metabolic derangement

TABLE 18.4	Adverse Neuropsychiatric Effects of Commonly Used Renal Transplant Medications
Medication	**Adverse Neuropsychiatric Reaction**
Cyclosporine	Anxiety, restlessness, delirium, visual hallucinations, parasthesias, tremors, seizures, ataxia, cortical blindness, impaired concentration
Tacrolimus, sirolimus	Insomnia, tremors, delirium, paranoia, akinetic mutism, impaired concentration, leukoencephalopathy
Penicillins, fluoroquinolones	Seizures, delirium, perceptual disturbances
Lamivudine	Headache, insomnia, fatigue
Ribavirin	Irritability, depression, suicidality, fatigue, insomnia, anxiety
Acyclovir, valacyclovir	Delirium, depression, perceptual disturbances
Ganciclovir, valganciclovir	Headache, seizures, nightmares, perceptual disturbances
Prednisone	Affective instability—ranging from depression to mania

(Adapted from Hafliger S. A primer on solid organ transplant psychiatry. In: Wyzynski AA, ed. *Manual of Psychiatric Care for the Medically Ill*. Washington, DC: American Psychiatric Association; 2005.) See also Chapter 6.

TABLE 18.5	Symptom Parallels between Depression and Uremia
Depression	**Uremia**
Poor concentration	Uremic encephalopathy
Irritability, Suicidality	Restlessness, akathisia, uremic encephalopathy
Somatization	Neuropathy, arthropathy
Decreased energy	Anemia, volume overload, uremia
Insomnia	Sleep apnea
Decreased appetite	Anorexia
Sexual dysfunction	Chronic kidney disease

depression (Table 18.5). Because most drug trials exclude patients with renal failure, there is little evidence to direct choice of antidepressant medications. However, studies specifically in the cardiac population have shown that selective serotonin reuptake inhibitors (SSRIs) are superior to placebo, and overall they are well tolerated.

When starting antidepressants in patients with renal disease, assuming there are no known interactions, it is still generally advisable to lower the starting dose by one-third. Starting at low dosages and titrating slowly minimizes the likelihood of common adverse effects such as nausea, restlessness, headache, grogginess, and sexual dysfunction. There is some evidence in a physically healthy population that improvement in the first 2 weeks may predict a more sustained benefit in 4 to 6 weeks. Medically ill patients often ultimately require higher doses to achieve full benefit.

Anxiety

Anxiety is prevalent across patients with severe medical illness and has a substantial negative impact on quality of life. Anxiety itself is a symptom, although when combined with other psychopathology and loss of function, it may be part of a diagnosable psychiatric disorder such as panic disorder, generalized anxiety disorder, obsessive compulsive disorder, or post-traumatic stress disorder.

Counseling, support groups, and psychotherapy are vital psychosocial interventions to reduce anxiety. For patients with panic disorder (a common diagnosis in ESKD), there is strong evidence that both cognitive behavioral therapy and psychoanalytically oriented psychodynamic psychotherapy are effective in achieving remission. The use of one type of therapy or another depends in large part on available clinical resources, funding, and patient preference. The pharmacologic approach to anxiety disorders rests largely on the judicious use of SSRIs. Unfortunately, these serotonin-based anxiolytics require 4 to 6 weeks to exert their full effects, and sometimes during that interval they actually exacerbate anxiety. One solution is to use a "bridging dose" of a benzodiazepine to provide immediate symptom relief. For this purpose, long-acting benzodiazepines, such as clonazepam, 0.5 mg twice daily, are preferred because their pharmacokinetics makes them less reinforcing than short-acting agents, and using them on a standing basis minimizes an inclination to self-medicate a wider range of symptoms. For acute phobic anxiety related to procedures or interventions, lorazepam, 1 mg every 8 hours, is effective and is favorable because it undergoes hepatic metabolism without active metabolites.

Psychosis

In the early history of organ transplantation, patients with psychotic disorders such as schizophrenia, schizoaffective disorder, and severe bipolar disorder were excluded because of concern about their ability to adhere to complicated immunosuppressive treatment regimens. A significant subset of patients on dialysis have been diagnosed with a psychotic disorder, however, and recognition that many patients with severe psychotic disorders can be perfectly adherent when appropriate supports are put in place has led to an incremental increase in organ allocation to this population. The physiologic and psychological stress of ESKD places the patient at high risk for decompensation, but a close relationship between psychiatric and medical teams can facilitate a smooth treatment course. For patients without a history of a psychotic disorder, a new-onset psychotic symptom represents delirium until proven otherwise. A comprehensive workup, including cerebral imaging and evaluation of metabolic, endocrine, infectious, autoimmune, and pharmacologic factors, must be undertaken. For patients with a history of illicit substance use, particularly stimulant use, a urine toxicology screen can be used to "rule in" substance-induced psychotic disorders.

Insomnia

Insomnia is commonplace among medically ill patients, and the many discomforts endured by patients with ESKD frequently lead to impairments in sleep. Nevertheless, treatment of insomnia begins with education on the importance of sleep hygiene. Patients should avoid stimulating agents such as caffeine after noon, and they should promote a relaxing environment in the hour before going to sleep. Sleep restriction, if possible, during the day should be introduced. Mid-day sun has been shown to increase melatonin. Underlying psychiatric (i.e., depression, anxiety) and medical (i.e., sleep apnea, hyperthyroidism, and restless legs syndrome) causes of insomnia must be identified because their treatment may resolve the symptom.

Benzodiazepines and benzodiazepine-like medications are generally avoided because they disturb sleep architecture (leading to decreased delta-wave restorative sleep) and may induce dependence. However, they are particularly helpful for patients with initial insomnia (difficulty falling rather than staying asleep), and used judiciously, they can provide substantial symptom relief. The medications mirtazapine and trazodone were developed as antidepressants. Their tendency to cause prominent sedation at low doses, coupled with their general tolerability, has led them to be used as effective sedatives more often than their use as antidepressants (the antidepressant dosages for these medications is multifold higher than their sedative dose range). Patients should be advised about the risk for weight gain with mirtazapine and of the rare but important risk for priapism with trazodone. Restless leg syndrome is a common cause of insomnia among renal patients, and addressing this is often sufficient to improve sleep.

Substance Use Disorders

Most patients are excluded from transplantation if they are actively abusing drugs or alcohol (see Chapter 8). Many programs require patients with a history of substance use disorder to demonstrate a fixed period—typically 6 months—of sobriety to demonstrate eligibility, though there is scant data underpinning the specificity of the timeline required.

Some previously sober individuals relapse under the stress of kidney transplantation, and still others succumb to self-medication of symptoms with alcohol and prescription or illicit drugs. The stigma associated with drug addiction leads many patients with a history of substance use disorders to expect misjudgment by medical professionals, and unfortunately, these expectations often frame the nature of their interactions. In turn, well-meaning but frustrated healthcare providers may become demoralized about their inability to help these patients and seek instead to discharge them form care or minimize interaction with them. Thus, a cycle is perpetuated in which these ill patients receive less rather than more treatment.

Treatment for substance use disorder can be divided into three groupings: self-help, psychosocial therapies, and psychopharmacologic interventions. Self-help groups such as alcoholics anonymous (AA) are free, ubiquitous, and offer vital support to those patients who are sufficiently self-motivated. Individual counseling or therapy can offer vital skills to patients who have been unable to stop using alcohol or drugs on their own. For patients whose lives are chaotic, or whose ambivalence prevents meaningful engagement in self-help groups, a structured intensive outpatient program or residential treatment may be necessary. Psychopharmacologic interventions are used first to assist with detoxification and second to aid patients' efforts to maintain sobriety. Table 18.6 reviews medications with U.S. Food and Drug

TABLE 18.6 Selected Psychotropic Medications and Renal Disease

Class	Drug	Typical Dose (mg)	Dose in ESKD (mg)	Half-Life (hours)	Half-Life in ESKD (hours)	Protein Bound (%)	Effect of Dialysis	Comments
SSRIs (selective serotonin reuptake inhibitors)	Citalopram	10–60	10–60	33–37	43–49	80	None	Increased QT prolongation with doses above 40 mg
	Escitalopram	10–30	10–30	22–32	30–43	56	—	Risk for reduced clearance with severe renal impairment
	Fluoxetine	20–60	20–60	24–96	40	95	None	May increase cyclosporine and tacrolimus as a P-450 3a4 inhibitor
	Paroxetine	20–60	10–30	17–25	11–55	95	—	May increase cyclosporine and tacrolimus as a P-450 3a4 inhibitor
	Sertraline	50–200	50–200	24–36	42–96	98	Minimally removed	Reduction in serum levels in hemodialysis, hypertension
SNRIs (serotonin and norepinephrine reuptake inhibitors)	Venlafaxine	37.5–225	37.5–112	4	6–11	30	None	50% reduction in dose for moderate/severe renal impairment
	Desvenlafaxine	50	25	11	23	30	None	50 mg every other day in severe renal impairment
	Duloxetine	60–120	Not recommended	8–17	—	90	—	Not recommended for patients with ESKD (requiring dialysis) or severe renal impairment (CrCl <30 mL/min)

(continued)

501

TABLE 18.6 Selected Psychotropic Medications and Renal Disease (*continued*)

Class	Drug	Typical Dose (mg)	Dose in ESKD (mg)	Half-Life (hours)	Half-Life in ESKD (hours)	Protein Bound (%)	Effect of Dialysis	Comments
TCAs (tricyclic antidepressants)	Amitriptyline	25–100 tid	25–100 tid	32–40	32–40	—	None	Associated with delirium
	Imipramine	25 tid	25 tid	6–20	—	—	None	Associated with delirium
Other antidepressants	Bupropion	100–450	100–300	10–21	—	85	—	Dose reduction recommended Risk for seizures with elevated levels
	Mirtazapine	15–45	7.5–22.5	20–40	—	85	—	Clearance reduced about 50% in renal disease
	Vilazodone	10–40	10–40	25	—	90	None	Care should be taken with P-450 3a4 substrates, dose should not exceed 20 mg with 3a4 inhibitors such as cyclosporin
	Trazodone	50–400	50–400	4–11	—	90	Mild removal	Risk for priapism
Psychostimulants	Methylphenidate	10–60	10–60	3	—	10–33	—	No active metabolites
	Lisdexamphetamine	10–70	10–30	9–11	—	—	—	Prodrug has half-life less than an hour
	Modafinil	100–400	—	7.5–15	22	60	—	Metabolized by 3A4

Mood stabilizers	Valproic acid	15–60 mg/kg	15–60 mg/kg	15–60 mg/kg	6–17	—	80–90	20% removed	Increased free levels in ESKD; use free levels when determining blood level for dosing
	Lithium	900–1,200	Not recommended		14–28	40	0	Yes	Administer single dose after dialysis (target serum trough levels of 0.8–1.0 mMol/L)
	Lamotrigine	100–200	50–100		13–30	42.9	55–56	20% removed	Needs to be re-titrated from 25 mg after discontinuing after five half-lives
Antipsychotics (dopamine antagonists)	Oxcarbazepine	300–600 bid	150–300		9–11	—	40	Yes	Not FDA approved for bipolar
	Chlorpromazine	50–400	50–400		11–42	11–42	90–99	None	Active metabolites
	Haloperidol	1–2 tid	1–2 tid		14–26	14–26	90	None	Active metabolites
	Aripiprazole	10–45	5–15		75–146	—	99	—	Substantial medication interactions with 2D6 or 3A4
	Ziprasidone	20–80 bid	20–80 bid		5–7	4.2	99	None	Inactive metabolites
	Risperidone	1–3 bid	0.5–1.5 bid		3–30	25	90	—	Clearance of active metabolites reduced by up to 60% with renal failure
	Olanzapine	5–20	5–20		32–38	32–38	93	—	Active metabolites
	Clozapine	12.5–450	—		8–12	—	97	—	Active metabolites
	Quetiapine	50–250 tid	50–250 tid		6	4.1	83	—	Active metabolites
	Lurasidone	20–120	20–80		18	—	99	—	Active metabolites

(continued)

TABLE
18.6

Selected Psychotropic Medications and Renal Disease (*continued*)

Class	Drug	Typical Dose (mg)	Dose in ESKD (mg)	Half-Life (hours)	Half-Life in ESKD (hours)	Protein Bound (%)	Effect of Dialysis	Comments
Benzodiazepines (GABA-A agonists)	Lorazepam (oral, IM, IV)	1–2 bid to tid	1–2 bid	9–16	32–70	85	Not removed	No active metabolites
	Clonazepam	0.25–1 bid to tid	0.25–1 bid to tid	18–80	—	85	Not removed	No active metabolites
	Alprazolam	0.25–1 tid	0.25–1 tid	9–19	9–19	80	Minimal removal	Active metabolites and increased free fraction of plasma protein bound drug in ESKD
	Temazepam	7.5–30	7.5–30	4–10	—	96	Not removed	No active metabolites
	Diazepam (oral, IM, IV)	5–40	5–40	92	37	98	Not removed	Elevated free serum levels in ESKD; increased free fraction of active metabolite in both ESKD and healthy
Other anxiolytic	Buspirone	10–30 bid	10–30 bid	2.4–2.7	2.7	95	No	Avoid use in severe renal insufficiency
Benzodiazepine receptor agonists (α-1 selective to GABA-A receptor)	Zaleplon	5–20	—	1	—	60	—	Not studied in ESKD
	Zolpidem	5–10	5–10	2–3	4–6	92	—	Increased free fraction
	Eszopiclone	1–3	1–3	6	—	55	—	FDA approved for extended use

504

Substance use medications	Dose (mg)	Renal dose adjustment	Half-life	Protein binding (%)	% renal excretion	Dialyzable	Comments
Naltrexone	50–150	—	5–10 days	—	—	—	—
Disulfiram	250–500	—	12 / 21 days	96	0	—	—
Acamprosate	333–666 tid	333 tid	3.2–13	—	8–34	—	Requires dose reduction but contraindicated with severe renal insufficiency
Topiramate	100–200 bid	50–100 bid	18–24	15–20	—	Yes	Associated with renal calculi in 1.5%–2% subjects
Buprenorphine	2–32	—	1.2–7.2	96	—	No	—
Methadone	20–200	Lower	23–50	71–88	—	—	Concern for QT prolongation at higher doses
Gabapentin	100–900 tid	25–50 tid	5–7	0	6.5–52	Yes	Dose adjustments for ESKD Needs to be dosed after dialysis

QD, dosing unless otherwise noted.

CrCl, creatinine clearance; ESKD, end-stage renal disease.

(Adapted from Micromedex 1.0. Available at: http://www.micromedexsolutions.com/ cited: 3/3/17).

Administration (FDA) approval for drug or alcohol use disorder. These drugs typically improve rates of sobriety by either reducing craving, diminishing the reinforcing effects of drug use, or pharmacologically replacing the drug of abuse with a legal and less harmful agent.

At the time of this writing, laws governing the use of cannabis are in a state of significant flux across the United States, with some states legalizing cannabis use, and others permitting for limited therapeutic applications. Smoked cannabis may expose immunocompromised patients to infectious agents such as aspergillus, but this risk has not been well documented. Ingesting cannabinoid agents orally has not been linked to adverse transplant outcomes, though theoretically if use rises to the level of a cannabis-use disorder, there may be increased risk of nonadherence. In the absence of clear data demonstrating a risk, it is prudent not to have cannabis use alone as an exclusive criterion for transplant candidacy. In July 2015, Governor Jerry Brown of California signed AB 258, the Medical Cannabis Organ Transplant Act, which prohibits discrimination against medical cannabis patients in the organ transplant process, unless a doctor has determined that medical cannabis use is clinically significant to the transplant process. Several other states have followed suit.

Pain Relief

The issue of pain is addressed here because when it occurs in the context of a current or past history of addiction, it can present a number of challenges. Patients manifesting drug-seeking behavior may simultaneously suffer from somatic pain. In fact, the term *pseudoaddiction* was coined to characterize the appearance of drug-seeking behavior among patients who simply have undertreated pain. Healthcare providers must walk the fine line of not undertreating pain while addressing manifest abuse behaviors. Putting aside moral or ethical considerations about drug use, abuse behaviors are concerning because they invariably lead down a path of nonadherence and consequent graft dysfunction and loss. Management of pain and addiction often requires an interdisciplinary approach, with a pain management service explicitly managing pain medications in collaboration with a psychiatric or psychological service to address risky behaviors. Interventions to help this population include: Maximizing use of nonopioid analgesics; minimal use of sedative hypnotic medications that induce dependence; preferential use of long-acting opioids in lieu of highly reinforcing short-acting agents; establishment of a clear treatment contract; and evaluation and treatment of underlying psychiatric disorders that compel self-medication.

Interpersonal Difficulties

The psychological impact of kidney transplantation is profound. Whereas all forms of illness undermine the fantasy of invulnerability that buoys the "sense of self," the significance of a failing organ system requiring replacement by donation is an enormous challenge for the psyche, and one that is best understood in the context of an individual's psychological, social, spiritual, and cultural background.

The patient with ESKD can adapt psychologically in ways that produce unintended consequences. For instance, those with long-standing illness and disability may adjust to being ill with maladaptive coping strategies that perpetuate a dependency on the "sick role." They may have difficulty with transitioning to a state of health and managing expectations from their families and transplant team. Patients who become acutely ill may minimize the seriousness of their medical illness, which may undermine adherence to medical care.

Family and friends may have mixed feelings about finding themselves in the unanticipated role of "caregiver." The tumultuous path from renal disease to renal failure, dialysis, and transplantation is beset with stress and disappointments. Even the strongest of relationships can waver in the face of such challenges, and relationships with preexisting problems often face a particularly turbulent course. Thus, patients must contend with both intrapersonal (having to do with their internal emotional life) and interpersonal (having to do with their relationships with others) difficulties. The pretransplantation psychosocial evaluation is intended to anticipate some of these challenges and initiate a plan to address them, but there is no way to fully defray the burden that patients have to bear. Caregiver burden can remain high after transplant.

Early attention to psychological reactions to medical illness can be critical. The fear of loss of bodily function can lead to impervious attitude and denial of care. Helplessness may lead to asserting autonomy and exerting control over treatment providers. Anger can leave the patient rejecting the team's recommendations. Over half a century ago, Kahana and Bibring defined seven archetypal personalities that remain useful to this day (see Table 18.7). These styles are not personality disorders but traits that can be activated under medical or psychosocial stress. Whatever the outward behavior or manifest personality of the patient, the first step in identifying and managing a style is to empathize with the underlying threat that the patient may be experiencing. Additional interventions are listed to help address the patient's behavior. A psychiatric liaison may further help with interpreting these struggles with the patient.

PSYCHOPHARMACOLOGY AND DRUG INTERACTIONS

Determining appropriate psychotropic agents requires an understanding of the pharmacokinetic and pharmacodynamic changes that occur before and after receipt of a kidney. Renal excretion, metabolism, medication dialyzability, protein binding, competitive inhibitions, and induction of P-450 systems must be taken into account. Moreover, a number of antirejection medications have important adverse neuropsychiatric effects (see Table 18.4 and Chapter 6).

The use of psychotropic medication prior to transplant should consider kidney excretion. Paroxetine, venlafaxine, desvenlafaxine, bupropion, and mirtazapine are antidepressants that require dose adjustments in ESKD. Duloxetine is not recommended for patients with severe renal impairment (CrCL < 30 mL/min). Hedayati has outlined a practical approach to the treatment of depression in ESKD (see Suggested Readings). Mood-stabilizing medications that are primarily cleared by the kidney require dose adjustments and include lithium, oxcarbamezapine, and lamotrigine. Since lithium is extensively cleared by dialysis, it needs to be dosed after each session. Lower doses are also required for gabapentin, pregabalin, topiramate, and acamprosate.

TABLE 18.7 Kahana and Bibring's Seven Personality Styles in the Medical Setting, their Meaning, and Interventions

Personality Style	Meaning	Interventions
Dependent, overdemanding (oral)	Threatened by abandonment	Set firm limits early. Provide regular short visits, identify most important needs, and follow-up plan.
Orderly, controlled (compulsive)	Fearing loss of control and desiring self-control	Offer control and choice where possible. Give choice between two healthy options in critical decisions.
Dramatizing, captivating (hysterical)	Requiring admiration and fearing loss of attention	Empathize with the patient's fear of losing medical attention, but set limits and gently correct unreasonable expectations.
Long-suffering, self-sacrificing (masochistic)	Feeling worthless and deserving punishment	Emphasize that recovery may be a slow, steady process, present recovery as a benefit for others; don't abandon.
Guarded, querulous (paranoid)	Inviting and fearing attack	Acknowledge complaints without arguing or ignoring; Correct reality distortions, gently question irrational thoughts.
Superiority, demeaning to others (narcissistic)	Fears loss of autonomy and needing to be invulnerable	Don't mistake patient's superior attitude for real confidence; Communicate best intentions for patient's care.
Aloof, uninvolved (schizoid)	Threatened by intrusion and desiring privacy	Accept the patient's unsociability; Reduce the patient's isolation as tolerated.

(Adapted from Nash SS, Kent LK, Muskin PR. Psychodynamics in medically ill patients. Harv Rev Psychiatry 2009;17(6):389–397.)

Antipsychotics such as risperidone, paliperidone, and lurasidone will also require lower doses.

Post-transplantation, the practitioner must consider the drug–drug interactions with immunosuppressive medications. The hepatic cytochrome p450 system has two iso-enzymes, 3A4 and 2D6, that are required for metabolism of cyclosporine and tacrolimus. Inhibitors can rapidly cause toxicity of these agents. Antidepressants listed according to decreasing order of CYP3A4 inhibition include fluvoxamine, nefazodone, fluoxetine, sertraline, TCAs, paroxetine, and venlafaxine. Introduction, dose adjustments, and discontinuation of these drugs require immunosuppressive drug-level monitoring and coordination between the treating psychiatrist and the transplant physician.

Table 18.6 details the concerns and dosing considerations for psychotropic medications in patients with ESKD and for those with a well-functioning kidney transplant.

OUTCOMES

Kidney transplantation can improve mental health in the broadest sense, and this alone is a powerful motivation to undergo transplantation for many patients. Collaborative mental healthcare is essential to help patients adjust to their new post-transplant reality and help maintain adherence. Patients with a kidney transplant tend to have lower rates of cognitive disturbance, anxiety, and depression than patients on hemodialysis and peritoneal dialysis. Transplant recipients perform better on processing speed, attention, short-term memory, and executive functioning, than do transplant candidates. Nonetheless, transplant patients face the constant specter of graft failure. Some patients will struggle with bodily integrity and physical adjustment to side effects from immunosuppression such as tremor and ataxia. Many patients will need to redefine their role with family members and adjust to increased autonomy and return to function. Depression can lead to poor adherence, whereas remission from depression and successful adaptation to transplantation have been shown to improve post-transplant outcomes.

Psychiatrists with subspecialty training in psychosomatic medicine, or who have worked with transplant patients, are well-suited to manage the mental health needs of patients post-transplant. Collaboration with medical providers, psychologists, social workers, nursing, and when appropriate, family members, is critical to providing well-integrated, and effective psychiatric care.

Selected Readings

Baghdady NT, Banik S, Swartz SA, et al. Psychotropic drugs and renal failure: translating the evidence for clinical practice. Adv Ther 2009;26:404–424.

Brar A, Babakhani A, Salifu MO, et al. Evaluation of non-adherence in patients undergoing dialysis and kidney transplantation: United States transplantation practice patterns survey. Transplant Proc 2014;46:1340–1346.

Dew MA, DiMartini AF, DeVito Dabbs AJ, et al. Preventive intervention for living donor psychosocial outcomes: feasibility and efficacy in a randomized controlled trial. Am J Transplant 2013;13:2672–2684.

Dew MA, Rosenberger E, Myakovsky L, et al. Depression and anxiety risk factors for morbidity and mortality after organ transplantation: a systemic review and mat-analysis. Transplantation 2015;100:988–1003.

Garcia MF, Bravin AM, Garcia PD, et al. Behavioral measures to reduce non-adherence in renal transplant recipients: a prospective randomized controlled trial. Int Urol Nephrol 2015;47:1899–1905.

Hedayati S, Yalamanchili V, Finkelstein FO. A practical approach to the treatment of depression in patients with chronic kidney disease and end-stage renal disease. Kidney Int 2012;81:247–255.

Iacoviello B, Shenoy A, Braoude J, et al. The Live Donor Assessment Tool: a psychosocial assessment tool for live organ donors. Psychosomatics 2015;56(3):254–261.

Maldonado JR, Sher Y, Lolak S, et al. The Stanford Integrated Psychosocial Assessment for Transplantation: a prospective study of medical and psychosocial outcomes. Psychosom Med 2015;77:1018–1030.

Messersmith EE, Gross CR, Beil CA, et al. Satisfaction with life among living kidney donors: a RELIVE study of long-term donor outcomes. Transplantation 2014;98:1294–1300.

Ozcan H, Yucel A, Avsar UZ, et al. Kidney transplantation is superior to hemodialysis and peritoneal dialysis in terms of cognitive function, anxiety, and depression symptoms in chronic kidney disease. Transplant Proc 2015;47:1348–1351.

Rodrigue JR, Vishnevsky T, Fleishman A, et al. Patient-reported outcomes following living kidney donation: a single center experience. J Clin Psychol Med Settings 2015;22(2–3):160–168.

19

Organ Transplant Law and Ethics

Alexandra Glazier

Organ transplantation exists at the intersection of life and death within the context of an explicitly rationed resource and thus creates a field ripe with legal and ethical issues. While the specific issues change over time as the technology of transplantation evolves, fundamentally the primary legal and ethical considerations are concentrated on two core areas: the permissibility of methods designed to obtain organs and increase organ donation, and the appropriate framework to allocate the transplant benefit. The urgency to increase the availability of organs together with clinical innovations results in the current ethical and legal issues that are the focus of this chapter. The international ramifications of these issues are discussed in Chapters 22 and 23 and on the website www.declarationofistanbul.org.

AVAILABILITY OF ORGANS: LEGAL AND ETHICAL CONSIDERATIONS

There are three primary ways to increase the availability of organs, and each has its own set of attendant legal and ethical considerations: increase the number of people who say "yes" to donation; increase the pool of suitable potential donors; and increase the number of organs that can be transplanted from the donor pool. The following section will look at some current, specific issues under this framework.

Increasing the Number of People Who Say "Yes" to Donation
Authorizing Deceased Donation through Donor Registries

One of the primary strategies to increase the number of donors in the United States has been the development and promotion of donor registries. The United States has always worked within an explicit "opt-in" system of donation versus "opt-out systems" (or "presumed consent"), where individuals are donors unless action is taken to negate that distinction. The legal framework for the opt-in system within the United States is set forth in the Uniform Anatomical Gift Act (UAGA)—the law governing organ donation that has been passed in every state.

The UAGA establishes gift law as the legal structure for organ donation. This choice of legal framework is important to understand as it is different than the informed consent legal paradigm that healthcare providers work within when providing medical care to patients. Informed consent requires a facilitated understanding of risks and benefits of a particular treatment or procedure. As a matter of law, the requirement to obtain informed consent is derived from the doctor/patient relationship. The legal principle of informed consent is, however, incongruent with deceased donation where there are neither risks nor benefits to the donor, *because the donor is deceased at the time the donation occurs.* Further, the decision to be a donor is made completely outside of a doctor/patient relationship. For these reasons, the law under the UAGA does not utilize an informed consent standard and instead follows gift law.

The legal underpinnings of gift law in the UAGA facilitated the development of donor registries. Adults can authorize an anatomical gift after death by registering as a donor. This is not an informed consent process, but rather conforms to legal gift law requirements to document the donor's legally binding intent to gift organs at death. The ability to register as a donor facilitates an individual's exercise of autonomy and comports with ethical principles of self-determination. When a donor has made his or her own legally binding donation decision, it is referred to a "first person authorization."

The law under the UAGA, since first enacted in 1968, has always provided for first person authorization as prioritized over a surrogate donation decision made by next of kin. However, moving away from traditional documents such as donor cards toward electronic designations in web-based donor registries ensures that the right people (Organ Procurement Organizations—OPOs) have the right information (donor registration) at the right time (when the patient dies); this has completely changed the practice of donation.

According to Donate Life America (www.donatelife.net), as of the early 2017, over 130 million people in the United States had registered as donors, representing over half of the adult population. This number has steadily increased over the past decade, and with further public education and registration campaigns, it is likely to continue to increase. The impact on actual donation rates is equally impressive with 50% of organ donors in 2016 having authorized their own donation via a registry. Further work to maximize the registration of those who would like to be donors will continue to positively impact donation rates consistent with respecting the individuals' right to make their own donation decisions.

Donation after Circulatory Death (DCD)—Timing of Approach to Families

Registering as a donor is an exercise of self-determination and constitutes legal consent for deceased donation. The donor registration may occur decades prior to death as compared with the next-of-kin permission that is sought at the time of death. This shift in the timing of consent for donation necessitates an examination of how and when families are being approached in cases of potential DCD (see Chapter 4). The traditional approach as recommended in a 2000 Institute of Medicine Report requires a "decoupling" or separation of the donation decision from the other end-of-life discussions. Decoupling donation from end-of-life decision making mitigates ethical concerns that an organ donation decision might hasten the withdrawal of support. By separating in time these two decisions, decoupling promotes an ethical framework to engage critical care providers in their support of organ donation. Decoupling has also resulted in greater rates of family consent.

At the time of a devastating brain injury, the decoupling approach was initially implemented because families were expected to make both the donation and the withdrawal of support decisions. As a result, the donation discussion was not initiated until after the decision to withdraw futile support to ensure that the decoupling principle was fulfilled. The advent of first person authorization, however, changes that sequence of decisions. Individuals who are registered donors have articulated their consent to donation long before end-of-life care is contemplated. Accordingly, in the circumstance of first person authorization, the donation decision was made well in advance of, and completely separate from, the discussion to withdraw support. Accordingly, the donation decision is, in cases of first person authorization, effectively decoupled from the end-of-life process. Because first person authorization provides a mechanism to completely separate these decisions, the protocol of approaching families to discuss donation only after a decision to withdraw must be reexamined. A delay of the donation discussion with the family until after withdrawal of support decision is made is no longer necessary to maintain the principle of decoupling.

The delay of a donation discussion may also be unjustified because it impedes fulfilling the substituted judgment standard—what would the patient want—as the central legal requirement for making a surrogate withdrawal of support decision. In cases of first person authorization, patients have already documented their intent and desire to be organ donors. The patient's status as a registered donor may in fact be relevant to the withdrawal decision. In order to honor the patient's donation decision, the withdrawal must be accomplished within timeframe and protocol that will allow for donation to proceed. Thus, it could be argued that the substituted judgment standard applicable to the surrogate decision to withdraw necessitates an awareness of the first person authorization decision by the care team and family at the time the withdrawal discussion occurs.

Financial Neutrality for Living Donors

One of the most significant debates in the field of donation and transplantation revolves around whether financial incentives for living organ donation should be permissible. Under the National Organ Transplant Act (NOTA), the buying and selling of organs is strictly illegal. Payment for reasonable expenses related to the donation of organs is, however, specifically expected out of the legal prohibition. This allows OPOs to be reimbursed for the reasonable costs of facilitating deceased donation and also permits the expenses of living donors to be covered.

The extent to which the law permits payment of living donor expenses has been continually debated from both ethical and legal perspectives. The principle of "financial neutrality" for the living donor is well supported ethically and practically (see Hays et al and Delmonico et al in Selected Readings), but in the context of possible federal criminal prosecution under NOTA for violations, there have been recent legislative efforts to better define what this means from a legal perspective. Specifically, the introduction of the Living Donor Protection Act in 2016 seeks to prohibit denial of coverage or increase in premiums of life or disability insurance for living organ donors; clarify organ donation surgery as qualifying as a serious health condition under the Family Medical Leave Act; and update educational materials on the benefits of live donor transplantation and the process/outcomes of live donation.

Parallel to these widely supported efforts are continual debates as to whether the prohibition in NOTA ought to be repealed in lieu of a market system that would allow direct payments to living donors for organs. The ethical arguments supporting payment for living donors range from the utilitarian (paying for organs will increase the availability of organs reducing the gap between supply and demand and potentially eliminate waitlist deaths for kidneys) to the normative (individuals should have the right to sell and direct use their own body parts). The arguments against lifting the legal prohibition are centered around the significance of the social harms that would result in developing a system that would be coercive to the poor who are assumed to be far more likely to sell a body part and the moral repugnance of permitting body part sales. Many also believe that permitting the development of a financial market in kidneys could in fact lower the availability of other organs or even kidneys by reducing altruistic donations. Finally, the experience worldwide is that kidney sales (legally permitted only in Iran) has in fact led to human rights violations in the form of human trafficking and resulted in significant medical risks with suboptimal outcomes to living donor and recipient.

An alternative for incentivizing donation that is less controversial than monetary payments provides allocation priority for those who have registered as donors. Such an alternative has been adopted in Israel (see Stoler et al. in Selected Readings). Providing some measure of potential future allocation priority to those (and their close family members) who are registered donors is not the same—ethically or legally—as paying for an organ. This has been demonstrated in the United States, for example, through ethical and legal support for kidney-paired exchange programs, and a priority granted for living donors if a transplant is later needed.

The ethical pillar of equity provides support for a system that ties the regulation of consent to organ donation to the regulation of access to transplantation. A nation that calls upon its population to be donors should provide fair access to organs if it expects that consent will be obtained. The reciprocal point also holds. Those that are eligible to receive transplants should be willing to donate. Referred to as "reciprocal altruism," there is a readily understood, simple, ethical parity to such a strategy. It would seemingly reduce inequities while simultaneously broaden access by increasing available organs for transplant over time.

Equity also demands the fair distribution of benefits and burdens of an organ procurement and allocation program. Granting some priority to those who have registered as donors in the allocation of available deceased organs can accomplish this synergy. It is not based on the moral character that some are more deserving than others. Rather, it is the idea that transplantation is a community endeavor that requires community obligation, because it can only be achieved through organ donation. Without organ donation, there can be no transplantation. This is not to suggest that consent and allocation should be tied to the point of over-riding critical factors such as medical need and utility. It is a concept for incentivizing participation in creating a community resource—organs for transplantation—for which everyone would have an opportunity to benefit.

Increasing the Pool of Clinically Suitable Donors: Ethical and Legal Considerations

Preserving the Option of Donation in a Critical Patient

Continuing to treat a patient in the face of unclear medical benefit in part for purposes of preserving the potential for organ donation raises a number of ethical concerns. One concern often articulated by the critical care community is whether such practices present an unacceptable conflict of interest for the healthcare provider who may treat patients within a context of futility for the possible benefit of other patients (those waiting for transplantation). In analyzing this ethical issue, first consider the definition of a conflict. A conflict of interest is generally defined as having three elements: (1) two incompatible interests (2) where the possibility of benefiting one's interest could influence the course of action (3) to the detriment of the other interest. Each of these three elements will be analyzed more fully below.

Two Incompatible Interests.   Continued critical care provided to patients with catastrophic brain injuries may serve multiple interests, but the two primary interests to examine are the patient and the potential organ transplantation recipients. Continued critical care in these cases serves two separate goals by potentially benefiting different patients. Continued critical care that will benefit donation may also medically benefit the patient: The two interests may be viewed as congruent rather than incompatible or in conflict. The physician's ethical duty to the patient is primary but not exclusive from other legitimate purposes (such as supporting the patient's family or providing donor management) to the extent that both interests can be served in a compatible manner. The responsibility for healthcare professionals to deliver care that might not medically benefit the patient is not unique to donation. Examples of this include maintaining a patient on mechanical support at the family's request whether to accommodate certain beliefs or to allow for travel to say "goodbye". These accommodations are usually a matter of days, not weeks or months similar to what preserving the option for donation might require. This is not viewed as incompatible with good patient care, but rather consistent with it.

Possibility of Benefiting One's Interest Could Influence Course of Action.   The second element in a conflict of interest is the possibility that benefiting one's interest will influence a course of action. Physicians manage multiple interests frequently including personal financial interest (payor arrangements) and hospital resource allocation (right of the last bed). There is nothing unique with balancing multiple interests when considering a course of patient care. The treating physician who continues critical care for patients with catastrophic brain injuries does not have the potential for personal or financial gain. The potential benefit from donation accrues to the patient, the donor's family, recipients, and society, not the treating physician.

To the Detriment of the Other Interest.   The final element in a conflict of interest is whether the first two elements lead to a course of action to the detriment of other interests. In the context of providing treatment to preserve the option of donation, there is no clear detriment to the patient because advocating for continuation of aggressive care rather than de-escalation of care may provide medical benefit and, in instances where the patient is a registered donor, promotes the patient's self-determination rights regarding organ donation.

In considering a patient's right to self-determination as it relates to organ donation and the goals of treatment, it is important to understand the broad support for organ donation. The US donation authorization rates are currently around 75%, and, as mentioned above, over 50% of adults are registered donors. This means that almost half of the adult patients in a critical care situation may have already made a legally binding donation decision prior to the hospital admission. Providing critical care to these patients in order to preserve the potential for organ donation supports the patient's autonomy rights and maximizes the utility of their gift through transplantation.

Autonomy considerations are equally compelling when patients are not registered as donors. Both law and ethics recognize that an incapacitated patient's self-determination rights can be exercised by a surrogate. Examples of this include the ability for surrogates to authorize withdrawal of care or to refuse treatment even if it is expected to result in the patient's death. The same principles apply for organ donation. The law provides a list of potential surrogate donation decision makers, which is broad enough to ensure a donation decision can be made. It would be ethically inappropriate to circumvent the donor's exercise of self-determination through a surrogate by medically undermining the potential for organ donation. The law also recognizes this interest by requiring that "measures necessary to ensure the medical suitability" of organs not be withdrawn until a surrogate decision maker has been approached about donation.

Preserving the option of donation is not only a potential benefit to the patient's exercise of autonomy. There are known benefits to the donor families' experience of grief that should be considered in evaluating the potential benefits. Alternatively, for those families who do not want donation, providing the opportunity to make that decision does not represent a harm.

In analyzing these elements and the underlying ethical principles, the primary interests at stake in aggressively treating a patient with a severe brain injury are compatible rather than in conflict.

DETERMINING DEATH: LEGAL DEFINITION AND ETHICAL DEBATE

Historically, the standard for defining death has been the permanent absence of breathing and circulation. Advances in modern medical care allowed certain physiologic functions to be artificially maintained for prolonged periods of time; mechanical ventilators breathe for patients and mechanical assist devices provide artificial circulation. Accordingly, traditional methods to determine death by absence of breathing and circulation were no longer clear or satisfactory.

To address concerns regarding the definition of death, a Presidential Commission was established. In their 1981 report, "Defining Death: A Report on the Medical, Legal and Ethical Issues in the Determination of Death," brain death was formally defined. This commission defined death as either "irreversible cessation of circulatory and respiratory functions; or irreversible cessation of all functions of the entire brain, including the brain stem." They further commented that "a determination of death must be made in accordance with accepted medical standards." This definition of death was reviewed and accepted by multiple national organizations including the American Medical Association, the American Bar Association, the National Conference of Commissioners on Uniform State Laws, the American Academy of Neurology, the American Academy of Pediatrics, the Society of Critical Care Medicine, and the Child Neurology Society. This definition was also adopted into the Uniform Determination of Death Act and has been accepted as law in every state in the country.

Brain Death: High-Profile Cases

Confusion often arises when brain death is compared to severe brain injury. Inexact descriptions of these two vastly different clinical and legal situations have led to misunderstanding of the important distinction between when patients are dead versus when patients have an altered level of consciousness commonly referred to as a coma. Patients with disorders of consciousness from a brain injury may exist in a coma or a persistent vegetative state. Importantly, these patients do not meet the legal criteria for death declaration because they still maintain some capacity of brain function, but their consciousness is not normal. These patients may respond to their environment when stimulated, they may breathe on their own or with mechanical ventilator assistance. They respond to painful stimuli, they may exhibit eye movements, cough, and other primitive reflexes. This is distinct from the brain dead patient who is completely unresponsive to the environment or stimulation and exhibits no brain activity or level of consciousness.

Under the law, patients who meet the medical criteria for brain death have experienced irreversible cessation of all functions of the entire brain, including the brain stem. If there is evidence of neurologic function such as cough and gag reflexes, pupillary reactivity or eye movements, spontaneous breathing, and evidence of electrical activity noted on an electroencephalogram or blood flow noted on a radionuclide cerebral blood flow study, the patient does not meet the legal standard and is not dead.

It is said that "hard cases make bad law." There are recent examples of this regarding brain death, the most notable of which is the case of Jahi McMath. In 2014, Jahi McMath was a 13-year-old who underwent a tonsillectomy. Shortly after the surgery, McMath reportedly suffered from cardiac arrest that led to a complete loss of brain function. McMath was subsequently declared dead on the basis of neurologic criteria. The patient's family, however, rejected the brain death diagnosis and ultimately filed court action to prevent the hospital from removing feeding and breathing tubes. Although the second medical opinion ordered by the court confirmed the brain death diagnosis, the court ultimately ordered the hospital to maintain the artificial support for a defined period in order to allow the family to transfer McMath out of state to a facility willing to continue medical intervention despite the fact that the patient had been declared consistent with medical and legal standards.

The court's actions allowing the prolonged artificial mechanical support of a legally dead patient was troubling and in conflict with the law. Once death is declared, there is no further legal or ethical duty to continue treatments including mechanical support unless organ donation is planned. The law has never required healthcare providers to provide treatment to deceased "patients." Leveraging legal avenues to keep the body of a decedent supported on artificial mechanical support raises difficult ethical issues regarding appropriate use of resources. It also undermines the public's understanding of the legal certainty of "brain death." There is no legal ambiguity; a patient who has been declared dead on the basis of irreversible cessation of all functions of the entire brain consistent with accepted medical standards is deceased under the law.

There are, however, a few states—notably New Jersey and New York—that provide families with the option to reject a death declaration on the basis of neurologic criteria if it is in conflict with sincerely held religious beliefs. This variation in legal standard has created havens in these states for situations such as the McMath case. As a result, there is a movement among some ethicists to reconsider the long-held assumption that a single legal definition of death is required for prudent public policy.

Given the recent cases that have occurred and the reinvigorated ethical debate on defining death, it is prudent for care providers to plan for future cases where there is disagreement between the family and the medical team regarding the declaration of death based on neurological criteria. A second opinion or another examination from a physician versed in determining death based on neurological criteria may help families understand and reinforce that death has occurred consistent with legal requirements. Communicating a consistent message that the patient has died in accordance with legal standards while being sensitive and sympathetic to the family who has suffered a loss is paramount but ultimately may not resolve deeply held differences and understanding of what constitutes death. It should be noted that medical and hospital staff are not at risk if they move forward with organ donation for a registered donor despite the objections of family members. The registration process has the power of a legally executed will.

Increasing the Number of Transplanted Organs per Donor
Clinical Innovation in Deceased Donation

Most efforts associated with clinical advances transplantation have been recipient focused. The future growth in the number of transplantable organs will, however, likely come from donor-focused innovations that increase the viability of organs donated for transplantation. The field of science surrounding donor management or *ex vivo* organ interventions remains in its infancy but has the potential to greatly increase the availability of organs for transplantation by maximizing each donation opportunity.

The need for innovation to the field of transplantation has brought focus to the legal and ethical considerations of conducting research on the clinical management of deceased donors or on repair of the donor organs. Professional confusion over how to apply well-understood principles for living human research subjects in the context of deceased donation has led to inconsistent practices and has been repeatedly cited as a barrier to conduct clinical research (see Glazier et al. in Selected Readings). This has been particularly complicated within the United States, given its legal and regulatory landscape. Issues that need to be addressed include the legally appropriate and ethical authorization to involve deceased donors in research; the application of privacy laws; the oversight and review of deceased donor research; and considerations of when a transplant recipient of organs that had been part of a research protocol becomes a human subject. The successful conduct of clinical research in the field of deceased donation and transplantation requires an understanding of the regulatory and legal nuances as well as identification of the primary ethical principles in order to adhere to preserve the public trust and transparency that are fundamental to donation and transplantation. Facilitation of these concepts will ultimately provide the professional and public support for innovative research designed to increase the availability of organs for transplantation.

ALLOCATING THE TRANSPLANT BENEFIT

There are many legal and ethical considerations related to allocation. The fundamental ethical principles of allocation include ensuring equity by balancing utility and justice. While these principles are well established, debates on how best to titrate those interests remain. In practical terms, the debate over allocation of deceased donor kidneys in the United States is expressed in the Kidney Allocation System (see Chapter 5) in effect since December 2014.

One current focus of debate is the appropriate role of geography in the national system of organ distribution. NOTA specifically requires that only medical criteria be used to allocate organs and the accompanying regulations state that geographic inequities must be minimized. With this federal directive, allocation and distribution polices have, over time, moved away from local geography as a priority. This, however, has resulted in some areas of the country considering legislation that would prohibit movement of organs outside of state boundaries raising an interesting legal issue of whether organ allocation is a matter of federal or state regulation.

The specific legal issue at play is whether the explicit preemption clause in the federal regulations under NOTA (which expressly nullifies inconsistent state laws or regulations regarding organ allocation) is constitutional. A federal agency may preempt state law only if and when it is acting within the scope of congressionally delegated authority. The legal analysis therefore hinges on whether Congress granted the Health and Human Services (HHS) administration "broad and preemptive authority" over organ allocation policy. Although never successfully litigated, arguments have been made in prior court cases that Congress did in fact intend to grant HHS exclusive authority over organ allocation and that is clearly expressed in the legislative history behind NOTA and the so-called Final Rule which, in the year 2000, established a regulatory framework for the structure and operations of the Organ Procurement and Transplantation Network (see Chapter 5).

The core of all this is the understanding of organs as a national resource rather than a local one. This is supported by the ethical directive to maximize utility and justice in the face of explicit rationing of a scare life-saving resource. The best way to meet those ethical directives—as codified in the federal law—is to do soon a national basis within the clinical limitations of organ transport. Restricting allocation to state lines or local designated service areas decreases the efficiency of the system both in terms of lives saved (utility) and fairness to those waiting (justice).

Selected Readings

Capron AM, Delmonico FL, Dominguez-Gil B, et al. Statement of the Declaration of Istanbul Custodian Group regarding payments to families of deceased organ donors. Transplantation 2016;100:2006–2009.

Danovitch GM. The high cost of organ transplant commercialism. Kidney Int 2014;85:248.

Delmonico FL, Martin D, Dominguez-Gil B, et al. Living and deceased organ donation should be financially neutral acts. Am J Transplant 2015;15:1187–1191.

Glazier A, Heffernan K, Rodrigue J. A framework for conducting deceased donor research in the United States. Transplantation 2015;99:2252.

Guidelines for the determination of death. Report of the medical consultants on the diagnosis of death to the President's Commission for the Study of Ethical Problems in Medicine and Biomedical and Behavioral Research. JAMA 1981;246:2184.

Hays R, Rodrigue J, Cohen D, et al. Financial neutrality for living organ donors: reasoning, rationale, definitions, and implementation strategies. Am J Transplant 2016;16:1973–1981.

Ross L, Thistlewaite J. The 1966 Ciba symposium on transplantation ethics: 50 years later. Transplantation 2016;100:1191–1197.

Ross L, Veatch, Parker W, et al. Equal opportunity supplemented by fair innings: equity and efficiency in allocating deceased donor kidneys. Am J Transplant 2012;12:2015.

Souter MJ, Blissitt PA, Blosser S, et al. Recommendations for the critical care management of devastating brain injury: prognostication, psychosocial and ethical management. A position statement for healthcare professionals from the neurocritical care society. Neurocritical Care 2015;23:4.

Stoler A, Askenazi T, Kessler J, et al. Incentivizing authorization for deceased organ donation with organ allocation priority: the first five years. Am J Transplant 2016;16:2639–2645.

Nutrition in Kidney Transplant Candidates

Mareena George and Susan Weil Ernst

Nutrition plays an integral role in the optimization of outcome in kidney transplant recipients in the pre- and post-transplantation phases of care. Dietary interventions may prevent or improve morbid conditions. As the field of transplantation has progressed, nutrition recommendations continue to evolve. Nutrition management across all three phases of transplantation, including pre-transplantation, acute post-transplantation, and long-term post-transplantation will be discussed in the sections to follow.

PRE-TRANSPLANTATION NUTRITION MANAGEMENT

While patients remain on dialysis, comorbidities often ensue, affecting transplant candidacy. Preexisting comorbidities may persist after transplantation. Efforts should be made to correct or improve nutrition-related concerns such as obesity, dyslipidemia, malnutrition, and bone mineral disorders. Optimization of nutritional status may enhance kidney transplantation outcomes.

Nutrition-Related Concerns
Obesity
Obesity is characterized as excessive body fat. It is associated with cardiovascular disease, diabetes, hypertension, and other chronic conditions. Though body mass index (BMI) is often used to classify patients as obese, it does not consider body fat distribution or musculature. The expression "obesity paradox" refers to the counterintuitive finding that obesity in patients with chronic kidney disease (CKD) appears to provide protective advantages and even survival benefit, such that recommendations for weight loss in transplant candidates should be made with great care. Any such recommendations should be made under the supervision of a CKD-trained dietitian.

BMI is often used, perhaps sometimes misused, when evaluating kidney transplant candidates. The topic is controversial. Though it has long been presumed that obese individuals (especially class II and III obese individuals with a BMI >35) have worse post-transplant outcomes, the reverse may in fact be true. Improvements in survival for obese patients post-transplant have also been described.

Post-transplantation, obesity is correlated with wound infection and dehiscence, incisional hernia, increased operation duration, new onset diabetes, increased length of hospital stay, delayed graft function, and hypertension. Potential kidney transplant recipients with obesity should be informed of the risks associated with obesity and counseled on lifestyle changes to aid in weight management.

Though the impact of obesity on the post-transplant course is controversial, it seems clear that BMI should not be solely relied upon as a determinant of transplant suitability, particularly for individuals with large lean body mass or musculature. Central obesity and weight distribution should also be considered together with physical fitness and cardiac risk factors. Waist circumference, waist-to-hip ratios, or body composition measurements may be used to better assess obesity in transplant candidates. Waist circumference >102 cm in men or >88 cm in women and waist-to-hip ratios >0.95 in men or >0.85 in women are considered risk factors for cardiovascular events. Fixed BMI limits are probably not justified as determinants of transplant candidacy though patients with a BMI of >40 should be approved for transplantation selectively. The topic is further discussed in Chapter 8.

Bariatric surgery may be considered to aid in weight loss. It has been shown to be the most effective method for weight loss. Bariatric surgery has been studied in the dialysis population and has been deemed to be safe. Ninety-day mortality following bariatric surgery in the pre- and post-kidney transplant population is comparable to that of the general population. Of note, there is a concern for alterations in pharmacokinetics among patients who have undergone bariatric surgery. Potential for malabsorption should be considered when choosing a bariatric procedure. Immunosuppression levels should be closely monitored.

Malnutrition and Frailty

Inferior transplant outcomes are observed with malnutrition. When evaluating effects of BMI on transplant outcomes, a J-shaped curve has been observed, showing worse outcomes with both underweight and morbidly obese patients. Low BMI ($<18.5 \text{ kg/m}^2$) has been associated with increased mortality and death-censored graft loss. In 2012, the Academy of Nutrition and Dietetics and the American Society of Parenteral and Enteral Nutrition reached a consensus in identifying malnutrition. Malnutrition can be diagnosed if an individual meets two of the following six criteria: insufficient energy intake, unintentional weight loss, loss of muscle mass, loss of subcutaneous fat, localized or generalized fluid accumulation that may sometimes mask weight loss, and diminished functional status.

In the chronically ill dialysis population, the serum albumin level is commonly measured as a nutrition marker. However, it may not be a reliable nutrition indicator during the acute phase of illness since its value may fall in the face of infection and inflammation. The albumin level has been shown to be a powerful predictor of mortality and morbidity in the dialysis population and in a large cohort of transplant patients, every 0.2 g/dL higher pre-transplant serum albumin was associated with 13% lower all-cause mortality, 17% lower cardiovascular mortality, 7% lower combined risk of death or graft failure, and 4% lower delayed graft function risk.

Similar to malnutrition, "frailty" refers to a manifestation of unintentional weight loss, sarcopenia, weakness, reduced activity, exhaustion, and slow ambulation. Regardless of age, frailty is a risk factor for adverse kidney transplant outcomes, such as increased length of hospital stay, early hospital readmissions following transplantation, delayed graft function, and mortality. Frailty and malnutrition should be considered when evaluating potential transplant candidates (see Chapter 8). Efforts should be made to optimize nutritional and functional status in the process of preparing for transplantation.

CKD-Associated Mineral and Bone Disorders

Alterations in metabolism of vitamin D, parathyroid hormone (PTH), and associated minerals occur as a result of CKD. Mineral and bone disorders are seen widely in CKD patients. Soft-tissue and vascular calcifications may lead to vascular complexities during the surgical operation. Severe vascular calcification may exclude patients as transplant candidates because of the absence of viable sites for vascular anastomosis. Additionally, following transplantation, use of steroids and calcineurin inhibitors contributes to decline in bone mineral density. In conjunction with renal osteodystrophy pre-transplant, risk of fracture and bone disease post-transplantation may be exacerbated. To minimize suboptimal outcomes, bone and mineral disorders should be addressed prior to transplantation.

Nutrition Assessment for the Transplant Candidate

Transplant candidates are required to be nutritionally assessed by a registered dietitian prior to transplantation according to the formal guidelines of the Centers for Medicare and Medicaid Services. The dietitian focuses on nutrition aspects of the patient's care, such as malnutrition, obesity, bone disease, metabolic parameters, and gastrointestinal issues.

The following aspects should be included as part of the nutrition assessment in the pre-transplantation candidate:

- History—comorbid conditions, medications, diet history/nutrition intake and adequacy, gastrointestinal issues, food allergies and dietary intolerances, weight history, functional status
- Anthropometric and nutrition-focused physical findings—body weight, weight changes, percent of standard body weight, height, body frame size, BMI, waist circumference, waist-to-hip ratio, fat distribution, triceps skinfold, muscle wasting, and micronutrient deficiencies
- Biochemical parameters—albumin, prealbumin, C-reactive protein, glucose, hemoglobin A1C, ferritin, transferrin saturation (TSAT), hemoglobin, PTH, vitamin D 25-hydroxy, calcium, phosphorus, potassium, lipid profile.

Additionally, factors such as adherence to phosphate binders, dietary restrictions, fluid restrictions, and dialysis treatments may help to determine a patient's adherence to their medical regime. The patient's laboratory data, interdialytic weight gains, and blood pressure records should be available for review. Poor adherence pre-transplantation may be an indication of non-adherence postoperatively, which may pose a risk to the patient as well as the outcome of the transplant (see Chapter 8).

POST-TRANSPLANTATION NUTRITION CARE

Immediate Post-Transplant Nutrition Requirements

The immediate post-transplantation period generally refers to the first 6 weeks postoperatively. Nutrition requirements during this acute period call for increased protein needs owing to the stress of surgery, administration of corticosteroids, and wound healing. Fluid and micronutrient requirements will vary depending upon graft function and biochemical parameters.

In this section, recommendations are listed per kilogram of actual body weight for underweight and normal weight individuals. For obese individuals, it is not unreasonable to use an adjusted weight to estimate nutrition needs. Table 20.1 summarizes post-transplant nutrient recommendations in the immediate transplant period.

Calories

Recommended energy intake is 30 to 35 kcal/kg of body weight or 1.3 to 1.5 × basal energy expenditure determined by the Harris–Benedict equation. Underweight patients are advised to consume the upper end of the calorie range, whereas the obese patients are advised the lower end of the range.

Protein

To overcome the effect of protein catabolism observed with use of corticosteroids, increased protein intake is required. Additionally, surgical stress and wound healing necessitate relatively high protein needs. Available studies involving post-kidney transplant protein

TABLE 20.1	Recommended Daily Nutrition Requirements in the Immediate Post-Transplantation Period
Nutrient	**Recommended Daily Requirement in the Immediate Post-Transplantation Period**
Calories	30–35 kcal/kg of body weight or 1.3–1.5 × basal energy expenditure
Protein	1.3–2 g protein/kg of body weight
Carbohydrate	50%–60% of daily energy requirements; limit simple sugars if hyperglycemia is present
Fat	25%–35% of daily energy requirements or remainder of calories
Fluids	Individualized; in the oliguric patient with DGF*, urine output + 500–700 mL to account of insensible losses
Sodium	Individualized; generally 2–4 g/day
Potassium	Individualized based on serum potassium levels; generally 2–4 g/day
Phosphorus	Individualized based on graft function and serum phosphorus levels; supplementation often required
Calcium	Individualized; generally 1,200–1,500 mg daily
Magnesium	Individualized based on serum magnesium levels; supplementation may be required

*DGF: Delayed Graft Function

requirements are limited. With the available evidence, it is reasonable to conclude that 1.3 to 2 g of protein per kilogram of body weight will lead to neutral or positive nitrogen balance.

Carbohydrate

Calories from carbohydrate sources should constitute about 50% to 60% of daily energy requirements. Dietary modifications controlling carbohydrate intake should be enforced in diabetics and hyperglycemic individuals. Recipients with diet controlled diabetes or those on oral glycemic agents prior to transplantation may require insulin postoperatively. Post-transplant diabetes (see Chapter 11) may occur as a result of corticosteroids, immunosuppression, preexisting obesity, post-transplant weight gain, and other non-modifiable risk factors, such as family history of diabetes, and ethnicity (see below). Persistent hyperglycemic individuals should be counseled by a registered dietitian on a carbohydrate-controlled diet and may require insulin.

Fat

Keeping in line with the National Heart, Lung, and Blood Institute Adult Treatment Panel III guidelines, 25% to 35% of total calories should come from fat. More importantly, in long-term post-transplant patient, dietary modifications addressing dyslipidemia are advised. Experimental evidence suggests that hyperlipidemia may promote transplant rejection.

Fluids

Fluid needs are dependent upon kidney function. Generally speaking, in a normovolemic recipient with a well-functioning graft, a reasonable minimum fluid intake is 2,000 mL/day. Oliguric individuals with delayed graft function should require the volume of urine output plus 500 to 750 mL to account for insensible losses. Variations should be determined by volume status and blood pressure, typically erring on the positive side, as urine output increases.

Sodium

In individuals who are hypertensive and who have extra-cellular fluid volume expansion, it is appropriate to limit daily sodium intake to 2 g/day. Although intake of sodium should be moderate, normotensive recipients who are edema free do not require sodium restriction. Hypotensive patients may be asked to increase sodium intake.

Potassium

Hyperkalemia is commonly observed in kidney transplant recipients. This may be resultant of diminished potassium excretion associated with calcineurin inhibitor use, suppression of aldosterone levels, impaired graft function, acidosis, or use of angiotensin-converting enzyme inhibitors, potassium-sparing diuretics, or potassium-containing phosphorus supplements. If hyperkalemia is present, potassium restriction is warranted. Hypokalemia is seen less often; however, it may occur with potassium-wasting diuretics and occasional cases of previously unrecognized adrenal adenomas.

Phosphorus

Hypophosphatemia is a common phenomenon that occurs postoperatively, especially in recipients with a well-functioning graft. Contributing factors include reduced intestinal absorption of phosphorus, reduced tubular phosphate reabsorption, increased phosphaturia as a result of increased levels of fibroblast growth factor-23 (FGF-23), and persistent hyperparathyroidism. Hypophosphatemia may persist even after PTH levels normalize, which supports the idea that post-transplant hypophosphatemia may be largely due to FGF-23, which accumulates in CKD. FGF-23 decreases the expression of type 1 sodium–phosphate co-transporter in the proximal tubule and accelerates phosphaturia. It also inhibits calcitriol synthesis by downregulating the expression of 1-alpha-hydroxylase.

Patients with hypophosphatemia should be encouraged to increase intake of phosphorus-containing foods. Often times, oral supplementation, and in some cases intravenous phosphate repletion, is necessary. Table 20.2 lists some available phosphorus supplementation preparations.

In the presence of delayed graft function with hyperphosphatemia, phosphate binders may be warranted. Of note, there is an interaction between both sevelamer- and calcium-based phosphate binders and mycophenolate, whereby mycophenolic acid levels may be lowered. Thus, caution should be used when both medications are prescribed.

Calcium

A decline in serum calcium is often observed postoperatively. The calcium then trends upward approximately 1 to 2 weeks after transplantation. Post-transplant hypocalcemia may be resultant of FGF-23-mediated suppression of calcitriol synthesis, impaired graft function, suppression of calcium reabsorption, low-bone turnover due to low serum PTH levels, or volume expansion triggered by high doses of corticosteroids and multiple transfusions. In some cases, calcium repletion is necessary as hypocalcemia may predispose patients to muscle cramps and arrhythmias. The recommended intake for calcium is 1,200 to 1,500 mg daily.

In patients with hypercalcemia, the underlying cause should be determined and treated accordingly. In these patients, vitamin D supplementation should be avoided.

TABLE 20.2	Commercially Available Phosphorus Supplementation Preparations		
Supplement or Preparation	**Phosphorus Content**	**Potassium Content**	**Sodium Content**
K-Phos neutral (tablet)	8 mmol (247 mg)	1.1 mEq (43 mg)	13 mEq (298 mg)
Neutra-Phos (capsule/packet)	8 mmol (247 mg)	7.1 mEq (278 mg)	7.1 mEq (164 mg)
Neutra-Phos K (capsule/ packet)	8 mmol (247 mg)	14.25 mEq (557 mg)	7.1 mEq (164 mg)
Potassium phosphate IV (mL)	3 mmol	4.4 mEq	0
Sodium phosphate IV (mL)	3 mmol	0	4 mEq

Vitamin D

A growing body of evidence demonstrates high prevalence of vitamin D deficiency and insufficiency in the kidney transplant population. Decline in bone mineral density may occur following transplantation owing to corticosteroid and immunosuppressant use, as well as persistent hyperparathyroidism. In the section to follow, mineral and bone disorders in the post-transplant patient will be discussed.

Magnesium

Hypomagnesemia commonly occurs following transplantation as a result of calcineurin inhibitor–induced magnesuria. Generally, oral supplementation is recommended when the magnesium levels are less than 1.5 mg/dL and intravenous supplementation when levels are less than 1.0 mg/dL. Magnesium supplementation should be administered 2 hours post mycophenolate administration to avoid a nutrient–drug interaction. Hypomagnesemia has been associated with impaired glucose metabolism and post-transplant diabetes, with improvement after supplementation.

Iron

Iron stores may be depleted in the post-transplant period as a result of surgical blood loss, frequent lab draws, and use of iron stores for erythropoiesis. Iron deficiency exacerbates anemia in the early post-transplant period. Preoperative evaluation of iron status and correction of iron deficiency immediately post-transplantation is indicated to reduce severity of anemia. As recommended by the KDIGO (Kidney Disease: Improving Global Outcomes) guidelines, intravenous iron therapy should be administered to individuals with transferrin saturation below 30% and ferritin less than 500 ng/mL.

Other Micronutrients

In patients undergoing dialysis, micronutrients may be lost during the dialysis process, in which case supplementation is warranted. The efficacy of routine supplementation of water-soluble vitamins after the patient no longer requires dialysis has not been well studied. In the past, there has been much attention on homocysteine, folic acid, vitamin B_{12}, and vitamin B_6 (pyridoxine). Elevated homocysteine levels are correlated with adverse cardiovascular outcomes. Hyperhomocysteinemia is also associated with low folic acid, vitamin B_{12}, and pyridoxine levels, and supplementation of these vitamins does lower homocysteine levels though has not been shown to reduce adverse cardiac outcomes.

Nutrition Support

Nutrition support encompasses oral, enteral, and parenteral nutrition therapy for individuals unable to maintain adequate nutrition intake through eating and drinking. In the typical uncomplicated transplant course, the patient is well enough to eat solid foods within the first 1 to 2 days postoperatively. Enteral and parenteral nutrition are not commonly indicated immediately following kidney transplantation. In some cases, nutrition support is warranted, especially in malnourished individuals or patients with complications, who may remain intubated or unable to utilize their gastrointestinal tract.

When to Feed Postoperatively

Feeding the patient by postoperative day 1 has been found to be safe and beneficial. Early postoperative feeding (defined as liquids or solid food within 24 hours) following surgery is associated with shorter time to presence of bowel sound, faster onset of flatus, reduced hospital length of stay, fewer infectious complications, and greater patient satisfaction. Along with early feeding, a bowel regimen may be helpful, as many individuals experience opioid-induced constipation postoperatively.

Choice of Feeding Modality

Oral Supplements

Protein needs are high in the immediate postoperative period. Optimal nutrition is essential for recovery. For individuals unable to meet nutrition requirements via diet alone, an oral nutrition supplement may be indicated to augment intake. Recipients with a well-functioning graft and acceptable electrolyte values may use a standard oral nutrition supplement. Those with delayed graft function, hyperphosphatemia, and/or hyperkalemia may require a kidney disease-specific nutrition supplement, or a supplement lower in potassium and phosphorus. Correctable causes for inadequate oral intake may include an overly restricted diet, unnecessarily slow progression to a solid food diet, or interference of meals due to schedules procedures, tests, or dialysis treatments.

Enteral Nutrition

Though tube feeding is rarely required following kidney transplantation, it may be deemed necessary if it is difficult to maintain adequate protein and calories via oral intake. If the gastrointestinal tract is functioning, tube feeding should be used over parenteral nutrition to maintain gut integrity, prevent intestinal bacterial overgrowth, and reduce risk of infection. In cases of delayed graft function, hyperkalemia, or hyperphosphatemia, a kidney disease–specific enteral formula may be appropriate. Otherwise, a standard formula may be used.

So-called "immune-modulating" formulas contain arginine, glutamine, omega-3 fatty acids, and antioxidants. Immunonutrients have been reported to reduce infectious complications in the perioperative oncology patient population, though their efficacy and safety in the kidney transplant population have not been substantiated. Their use is not recommended.

Parenteral Nutrition

Inability to absorb adequate nutrients through the gastrointestinal tract for a period greater than 5 days mandates use of parenteral nutrition. A central venous catheter is needed for total parenteral nutrition (TPN). In instances where parenteral nutrition is required for a short period, under 2 weeks, peripheral parenteral nutrition, or PPN, may be used. To avoid thrombophlebitis, the osmolarity of PPN admixtures should not exceed 900 mOsm/L. Thus, PPN requires significant volume to maintain a safe osmotic load to the peripheral vein. Protein and energy requirements are dependent on a number of factors such as whether the patient is catabolic, under physical stress, or dialysis dependent.

Post-Transplant Nutrition Concerns
Nutrient–Drug Interactions
Potential food–drug interactions should be avoided. The following fruits interfere with the metabolism of immunosuppressant medication: grapefruit, pomelo, seville orange (also known as bitter orange), pomegranate, and star fruit. Furanocoumarin derivatives found in grapefruit, pomelo, and seville orange have been found to inhibit cytochrome P-450 CYP3A4 isozyme and P-glycoprotein. Contents of pomegranate and star fruit also have an inhibitory effect on the catalytic activity of CYP3A4. Therefore, ingestion of these fruits will lead to elevated tacrolimus, cyclosporine, or sirolimus levels. Additionally, star fruit should be avoided in individuals with impaired renal function, as ingestion has been associated with neurological symptoms and death. Table 20.3 lists nutritional side effects of immunosuppressive agents.

Herbal Supplements
Use of herbal or botanical supplements for therapeutic or medicinal purposes has become a common trend. In the United States, dietary supplements do not require approval from the FDA prior to being marketed. This poses a serious risk for consumers as many products available on the market lack safety and efficacy. In addition to lacking scientific evidence, dietary supplements may vary in composition and

TABLE 20.3	Nutritional Side Effects of Immunosuppressive Agents
Agent	**Side Effect**
Corticosteroids	Polyphagia, glucose intolerance, hyperlipidemia, osteoporosis, gastritis and peptic ulcer disease, fluid retention, hypertension, protein catabolism, altered mood
Tacrolimus	Anemia, leukocytosis, hypertension, hyperglycemia, hyperkalemia or hypokalemia, hyperuricemia, hypomagnesemia, nausea, abdominal pain, gas, vomiting, anorexia, constipation, diarrhea, leukopenia
Cyclosporine	Nephrotoxicity, neurotoxicity, hypertension, glucose intolerance, hyperlipidemia, hyperkalemia, hypomagnesemia, hyperuricemia, gingival hypertrophy
Sirolimus	Hypertriglyceridemia, hypercholesterolemia, thrombocytopenia, leukopenia, hypokalemia, delayed wound healing (at high doses); diabetogenic
Azathioprine	Leukopenia, thrombocytopenia, megaloblastic anemia, nausea and vomiting, hepatic dysfunction
Mycophenolate mofetil	Anorexia, nausea, epigastric pain, gas, diarrhea, abdominal pain
Thymoglobulin	Chills, fever, leukopenia, thrombocytopenia, hyperglycemia (rare), diarrhea, nausea, vomiting

concentration and may be contaminated or purposely adulterated. There have been reports of heavy metals such as lead, mercury, and arsenic, as well as pharmaceutical drugs, found in botanical supplement preparations. Additionally, the majority of existing supplements have not been well studied in the kidney transplant population. Bearing this in mind, kidney transplant recipients should be advised to avoid herbal supplements.

According to a national health survey, the top 10 most common dietary supplements include fish oil, glucosamine, echinacea, flaxseed oil, ginseng, ginkgo biloba, chondroitin, garlic supplements, co enzyme Q-10, and fiber. Surveys reveal that the majority of individuals do not disclose use of dietary supplements to healthcare providers. This is concerning as many supplements have the potential to interfere with medications. For example, St. John's Wort, which is used to treat depression, induces CYP3A4 and upregulates P-glycoprotein expression, thereby causing subtherapeutic tacrolimus or cyclosporine trough levels. Herbal preparations with concentrated amounts of furanocoumarins or various flavonoids such as naringin, naringenin, catechins, and quercetin should be avoided as they have been shown to have inhibitory effects on CYP3A4.

In the kidney transplant population is the use of botanicals that may cause hyperkalemia. Some of which include noni juice, dandelion, stinging nettle, horsetail, and alfalfa. Dandelion, stinging nettle, and alfalfa may have a diuretic effect. Additionally, licorice root (*Glycyrrhiza glabra*) has been known to have an aldosterone-like effect, causing sodium and fluid retention.

Multiple supplements on the market claim to boost the immune system. In theory, while transplant recipients are on immune-suppressing medication, taking an immune-enhancing supplement is counterintuitive and therefore should be avoided until further research validates safety and efficacy of use in the transplant population.

Probiotics

Probiotics have gained much attention over the past decade and use of pre- and probiotics have become increasingly widespread. Probiotics are microorganisms, which confer health benefits to the host such as improving gastrointestinal barrier function, maintaining optimal pH at the mucosal barrier, and regulating immune response to infectious organisms. Prebiotics are non-digestible carbohydrates that promote the growth of beneficial bacteria. In the liver transplant population, a combination of prebiotics and probiotics either before or shortly after liver transplantation resulted in a significant reduction of overall infection rates.

It is important to point out that there are numerous species and strains of bacteria. Safety and efficacy must be evaluated separately for each strain or combination of strains. Data remain inconclusive, and accordingly, the risks and benefits must to be considered very carefully when pondering use of a probiotic. Caution should be taken against use of *Saccharomyces boulardii*, a yeast not normally found in gut microflora. There have been cases of fungemia after use of *S. boulardii*, and thus it should be avoided in the immunocompromised patient.

Alcohol

Presently, there are no formal recommendations from KDIGO regarding alcohol consumption in the kidney transplant population. In practice, kidney transplant recipients are typically advised to avoid alcohol consumption in the early transplant period to prevent potential medication interactions and promote adherence to the medication regimen. Alcohol abuse is rare following kidney transplantation. Moderate alcohol consumption (10 to 30 g/day) has been associated with a lower risk of post-transplant diabetes and metabolic syndrome. Individuals with liver disease should avoid alcohol, but alcohol in moderate quantities is not nephrotoxic. Patients are often misinformed regarding the toxicity of alcohol and should not be concerned about use in moderation if they so desire. Prescribed medications should be screened for drug and alcohol interactions, and the transplant recipient should be educated accordingly.

Food Safety

Immunosuppressed kidney transplant recipients have an increased risk for contracting food-borne illness. Food pathogens, which may lead to serious illness in immune compromised patients, include: *Listeria monocytogenes*, *Salmonella*, *Campylobacter jejuni*, *Vibrio vulnificus*, *Cryptosporidium*, noroviruses, and *Toxoplasma gondii*. In severe cases of life-threatening illness, immunosuppression may need to be withdrawn. To mitigate risk, recipients should be educated on safe food handling and preparation techniques, proper hand washing, and food storage. Additionally, avoidance of high-risk foods should be stressed. "High-risk" foods that serve as a vehicle for pathogens include unpasteurized milk and soft cheeses, raw or undercooked meat, poultry, eggs, and seafood, cured or processed deli meat that has not been reheated, and raw sprouts. It is prudent for transplant recipients to observe food safety practices outlined by the US Department of Agriculture. Patient resources regarding food safety are available at: http://www.fda.gov/downloads/Food/FoodborneIllnessContaminants/UCM312793.pdf.

PTDM/NODAT

The terms "Post-Transplant Diabetes" (PTDM) and "New Onset Diabetes After Transplant" (NODAT) are interchange (see Chapter 11). Many, but not all, cases of NODAT actually have evidence of pre-transplant diabetes or risk factors for diabetes. NODAT is defined using the same criteria as for non-transplant patients (symptoms of diabetes plus random plasma glucose ≥ 200 mg/dL, fasting plasma glucose ≥ 126 mg/dL, or 2-hour plasma glucose ≥ 200 mg/dL during an oral glucose tolerance test). Adverse associations observed with NODAT include negative impact on patient survival, decreased long-term allograft survival, increased infections, and diabetic complications. Non-modifiable risk factors for NODAT include age, family history, African American or Hispanic ancestry, male donor, autosomal-dominant polycystic kidney disease, HLA mismatches, acute rejection history, hepatitis C virus infection, and *Cytomegalovirus* infection. Modifiable risk factors include weight gain, obesity, and use of glucocorticoids, calcineurin inhibitors (tacrolimus more than cyclosporine), and mTOR inhibitors (see Chapter 6). In the registration studies for belatacept, the incidence of post-transplant diabetes was 5% compared to 10% for those receiving cyclosporine (see Chapter 6).

Dietary counseling is central in managing glycemic control. Referral to a registered dietitian and certified diabetes educator should be established. Weight management, exercise, and dose adjustment of corticosteroids are also important considerations. Insulin or oral glycemic agents are often indicated when euglycemia is unattainable hypoglycemic diet and lifestyle changes alone.

Weight Gain

Weight gain following transplantation is common. The average weight gain is approximately 10% of body weight within the first year post-transplantation and is predominantly adipose tissue rather than muscle mass. Excessive caloric intake commonly occurs due to an enhanced appetite related to corticosteroids, liberation of dietary restrictions, and an increased sense of well-being. Although weight gain may be beneficial in underweight or malnourished individuals, weight gain in overweight and obese recipients should be avoided. As with the general population, obesity may contribute to dyslipidemia, cardiovascular disease, diabetes, and hypertension.

Interventions may include frequent dietary counseling, an exercise program, and behavior modification. Lifestyle interventions and counseling by a dietitian should be initiated early on; frequent follow up is imperative for efficacious outcomes. Severely obese individuals may consider bariatric surgery. Early experience suggests that it is safe and highly effective in transplant recipients.

Bone Disease

Decline in bone mineral density occurs in the first 12 months following transplantation, with the most rapid decline occurring during the first 6 months. Kidney transplant patients are at an increased risk for bone fractures as compared to individuals on dialysis. Factors affecting bone mineral density include preexisting bone disease, glucocorticoids, immunosuppressant medication, and alterations in calcium, vitamin D, and phosphorus. Glucocorticoids may induce suppression of bone formation by increasing osteoclast resorption as well as osteoclastogenesis, decreasing osteoblast activity, and reducing intestinal absorption of calcium. Bone biopsy remains to be the gold standard for classification of post-transplant bone disease. Though not always feasible, bone biopsy is an important consideration to assist in selecting appropriate therapy, especially in individuals with fractures or unexplained hypercalcemia. Adynamic bone disease is the most commonly found bone abnormality and may be exacerbated by bisphosphonates.

Much of the literature on prevention of bone loss shows some benefit to the use of vitamin D or analogues with or without calcium supplementation, as well as bisphosphonates. KDIGO and KDOQI (Kidney Disease Outcomes Quality Initiative) recommendations for evaluation and treatment for bone disease in the transplant population are available. Recipients are encouraged to acquire calcium and vitamin D via dietary sources to meet recommended daily intake requirements, and exercise should be encouraged. Resistance training has been shown to be effective in improving bone mineral density in non-kidney solid organ transplant recipients; there are no published data to date in the kidney transplant population.

Cardiovascular Disease/Dyslipidemia

Cardiovascular disease continues to be the leading cause of mortality among kidney transplant recipients. Contributing factors of cardiovascular disease include dyslipidemia, obesity, diabetes, hypertension, advanced age, male sex, and smoking. Dyslipidemia affects the majority of adult recipients and is defined as the presence of one or more of the following: total serum cholesterol >200 mg/dL, LDL-cholesterol >130 mg/dL, triglycerides >150 mg/dL, or HDL-cholesterol <40 mg/dL. Dyslipidemia may be influenced by use of cyclosporine, sirolimus, corticosteroids, excessive alcohol intake, obesity, nephrotic syndrome, chronic liver disease, and physical inactivity. It may make the transplant more susceptible to episodes of rejection.

Dietary interventions should be aimed to reduce risk of cardiovascular illness. Inclusion in the diet of whole grains, legumes, nuts, seeds, vegetables, fruits, monounsaturated fatty acids, and limiting saturated and trans fats has been found to be beneficial in reducing levels of cholesterol and triglycerides. Recommendations from the therapeutic lifestyle changes (TLC) diet for adults with CKD suggest less than 7% of calories to be derived from saturated fat, less than 200 mg of cholesterol intake per day, and 25% to 35% of calories should be obtained from fat. The TLC diet also emphasizes incorporating 20 to 30 g of fiber, with 5 to 10 g coming from soluble fiber. Physical activity is particularly important and should be repeatedly stressed. Overweight individuals should aim to lose weight. Weight loss may lower LDL and total cholesterol.

Hypertension

Most kidney transplant recipients have hypertension or are on antihypertensive medications at some time in their course. Elevated blood pressure puts individuals at risk for cardiovascular morbidity and mortality, and chronic allograft injury. Dietary sodium restriction has been shown to lower blood pressure in the CKD population and sodium intake is positively correlated with blood pressure in the CKD, and kidney transplantation population. Hence control of sodium intake may lead to improvement in blood pressure in transplant recipients. Sodium intake recommendations should be individualized, as not all transplant recipients require a salt restricted diet. Weight loss and exercise also may play a role in lowering of blood pressure. The Dietary Approaches to Stop Hypertension (DASH) diet, which emphasizes fruits, vegetables, low-fat dairy products, and whole grains, has been effective in improving blood pressure in the non-transplant population but has not been proven to be effective in renal transplant recipients who were counseled on the DASH diet.

Progression of Renal Disease in Kidney Transplant Patients

Nutrition therapy for individuals with a long-term failing kidney transplant has not been well studied, though available literature suggests that protein restriction may reduce proteinuria. Although the ideal amount of protein intake for long-term kidney transplant recipients remains unclear, a daily intake of 0.6 to 0.9 g of protein per kilogram of body weight has been suggested. There is evidence that red meat may increase the risk of ESKD.

Nutrition Requirements in the Long-Term Post-Transplantation Period
Macronutrients
Caloric requirements should be aimed to maintain desirable body weight. For overweight individuals requiring weight reduction, a reasonable caloric intake would be 25 Cal/kg of ideal body weight.

The ideal long-term protein requirement remains to be determined and are discussed above. In individuals with progression of kidney disease, protein restriction may be advised.

Carbohydrate food sources should be obtained primarily from complex carbohydrates, rich in fiber. Fiber-rich foods may assist with improvement of glucose and cholesterol levels. Limitation of simple sugars is advised for optimal glycemic control, especially in individuals with diabetes.

Fat should comprise up to 35% of total calories. Limitation of saturated fats and avoidance of trans fats may improve dyslipidemia. Optimal food sources of fatty acids include monounsaturated and polyunsaturated fatty acids. Balanced ratios of omega-3 and omega-6 fatty acids may reduce inflammation.

Sodium
As previously stated, the majority of kidney transplant patients are hypertensive. These individuals should limit sodium intake to 2 g daily. In normotensive, non-edematous recipients, a strict low-sodium diet is unnecessary. As kidney function declines, a sodium-restricted diet may be advised. Chronically hypotensive patients, without severe cardiac or liver disease or nephrotic-range proteinuria, should be encouraged to eat a high-salt diet or may prefer salt in tablet form.

Potassium
Hyperkalemic individuals should limit potassium intake 2 to 4 g daily. Otherwise, potassium is generally not restricted. Potassium recommendations under "Immediate Post Transplant Nutrition Requirements" continue to apply in this setting.

Calcium, Phosphorus, Vitamin D
Recommended calcium intake ranges from 800 to 1,500 mg/day. This amount includes dietary and supplement sources. Calcidiol, or 25-hydroxyvitamin D, levels should be measured, and insufficiency or deficiency should be treated accordingly. Type of vitamin D therapy remains unclear. It is reasonable to use calcitriol in individuals with a GFR below 30 mL/min. Hypophosphatemia and hypercalcemia may persist. Though not entirely explained by PTH levels, residual hyperparathyroidism should be addressed. In chronic allograft nephropathy, hyperphosphatemia and other manifestations of renal bone mineral disorders should be treated using guidelines for stage 3 and 4 CKD.

Magnesium

Renal loss of magnesium due to inhibited uptake of magnesium in the distal convoluted tubule is the most potent cause of hypomagnesemia. It may persist in the long-term post-transplantation period, and supplementation may be required. As mentioned previously, hypomagnesemia has been associated with impaired glucose metabolism.

Vitamins

There is a lack of evidence to suggest routine multivitamin supplementation in the kidney transplant patient. The bulk of micronutrient literature in this population exams the effect of vitamin B_{12}, folic acid, and pyridoxine on homocysteine levels as well the effect of vitamin D supplementation on bone and mineral disorders. As previously mentioned, supplementation of vitamin B_{12}, folate, and pyridoxine does lower homocysteine levels, but adverse cardiac outcomes are not reduced. Emphasis on a well-balanced and varied diet incorporating an array of micronutrients should be stressed. Individuals who have undergone bariatric surgery should continue on a multivitamin to avoid potential micronutrient deficiencies.

Exercise

Exercise may reduce the risk of cardiovascular morbidity, control weight, and improve blood pressure, insulin sensitivity, and lipids. Recommended daily physical activity for the general population is 30 minutes of moderate to vigorous exercise 5 days per week. There are currently no specific guidelines for exercise in the renal transplant recipient. Research indicates that the majority of kidney transplant recipients do not meet these recommendations. Healthcare providers should encourage physical activity on a routine basis as this has been shown to be the most effective strategy.

NUTRITION RECOMMENDATIONS FOR THE PREGNANT TRANSPLANT RECIPIENT

Recommended caloric intake for the pregnant transplant recipient is 25 to 35 Cal/kg of body weight plus 300 Cal daily in the 2nd and 3rd trimester. Protein intake should be 1 to 1.2 g/kg of body weight plus 10 to 25 g of protein per day. Micronutrient requirements are the same as for a non-transplant pregnant female. Prenatal vitamins are advised, especially in early pregnancy. Folic acid intake should be at least 400 μg daily.

NUTRITION CONSIDERATIONS DURING ACUTE REJECTION EPISODES

During acute rejection episodes, provision of optimal protein and calorie intake is the primary nutritional concern. High-dose steroids produce a dose-related increase in protein catabolic rate, leading to catabolism. Protein intake providing 1.5 g/kg is appropriate.

NUTRITION CONSIDERATIONS FOR THE BARIATRIC KIDNEY TRANSPLANT RECIPIENT

Bariatric surgical procedures include Roux-en-Y gastric bypass, sleeve gastrectomy, gastric banding, and biliopancreatic diversion with duodenal switch. Bariatric surgery is the most effective method for weight loss. Micronutrient deficiencies may arise following bariatric procedures, especially depending upon the type of procedure. The majority of vitamins and minerals are absorbed in the small intestine. The Roux-en-Y gastric bypass, whereby most of the stomach, the duodenum, and much of the jejunum are bypassed, may lead deficiencies in folic acid, vitamin B_{12}, iron, and calcium, among other vitamins and minerals. The duodenal switch creates a sleeve gastrectomy with a small portion of the duodenum intact while much of the small intestine is bypassed leading to fat-soluble vitamin deficiencies, as well as iron and calcium deficits.

Following the surgery, dumping syndrome may occur, especially with the Roux-en-Y procedure as the pylorus is bypassed. To minimize risk of dumping syndrome, individuals should avoid simple sugars and high-fat foods. Fluid intake should be emphasized to avoid dehydration. To avoid long-term complications of micronutrient deficiencies, vitamin and mineral levels should be monitored annually. Practitioners should be vigilant in assessing for signs and symptoms of micronutrient deficiencies in patients with a history of bariatric surgery. Following kidney transplantation, bariatric patients should continue on a daily multivitamin supplement that includes 100% to 200% daily values of micronutrients.

Selected Readings

Alshayeb H, Josephson M, Sprague S. CKD–mineral and bone disorder management in kidney transplant recipients. Am J Kidney Dis 2013;61:310–325.

Beindorff ME, Ulerich LM. Nutrition management of the adult renal transplant patient. In: Byham-Gray L, Stover J, Wiesen K, eds. A Clinical Guide to Nutrition Care in Kidney Disease. 2nd ed. Chicago: Academy of Nutrition and Dietetics, 2013:87–101.

Chadban S, Chan M, Fry K, et al. Nutritional management of dyslipidaemia in adult kidney transplant recipients. Nephrology 2010;15:S62–S67.

Chan M, Chadban S. Nutrition management of kidney transplant recipients. In: Kopple JD, Massry SG, Kalantar-Zadeh K, eds. Nutritional Management of Renal Disease. 3rd ed. London: Elsevier, 2013:563–580.

Corey R, Rakela J. Complementary alternative medicine: risks and special considerations in pretransplant and posttransplant patients. Nutr Clin Pract 2014;29: 322–331.

Dontje ML, de Greef MHG, Krijnen WP, et al. Longitudinal measurement of physical activity following kidney transplantation. Clin Transplant 2014;28:394–402.

Dounousi E, Leivaditis K, Eleftheriadis T, et al. Osteoporosis after renal transplantation. Int Urol Nephrol 2015;47:503–511.

Heng A, Montaurier C, Cano N, et al. Energy expenditure, spontaneous physical activity and with weight gain in kidney transplant recipients. Clin Nutr 2015;34:457–464.

Hirukawa T, Kakuta T, Nakamura M, et al. Mineral and bone disorders in kidney transplant recipients: reversible, irreversible, and de novo abnormalities. Clin Exp Nephrol 2015;19:543–555.

Jamal MH, Cocelles R, Daigle CR, et al. Safety and effectiveness of bariatric surgery in dialysis patients and kidney transplantation candidates. Surg Obes Relat Dis 2015;11:419–423.

Kalanter-Zadeh K, von Visger J, Foster C. Overcoming the body mass index as a barrier in kidney transplantation. Am J Transplant 2015;15:2285–2287.

Krishnan N, Higgins R, Short A, et al. Kidney transplantation significantly improves patient and graft survival irrespective of BMI: a cohort study. Am J Transplant 2015;15:2378–2386.

Lew Q, Jafar T, Koh H, et al. Red meat intake and risk of ESRD. J Am Soc Nephrol 2017;28:304–312.

McAdams-DeMarco MA, Law A, King E, et al. Frailty and mortality in kidney transplant recipients. Am J Transplant 2015;15:149–154.

Molnar MZ, Kovesdy CP, Bunnapradist S, et al. Associations of pretransplant serum albumin with post-transplant outcomes in kidney transplant recipients. Am J Transplant 2011;11:1006–1015.

Molnar MZ, Naser MS, Rhee CM, et al. Bone and mineral disorders after kidney transplantation: Therapeutic strategies. Transplant Reviews 2014;28:56–62.

Obayashi P. Food safety for the solid organ transplant patient: preventing foodborne illness while on chronic immunosuppressive drugs. Nutr Clin Pract 2012;27:758–766.

Van den Berg E, Geleijnse JM, Brink EJ, et al. Sodium intake and blood pressure in renal transplant recipients. Nephrol Dial Transplant 2012;27:3352–3359.

Van Laecke S, Van Biesen W. Hypomagnesaemia in kidney transplantation. Transplant Rev 2015;29:154–160.

Wee PM. Protein energy wasting and transplantation. J Renal Nutr 2013;23:246–249.

Wissing K, Pipeleers L. Obesity, metabolic syndrome and diabetes mellitus after renal transplantation: prevention and treatment. Transplant Rev 2014;28:37–46.

21 Psychosocial and Financial Aspects of Kidney Transplantation

Mara Hersh-Rifkin

The diagnosis of advancing kidney disease is life changing, not only for the patient, but also for family members. Many questions and concerns may arise that can be addressed by the social worker who is highly invested in patient care and treatment, including the following:

- What treatment choice is best for me?
- How will my life change because of my illness?
- How will my illness affect my family?
- How will I pay for my treatments?
- Will I be able to continue working and return to my daily activities?

ROLE OF THE TRANSPLANTATION SOCIAL WORKER

Clinical social workers, who are licensed and have a Master's degree in social work, play a key role before and after kidney transplantation. Once patients are referred to the transplant center, they are scheduled for a pretransplantation psychosocial evaluation to afford the patient, caregiver, and family members an opportunity to obtain sufficient information to maximize the possibility of a successful outcome. In the United States, the Center for Medicare Services (CMS) guidelines for social services state that the transplant center must make social services available by qualified social workers to all transplant recipients, living donors, and their families.

The transplantation social worker assesses important psychosocial factors which could significantly affect the outcome of the transplant, including adequacy of social support, adherence, substance use history, psychiatric status, access to resources, and the ability to understand and cope with changes in health status, prognosis, and treatment options. If a patient is experiencing a significant psychosocial problem, the patient may not be approved for transplantation until this issue is addressed. Table 21.1 identifies the areas that should be covered in a comprehensive psychosocial assessment, and the availability of community resources.

When a patient is admitted to the hospital for kidney transplantation, the inpatient clinical social worker assists both the patient and family in coping with the emotional, psychosocial, and financial aspects of post-transplantation care. Once discharged from the hospital, outpatient clinical social work services are available to patients and their family members. The transplantation social worker can help patients understand and cope with their feelings and adjust to a new way of life with a kidney transplant. They can assist patients in resolving issues

TABLE 21.1	Major Areas Covered in Psychosocial Assessment

Illness Assessment

1. Illness history and impact on patient's functioning, understanding, reaction, and adjustment
2. Patient's knowledge of transplantation, process of being referred to transplant center, understanding of the assessment process for candidacy, feelings about transplantation

Patient Assessment

Personal
  Age, life cycle stage
  Physical functioning
  Intellectual functioning
  Emotional functioning
  Sexual functioning
  Major stressful events
  Coping style and approaches
  Religious beliefs and faith
  History of substance abuse
  Ability to comply with medical regime

Educational
  Level of education attained

Type of Occupation
  Length of employment
  Stability of present or recent job

Financial
  Sources of income and other resources, their adequacy for current lifestyle, and their adequacy for transplantation and for future medical needs

Support System Assessment

Family
  Composition—spouse and children; age, education, occupation; needs, availability
  Role structure—effect of illness on roles
  Interactions—patterns and quality of communication
  Functioning—quality of family life
  Problem-solving approach and skills

Social
  Extended family—quality of contacts
  Friends, neighbors, colleagues—quality of relationships
  Others—religious, cultural, and social affiliations

Environmental
  Housing and transportation
  Need for relocation
  Need for travel alternatives

surrounding employment, finances and insurance, issues with sex and intimacy, and concerns about death and dying. In this chapter, many of the specific recommendations regarding employment, finances, and insurance relate to the care of transplant recipients residing in the United States.

The clinical social worker on the transplant team is an expert on community resources and can refer patients and family members to the appropriate resources they might need, such as disability insurance, Social Security, vocational rehabilitation, home care and medical equipment, support groups, and financial resources.

PSYCHOSOCIAL BENEFITS OF TRANSPLANTATION

Although kidney transplant surgery is a major surgery with significant time needed for recovery, in comparison with ongoing dialysis it offers patients with kidney failure the opportunity to live a longer and more satisfying life. Many patients who have been on dialysis and receive a transplant report having increased energy and stamina, along with fewer comorbidities with a transplant than if they remained on dialysis. While dialysis is a lifesaving treatment, it provides only approximately 15% of the work a functioning kidney does, and because of its impact on the body, can lead to nerve damage, bone disease, and increase the risk of infection. Transplantation not only affords better physical health, but relieves many of the barriers patients face in employment, education, and interpersonal relationships.

An obvious benefit of kidney transplantation is the freedom from the time and logistical constraints of dialysis. Successful transplantation permits much more personal time for an individual who no longer requires dialysis treatments for several hours 3 times a week at a dialysis facility, or home hemodialysis, or peritoneal dialysis. Advances in home hemodialysis have allowed individuals more freedom to dialyze at home on their own schedules, but all these treatments remain time consuming. There are also significant psychosocial stressors associated with dialysis, including issues surrounding machine dependence, the ability to maintain full-time employment, loss of spontaneity, and reduced time for family activities.

Transplantation permits greater flexibility and allows for travel without the need to arrange transient hemodialysis treatments in other cities ahead of time, enabling the recipient the freedom to plan a vacation or take urgent business trips. Many patients have reported that they have not taken an extended trip since commencing dialysis because of inconvenience and concerns about being too far away from their home dialysis centers, or dialyzing in an unfamiliar setting. There is also greater dietary flexibility (see Chapter 20) after kidney transplantation. Dialysis patients can find it difficult to follow the dietary restrictions necessitated by being on dialysis, which may include fluid, phosphorous, and potassium restrictions.

The time alone saved in being off dialysis is about 600 h/yr. This can result in increased earning potential and increased family and personal time. The long-term complications of dialysis may be avoided (see Chapter 1), and many patients view a transplant as a symbol of freedom and restored health.

Ideally, after receiving a kidney transplant, patients are able to return to normal functioning by going back to work or school, no longer needing disability payments to maintain a household. Patients are encouraged to engage in vocational rehabilitation while they are on dialysis because the waiting time for a deceased donor transplant may be years, during which time they may complete training courses or school programs. Social Security offers programs for vocational training and trial work programs that patients can take advantage of while they are receiving disability benefits, and assists with job placement to help individuals get back into the workforce when they are medically able to do so.

Financial Benefits of Transplantation

Relative to individuals who are suffering from other medical conditions, patients with chronic kidney disease in need of dialysis or transplantation receive special treatment in the United States healthcare system. Since 1972, patients with kidney failure have been eligible for subsidized public health insurance conditional only on their disease status, regardless of age, income, or functional status. This federal Medicare program, which otherwise provides coverage only to individuals who are 65 years and older and those with other qualifying disabilities such as blindness or terminal cancer, also covers patients with Chronic Kidney Disease (CKD) Stage V. Individuals who are in need of kidney transplantation are eligible for Medicare at the time of the transplantation as well as before transplantation if they are on dialysis. Medicaid, insurance for low-income individuals, also pays for the cost of dialysis and transplantation, and is often a supplement to Medicare in the low-income CKD population.

Successful kidney transplantation is substantially less costly than maintenance dialysis. Transplantation costs Medicare an average $106,400 for the first year, with Medicare spending about $17,000 for a functioning transplant in subsequent years. Medicare spends on average $87,000 per year on each in-center hemodialysis patient, and $67,000 on home peritoneal dialysis care per patient.

Long-term success of kidney transplantation requires lifetime coverage of immunosuppressive drugs. Medicare drug coverage ends after 3 years for these drugs, a policy that differs from most developed countries which afford lifetime drug coverage for transplant recipients. Transplant recipients younger than age 65 and no longer viewed as disabled, lose their Medicare coverage based on the rationale that younger recipients will reenter the work, force and gain private insurance. The continuation of current limitations on the coverage of immunosuppressive medications is actually costing the healthcare system in the long run. Studies have shown that it is far more cost effective to continue the coverage of immunosuppressive drugs for kidney transplant patients beyond the current 3 years then it is to pay for the resumption of dialysis for the same population.

In the United States, despite decades of legislative history and clinical data revealing gaps in coverage for post-transplant care entitlements, extending the duration of coverage for immunosuppressive medications was not included in the Affordable Care Act of 2010 (ACA). Beginning in 2014, however, patients with a kidney transplant who are no longer entitled to Medicare payments for their immunosuppressive medications now have access to extended coverage under ACA private health plans, offered through exchanges to cover essential health benefits (EHB). The 2012 benchmark standards require all plans available in exchanges to cover drugs in the immunosuppressive class. This means that potentially multiple anti-rejection medications and products must be covered by state exchanges, including many common immunosuppressive drugs used by kidney transplant recipients. Transplantation social workers can play an important role in assisting transplant recipients and their families to cope with the financial impact of paying for immunosuppressive medications. By directing them to plans within individual states that may be the most beneficial for them, transplantation social workers positively impact the lives of patients who are facing the financial burden of high co-pays for their medications. Additionally, transplantation social workers can direct patients to various financial assistance programs to help pay for their medications or medication co-pays. The expansion of the Medicaid program under the ACA allows individuals who remain financially eligible to continue coverage for as long as necessary, although most must opt into Health Maintenance Organizations (HMO), sometimes making it a challenge if their transplant center is out of network in regard to service providers. Threats to the ACA following the US Presidential election of 2016, must be regarded with great concern and vigilance.

Psychosocial Risks of Transplantation

There are a number of psychosocial risks and complications associated with kidney transplantation, just as there are with chronic dialysis. The transplantation social worker can offer support for the patient, family, and significant others with issues that can have a negative effect on transplant results, such as reluctance to leave the dependent "sick role," and concerns many recipients have about reentering the workforce. The acceptance of change of health status is often difficult for family members who have had to redefine roles within the family and recognize the effective autonomy skills of the transplant recipient.

Although patients are educated about medication side effects, until they are faced with them, it is uncertain how they will cope. Patients who have a prior psychiatric history of anxiety or depression are particularly susceptible to an exacerbation of their symptoms when immunosuppressive therapy begins, although patients with no prior history are also at risk (see Chapter 18). Both patients and family members should be comforted by the assurance that such symptoms are generally temporary and treatable. The physical side effects of some transplant medications such as diarrhea, insomnia, and weight gain may affect body image in a manner that is not always easily detectable, and sensitive probing may be required. Side effects are almost inevitable after transplantation and can cause medication noncompliance, especially in young adults. Patients should be systematically questioned about their attitude toward their side effects. Patients can ameliorate some of the side effects of medications with careful attention to diet and exercise, and team members should promote empowerment to do so, rather than promote an expectation of inevitability.

Multiple lifestyle changes occur for the transplant recipient. Their place may change within their family system and work environment. Their capacity to reenter the workforce after many years may be changed. There may be a risk for losing financial support, such as disability income. Personal relationships may be at risk, and post-transplantation stress may lead to divorce and separation. Sexual functioning may change after transplantation (see Chapter 11) and engender new hopes and fears. The newly found post-transplantation freedom may be a threat to patients whose identity has been associated with their "sick role" as a dialysis patient. Some dialysis patients create a social network at their dialysis units, and transplantation can disrupt this connection.

The shift to health may be difficult, and an identity crisis may occur. Counseling and support groups can aid in this transition. Participation in transplant community activities, such as participation in the Transplant Games or run/walks that raise money for transplant research and patient assistance funds offer the newly transplanted patient an opportunity to establish new relationships. This may ease the transition for patients to a lifestyle that does not surround dialysis treatments; this is especially salient for recipients who may have had little social support outside of their dialysis units.

Employment after kidney transplantation is an important marker of restored health. It has been shown that employment has a strong independent association with both patient and graft survival. Transplant patients can often find assistance by contacting their City and State Personnel Departments/Job Service Centers, Federal Job Information Centers, Veterans Action Centers, Job Corps, and Local or Regional Offices of Vocational Rehabilitation (Rehabilitation Services Administration). These agencies can provide direct assistance with job placement and training, and help individuals who have been out of the work force secondary to illness by assisting with interviewing and resume skills and developing relationships with prospective employers. Trial work periods offered through Social Security can help newly transplanted patients reenter the workforce without losing financial benefits for up to 1 year. Healthcare reform has enabled transplant recipients to obtain health insurance that is not tied to employment, but concern related to loss of financial support after successful transplantation remains.

Many patients live in fear of suffering rejection episodes and losing their transplants, or experiencing other catastrophic complications. These fears are not irrational, although they may be exaggerated; they can be best addressed by an open and factual discussion of the extent of the risk at all phases of treatment. Patients may also suffer feelings of guilt at having received a kidney at the expense of someone else. Patients should be assured that these are common feelings and reminded that they are deserving beneficiaries of the wishes of the donor and the donor's loved ones.

NONADHERENCE AND NONCOMPLIANCE

The terms *nonadherence* and *noncompliance* are used to indicate failure of transplant recipients to behave in a manner that best promotes the function of their transplant.

Kidney transplant patients are required to take lifelong immunosuppressive medication to prevent graft rejection. Nonadherence to immunosuppressive medication is a common issue and is multifactorial. Dosage and timing of these medications is crucial. Failure to take the medication as prescribed is a risk factor for (late) acute rejection, (late) graft failure/loss, and even death. Noncompliance with medical therapies affects treatment outcomes in CKD as well as many other chronic diseases. A series of variables have been linked to medication noncompliance (Table 21.2), and each is evident in transplant immunosuppressant regimens. Occasional noncompliance and "forgetfulness" are widespread, although their clinical significance is difficult to assess. Both multiple and late episodes of acute rejection predict subsequent graft loss (see Chapter 11), and medication noncompliance significantly enhances the risk for both. Noncompliance greatly increases the risk for graft loss and is a contributing factor in more than one-third of cases of graft loss.

Estimates of the frequency of nonadherence among renal transplant recipients vary widely, but it is safe to assume that approximately one-third of all patients will manifest nonadherence each year. A number of patient-, practitioner-, and program-related factors have been shown to be related to adherence after renal transplantation. The number and frequency of medication, as well as the relationship, communication, and trust between the patients and healthcare provider, are likely to influence adherence. Nonadherence is particularly a problem among adolescent transplant recipients. Rates of nonadherence have also been found to be related to factors such as level of social support, education, and socioeconomic status. Nonadherence prior to transplantation is an independent predictor of nonadherence after transplantation.

Few patients consciously decide to behave in such a manner. For most, noncompliant or nonadherent behavior evolves gradually as a consequence of many interacting variables. Leading barriers to medication-taking were not remembering to refill prescriptions and changes to medication prescriptions or dosages, an occurrence all newly transplanted patients must face. Medication nonadherence is a common problem in organ transplantation patients with severe consequences for the patients' health. Some studies into attitudes about medication nonadherence in the posthospitalization period have shown that educational interventions in the crucial outpatient recovery period have improved compliance. Transplant centers, nephrologists, and social workers should routinely assess whether kidney recipients encounter new or additional barriers, and provide intervention targeted at assisting patients develop strategies to overcome them.

TABLE 21.2	Attributes of Pharmacologic Therapies that Increase the Risk for Noncompliance

Multiple medications
Prolonged duration of therapy
Short dosing intervals
Palatability of medication
Definable adverse effects
Financial expense
Beliefs about severity of illness
Failure to understand treatment regimen
Increasing intervals between contacts with providers

(Adapted from Cramer JA. Practical issues in medication compliance. Transplant Proc 1999;31(suppl 4A):7S–9S.)

Several demographic variables appear to affect the likelihood of noncompliance. Diabetic patients, accustomed to the demands of living with chronic illness, are less likely to have problems with compliance after transplantation. Younger patients, particularly adolescents, and those with a limited educational background are more likely to be noncompliant (see Chapter 17). Psychiatric illness and a history of substance abuse also increase risk. As addressed in the Financial Aspects of Transplantation section, noncompliant behavior is often attributable to either financial hardship or the relative inability to procure appropriate medication when no funds are available. Low socioeconomic status is a strong predictor of noncompliance and poorer long-term outcomes in renal transplantation. Knowledge of these demographic risk factors, however, is of only limited benefit in dealing with individual patients. It does little to facilitate identification of noncompliant behavior early enough to allow remedy, nor does it provide insight into what that remedy should be.

The interventions required to alter noncompliant behavior vary from patient to patient. At the very least, transplant recipients must have access to immunosuppressants, the annual cost of which may exceed that of housing for many patients (Table 21.3). There is a significant risk for late rejection and graft loss for patients who discontinue immunosuppressant medications because of financial hardship; when patients are provided with drugs, outcomes improve dramatically. The extension of Medicare coverage for immunosuppressant medication

TABLE 21.3	Maintenance Immunosuppression Costs Associated with Typical Dosing Regimens			
Medication	**Dose/Day (mg)**	**Formulation**	**AWP*/30 days ($)**	**AWP/yr ($)**
Azathioprine	100	Generic	79	944
Belatacept	350[†]	Brand (Nulojix)	1,551	18,612
Cyclosporine, modified	300	Brand (Neoral)	736	8,832
		Generic	495	5,940
Everolimus	1.5	Brand (Zortress)	1,576	18,912
Mycophenolate mofetil	2,000	Brand (Cellcept)	2,057	24,684
		Generic	942	11,304
Mycophenolic acid	1,440	Brand (Myfortic)	1,294	15,528
		Generic	1,097	13,164
Prednisone	5	Generic	22	264
Sirolimus	2	Brand (Rapammune)	5,225	62,700
		Generic	3,150	37,800
Tacrolimus	8	Brand (Prograf)	1,379	16,548
		Generic	1,070	12,840
Tacrolimus, extended release	8	Brand (Astagraf XL)	1,142	13,700
	6	Brand (Envarsus XR)	840	10,083

*Average Wholesale Price.
[†]Given as a monthly infusion (Red Book Online, accessed October 10, 2015). Price is rounded to the nearest dollar using a single dosage form. AWP is a measurement of the price paid by retail pharmacies to purchase drug products from wholesale distributors. Actual institutional and/or patient costs may vary.

from 1 to 3 years was shown to attenuate income-related differences in long-term graft survival. The introduction of Health Care Reform and provisions within the ACA should improve graft survival by providing more options for medication coverage for the kidney transplant population of the United States (please refer to the Financial Benefits of Transplantation section for details).

In addition to ensuring financial access to proper medications, other interventions might improve patient compliance. Drug regimens should be simplified, with perhaps optimal compliance as a more compelling goal than optimal pharmacokinetics. Patients should be helped to develop daily routines that foster compliance. Use of pill boxes, time alarms, and receiving reminders from others facilitates compliance. New technology and lower costs have made the use of cellular telephone reminders commonplace for transplant recipients.

DISABILITY INSURANCE FOR TRANSPLANT RECIPIENTS IN THE UNITED STATES

State Disability Insurance

In some states, state disability insurance (SDI) is available for patients who are employed and are paying state income taxes. Patients are also eligible to apply if they are unable to work because of disabilities that are not work related (e.g., while they are receiving medical treatments or recovering from illness, surgery, or non–work-related accidents). SDI eligibility begins 1 week after the patient stops work for any of the above reasons, and continues for a maximum of 1 year, or until the patient is able to return to work, or until their SDI funds run out (usually up to 12 months). Patients who continue to be disabled after 1 year need to apply for long-term disability. The maximum financial benefit is based on the individual's earned highest quarter wage. It is often supplemented by employer disability plans to approximate the original salary.

For transplant recipients, the estimated amount of time off work is 2 to 3 months, although some patients may return to work sooner. Because transplant recipients require close medical follow-up in the first 2 to 3 months, it is generally recommended that they do not return to work before 2 months after transplantation. Some patients are unable to cope financially on SDI for more than 1 month, and request to return to work sooner. A decision needs to be made about whether the patient is medically stable and can be cleared to return to work.

Family members who care for transplant recipients during their recovery may be eligible for up to 12 weeks of leave per calendar year through family medical leave (FMLA); this may be paid or unpaid leave, depending on their employer, whether they paid into SDI, or if they have a private disability benefit. Individuals are encouraged to investigate SDI eligibility, private disability benefits, and FMLA benefits in advance of kidney transplantation, so they can be educated and more prepared financially after transplantation.

Social Security Disability Income

Social Security disability income (SSDI) is long-term disability program for patients who are considered "permanaently" disabled for at least 1 year. Patients who run out of temporary disability and yet are still unable to return to work often apply for SSDI, even before 1 year of becoming disabled, because the eligibility process can take several months.

Social Security payments are monthly and are based on a patient's individual earnings in the highest quarter. Patients with CKD who are on dialysis or who have undergone transplantation are eligible for SSDI if they have paid Federal Insurance Contributions Act (FICA) taxes. Patients are encouraged to continue working even after starting dialysis because they may be able to have flexible work hours or reduce their work schedule to part-time. Patients may choose home hemodialysis or peritoneal dialysis so as not to interrupt their work schedules by having to go to a hemodialysis center several times a week.

Some patients continue on SSDI, particularly if they have disabling conditions in addition to CKD (e.g., diabetes, retinopathy, blindness, or other physical disabilities).

Consolidated Budget Reconciliation Act of 1985

When someone loses job-based insurance, they may be offered continuation of coverage by their former employer. The Consolidated Budget Reconciliation Act (COBRA) of 1985 provides additional help to employees and their dependents that would normally lose their health insurance coverage because of job loss, divorce, or the death or retirement of a spouse. This is a federal law that requires companies with 20 or more employees to extend their insurance coverage to employees and their dependents for 18 months (up to 36 months) when benefits would otherwise end. Although patients may receive extended coverage through COBRA, they are still fully responsible for premium payments to the group health plan.

An employee covered by a group health plan may continue coverage for up to 18 months if the employee left work voluntarily or involuntarily (for reasons other than misconduct), or the working hours are reduced beyond the minimum amount to qualify for health benefits. Patients considered disabled under Social Security guidelines at the time work is discontinued can choose to continue their health coverage for up to 29 months, after which time they become eligible for Medicare. They must show that they are insurable in order to continue coverage. If a person leaves work because of disability, they may be able to keep their life insurance policy if there is a disability waiver. The insurer must be notified and proof of disability provided. Under provisions in the ACA (see Financial Benefits of Transplantation), patients who choose not to take COBRA coverage, can enroll in a Marketplace Plan instead. Losing job-based coverage qualifies you for a Special Enrollment Period that allows 60 days to enroll in a health plan, even if it is outside the annual Open Enrollment Period (usually November through January).

Recipients already enrolled in COBRA have options in the Marketplace; this will depend on the time of year and if the COBRA benefit is running out.

Family Medical Leave Act

The Family Medical Leave Act (FMLA) requires employers to provide up to 12 weeks of unpaid job-protected leave to "eligible" employees for certain family and medical reasons that make the employees unable to perform their work. Employees are eligible if they have worked for an employer for at least 1 year (minimum of 1,250 hours over the previous 12 months).

The employee may be required to provide advance leave notice and medical certification. Leave may be denied if requirements are not met. The employee ordinarily must provide 30 days' advance notice when leave is "foreseeable." An employer may require a medical documentation (and may require a second opinion at the employer's expense) to support a request for leave because of a serious health condition. For the duration of FMLA leave, the employer must maintain the employee's health coverage under any "group health plan." Upon return from FMLA leave, most employees must be restored to their original or equivalent positions with equivalent pay, benefits, and other employment terms. The use of FMLA leave cannot result in the loss of any employment benefit that accrued before the start of an employee's leave. The U.S. Department of Labor is authorized to investigate and resolve complaints of violations. An eligible employee may bring a civil action against an employer for violations.

Vocational Rehabilitation

Successful kidney transplantation enhances the physical and mental quality of life for many individuals. With improved health and stamina, transplant recipients may be more willing to reenter the workforce, enter a vocational training program, or return to school. Many transplant patients are not working at the time of the transplantation for various health reasons. They may be eligible for vocational rehabilitation, as are patients who are unable to return to their prior employment because their job responsibilities are in conflict with transplant-related restrictions.

Vocational rehabilitation is a service that provides people with disabilities the tools they need to be able to return to work, enter a new line of work, maintain work, or start work for the first time. After transplantation, it is important that the patient enter a rehabilitation program as soon as the patient is able to work in order to protect their disability coverage. The Social Security Administration (SSA) can help people with disabilities get the vocational rehabilitation services they need. SSDI recipients are entitled to test their ability to work with a trial work period and continue to receive full benefits regardless of whether they make more than what is considered the "substantial gainful activity" amount for a 9-month trial work period. For 2015, the Social Security Administration considers any month where a person has a monthly income of more than $780 a trial work month. If patients are self-employed, any month where they work more than 80 hours (or earn more than $780) is considered a trial work month.

There are other public and private agencies to help transplant recipients find jobs. Some of these agencies can help patients decide what they want to do, write a resume and practice interviewing so they feel more confident. This includes: Local or Regional Offices of Vocational Rehabilitation (Rehabilitation Services Administration), city and state personnel departments/job service centers, federal job information centers, veterans action centers, YMCA job banks, Job Corps, and employment agencies. Guidance counselors at local schools or colleges can also help transplant patients, and some agencies may help pay for training.

Selected Readings

De Pasquale C, Veroux M, Indelicato L, et al. Psychopathological aspects of kidney transplantation: efficacy of a multidisciplinary team. World J Transplant 2014;4:267–275.

Faraldo MF, Garcia M, Bravin AM, et al. Behavioral measures to reduce non-adherence in renal transplant recipients: a prospective randomized controlled trial. Int Urol Nephrol 2015;47:1899–1905.

Ganji S, Ephraim PL, Ameling JM, et al. Concerns regarding the financial aspects of kidney transplantation: perspectives of pre-transplant patients and their family members. Clin Transplant 2014;28:1121–1130.

Garcia MF, Bravin AM, Garcia PD, et al. Behavioral measures to reduce non-adherence in renal transplant recipients: a prospective randomized controlled trial. Int Urol Nephrol 2015;47:1899–1905.

Gordon EJ, Gallant M, Sehgal AR, et al. Medication-taking among adult renal transplant recipients: barriers and strategies. Transpl Int 2009;22:534–545.

Greene GM. Description of a psychosocial assessment instrument and risk criteria to support social work recommendations for kidney transplant candidates. Soc Work Health Care 2013;52:370–396.

James A, Mannon RB. The cost of transplant immunosuppressant therapy: is this sustainable? Curr Transplant Rep 2015;2:113–121.

Purnell TS, Auguste P, Crews DC, et al. Comparison of life participation activities among adults treated by hemodialysis, peritoneal dialysis, and kidney transplantation: a systematic review. Am J Kidney Dis 2013;62:953–973.

Salter M, Gupta N, King E, et al. Health-related and psychosocial concerns about transplantation among patients initiating dialysis. Clin J Am Soc Nephrol 2014;9: 1940–1948.

Tielen M, Exel JB, Laging M, et al. Attitudes to medication after kidney transplantation and their association with medication adherence and graft survival: a 2-year follow-up study. J Transplant 2014;2014:675301.

Tzvetanov I, D'Amico G, Walczak D, et al. High rate of unemployment after kidney transplantation: analysis of the United Network for Organ Sharing database. Transplant Proc 2014;46:1290–1294.

22

Kidney Transplantation in the Developing World

Elmi Muller and Rudolph A. García-Gallont

The worldwide promotion of organ donation and transplantation activities are consistent with the principles outlined in the Declaration of Istanbul (see Chapter 23), the World Health Assembly Resolution on Human Organ and Tissue Transplantation, and the Madrid Resolution on government accountability to achieve self-sufficiency in organ donation and transplantation (see Selected Readings). "Self-sufficiency" in this context refers to the necessity for countries or regions to address the needs of their residents for solid-organ transplants from within their own populations, rather than attempting to "export" those needs to other countries whose own populations typically have needs that go unaddressed.

The Global Observatory on Donation and Transplantation (GODT at www.transplant-observatory.org) and its annual newsletter (see Selected Readings) maintained by the World Health Organization (WHO) and the Spanish-based Organization Nationale Transplantation (ONT) are invaluable resources for worldwide information on transplant activities. Figure 22.1 illustrates the gross inequalities in both living donor and deceased donor kidney transplant activities across the globe.

Examples from Central and Eastern Europe and South America have demonstrated the impact of local leadership on the development of organ donation and transplantation programs, and illustrate the supportive role that professional societies can play in these developments. The South East Europe Initiative on Deceased Organ Donation (Macedonia, May 2011) and The Croatian Regional Health Development Centre in Organ Donation and Transplantation are two such examples of active and successful partnerships between clinicians, governments, and professional societies, which might in turn be applied to other developing countries. It is the role of professional societies and clinicians to approach governments and to advocate for appropriate legislative frameworks and for the allocation of resources to transplantation, especially in settings where dialysis availability is rapidly outpacing the development of kidney transplantation.

ESSENTIAL REQUIREMENTS FOR A TRANSPLANT PROGRAM IN THE DEVELOPING WORLD

International Oversight

For Health Systems in most developed countries, access to transplantation is available as part of the normal services rendered to the population: this is not the case in the developing countries. In many of these countries, even basic needs in public health remain unmet,

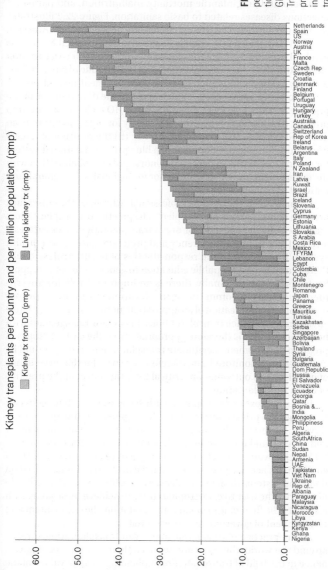

Kidney transplants per country and per million population (pmp)

- Kidney tx from DD (pmp)
- Living kidney tx (pmp)

Netherlands
Spain
US
Norway
Austria
UK
France
Malta
Czech Rep
Sweden
Croatia
Denmark
Finland
Belgium
Portugal
Uruguay
Hungary
Turkey
Australia
Canada
Switzerland
Rep of Korea
Ireland
Belarus
Argentina
Italy
Poland
N Zealand
Iran
Latvia
Kuwait
Israel
Brazil
Iceland
Slovenia
Cyprus
Germany
Estonia
Lithuania
Slovakia
S Arabia
Costa Rica
Mexico
TFYRM
Lebanon
Egypt
Colombia
Cuba
Chile
Montenegro
Romania
Japan
Panama
Greece
Mauritius
Tunisia
Kazakhstan
Serbia
Singapore
Azerbaijan
Bolivia
Thailand
Syria
Bulgaria
Guatemala
Dom Republic
Russia
El Salvador
Venezuela
Ecuador
Georgia
Qatar
Bosnia &...
India
Mongolia
Philippiness
Peru
Algeria
SouthAfrica
China
Sudan
Nepal
Armenia
UAE
Tajikistan
Viet Nam
Rep of...
Ukraine
Albania
Paraguay
Malaysia
Nicaragua
Morocco
Libya
Kyrgyzstan
Kenya
Ghana
Nigeria

FIGURE 22.1 Kidney transplants per country and per million population (pmp). (Data from the WHO-ONT Global Observatory on Donation and Transplantation. The 2014 data are provided by national health authorities in WHO Member States whenever transplantation programmes do exist.)

and the timely diagnosis and initial treatment of organ failure may be a challenge. In most developing countries, a low Human Development Index (HDI, a composite statistic of life expectancy, education, and income per capita indicators) will correlate with limited health resources and lack of unavailability of transplantation to its population. In these countries, most of the population is not covered by health insurance, and therefore depend on a public health system that will often still prioritize resources to other more pressing problems like high perinatal and infantile mortality, malnutrition, and parasitic/infectious diseases related to basic sanitation. Figure 22.2 illustrates the relationship between HDI and transplant activity in Latin America.

The WHO, which is the public health arm of the United Nations, is involved in every region of the globe and works to achieve a common global attitude toward transplantation via a multitude of partnerships with key bodies, including health authorities, scientific and professional societies, and experts. With respect to the development of the practice of deceased organ donation, the WHO endorses a four-step process: (i) adoption of the Critical Pathway for organ donation from deceased persons (see Chapter 4, Part I); (ii) the drafting of a legal framework; (iii) the development of a blue print of a national system for organ donation from deceased donors; and (iv) collaboration with the government and the private sector for regional, sub-regional, and national implementation.

Ultimately, it is the medical professionals who are at the crossroads between donor, patient, and recipient. The practice of transplantation, and especially deceased donor organ transplantation, necessitates a level of trust in the transparency and professionalism of the health system. In addition to the responsibilities of health professionals, there is also a need for public education to generate societal support for transplantation. Finally, there is an important role for governments in terms of commitment to allocation of resources, proper oversight, and the creation of an appropriate normative and legislative environment in which transplantation can operate. Engagement with health authorities is therefore appropriate from the earliest stages of program development. Legitimate transplantation activity should be examined and monitored, and therefore registries for the surveillance of practices and outcomes are critical from the outset of the practice of organ transplantation.

In the context of developing health systems, it is often necessary to engage the private sector in the development of transplantation services; however, such arrangements mandate complete transparency and specific and effective oversight from health authorities. Universal health coverage is a current major objective of the WHO, with an emphasis on access, quality, and financial protection for all, based on financing systems designed to deliver cost-effective services that do not expose the user to catastrophic costs. To achieve these goals with respect to the financing of organ transplantation, the engagement and commitment of governments are essential.

As the practice of tissue, cell, and organ transplantation spreads around the world, there is a greater need than ever for global governance in the field of transplantation, upholding societal values of the

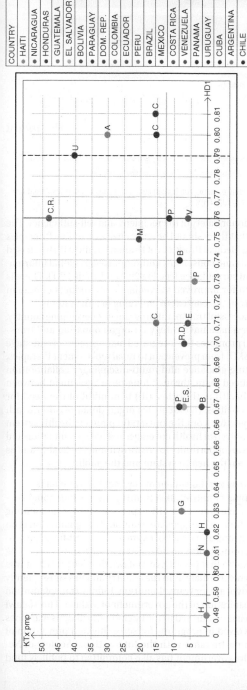

COUNTRY	KTx pmp
● HAITI	0
● NICARAGUA	0
● HONDURAS	0
● GUATEMALA	7.5
● EL SALVADOR	7.1
● BOLIVIA	2.8
● PARAGUAY	8.9
● DOM. REP.	7.4
● COLOMBIA	15.6
● ECUADOR	6.4
● PERU	4.3
● BRAZIL	7.3
● MEXICO	21.1
● COSTA RICA	47.6
● VENEZUELA	6.5
● PANAMA	12.3
● URUGUAY	40.6
● CUBA	15.5
● ARGENTINA	30.6
● CHILE	15.2

FIGURE 22.2 In developing areas of the world (as exemplified for Latin America), kidney transplantation activity (KTx) grossly correlates with the Human Development Index (HDI) of each country, reflecting budgets dedicated to Health Programs, access to Health Services, and development of specialized attention to the population. Increasing HDI is accompanied by increase in KTx activity. Data are from 2015.

See Cusumano et al. in Selected Readings.

553

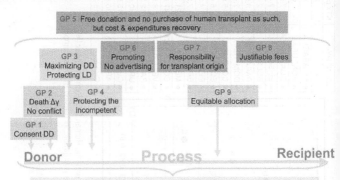

FIGURE 22.3 WHO guiding principles on human cell, tissue, and organ transplantation. (Courtesy of Jose R. Nuñez MD, PhD)

protection of the donor, safety of the recipient, and self-sufficiency. The WHO recognizes that there should be generalizable Guiding Principles (GPs) surrounding Medical Products of Human Origin (MPHO), based on global standards and consensus, and supported by global information standards and surveillance (see Fig 22.3 and Table 22.1). There is considerable room for improved surveillance of products of human origin, particularly in the context of emerging health systems.

To develop a successful transplant program in a developing country, there is a need for a national strategy for organ donation and transplantation that: (i) promotes the integrated management of end-stage kidney disease (ESKD) from prevention to renal replacement therapies, (ii) relies on existing guidance and multi-disciplinary collaboration with a more advanced team, through long-term agreement between institutions and health authorities; (iii) is mindful of the need for transparency of activities; (iv) identifies organ donation after death as a long-term objective from the outset; (v) pioneers health system development and universal health coverage; and (vi) uses donation and transplantation as an opportunity to create dynamics in health, and as an interface between the health system and the public.

National Oversight by and Commitments by Local Governments

In several developing countries, health ministries or individual government officials have independently expressed interest in pursuing organ transplantation. In Ethiopia, for example, transplantation is on the government agenda as a result of expressed interest from government ministers in transplantation taking root locally, with the training of local professionals a first priority. In Malawi, the vice president was the first person to receive dialysis in the country and has subsequently become a vocal advocate for transplantation. Kidney transplantation is considered an aspiration of the government of Malawi. The Malawi Ministry of Health has committed to the upgrading of dialysis machines and is actively involved in programs for screening and prevention of kidney disease in partnership with the International Society of Nephrology (ISN). The government has also committed to publicly fund

TABLE 22.1	Global Governance Tools for Medical Products of Human Origin (MPHO)

A Global Set of Principles

1. Transparency and openness to scrutiny indispensable while confidentiality and anonymity when required must be preserved;
2. Prohibition of financial gain on the human body and its parts as such and when not forbidden (e.g., plasma and gametes in some countries) mandating full transparency;
3. Responsibility for the provision of MPHO placed with authorities and through them the individual citizen and resident;
4. Genuine consent of donors and recipients;
5. Protection of the incompetent;
6. Equity as a goal, in the burden of donation and in allocation of MPHO;
7. Use of MPHO justified by evidence and absence of comparable alternative;
8. Traceability and accountability mandated throughout the process, from donors to recipients, including long-term outcomes and vigilance and surveillance under the oversight of national competent authorities;
9. Duty to constantly optimize the safety, quality, and efficacy of procurement, process, and clinical application of MPHO.

Global Use of ISBT 128*
Global governance function with national competent authorities
- Global harmonization (Global Terminology→ Global code . . .etc)
- Unique donation identifier
Allow: easier information transfer + traceability + interoperability across MPHO, and between countries in routine and emergency + cost containment[†]

Global Vigilance and Surveillance
Notify project for Vigilance and Surveillance of medical products of human origin
Global collaboration for V&S of MPHO
- To support operation and oversight
  - Donor selection and management
  - Recipient management
  - Quality system—risk assessment and management
- To establish transparency for trust

*A global standard for the identification, labelling, and information transfer of MPHO
See Warwick et al. in Selected Readings

transplantation in the future. In the interim, the Malawi government is seeking to send patients to India at a cost of $30,000 per living donor transplant, with patients returning to Malawi with a personal supply of immunosuppression.

In Cameroon, there has been a rapid expansion of dialysis availability. The government is now eager to move ahead with transplantation, beginning with a legislative framework. Currently, the government of Cameroon pays for patients to undergo transplantation abroad, providing financial aid unless that patient has private insurance. Many patients relocate to France for transplantation. The experience of Cameroon suggests that where government has undertaken to fund dialysis, there may be greater incentive to pursue kidney transplantation if transplantation can be demonstrated to be cost saving.

There is strong political will to support patients with chronic kidney disease in Zambia. New dialysis units are being opened, and the government is developing a health insurance scheme that would cover the costs of dialysis and potentially transplantation. There is also strong political will to enact legislation with respect to organ donation and transplantation. Pubic health insurance has been proposed, which will have implications for the funding of future transplantation programs.

Nigeria and Ghana represent good examples of resource-rich developing countries facing formidable economic and political challenges with an increasingly sophisticated population whose needs for transplantation may go unanswered. As of 2015, there were 10 centers in Nigeria performing living donor transplantation. There is no national transplant database and deceased donor transplantation is not performed. A national health bill providing a framework for transplantation was signed into law in 2014 but has not yet been implemented. In Nigeria, as in many developing countries, patients with financial resources often travel abroad for transplantation, preferably through legitimate "travel for transplant" but sometimes, unfortunately, through "transplant tourism" (see Chapter 23).

The experience of Tunisia illustrates the scale of the transition from provision of living donor transplantation to provision of deceased donor transplantation. Despite a well-developed living donor transplantation program in Tunisia, established in 1986, deceased donor transplantation is not yet available. Barriers to the initiation of deceased donor transplantation in Tunisia were identified as an absence of legislation on brain death, and the lack of infrastructure, personnel, and capacity for coordination required to support deceased donation. Whereas living donor transplantation might be successfully driven by a motivated individual and a single institution, deceased donor transplantation requires dialysis programs, tissue typing and crossmatching facilities, an organ procurement program, an on-call surgical team, capacity to fund this infrastructure, and an appropriate legislative framework. Moreover, a significant level of regional and national organization is required. The historical experience of the United States was that deceased donation gained momentum only when it was separated from the hospital and placed under an independent coordinating authority. There is also the need to contend with the public perception of deceased donation—it will be easier to commence deceased donation in the context of an established living donor program with acceptable and consistent recipient outcomes. Therefore, in advocating for deceased donor transplantation, the requirements in terms of resources, infrastructure, track-record, and capacity for coordination need to be realistically acknowledged.

In Latin America, organ donation rates and transplant activities differ greatly in the various regions. Colombia, Brazil, and Argentina have well-developed programs and derive more than 80% of their transplanted organs from deceased donors, whereas Mexico, Bolivia, and the Central American region have living donors as the main source.

The major problem in the developing world is the limited number of patients having access to dialysis and the high cost to sustain chronic dialysis programs. In many countries, dialysis is not funded by the state sector and the fact that patients pay for dialysis results in inadequate dialysis for these patients. In many ways, transplantation will provide a good quality of life and better clinical outcome for the same or less money. Therefore, developing countries would be advised to develop transplantation programs rather than dialysis programmes. Countries that start transplantation programs should have the ability to dialyze these transplant candidates pre- and immediately postoperatively as a minimum requirement.

Clinical Requirements

Resource requirements differ for living versus deceased donor transplantation. In the developing world, difficult questions need to be addressed: at what stage is it appropriate for a developing country to consider deceased donor organ transplantation? What is a sufficient level of dialysis availability? Should deceased donor transplantation be contemplated in parallel with the development of living donor transplantation? To what extent is it necessary to consolidate experience with living donor transplantation prior to commencing deceased donor transplantation? What are the minimum requirements in terms of ICU beds and trained personnel that remain on the agenda in the developing world?

To perform organ transplantation, there are certain basic surgical requirements which are probably equivalent to those for general surgery or orthopaedic surgery. At a bare minimum, a self-retaining retractor is probably essential, but aside from this self-retaining retractor to facilitate the extraperitoneal approach, a routine kidney transplant could be done with a general laparotomy set. Laparoscopic donor nephrectomy (see Chapter 7) has been recommended as a strategy to minimize the overall health and financial cost to the living donor—decreased morbidity, length of hospitalization, and faster return to work. However, the cost of equipment used in a standard technique may prohibitively expensive and surgical training and experience may be limited. When general surgical laparoscopic procedures are available, specialized training may lead to the introduction of laparoscopic donor nephrectomy to great advantage. For example, laparoscopic kidney donation is now practised routinely in Guatemala City after training by a surgical team from UCLA in Los Angeles.

A dedicated anaesthesiologist is essential as this person needs to be familiar with transplant "friendly" muscle relaxants, vasoactive drugs, and anaesthetic agents. Essential monitoring equipment, airway equipment, and intravenous and monitoring catheters (more rigorous for pediatric transplant) should be available at all centers. Ultrasound equipment and expertise are essential to assess graft anatomy and function (see Chapter 14).

Though the surgical aspects of kidney transplantation are obviously important, they are not the rate-limiting step. Multiple programs in resource-limited countries have demonstrated excellent initial results: it is long-term follow-up (and necessary resources) that is a significant problem. Successful programs have started with living donors and only after establishment of a successful program have they slowly transitioned to deceased donation. Most have started with surgeons trained at large transplant centers with continued support from a "sister" institution in the developed world.

Laboratory Requirements

The laboratory requirements for living donor transplantation are significantly different from the requirements for deceased donor transplantation. In terms of minimal laboratory requirements, the question is whether people are suitable for transplantation if they are ABO matched and have negative donor-specific HLA antibodies, or whether they should be HLA matched as well. In living donation, ABO typing and matching are essential. In terms of HLA typing, a combination of crossmatch and solid-phase assays is available and probably ideal. A factor that will affect outcomes is the presence of donor-specific HLA antibodies—well-matched donors and recipients certainly have better outcomes than completely mismatched patients. In the case of deceased donation, these tests need to be provided on an on-call basis. Typing of all donors for A, B, Bw, C, DR, and DQ by molecular method, and the availability of solid-phase assays would be ideal in this setting. Furthermore, a strategy should be available to streamline organ allocation and prevent prolonged ischaemic time: something like a calculated PRA combined with unacceptable antigens. This would mean a virtual crossmatch, where the presence of donor-specific antibodies would predict a positive crossmatch.

Tissue-typing laboratories are still not established in many developing countries and good pathology training programmes do not currently exist. However, for countries performing living-related donation only, it should be an option to establish one or two central high-throughput laboratories based on regional collaboration, where local expertise gets pooled and shared. This would be a viable option for countries with small transplant numbers as well. Tissues typing could be tailored to the local setting, but it should also be possible to build up expertise and to gradually build up more extensive tissue typing facilities. Basic tissue typing might be done locally with outsourcing of some of the more complicated tests to more sophisticated centers in the developed world particularly in the face of frequently transfused and multiparous patients who may be sensitized.

Infectious Disease Requirements

Infection control is essential to good transplant outcomes in all circumstances (see Chapter 12) but is particularly important in the developing world. It must include screening and vaccination prior to transplantation, and prevention of disease post-transplantation. Infections are the most common post-transplant complication in the developing world. Not only do we need to think about common bacterial and viral infections but also about reactivation of diseases like tuberculosis. There is also the issue of donor-derived infections like Chagas, strongyloides, schistosoma, malaria, and babesia.

Standard screening includes the facilities to test for: HIV, Hepatitis B and C, CMV, Syphilis, Varicella, EBV, Measles, mumps and rubella, toxoplasmosis, and tuberculosis in all recipients. Donors should complete similar screening. In terms of vaccination, a hepatitis B, Pneumovax, Tetanus, and Yellow fever vaccination would be strongly recommended preoperatively. Postoperative prophylactic therapy should probably include antivirals, TMP/SMX, antifungals, as well as tuberculosis, strongyloides, and malaria prophylaxis.

Some emerging and reemerging diseases in Africa and Latin America are not controllable or treatable in the immunosuppressed patient, and higher rates of parasitic disease might occur in these patients. Tuberculosis is also highly prevalent in many countries of the developing world; therefore, tuberculosis chemoprophylaxis and screening should be a priority. Optimal duration of prophylactic therapy varies widely and should be tailor-made to each individual region. Comorbidities, particularly diabetes, also increase the risk of infection and might be more prevalent in the developing world.

THE NEED FOR KIDNEY TRANSPLANTATION IN THE DEVELOPING WORLD

The demand for sophisticated medical care in the developing world is growing. Economic growth and corresponding increases in health expenditures mean that we can confidently anticipate increased demand for organ transplantation. The WHO has a role to play in fostering these anticipated developments in accordance with the Guiding Principles on Human Cell, Tissue and Organ Transplantation (see Table 22.1).

Although the availability of renal replacement therapy is lower in Africa than in any other regions of the world, the true scale of the unmet need for treatment of ESKD is unknown. Ideally, population-based studies, death registration data, and dialysis and transplant registries would enable quantitative estimation of the underlying burden of ESKD and its risk factors in the population. Yet, although such data are largely unavailable, the underlying burden of ESKD in Africa is likely to exceed that of high-income countries: firstly, because the underlying prevalence of risk factors associated with organ failure is known to be very high, given the increasing rates of noncommunicable diseases in the region; in particular, diabetes and hypertension, combined with undiminished rates of infection-related nephropathies.

The nature of the primary causes of ESKD and the limited capacity for secondary prevention in patients living in developing countries result in more rapid progression to organ failure than experienced high-income countries. Glomerular nephropathies and hypertension are the leading causes of treated ESKD in sub-Saharan Africa. Diabetes is a less frequently diagnosed cause of ESKD in sub-Saharan Africa than it is in the high-income countries, though this will likely change given the projections that the number of adults in Africa with diabetes will double by 2030. HIV-related nephropathy is also likely to be responsible for a significant burden of ESKD in Africa. Hypertension, diabetes, and HIV in the African region have been estimated to produce an annual incidence of ESKD potentially exceeding 900 cases per million adults.

Estimating the burden of ESKD in the developing world is a necessity to effectively advocate for the allocation of resources to organ donation and transplantation. "Need" may be defined as "the population's ability to benefit from organ transplantation," and has three aspects: (i) the underlying burden of organ failure and its risk factors, irrespective of current treatment availability or eligibility criteria; (ii) the cost and efficacy of treatment (cost will constrain the number of people able to benefit from transplantation, and transplantation outcomes must be acceptable) and; (iii) comparison to the existing provision of services.

For those considered medically suitable for transplantation, demand for transplantation will be tightly constrained by the availability of specialist physicians and surgeons, pathology facilities, capacity to achieve acceptable graft outcomes, cultural and religious attitudes toward organ donation, trust in the health system, and the extent to which patients are able to meet the costs of surgery and ongoing immunosuppression. Continuing demographic, epidemiologic, and economic shifts will have implications for the future incidence of organ failure in the developing world and/or the level of demand transplantation.

LIMITING FACTORS FOR TRANSPLANT PROGRAMS IN THE DEVELOPING WORLD

Dialysis as a Logistically Easier Treatment Option

Renal Replacement Therapy is not widely available in the developing world and often dialysis is a limited resource in developing countries. Referral of a patient diagnosed with ESKD to a dialysis center offers an immediate survival benefit and there is currently a significant increase of dialysis units in the developing world. Dialysis services are available through companies that mount complete units with almost no initial investment for the healthcare provider, but subject to a minimum number of procedures to be performed on each machine per month. This means that dialysis is often available without the option of getting an organ transplant.

The increase of ESKD owing to known causes (hypertension, diabetes, and regional entities such as "Mesoamerican nephropathy") guarantees a huge influx of patients to the treatment centers, with expenses for consumables usually covered by public health, even in many poor countries. This initial ease of access to dialysis therapy, does, nevertheless not signify an optimal treatment, and many patients are chronically underdialyzed, and have constant catheter infections and exhaustion of access sites.

The lack of adequate technical planning for subsequent clinical steps, like policies for establishment of vascular accesses or the timely referral for transplantation, causes enormous crowding and high morbidity and mortality in many programs in the developing world. The relative ease of access to dialysis contrasts with the limited access to immunosuppressive therapy after transplantation, where most patients have to cover the cost for their medication.

Many developing countries also lack the organization needed to run efficient programs of deceased donation. In these societies, where there might be little or no information on organ donation and frequent refusal for both living as well as deceased organ donation, dialysis has become an easier strategy and is often driven without further consideration to transplantation as a treatment option. Hospitals with limited capacity for training or a limited budget might have little impetus to identify, report, or maintain a deceased donor.

Because of ICU bed shortages, limited or untrained surgeons, scarce or centralized transplantation facilities, and a lack of transparent and safe allocations systems, transplantation is often not available as a treatment option in developing countries. Furthermore, tissue typing laboratories are scarce, sometimes regionally shared by two or more countries and available on working days only, and therefore having limited suitability only for elective living donation. In some countries, distrust in fair distribution of the few available organs, owing to publicized cases of transplant tourism and organ trafficking, further contribute to keep deceased donation rates low or nonexistent.

Many of the above-mentioned facts historically favoured dialysis above transplantation for the treatment of ESKD. Where there are kidney transplant programs in developing countries, they often only offer living donation as a treatment option. The responses of health authorities to this problem are influenced by the degree of development of their health systems, their preferred policies, adequate or inadequate planning, and financial status.

Transplantation is often not available in remote and rural areas, and in many developing countries there are large differences between clinical options for patients with ESKD in urban in contrast with rural areas. In Brazil, for example, there is high transplantation activity existing in big cities such as Sao Paulo, but no availability of transplantation in the rural areas.

Brain-Death Legislation

All countries with well-developed deceased donor organ transplant programs have national brain-death legislation (see Chapters 4 and 19) and national or regional mechanism for organ recovery and distribution (see Chapter 5). The lack of development of robust deceased donation in the developing world is often ascribed to negative public attitude and cultural barriers to deceased donation, though the true barrier is actually lack of legislation and infrastructure and governmental determination to address their absence. Living donation may then seem to be a viable and easier option in many countries. When new programs are started, protection and advocacy for the living donor according to the Principles of the Declaration of Istanbul (see Chapter 23) and standard international practice (see Chapter 7) is a core requirement. Countries with high rates of living donation have typically neglected the more complex requirements for deceased donation.

An option for developing countries that want to start deceased donor transplant program but have yet to introduce and promulgate donation after brain death, is donation after circulatory death (DCD) (see Chapter 4, Part I). Since death as determined by circulatory criteria is the more traditional way of determining death, it may be more likely to be accepted than brain death, and DCD has fewer resource requirements compared with donation after brain death. Family consent tends to be higher for DCD since brain-dead donors still have a beating heart, which is harder for the family to understand. In high-income countries, DCD is complementary to donation after brain death, as there are adequate numbers of ICU beds, an unlikely resource in the developing world.

The current experience in Cape Town, South Africa involves no machine perfusion and only Maastricht type III donors are used (see Chapter 4). If consent from a potential DCD family member is obtained, ventilation is stopped after the team has prepared the theater. The warm ischemic time is about 20 minutes.

Spatial Distribution of Transplant Centers

Not surprisingly, the majority of dialysis and transplant centers in the developing world, where these exist, tend to be located in major urban centers or capital cities, with major implications for access to treatment. In Nigeria, for example, attempts have been made to address this issue. The size and diversity of the country mean that patients cannot be expected to travel long distances to receive treatment. Although 20 of 76 of dialysis centers are located in Lagos, centers have also been established across a range of geographic areas. Transplant centers located in various regions are currently performing living donor kidney transplantation; however, individual center volumes are low. The dispersion of transplantation activities in Nigeria highlights potential trade-offs between access and volume for emerging transplant programs.

Cost

Challenges noted from existing partnerships with individual centers in Africa and elsewhere include limited availability of necessary surgical instruments for visiting surgeons (e.g., microvascular instruments), poor long-term transplant outcomes owing to inability to meet the costs of maintenance immunosuppression, lack of monitoring and surveillance of transplant outcomes ("you can't improve what you don't measure"), the absence of a physician or surgeon "champion" of transplantation, and histologic capacity.

Another issue may be difficulty in establishing tertiary care in settings where traveling to another country to receive high-level medical care is standard practice. On-the-ground "fact finding" is an important first step in establishing a sister link, to determine whether linkage is likely to be successful, what the major challenges are likely to be, what resources are required as a priority, and what the needs of the population are (e.g., how many patients are on dialysis). It is also important for the success of sister programs that partnership teams become close and establish camaraderie.

The cost and sustainability of immunosuppression for transplanted patients remain a problem in many developing countries. A system where these drugs are freely available at a reasonable price to the patient before transplantation programs can be started must be in place. Since many of the transplants will be from living donors at low immunologic risk, it is often possible to develop low-intensity immunosuppressive protocols using low-cost drugs, most of which are now available as less-expensive generic alternatives (see Chapter 6).

Selected Readings

Busic M, Spasovski G, Zota V, et al. South East European Health Network Initiative for organ donation and transplantation. Transplantation 2015;99:1302–1304.

Cusumano A, Rosa-Diex G, Gonzalez-Bedat M. Transplant registry: experience and contributions to end-stage renal disease epidemiology. World J Nephrol 2016;5:389–397.

Garcia-Garcia G, Jha V. Chronic kidney disease in disadvantaged populations. Transplantation 2015;99:13–16.

García-Gallont R, Matesanz R, Delmonico FL. Organ donation and transplantation in Central America. Transplantation 2015;99:459–460.

Jha V, Arici M, Collins A, et al. Understanding kidney care needs and implementation strategies in low-and middle-income countries: conclusions from "Kidney

Disease: Improving Global Outcomes" (KDIGO) controversies conference. Kidney Int 2016;90:1164–1174.

Katz I. International aid and medical practice in the less-developed world: doing it right, what can renal organizations learn? Kidney Int 2005;(68, suppl 90):S60–S65.

Moosa R. Kidney transplantation in the developing world. In: Morris P, Knechtle S, eds. Kidney Transplantation: Principles and Practice. New York, NY: Grune & Stratton, 2013: 643–676.

Muralidharan A, White S. The need for kidney transplantation in low- and middle-income countries in 2012: an epidemiological perspective. Transplantation 2015;99:476–481.

ONT Newsletter 2016. http://www.ont.es/publicaciones/Documents/NEWSLETTER% 202016%20NIPO.pdf

Radhakrishnan J, Remuzzi G, Saran R, et al. Taming the chronic kidney disease epidemic: a global view of surveillance efforts. Kidney Int 2014;86:246–250.

Ready A, Nath J, Milgord D, et al. Establishing sustainable kidney transplantation programs in developing world countries: a 10-year experience. Kidney Int 2016;90:916–920.

Rizvi A, Zafar M, Jawad F, et al. Long-term safety of living kidney donation in an emerging economy. Transplantation 2016;100:1284–1293.

Ulasi I, Ijoma C. Organ transplantation in Nigeria. Transplantation 2016;100:695–697.

Warwick R, Chapman J, Pruett T, et al. Globally consistent coding systems for medical products of human origin. Bull World Health Organ 2013;91:314–314A.

23

The Declaration of Istanbul on Organ Trafficking and Transplant Tourism

Gabriel M. Danovitch

INTRODUCTION

The phenomenon of human organ trafficking was first recognized in the 1990s. Originally a hidden and limited activity in the back streets of a handful of developing countries, it later became a widespread, and sometimes brazen, activity that involved potential recipients traveling to clinics around the world to receive a kidney from poor, and poorly paid, "donors." By the first years of the new millennium, it had become a pervasive phenomenon that was estimated by the World Health Organization (WHO: whose primary role is to direct and coordinate international health within the United Nations' system) to account for as much as 10% of all organs transplanted worldwide. The WHO designated "hot-spots" of organ trafficking activity in India, Pakistan, Egypt, Colombia, and the Philippines, where the source of organs was from the living, and China, where the source of organs was executed prisoners. The main "exporters" of transplant recipients, unfortunately named "transplant tourists," were wealthy countries of the Persian Gulf, and included Japan, Israel, and other developed economies.

In 2004, the World Health Assembly (WHA), the decision-making body of the WHO, issued a revision of its 1991 "Guiding Principles for Human Organ Transplantation" that made clear that the buying and selling of organs for transplantation was to be condemned, and it asked its member nations to take steps to bring the phenomenon to an end. The transplant community itself, whose profession and expertise were being used at the expense of the exploited donors, had not yet expressed its response to the problems in a coordinated manner.

In May 2008, the two leading international professional organizations for transplantation and nephrology, The Transplantation Society (TTS) and the International Society of Nephrology (ISN), convened an international summit meeting on organ trafficking and transplant tourism in Istanbul that brought together more than 150 professionals with a variety of backgrounds from 78 member countries of the United Nations that offered organ transplant services of some degree. Istanbul was selected as the venue because it straddles Asian and European cultural and religious traditions. The text of the **Declaration of Istanbul on Organ Trafficking and Transplant Tourism** (DoI) was published simultaneously in several international medical journals and is reproduced in full following this introduction. The DoI consists of *preamble*, *definitions* of critical terms (organ trafficking, transplant commercialism, and transplant tourism), a set of *principles* to guide professional conduct and government policy, and a series of *proposals* applying those principles to particular problems in transplantation. The DoI has been endorsed by over 130 national and international professional organizations including the Council of Europe and the Vatican, has entered the legislation of several governments, and has influenced policies of health ministries. Major international medical journals and organizations have been lobbied successfully to apply an "academic veto" on submissions that include data obtained from transplants involving organ trafficking or the use of organs from executed prisoner in China.

In order to promote and sustain the DoI, the Declaration of Istanbul Custodian Group (DICG) was established, comprised representatives from the two parent organizations, TTS and ISN, and other interested individuals. A website www.declarationofistanbul.org was developed that contains translations of the DoI in multiple languages, a downloadable patient-orientated educational pamphlet entitled "Thinking of Buying a Kidney: STOP," in multiple languages, a bibliography of relevant articles, and a news section of relevant material from the international press. Though the DoI deals mainly with living organ donation, the DICG has expressed its firm objection to payments to the families of deceased donors (see Capron et al. in Selected Readings) and it strongly supports the principle of "financial neutrality" for organ donors (see Delmonico F, Martin D, et al. in Selected Readings). Though the DoI specifically promotes the availability of health insurance for all organ donors, it must be emphasized that in those countries where universal health insurance is not available, the provision of general health insurance to donors should be related to the donation itself rather than broadly applied in a manner that would represent a significant and its complications potentially coercive financial incentive for uninsured living donors. The DICG also remains alert to counter recurrent calls by a vocal minority to permit payments (other than those required to maintain financial neutrality), in one form or the other, to organ donors or their families.

In the years that have followed the DoI, there has been much progress and some setbacks related to its core mission (see Danovitch et al. in Selected Readings). Colombia, a country that once permitted nearly 20% of its deceased donor organs to be transplanted into foreigners, has essentially put an end to the practice. Progress, albeit fragile, has been made in Pakistan and India. Israel, once an "exporter" of transplant recipients, has implemented radical changes in policy (see Chapters 5 and 19) that has nearly eliminated the practice. China, after much international pressure, and widespread repugnance over its policy of "donation by execution," has made the practice illegal and appears to be replacing it by ethically acceptable deceased donation practices. Time will tell if progressive forces in China will gain sway and bring this abhorrent practice to an end, allow the country to be welcomed into the international transplant community. As of this writing, Egypt remains a major location for organ trafficking and reports of trafficking activities continue to come from Pakistan, Turkey, India, Sri Lanka and Nepal.

The positive changes that have taken place in Colombia and Israel, for example, are a manifestation of the impact of a combination of professional pressure, governmental support, and legislation. A call has been made for governmental accountability to achieve "self-sufficiency" in organ donation and transplantation so that each country or geographical region addresses the need of its own population from within its own population. The 2011 "Madrid Resolution" articulates specific processes by which this goal can be reached. Madrid was also the site, in 2016, of an international conference designed to help differentiate between legitimate "travel for transplant" and transplant tourism, and to better define the "prospective" and "retrospective" response to the phenomenon. The conclusion of this conference will be published in late 2017.

In February 2017 the Pontifical Academy of Sciences (PAS) at the Vatican held an international summit on organ trafficking and transplant tourism that expressed abhorrence for these practices and suggested a series of responses. The statement of the summit is available on the website of the PAS at http://www.pas.va/content/accademia/en/events/2017/organ_trafficking/statement.html

Selected Readings

Capron A, Delmonico F, Dominguez-Gil et al. Statement of the declaration of Istanbul custodian group regarding payments to families of deceased organ donors. Transplantation 2016;100:2006–2009.

Danovitch G, Delmonico F. A path of hope for organ transplantation in China? Nephrol Dial Transplant 2015;30:1413–1414.

Delmonico F, Martin S, Dominguez-Gil, et al. Living and deceased organ donation should be financially neutral acts. Am J Transplant 2015;15:1187–1191.

Delmonico F, Domínguez-Gil B, Matesanz R, et al. A call for government accountability to achieve national self-sufficiency in organ donation and transplantation. Lancet 2011;378:1414–1418.

Martin D, Van Assche K, Dominguez-Gil B, et al. Prevention of transnational transplant-related crimes-what more can be done? Transplantation 2016;100:1776–1784.

World Health Organisation (WHO). The Madrid Resolution on organ donation and transplantation. Transplantation 2011;91:S29–S31.

Full Text of the Declaration of Istanbul

PREAMBLE

Organ transplantation, one of the medical miracles of the 20th century, has prolonged and improved the lives of hundreds of thousands of patients worldwide. The many great scientific and clinical advances of dedicated health professionals, as well as countless acts of generosity by organ donors and their families, have made transplantation not only a life-saving therapy but also a shining symbol of human solidarity. Yet these accomplishments have been tarnished by numerous reports of trafficking in human beings who are used as sources of organs and of patient-tourists from rich countries who travel abroad to purchase organs from poor people. In 2004, the WHO called on member states "to take measures to protect the poorest and vulnerable groups from transplant tourism and the sale of tissues and organs, including attention to the wider problem of international trafficking in human tissues and organs" (1).

To address the urgent and growing problems of organ sales, transplant tourism and trafficking in organ donors in the context of the global shortage of organs, a Summit Meeting of more than 150 representatives of scientific and medical bodies from around the world, government officials, social scientists, and ethicists was held in Istanbul from April 30 to May 2, 2008. Preparatory work for the meeting was undertaken by a Steering Committee convened by the TTS and the ISN in Dubai in December 2007. That committee's draft declaration was widely circulated and then revised in light of the comments received. At the Summit, the revised draft was reviewed by working groups and finalized in plenary deliberations.

This Declaration represents the consensus of the Summit participants. All countries need a legal and professional framework to govern organ donation and transplantation activities, as well as a transparent regulatory oversight system that ensures donor and recipient safety and the enforcement of standards and prohibitions on unethical practices.

Unethical practices are, in part, an undesirable consequence of the global shortage of organs for transplantation. Thus, each country should strive both to ensure that programs to prevent organ failure are implemented and to provide organs to meet the transplant needs of its residents from donors within its own population or through regional cooperation. The therapeutic potential of deceased organ donation should be maximized not only for kidneys but also for other organs, appropriate to the transplantation needs of each country. Efforts to initiate or enhance deceased donor transplantation are essential to minimize the burden on living donors. Educational programs are useful in addressing the barriers, misconceptions, and mistrust that currently impede the development of sufficient deceased donor transplantation; successful transplantation programs also depend on the existence of the relevant health system infrastructure.

Access to healthcare is a human right but often not a reality. The provision of care for living donors before, during, and after surgery—as described in the reports of the international forums organized by the TTS in Amsterdam and Vancouver (2,3) is no less essential than taking care of the transplant recipient. A positive outcome for a recipient can never justify harm to a live donor; on the contrary, for a transplant with a live donor to be regarded as a success means that both the recipient and the donor have done well.

This Declaration builds on the principles of the Universal Declaration of Human Rights (4). The broad representation at the Istanbul Summit reflects the importance of international collaboration and global consensus to improve donation and transplantation practices. The Declaration will be submitted to relevant professional organizations and to the health authorities of all countries for consideration. The legacy of transplantation must not be the impoverished victims of organ trafficking and transplant tourism but rather a celebration of the gift of health by one individual to another.

DEFINITIONS

Organ trafficking is the recruitment, transport, transfer, harboring, or receipt of living or deceased persons or their organs by means of the threat or use of force or other forms of coercion, of abduction, of fraud, of deception, of the abuse of power or of a position of vulnerability, or of the giving to, or the receiving by, a third party of payments or benefits to achieve the transfer of control over the potential donor, for the purpose of exploitation by the removal of organs for transplantation (5).

Transplant commercialism is a policy or practice in which an organ is treated as a commodity, including by being bought or sold or used for material gain.

Travel for transplantation is the movement of organs, donors, recipients, or transplant professionals across jurisdictional borders for transplantation purposes. Travel for transplantation becomes transplant tourism if it involves organ trafficking and/or transplant commercialism or if the resources (organs, professionals, and transplant centers) devoted to providing transplants to patients from outside a country undermine the country's ability to provide transplant services for its own population.

PRINCIPLES

1. National governments, working in collaboration with international and nongovernmental organizations, should develop and implement comprehensive programs for the screening, prevention, and treatment of organ failure, which include:
   a. The advancement of clinical and basic science research;
   b. Effective programs, based on international guidelines, to treat and maintain patients with end-stage diseases, such as dialysis programs for renal patients, to minimize morbidity and mortality, alongside transplantation programs for such diseases;
   c. Organ transplantation as the preferred treatment for organ failure for medically suitable recipients.

2. Legislation should be developed and implemented by each country or jurisdiction to govern the recovery of organs from deceased and living donors and the practice of transplantation, consistent with international standards.
   a. Policies and procedures should be developed and implemented to maximize the number of organs available for transplantation, consistent with these principles;
   b. The practice of donation and transplantation requires oversight and accountability by health authorities in each country to ensure transparency and safety;
   c. Oversight requires a national or regional registry to record deceased and living donor transplants;
   d. Key components of effective programs include public education and awareness, health professional education and training, and defined responsibilities and accountabilities for all stakeholders in the national organ donation and transplant system.
3. Organs for transplantation should be equitably allocated within countries or jurisdictions to suitable recipients without regard to gender, ethnicity, religion, or social or financial status.
   a. Financial considerations or material gain of any party must not influence the application of relevant allocation rules.
4. The primary objective of transplant policies and programs should be optimal short- and long-term medical care to promote the health of both donors and recipients.
   a. Financial considerations or material gain of any party must not override primary consideration for the health and well-being of donors and recipients.
5. Jurisdictions, countries, and regions should strive to achieve self-sufficiency in organ donation by providing a sufficient number of organs for residents in need from within the country or through regional cooperation.
   a. Collaboration between countries is not inconsistent with national self-sufficiency as long as the collaboration protects the vulnerable, promotes equality between donor and recipient populations, and does not violate these principles;
   b. Treatment of patients from outside the country or jurisdiction is only acceptable if it does not undermine a country's ability to provide transplant services for its own population.
6. Organ trafficking and transplant tourism violate the principles of equity, justice, and respect for human dignity and should be prohibited. Because transplant commercialism targets impoverished and otherwise vulnerable donors, it leads inexorably to inequity and injustice and should be prohibited. In Resolution 44.25, the WHA called on countries to prevent the purchase and sale of human organs for transplantation.
   a. Prohibitions on these practices should include a ban on all types of advertising (including electronic and print media), soliciting, or brokering for the purpose of transplant commercialism, organ trafficking, or transplant tourism.
   b. Such prohibitions should also include penalties for acts—such as medically screening donors or organs, or transplanting

organs—that aid, encourage, or use the products of organ trafficking or transplant tourism.
   c. Practices that induce vulnerable individuals or groups (such as illiterate and impoverished persons, undocumented immigrants, prisoners, and political or economic refugees) to become living donors are incompatible with the aim of combating organ trafficking, transplant tourism, and transplant commercialism.

PROPOSALS

Consistent with these principles, participants in the Istanbul Summit suggest the following strategies to increase the donor pool and to prevent organ trafficking, transplant commercialism, and transplant tourism and to encourage legitimate, life-saving transplantation programs.

To respond to the need to increase deceased donation:

1. Governments, in collaboration with healthcare institutions, professionals, and nongovernmental organizations, should take appropriate actions to increase deceased organ donation. Measures should be taken to remove obstacles and disincentives to deceased organ donation.
2. In countries without established deceased organ donation or transplantation, national legislation should be enacted that would initiate deceased organ donation and create transplantation infrastructure, so as to fulfill each country's deceased donor potential.
3. In all countries in which deceased organ donation has been initiated, the therapeutic potential of deceased organ donation and transplantation should be maximized.
4. Countries with well-established deceased donor transplant programs are encouraged to share information, expertise, and technology with countries seeking to improve their organ donation efforts.

To ensure the protection and safety of living donors and appropriate recognition for their heroic act while combating transplant tourism, organ trafficking, and transplant commercialism:

1. The act of donation should be regarded as heroic and honored as such by representatives of the government and civil society organizations.
2. The determination of the medical and psychosocial suitability of the living donor should be guided by the recommendations of the Amsterdam and Vancouver Forums (2,3).
   a. Mechanisms for informed consent should incorporate provisions for evaluating the donor's understanding, including assessment of the psychological impact of the process;
   b. All donors should undergo psychosocial evaluation by mental health professionals during screening.
3. The care of organ donors, including those who have been victims of organ trafficking, transplant commercialism, and transplant tourism, is a critical responsibility of all jurisdictions that sanctioned organ transplants utilizing such practices.

4. Systems and structures should ensure standardization, transparency, and accountability of support for donation.
   a. Mechanisms for transparency of process and follow-up should be established;
   b. Informed consent should be obtained both for donation and for follow-up processes.
5. Provision of care includes medical and psychosocial care at the time of donation and for any short- and long-term consequences related to organ donation.
   a. In jurisdictions and countries that lack universal health insurance, the provision of disability, life, and health insurance related to the donation event is a necessary requirement in providing care for the donor;
   b. In those jurisdictions that have universal health insurance, governmental services should ensure donors have access to appropriate medical care related to the donation event;
   c. Health and/or life insurance coverage and employment opportunities of persons who donate organs should not be compromised;
   d. All donors should be offered psychosocial services as a standard component of follow-up;
   e. In the event of organ failure in the donor, the donor should receive:
      i. Supportive medical care, including dialysis for those with renal failure, and
      ii. Priority for access to transplantation, integrated into existing allocation rules as they apply to either living or deceased organ transplantation.
6. Comprehensive reimbursement of the actual, documented costs of donating an organ does not constitute a payment for an organ, but is rather part of the legitimate costs of treating the recipient.
   a. Such cost reimbursement would usually be made by the party responsible for the costs of treating the transplant recipient (such as a government health department or a health insurer);
   b. Relevant costs and expenses should be calculated and administered using transparent methodology, consistent with national norms;
   c. Reimbursement of approved costs should be made directly to the party supplying the service (such as to the hospital that provided the donor's medical care);
   d. Reimbursement of the donor's lost income and out-of-pocket expenses should be administered by the agency handling the transplant rather than paid directly from the recipient to the donor.
7. Legitimate expenses that may be reimbursed when documented include:
   a. The cost of any medical and psychological evaluations of potential living donors who are excluded from donation (e.g., because of medical or immunologic issues discovered during the evaluation process);

b. Costs incurred in arranging and effecting the pre-, peri-, and postoperative phases of the donation process (e.g., long-distance telephone calls, travel, accommodation, and subsistence expenses);

c. Medical expenses incurred for postdischarge care of the donor;

d. Lost income in relation to donation (consistent with national norms).

References

1. World Health Assembly Resolution 57.18, Human organ and tissue transplantation, 22 May 2004, http://www.who.int/gb/ebwha/pdf_files/WHA57/A57_R18-en.pdf.

2. The Ethics Committee of the Transplantation Society. (2004). The consensus statement of the Amsterdam forum on the care of the live kidney donor. Transplantation 78(4):491–492.

3. Pruett TL, Tibell A, Alabdulkareem A, et al. The ethics statement of the Vancouver forum on the live lung, liver, pancreas, and intestine donor. Transplantation 2006;81(10):1386–1387.

4. Universal Declaration of Human Rights, adopted by the UN General Assembly on December 10, 1948, http://www.un.org/Overview/rights.html.

5. Based on Article 3a of the Protocol to Prevent, Suppress and Punish Trafficking in Persons, Especially Women and Children, Supplementing the United Nations Convention Against Transnational Organized Crime, http://www.uncjin.org/Documents/Conventions/dcatoc/final_documents_2/convention_%20traff_eng.pdf.

Full text of Declaration reprinted from International Summit on Transplant Tourism and Organ Trafficking. The Declaration of Istanbul on organ trafficking and transplant tourism. *Kidney Int.* 2008;74:854–859, with permission from Elsevier.

Page numbers followed by *f* denote figures, those followed by *t* denote tables.